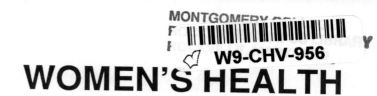
WOMEN'S HEALTH

Readings on Social, Economic, and Political Issues

Second Edition

Edited by

Nancy Worcester and Mariamne H. Whatley
Women's Studies Program
University of Wisconsin — Madison

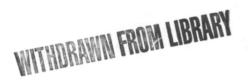

KENDALL/HUNT PUBLISHING COMPANY

KENDALL/HUNT PUBLISHING COMPANY
4050 Westmark Drive   Dubuque, Iowa 52002

AB F 8805

Copyright © 1988, 1994 by Kendall/Hunt Publishing Company

ISBN 0-7872-1368-3

Printed in the United States of America
10 9 8 7 6 5 4 3

Contents

Acknowledgments

Each woman who has worked as a part of the Women's Studies 103 teaching team of the University of Wisconsin-Madison has made her own contributions to the course. This reader reflects the input of all the women who have worked as Teaching Assistants for WS103 since the course was first taught in 1978.

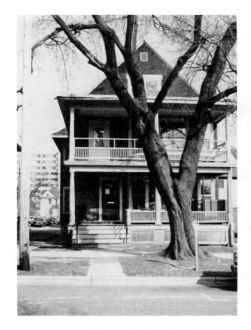 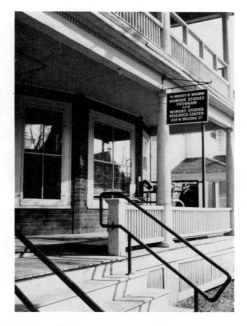

Women's Studies Building, University of Wisconsin—Madison

Introduction

Women cannot have control over our own lives until we have control over our bodies; thus understanding and gaining control over our bodies and our health is essential to taking control of our lives. Consequently, activism around women's health issues has been a central part of the struggles, by women and men, for improving the role of women in society.

The readings in this book are a representation of the exciting range of excellent resources now available on women's health issues. The resource information at the end of the book summarizes many of the sources for the material used in this book and thus serves as a partial list of the periodicals and magazines which regularly feature women's health topics. These articles are examples of the amazing range of women's health writing and organizing being done throughout the world by individuals and groups actively striving for health care systems more appropriate to women's needs.

This collection of readings is designed specifically for use as a part of the women's health course, *Women Studies 103: Women and Their Bodies in Health and Disease,* which is taught to 320-400 students each semester, in the Women's Studies Program at the University of Wisconsin-Madison. (We are delighted to hear that the book is also being used in many other women's health courses throughout the country!) Readings and worksheets are particularly chosen or written to stimulate thought and analysis in preparation for discussion sections. Selections have been made to complement, rather than overlap, material covered in the other books which are required for the course: *Biology of Women* by Ethel Sloane, published by Wiley, *The Black Women's Health Book* edited by Evelyn C. White, published by Seal Press, and *The New Our Bodies, Ourselves* by the Boston Women's Health Book Collective, published by Simon and Schuster.

This is the second edition of this book. Reflecting the rapidly changing area of women's health, the tremendous interest shown in women's health in recent years by both health care providers and consumers, and the new national debates, this book contains a very different range of articles than was available for the first edition. In an effort to provide an historical context to many present debates, we have deliberately added not only new articles but also those with an historical perspective, as well as older articles which we often refer to as "classics." A new goal for this book is to have students learn to value and use women's health "classics" as a part of studying present day issues and developing their own analysis. Often in the field of women's health, earliest articles written on a topic do an excellent job of identifying the crucial issues. Once that basic analysis has been written, other women's health writers are more likely to write an article which serves to update the information rather than writing an article very similar to the first one. When researching a women's health topic, students are encouraged to read both the "classics" and the most recent information to get the clearest overview of both the fundamental issues and which aspects of the area have and have not changed.

This collection will be regularly updated. We work towards having an anti-racist, cross-cultural perspective on topics, and are eager to find articles which make the connections between social, economic, scientific and political issues and women's mental and physical health. We hope our next book will be even better in looking at health issues related to poverty, ageism, racism, anti-semitism, heterosexism, fatphobia, and what it means to be differently abled. Readers' suggestions or reactions to articles are welcome and valued.

1

Women and the Health Care System

The role of women in the health care system reflects the role of women in society. Men tend to be "at the top", having status and power, and making decisions which greatly influence others' lives. Women have less status and little role in decision-making, but carry the responsibility for daily servicing and caring. Mirroring the family, we see the doctor as father, the nurse as mother, and the patient often is treated as a child. Since the late 1960's, modern women's health movements have critiqued curative medical systems based on the values of the male medical establishment, organized for fundamental changes in the system, and worked for the empowerment of women, as consumers and as health care providers, to be more involved in health care decisions for themselves and the system.

In "When Yogurt Was Illegal", the Boston Women's Health Book Collective (the group which produced and constantly updates *Our Bodies, Ourselves,* now translated into many languages and continuing to be "the bible" of women's health movements internationally) briefly summarizes many of the key issues, victories and challenges around which women's health activists in the USA have been organizing for the last twenty-five years.

The classic "Sexism in Women's Medical Care" shows how sexism in medical practice is rooted in the socialization of women to be passive patients and the socialization of doctors (men and women) to have a lack of respect for women and their right to information about their own bodies. Mary Halas sets the scene for why it is essential for women to take a more involved role in their own health care. Adriane Fugh-Berman's more recent "Tales Out of Medical School" vividly describes some of the traumas still facing women trying to become doctors today and reminds us that simply getting more women into medicine will do little to make the health system more appropriate for women (or men) until the medical school socialization of doctors is changed.

Increasingly, many women's health activists like Adriane Fugh-Berman are simultaneously critiquing the delivery of health care both from outside, as consumers, and from inside the health system as health care workers. The next three papers represent some of the changes and debates which are taking place as health care practitioners/activists work to make the system more appropriate for women. Judy Schmidt's "The Gynecologic Exam and the Training of Medical Students: An Opportunity for Health Education" gives an example of a training program which consciously aims to educate physicians to be "patient-orientated" so they can communicate with their patients. The debate between doctors Karen Johnson ("PRO: Women's Health: Developing a New Interdisciplinary Specialty") and Michelle Harrison ("CON: Women's Health as a Specialty: A Deceptive Solution") is quite a new phenomenon of the 1990's. The writing and debates of the 70's and 80's focused largely on why the health system was not adequately serving women and *why* women's health needed to be taken seriously. Now that the medical system has "discovered" women's health, the debate has changed to *how* it should take women's health seriously.

Readers will want to read these articles carefully and monitor the health system's changing (or non-changing) response to the issues of women's health. For the most part, the medical establishment does not deserve congratulations for how it has listened and responded to the issues raised by women's health movements. A clear pattern has emerged. When possible, the medical establishment has ignored women's health movements. When a demand could not be ignored, the medical response has been to coopt the move for change without making fundamental changes. For example, converting hospital-run services into a "women's health center" by painting the walls pink, buying several paintings by women artists, ordering a few women's health books, hiring a couple women doctors, and only superficially imitating the feminist women's health centers run by women, for women, did little to transform the dynamics of the doctor-patient relationship. Health institutions are now acting on what the drug companies have known for years—marketing products or services to normal, healthy women opens up huge markets ready to be exploited. There is enormous potential for what the medical "discovery" of women's health can mean, but activists need to remain diligent in making certain that women's health is no longer medically defined merely as issues related to gynecology but is redefined as encompassing all aspects of women's bodies and the social, economic factors (including our interactions with the health system) which impact upon our health. But, in asking for wider definitions of women's health, we also have to be careful that we are not encouraging yet more aspects of women's lives to become medicalized!

At the core of discussions on women's health is the question of who does and does not have access to the health system. The national debate on health reform (although seldom focusing on women and too often leaving out women's voices) is basically a women's health debate because women are overwhelmingly the health care providers and consumers who have the most to gain by meaningful change. The next two articles provide the type of information people need in order to appreciate and participate in decisions about how to move out of our present health care crisis. "The Health Insurance Conspiracy" provides very basic information on the problem that "insurance is the key to US health care." The names of the players in Washington, D.C. and their specific "health reform bills" constantly change, but this article outlines the key components of three very different types of "prescriptions for change" which are the core of most packages which are introduced into the House and Senate as specific health-reform bills. Everyone concerned about women's health should be informed about how differently each of the three types of "prescription for change" would impact on women and make sure that policy makers know their views. This issue is too important to leave to politicians and lobbyists! Recurring resistance to meaningful health care reform often gets framed, always by people who presently have decent health insurance coverage, as the fear of having health care rationed in this country. Adriane Fugh-Berman's "Health Care Rationing" clarifies the situation and the question which must be asked. Health care is already rationed in this country. Do we want to keep our present system (which uses income and access to health insurance as the rationing determinant) or is it time to move to a fairer, more health-promoting system which establishes a standard of care to which everyone is entitled?

"Women in Prison, Women in Danger" talks about the type of literal barriers to health care which are almost always left out of the debates about access to the health care system and taking control of one's body. Having taught women's health courses in prison, we have become aware of the physical and mental health hazards which many women face in prison. We have been impressed with how many women in prison, against all odds, were still trying to take care of health needs for themselves and their families—teaching each other yoga so they could find a healthy way to relieve stress in the confines of their cells, asking specific questions about contraceptives and STDs so they could share this information with their teenagers in the next phone call, trying to organize for an additional source of vitamin C so that if they missed orange juice at breakfast they had not missed the day's only vitamin C source. Seeing the physical bars which kept women in prison from taking care of their health issues was a thought-provoking reminder to us to be more aware of the less visible bars which keep millions of women from being able to maximize on their health.

The last articles in this chapter represent a range of ways that women have been working to empower themselves individually and collectively to address some of their own health needs. Another classic, "How to Tell Your Doctor a Thing or Two," published by Bread and Roses Women's Health Center (a feminist health center, *by* women, *for* women) is representative of how women's health movements have encouraged women to be a different kind of patient. In this article, Morton Hunt identifies changes in medical practices which have caused a deterioration in doctor-patient relationships and proposes a seven-point program for becoming a more active patient. In an article reminiscent of women researching topics for the original *Our Bodies, Ourselves,* Louise Marsden's "More than One Womb" shares what she learned about the wide range of "normal" variations in female anatomy as she pored over medical books to figure out her own anatomy. Building on a key women's health issue, "the politics of information" (who does and does not have access to information and who benefits and who loses when women do not have the information they need for health care decision-making?), this article questions whether women are not told about possible variations in female reproductive anatomy because the mystification prevents them from having control over their bodies and their lives, and she goes on to ask for a healthier definition of "normal" for women's bodies (and women's lives.)

Self-help groups around the country, devoted to many approaches to a wide range of issues, have been one of the most radical parts of the women's health movement. Discovering for themselves what is appropriate for their own situations, and often sharing this with others through talks, pamphlets, and experimental projects, self-help groups have provided us with totally new models of what appropriate (including culturally appropriate) health care can be. The final article, "Self-Help Health Education: Models from Diverse Communities," introduces us to six groups presently using the self-help approach to serving women in their communities.

When Yogurt Was Illegal
by The Boston Women's Health Book Collective

Imagine your best friend confiding in strictest secrecy that she is taking a trip to Puerto Rico to get an abortion, illegal on the U.S. mainland. Another friend enthusiastically tells you about a terrific new minipill that doesn't make you gain weight the way the regular birth control pill does. Your doctor says he'll fit you with a diaphragm after your honeymoon, not before. The obstetrician tells your sister that natural childbirth is kooky and dangerous and that it is better to take a little something to forget what happens. Welcome to 1969.

In your search to find a good ob/gyn you hear that a group of women is trying to compile a referral list. But one woman's guru is another woman's disaster. The group, meeting around a kitchen table (interrupted by visits from the resident toddler), makes a list of questions to ask and topics to investigate. Each woman volunteers to research one subject and report back. The women go to the library, and they interview professionals about anatomy and physiology, sexuality, birth control, pregnancy, childbirth, postpartum, abortion, and other topics. They find that they have heard different opinions, stated as fact, from their doctors. Then they discover astonishing medical facts hardly known to U.S. women; for instance, that women in Europe still use midwives—sometimes giving birth at home—and incredibly, their birth outcomes are better than in the U.S. This provokes discussions on sexuality in a new and serious way—the women compare notes about faking orgasms to please partners, penile thrusting as a poor method of producing orgasms, lesbianism. Other women hear about these exciting discussions and want to know more. Courses start. Piles of uncollated, photocopied pages, lined up on the floor outside the discussion rooms, keep disappearing. When the group takes the papers to be printed at a local radical press, the men don't think the papers are "political," but the press *women* insist they take it on.

In 1970, about a year and half after that initial kitchen table discussion in Boston, the first printing of *Women and Their Bodies* appeared. It cost 75 cents. On the second printing the name was changed to *Our Bodies, Ourselves,* which went on to sell 250,000 copies by word of mouth even before the first commercial edition appeared.

Women took to heart the idea that we are the best experts on ourselves. In 1970 a few feminists disrupted congressional hearings on the birth control pill. They were fed up with the testimony presented by medical professionals and drug company representatives while women who suffered problems with the high-dose estrogen pill were

being ignored. As pressure from women mounted, the Food and Drug Administration agreed on an insert listing possible side effects of the pill, to be placed in every package of oral contraceptives. And women realized that if they were going to influence government policy, they needed a presence in Washington. In 1976, the National Women's Health Network (NWHN) began. Still strong today, the network monitors federal health policies and regulations, and its members testify at public hearings.

Meanwhile, the self-help movement started in California, with women looking at their own cervixes. Carol Downer, one of the founders of the Feminist Women's Health Center, was even arrested for using yogurt to treat a vaginal yeast infection. Other women, with the help of some supportive health professionals, started dozens of women-controlled health centers across the U.S. Most offered self-help groups, with support groups dealing with such experiences as premenstrual syndrome and menopause. They were so successful that competing clinics sprang up to serve the same needs (but not necessarily to promote self-reliance or offer alternatives to allopathic medicine). Between 20 and 30 women-controlled health centers remain today, a model of care duplicated only in rhetoric by other clinics and hospitals.

By the mid-1970s articles began to appear in medical journals on how to manage the "new breed of women" who asked questions and demanded to know why they were getting a particular treatment. Several medical schools invited members of the Boston Women's Health Book Collective to speak, and even used *Our Bodies, Ourselves* as a text.

Women's health groups in the 1970s were predominantly young, white, and middle-class. Many women of color were frustrated in some of the organizations that failed to address *their* concerns adequately—for example, in their efforts to get federal regulations to curb the high incidence of sterilization abuse against poor women, especially women of color. The 1980s witnessed the emergence of organizations run by and for women of color. In 1981 Byllye Avery, then one of the few women of color on the NWHN board of directors, began to meet with other African American women to create the National Black Women's Health Project (NBWHP). In 1983 the first national conference on black women's health, co-sponsored with the NWHN, drew almost 2,000 women to Spelman College, Atlanta. The project now boasts 150 chapters in 31 states—and in Africa and the Caribbean.

The National Latina Health Organization, the Native American Women's Health Education Resource Center, and the Asian Health Project also adopted an empowerment model similar to that of the NBWHP. They emphasize

From *Ms. Magazine,* July/August 1992, pp. 38-39. Copyright © 1992 by Ms. Magazine. Reprinted by permission.

women organizing at the community level with a commitment to self-help. Current efforts to build bridges among women of different classes—an inevitable challenge as laywomen work collaboratively—may have significant impact on the ability of these groups to influence public policy.

Over the past 20 years, these groups have made a tremendous difference in the lives of individual women. They've had an impact on policy. Abortion is currently legal, though in jeopardy. Midwives and nurse practitioners are now legitimate, though not as common as they should be. Women are more accepted in medical schools, especially in ob/gyn. If a women has breast cancer, she doesn't automatically have to have a mastectomy. The birth control pill no longer contains so much estrogen. Tampons have standard absorbency labeling so a woman can reduce her risk of toxic shock syndrome. Diethylstilbestrol (DES) is no longer given during pregnancy. The Dalkon Shield is off the market and IUDs come with a more thorough consent form. Silicone-filled breast implant use is severely restricted—at least for the time being.

Congressional hearings on breast cancer, osteoporosis, and other problems not related to our reproductive functioning reflect years of work to gain recognition for women's health needs beyond our childbearing potential. The Women's Health Equity Act—an omnibus package of 22 different bills dealing with research, services, and prevention in such areas as breast and ovarian cancer, sexually transmitted diseases, contraceptive research, infertility, adolescent pregnancy, and osteoporosis—is gaining momentum in Congress. Increased funding is not far behind, although *what* gets funded will be critically important. Currently, the National Institutes of Health is carrying out the Women's Health Research Initiative, an estimated half-billion-dollar program of research over the next decade.

But challenges persist. Abortion is no longer accessible to many women and it is common for medical students to graduate without even learning the procedure. The full range of reproductive care is still not an option if you are poor. Reproductive technology and surgical intervention during childbirth are increasing. We still don't have important answers to the long-term effects of hormones, especially when used around the time of menopause. Women continue to be excluded from clinical trials of many drugs. HIV/AIDS is a great—and growing—threat to women. The FDA refuses to regulate medical devices and drugs unless there is tremendous pressure to do so. When products like Depo Provera are considered too dangerous for sale in this country, they are dumped abroad. The structure of medical education remains as inhospitable to teaching *caring* as ever. The medical profession retains its stranglehold, still marginalizing acupuncture, chiropractic, and other alternative therapies that often meet women's needs in unique ways. A national health program is still years away.

We have made great strides in two decades. But we have a long road to travel before women truly control our own health and medical care.

Contact the following national organizations for information or to find other feminist health groups:

Asian Health Project, 3860 West King Blvd., Los Angeles, Calif. 90008; (213) 295-6571.

National Black Women's Health Project, 1237 Ralph Abernathy Blvd., S.W., Atlanta, GA. 30310; (404) 758-9590.

National Latina Health Organization, P.O. Box 7567, Oakland, Calif. 94601; (510) 534-1362.

National Women's Health Network, 1325 G St., N.W., Washington, D.C. 20005; (202) 347-1140.

Native American Women's Health Education Resource Center, P.O. Box 572, Lake Andes, S.D. 57356; (605) 487-7072.

Ω

Sexism in Women's Medical Care

by Mary A. Halas

A twenty-seven-year-old woman complained that her health had taken a sudden unexplained change for the worse. She had a diffuse sense of not being well, with pains in various parts of her body, weakness, and fatigue. Her gynecologist gave her a physical exam and pronounced her fine. As the symptoms continued, she returned to her physician and also went to several other doctors—meeting reactions of disbelief and even ridicule with increasing frequency. Eventually one specialist recommended she see a counselor, because she obviously had no real physical problems.

That recommendation turned out to be a good one. After a few sessions the counselor concluded that the woman was in good mental health and concentrated on supporting

Reprinted with permission from Frontiers: A Journal of Women's Studies, Vol. IV, No. 2, 1979. Copyright © 1979 by Frontiers Editorial Collective.

her to continue seeking medical attention to evaluate the sudden change in her physical health.

Finally, months after her symptoms appeared and weeks after her last visit to her gynecologist, the woman had an appointment with a female physician who listened to an exhaustive list of her symptoms and concerns, and gave her an extremely thorough physical examination.

The results: the woman had a large lump in her left breast; after surgery two days later the lump was diagnosed as cancer. No one will ever know whether the lump was already there during her gynecologist's hurried and skeptical exam, but it is certain that the woman might have had a better chance of finding the lump herself if her doctor had ever taught her how to examine her own breasts. According to the woman's oncologist, there is a 70 percent chance that the cancer will recur, because of its type and size at the time of discovery.

Fortunately, the woman's counselor knew that sexism in the medical care system poses particular problems for women. Many physicians see women's physical complaints as trivial, neurotic disorders best treated with placebos or symptomatic therapy. A therapist who had conducted a prolonged analysis of the possible psychological causes of this woman's complaints or had considered the symptoms to be evidence of emotional disturbance would have put her life in even further jeopardy.

The medical needs of women and their problems in getting good health care are key issues. First, many women have psychosomatic illnesses, and counselors get many legitimate referrals from doctors who recognize that there needs to be a psychological as well as medical component to healing women's medical problems. Second, therapists get *too many* referrals from doctors, as the case of the woman with undetected breast cancer illustrates. Serious, treatable problems often progress to irreversible damage or death while a woman is trying to convince her doctor that her problems are not all in her head.

Before the advent of modern medical technology and the professionalization of medicine, women were the primary healers as "witches" and herbalists, and female midwives were the sole practitioners of physical care for women's special concerns—childbirth and gynecology. Now, however, the situation is radically reversed. Although women are the largest single group of health care consumers, 93 percent of all doctors are male, and 97 percent of all gynecologists are male.[1]

Women's experience in obtaining health care is different from men's in that women almost always are putting their bodies in the hands of someone of the opposite sex for medical care. In addition, women make 25 percent more visits to the doctors than men. They also take 50 percent more prescribed drugs than men and are admitted to hospitals more frequently.[2]

Sex-role stereotyping in the socialization of women has skewed the kind of medical care they seek. Women learn to identify themselves in terms of their reproductive potential, and the medical system reinforces this behavior.

For example, a majority of women turn to the specialist obstetrician/gynecologist, not as a source of care for specialized problems, but as a first-line source for all medical care—rather than choosing a general practitioner or internist for routine care. A study which Helen Marieskind presented at a 1974 meeting of the American Association of Obstetricians and Gynecologists found that 86 percent of the women in the study saw no doctor other than an obstetrician/gynecologist on a regular, periodic basis.

Socialization of Women as Patients

The socialization of women to be passive recipients of medical care—especially from men—militates against their receiving adequate care. The attitude with which women seek medical care within the male-dominated system is one of subservient dependence on all-knowing authority. This dependence on all-powerful doctors and women's relinquishing of responsibility for their health to male doctors is the result of physician behavior that reduces the patient's sense of autonomy.

For example, a woman having a routine gynecological exam is ushered into the examining room without meeting the physician first in his office and is instructed to take off her clothes. Vulnerable, naked, and draped with a white sheet, she waits an indeterminate period for the doctor to enter. Once he arrives and her feet are in the examining table stirrups, she is literally helpless in his hands and feels this way—naked, supine, being manipulated with fingers and tools in her body by a male hidden behind a sheet. This dependence on male doctors works against women patients' interests. A patient's stereotyped respect for a doctor's wisdom and competence does not make a poor doctor into a good one.

Dependence on doctors also eliminates the woman's own desires and needs from decision-making about her care. Most medical care involves various levels of benefits and risks and choices about them, even when doctors do not allow patients to make those choices. Lack of information about their bodies, plus the dependent, fearful relationship with their physicians, make it difficult for women to find out what is really wrong with them physically and what methods of treatment are possible. In a study on doctor-patient communication, Barbara Korsch and Vida Negrete found that the use of medical jargon which is unintelligible to patients, plus doctors' frequent disregard for patients' concerns and perspectives, were obstacles to effective care.[3]

A logical result of this confusion and failure in doctor-patient communication is that only 42 percent of the women in this study carried out all the medical advice they received; 38 percent complied in part; and 11 percent did not follow instructions at all.

In gynecology and obstetrics the level of communication can be even poorer, because of an attitude generated by the fact that many of the visits are from healthy women. The attitude is that if there is nothing wrong, then there is nothing to tell. In 1970 hearings before the U.S. Senate, a

5

physician who did research on oral contraceptives opposed labeling for these drugs which would inform women of the risks. He said, "A misguided effort to inform such women leads only to anxiety on their part and loss of confidence in the physician.... They want him [the doctor] to tell them what to do, not to confuse them by asking them to make decisions beyond their comprehension.... The idea of informing such a woman is not possible."[4]

One would hope that this individual doctor's attitude represents an extreme case. However, in general many doctors neglect to give women information they do not ask for, and treat them as if they are not capable of understanding the basis of decisions and treatment. In the view of much of the medical profession, women cannot even be trusted with information about their own conditions or medication.

A graphic illustration of this point is the years-old controversy still raging over the government's proposal to require patient education leaflets on all prescription drugs. In response to tremendous pressure from Congressional advocates and the Food and Drug Administration, the major medical associations reluctantly have endorsed the abstract concept of such leaflets but continue to oppose specific applications.

The specter the medical associations raise in their congressional testimony on patient package inserts for drugs is that if patients are told all that can go wrong with a drug, a disease, or an operation, their hypochondriacal minds will ensure that all these things do go wrong. It is significant that it was a consumer group, the Center for Law and Social Policy, which sparked the government initiative on patient package inserts through a petition—and not the medical profession.

An example in which doctors have not given women information that can have life and death consequences for themselves and their children involves the hormone diethylstilbestrol (DES). During the 1950's many thousands of pregnant women received DES without being informed what the medication was. No one knew until fifteen years later that this drug greatly increased the risk of cancer in their children.

In October 1978, after years of press coverage of DES-caused cancer, the government issued a special letter and bulletin to the country's doctors because of the finding that some doctors were still prescribing DES for pregnant women and many others still were not informing their patients who had taken the drug of possible risks.[5]

Socialization of Doctors

Where do doctors get this lack of respect for a woman's right to information about health care and for her ability to participate intelligently in her medical care? Mary Howell describes the process of professionalization of doctors in medical school—where they learn attitudes about work and patients—as strongly colored by a demeaning regard for women.[6] Medical schools teach discrimination against women as patients, Howell says, through lack of

focus on diseases specific to women, in misogynic comparisons made between male and female patients with similar health problems, and in instructions regarding the appropriate behavior of doctors toward women patients.

In their classes, medical students learn both implicitly and explicitly that women patients have uninteresting illnesses, are unreliable historians of their health, and are beset by such emotionality that their symptoms are unlikely to reflect real disease.

Pauline Bart and Diana Scully reviewed twenty-seven gynecology textbooks published between 1943 and 1972 and found that at least half of the writers stated women are inherently frigid, have less sex drive than men, or are interested in sex only for procreation.[7] Two authors urged physicians to encourage women to simulate orgasm to please their husbands. The core of the female personality as described in these textbooks is narcissistic, masochistic, and passive.

Another much-used vehicle for the socialization of doctors in their attitudes toward women is drug advertisements in medical journals. Many of these ads serve to reinforce the prejudices against women. They teach doctors that women's physical complaints are trivial; their illnesses are irritating to others; and that women are emotional, have psychosomatic illnesses, and are bothersome to doctors.

Many ads for tranquilizers and antidepressants in particular suggest these products as treatment of choice before psychotherapy or social action for life situations and problems beyond the traditional concepts of illness and disease.

In a 1971 review of medical journals, Seidenberg found that misogynic statements in drug advertisements resonate with the bias of the intended observer—the male doctor. He targeted in particular advertisements that recommended doctors use drugs to adjust women to their lot when they are discontented with a humdrum environment. One caption accompanying a portrayal of a woman behind the bars of broom and mop handles read, "you can't set her free, but you can help her feel less anxious."[8]

In 1979 men are beginning to appear more frequently in drug advertisements as patients, but the difference in portrayal of men and women is still striking. Men on antidepressant medications are depicted as, "Alert on the job," and "functioning effectively in daily activities" (Pamelor). Women needing antidepressant medications, however, appear in drug ads as helpless patients under a doctor's care because, "Everything I saw was negative" (Norpramin).

The insidious effects of the sexist bias doctors learn in medical school, the professional literature they read, and the drug advertising they are exposed to are broad-ranging. The bias affects decision-making about individual patients and perpetuates misinformation about women's psychic and physiological processes. Negative consequences of these medical myths about women include the justification of limited opportunities for education, employment, and participation in the political process.

The following three specific issues are examples of sexism in medical care. All pose particular threats to women's well-being and as such are illustrations of medical care delivery to women.

Contraceptive Methods. Every woman has a right to make a free and informed choice about birth control for herself. The information about methods and the freedom of choice are key, because there is no completely satisfactory method of birth control. Each method has a unique range of benefits and risks which will differ for women of various medical histories, personal preferences, income, and health habits.

There are widespread misunderstandings about the risks and failure rates of various methods of contraception.[9] Some of this is caused by unethical advertising by pharmaceutical firms. In addition, the biases of clinics or individual doctors frequently deprive women of complete information on which to base their choices. Planned Parenthood prides itself on giving women unbiased information so they can make choices, but many women have already made up their minds about a method before they come into the clinics. According to the Washington, D.C. Public Interest Research Group, the popularity of the Pill is based on its convenience, and fewer women would expose themselves to its many risks if they took these into account in making their choices. Much of the pro-Pill reasoning is fallacious, especially the comparison of risks of the Pill with risks of pregnancy. Such comparisons assume that women not taking oral contraceptives will become pregnant, whereas they could use other safer contraceptive methods; furthermore, many of the necessary studies on the Pill's long-term safety have not been done, and many complications are never reported, so that valid comparisons between the risks of pregnancy and oral contraceptives cannot be made.

Estrogen Use in Menopause. Uterine cancer used to be rare—about one in 1,000 postmenopausal women who had not had their uteruses surgically removed. Since 1970, however, the incidence of uterine cancer in women over fifty years of age increased dramatically—by 50 percent for invasive cancer and by 100 percent for localized cancer.[10] It is not a coincidence that in the last ten to fifteen years the use of estrogen has at least tripled, and recent studies have concluded that there is a causal connection, and that the major cause of the increasing rate of uterine cancer in the United States is estrogen therapy. The sharpest rise in uterine cancer rates is among white upper- and middle-class women, who are most likely to take estrogens. Fifty percent of all postmenopausal women have taken estrogens, and approximately half of these women have taken estrogen for more than ten years. The longer the estrogen treatment and the higher the dose, the higher the incidence of uterine cancer. There are strong social pressures causing the high use of estrogen. Unsupported claims that estrogen will retard the aging process, plus the sexism that devalues older women, combine to create strong consumer demand for the drug. This demand reinforces physicians' entrenched prescribing habits, despite new scientific findings.

Six million women are using estrogens, many of them in hopes that the drug will keep them "feminine forever." This attitude, created in large part by irresponsible drug company advertising, is not going to evaporate soon. Also resistant to change are the time-hallowed doctors' attitudes toward menopause as a disease rather than as a normal physiological process.

Psychoactive Drugs: Use of legitimate psychoactive drugs among women is an important issue. An estimated one to two million people in the U.S. from all walks of life and social strata have abuse problems with prescription drugs, according to the National Institute of Drug Abuse's February and April 1978 *Capsules* press releases.

Almost twice as many women as men have had tranquilizers, sedatives, and stimulants prescribed for them. In many cases, there is no medical reason for use of the drugs, but they become a chemical support system to adjust a woman to a frustrating or unfulfilling marriage, divorce, lifestyle, or work situation. Psychoactive drugs become both a substitute and a barrier to use of counseling or other measures to combat or alter the distressing situation or the individual's response to it.

Chemical crutches for women are nothing new. In the 1800's it was common medical custom to prescribe then-legal opium for "female troubles."[11] A wide spread pattern of opium abuse grew among women-outnumbering male opium-eaters three to one in the late nineteenth and early twentieth centuries. In the drug pattern of the 1970's, general practitioners write most of the tranquilizer prescriptions and for Valium alone, there were fifty-seven million prescriptions between May 1976 and April 1977.[12]

Doctors get their education about psychoactive drugs primarily from drug companies. A survey of seventy-two medical schools found that only 20 percent had any courses in psychopharmacology, and the average time on the subject was seventeen hours in four years.[13] Medical advertising for drugs typically portrays women as frustrated, anxious, neurotic, and depressed.

Tranquilizers, sedatives, and stimulants are addictive, and in conjunction with alcohol they can be deadly. Persons who take excessive doses of either sedatives or certain tranquilizers for extended periods of time will experience dramatic withdrawal symptoms including convulsions, tremor, abdominal and muscle cramps, vomiting, and sweating.[14]

Alarming information that only recently has come to light is that some patients will experience withdrawal from such drugs as Librium and Valium when they have been taking normal therapeutic doses, with no abuse.[15] These symptoms include tremors, agitation, fear and anxiety, stomach cramps, and sweating. Since these symptoms of withdrawal so closely resemble the anxiety manifestations for which women in particular originally receive these drugs, and since so many millions of women are taking these drugs, they represent a complex problem for counselors.

Sexism in medical practice is rooted in the socialization of women to be passive recipients of care from authoritarian male doctors, plus doctors' socialization which trivializes women's medical problems and fosters attitudes that demean women patients. The results are that many women suffer needlessly from treatable organic problems labeled as psychogenic, experience irreparable damage or death because of ignored symptoms, or unwittingly fall into drug dependence due to doctors' attempts to "help" women adjust through drugs to an uncomfortable sex-typed role.

The implications are clear—it is vital for women to become informed partners in their own medical care. This will involve learning about key medical issues concerning women and developing skills to assert their rights in the sexist dynamics that pervade the health care of women. Useful tools in this task will be information sharing and assertiveness training to assist women in getting information on their own and getting responses they want from professionals. Some authors suggest limiting the practice of women's medicine (obstetrics/gynecology) to women practitioners. At some future date that may be thinkable or possible; at present, however, since 97 percent of all obstetrician/gynecologists are male, women are faced with the art of the possible in dealing with sexism in their medical care.

Notes

1. Linda Bakiel, Susan Daily, and Carolyn Kott Washburne, ed., *Women in Transition: A Feminist Handbook on Separation and Divorce* (New York: Scribners, 1975), p. 392.
2. Boston Women's Health Collective, *Our Bodies Ourselves* (New York: Simon and Schuster, 1976), p.337.
3. Barbara H. Korsch and Vida F. Negrete, "Doctor-Patient Communication." *Scientific American*, 227 (1972), 66-72.
4. Gena Corea, *The Hidden Malpractice* (New York: Marron Co., 1977), p.77.
5. Food and Drug Administration, "Alert on DES," *FDA Drug Bulletin*, 8, (1978), p.3.
6. Mary Howell, "What Medical Schools Teach About Women, *New England Journal of Medicine*, 291 (1974), 304-07.
7. Pauline Bart and Diana Scully, "A Funny Think Happened on the Way to the Orifice," *American Journal of Sociology*, 28 (1973), 1045-50.
8. R. Seidenberg, "Drug Advertising and Perceptions of Mental Illness," *Mental Hygiene*, 55 (1971), 21-31.
9. *Our Bodies Ourselves*, p. 185.
10. Food and Drug Administration, "Estrogens and Endometrial Cancer," *FDA Drug Bulletin*, 6 (1976), 2-3.
11. Annabel Hecht, "Women and Drugs," *FDA Consumer*, October 1978, pp. 7-12.
12. Jody Forman-Sher and Jonica Homiler, "An Overview of the Problem of Combined Drug/Alcohol Dependencies Among Women," paper presented at the International Conference on Alcoholism and Addictions, Zurich, Switzerland, June 1978.
13. Ann H. Clark, *National Consumers League Position on Minor Tranquilizers,* paper presented at the public hearing before the Food and Drug Administration, Rockville, Maryland, March 1978.
14. David Haskell, "Withdrawal of Diazepam," *Journal of the American Medical Association*, 233 (1975), 135.
15. Arthur Rifkin, Frederick Quitkin, and Donald Klein, "Withdrawal Reactions to Diazepam," *Journal of the American Medical Association*, 236 (1976), 2173.

Ω

Tales Out of Medical School
by Adriane Fugh-Berman, M.D.

With the growth of the women's health movement and the influx of women into medical school, there has been abundant talk of a new enlightenment among physicians. Last summer, many Americans were shocked when Frances Conley, a neurosurgeon on the faculty of Stanford University's medical school, resigned her position, citing "pervasive sexism." Conley's is a particularly elite and male-dominated subspecialty, but her story is not an isolated one. I graduated from the Georgetown University School of Medicine in 1988, and while medical training is

From *The Nation*, January 20, 1992. Copyright © 1992 by The Nation Company, Inc. Reprinted by permission.

Adriane Fugh-Berman, M.D., is on the board of the National Women's Health Network. She practices general medicine in Washington, D.C.

a sexist process anywhere, Georgetown built disrespect for women into its curriculum.

A Jesuit school, most recently in the news as the alma mater of William Kennedy Smith, Georgetown has an overwhelmingly white, male and conservative faculty. At a time when women made up one-third of all medical students in the United States, and as many as one-half at some schools, my class was 73 percent male and more than 90 percent white.

The prevailing attitude toward women was demonstrated on the first day of classes by my anatomy instructor, who remarked that our elderly cadaver "must have been a Playboy bunny" before instructing us to cut off her large breasts and toss them into the thirty-gallon trash can marked "cadaver waste." Barely hours into our training, we were already being taught that there was nothing to be learned from examining breasts. Given the fact that one out of nine American women will develop breast cancer in her lifetime, to treat breasts as extraneous tissue seemed an appalling waste of an educational opportunity, as well as a not-so-subtle message about the relative importance of body parts. How many of my classmates now in practice, I wonder, regularly examine the breasts of their female patients?

My classmates learned their lesson of disrespect well. Later in the year one carved a tick-tack-toe on a female cadaver and challenged others to play. Another gave a languorous sigh after dissecting female genitalia, as if he had just had sex. "Guess I should have a cigarette now," he said.

Ghoulish humor is often regarded as a means by which med students overcome fear and anxiety. But it serves a darker purpose as well: Depersonalizing our cadaver was good preparation for depersonalizing our patients later. Further on in my training an ophthalmologist would yell at me when I hesitated to place a small instrument meant to measure eye pressure on a fellow student's cornea because I was afraid it would hurt. "You have to learn to treat patients as lab animals," he snarled at me.

On the first day of an emergency medicine rotation in our senior year, students were asked who had had experience placing a central line (an intravenous line placed into a major vein under the clavicle or in the neck). Most of the male students raised their hands. None of the women did. For me, it was graphic proof of inequity in teaching; the men had had the procedure taught to them, but the women had not. Teaching rounds were often, for women, a spectator sport. One friend told me how she craned her neck to watch a physician teach a minor surgical procedure to a male student; when they were done the physician handed her his dirty gloves to discard. I have seen a male attending physician demonstrate an exam on a patient and then wade through several female medical students to drag forth a male in order to teach it to him. This sort of discrimination was common and quite unconscious: The women just didn't register as medical students to some of the doctors. Female students, for their part, tended (like male ones) to gloss over issues that might divert attention, energy or focus from the all-important goal of getting through their training. "Oh, they're just of the old school," a female classmate remarked to me, as if being ignored by our teachers was really rather charming, like having one's hand kissed.

A woman resident was giving a radiology presentation and I felt mesmerized. Why did I feel so connected and involved? It suddenly occurred to me that the female physician was regularly meeting my eyes; most of the male residents and attendings made eye contact only with the men.

"Why are women's brains smaller than men's!" asked a surgeon of a group of male medical students in the doctors' lounge (I was in the room as well, but was apparently invisible). "Because they're missing logic!" Guffaws all around.

Such instances of casual sexism are hardly unique to Georgetown, or indeed to medical schools. But at George-town female students also had to contend with outright discrimination of a sort most Americans probably think no longer exists in education. There was one course women were not allowed to take. The elective in sexually transmitted diseases required an interview with the head of the urology department, who was teaching the course. Those applicants with the appropriate genitalia competed for invitations to join the course (a computer was supposed to assign us electives, which we had ranked in order of preference, but that process had been circumvented for this course). Three women who requested an interview were told that the predominantly gay male clinic where the elective was held did not allow women to work there. This was news to the clinic's executive director, who stated that women were employed in all capacities.

The women who wanted to take the course repeatedly tried to meet with the urologist, but he did not return our phone calls. (I had not applied for the course, but became involved as an advocate for the women who wanted to take it.) We figured out his schedule, waylaid him in the hall and insisted that a meeting be set up.

At this meeting, clinic representatives disclosed that a survey had been circulated years before to the clientele in order to ascertain whether women workers would be accepted; 95 percent of the clients voted to welcome women. They were also asked whether it was acceptable to have medical students working at the clinic; more than 90 percent approved. We were then told that these results could not be construed to indicate that clients did not mind women medical students; the clients would naturally have assumed that "medical student" meant "male medical student." Even if that were true, we asked, if 90 percent of clients did not mind medical students and 95 percent did not mind women, couldn't a reasonable person assume that female medical students would be acceptable? No, we were informed. Another study would have to be done.

We raised formal objections to the school. Meanwhile, however, the entire elective process had been postponed by the dispute, and the blame for the delay and confusion was placed on us. The hardest part of the struggle, indeed, was dealing with the indifference of most of our classmates—out of 206, maybe a dozen actively supported us—and with the intense anger of the ten men who had been promised places in the course.

"Just because you can't take this course," one of the men said to me, "why do you want to ruin it for the rest of us?" It seemed incredible to me that I had to argue that women should be allowed to take the same courses as men. The second or third time someone asked me the same question, I suggested that if women were not allowed to participate in the same curriculum as the men, then in the interest of fairness we should get a 50 percent break on our $22,500 annual tuition. My colleague thought that highly unreasonable.

Eventually someone in administration realized that not only were we going to sue the school for discrimination but that we had an open-and-shut case. The elective in sexually transmitted diseases was canceled, and from its ashes arose a new course, taught by the same man, titled "Introduction to Urology." Two women were admitted. When the urologist invited students to take turns working with him in his office, he scheduled the two female students for the same day—one on which only women patients were to be seen (a nifty feat in a urology practice).

The same professor who so valiantly tried to prevent women from learning anything unseemly about sexually transmitted diseases was also in charge of the required course in human sexuality (or, as I liked to call it, he-man sexuality). Only two of the eleven lectures focused on women; of the two lectures on homosexuality, neither mentioned lesbians. The psychiatrist who co-taught the class treated us to one lecture that amounted to an apology for rape: Aggression, even hostility, is normal in sexual relations between a man and a woman, he said, and inhibition of aggression in men can lead to impotence.

We were taught that women do not need orgasms for a satisfactory sex life, although men, of course, do; and that inability to reach orgasm is only a problem for women with "unrealistic expectations." I had heard that particular lecture before in the backseat of a car during high school. The urologist told us of couples who came to him for sex counseling because the woman was not having orgasms; he would reassure them that this is normal and the couple would be relieved. (I would gamble that the female half of the couple was anything but relieved.) We learned that oral sex is primarily a homosexual practice, and that sexual dysfunction in women is often caused by "working." In the women-as-idiots department, we learned that when impotent men are implanted with permanently rigid penile prostheses, four out of five wives can't tell that their husbands have had the surgery.

When dealing with sexually transmitted diseases in which both partners must be treated, we were advised to vary our notification strategy according to marital status. If the patient is a single man, the doctor should write the diagnosis down on a prescription for his partner to bring to her doctor. If the patient is a married man, however, the doctor should contact the wife's gynecologist and arrange to have her treated without knowledge of what she is being treated for. How to notify the male partner of a female patient, married or single, was never revealed.

To be fair, women were not the only subjects of outmoded concepts of sexuality. We also received anachronistic information about men. Premature ejaculation, defined as fewer than ten thrusts (!). was to be treated by having the man think about something unpleasant, or by having the woman painfully squeeze, prick or pinch the penis. Aversive therapies such as these have long been discredited.

Misinformation about sexuality and and women's health peppered almost every course (I can't recall any egregious wrongs in biochemistry). Although vasectomy and abortion are among the safest of all surgical procedures, in our lectures vasectomy was presented as fraught with long-term complications and abortion was never mentioned without the words "peritonitis" and "death" in the same sentence. These distortions represented Georgetown's Catholic bent at its worst. (We were not allowed to perform, or even watch, abortion procedures in our affiliated hospitals.) On a lighter note, one obstetrician assisting us in the anatomy lab told us that women shouldn't lift heavy weights because their pelvic organs will fall out between their legs.

In our second year, several women in our class started a women's group, which held potlucks and offered presentations and performances: A former midwife talked about her profession, a student demonstrated belly dancing, another discussed dance therapy and one sang selections from *A Chorus Line*. This heavy radical feminist activity created great hostility among our male classmates. Announcements of our meetings were defaced and women in the group began receiving threatening calls at home from someone who claimed to be watching the listener and who would then accurately describe what she was wearing. One woman received obscene notes in her school mailbox, including one that contained a rape threat. I received insulting cards in typed envelopes at my home address; my mother received similar cards at hers.

We took the matter to the dean of student affairs, who told us it was "probably a dental student" and suggested we buy loud whistles to blow into the phone when we received unwanted calls. We demanded that the school attempt to find the perpetrator and expel him. We were told that the school would not expel the student but that counseling would be advised.

The women's group spread the word that we were collecting our own information on possible suspects and that any information on bizarre, aggressive, antisocial or misogynous behavior among the male medical students should be reported to our designated representative. She was inundated with a list of classmates who fit the bill. Finally, angered at the school's indifference, we solicited the help of a prominent woman faculty member. Although she shamed the dean into installing a hidden camera across from the school mailboxes to monitor unusual behavior, no one was ever apprehended.

Georgetown University School of Medicine churns out about 200 physicians a year. Some become good doctors despite their training, but many will pass on the misinformation and demeaning attitudes handed down to them. It is a shame that Georgetown chooses to perpetuate stereotypes and reinforce prejudices rather than help students acquire the up-to-date information and sensitivity that are vital in dealing with AIDS, breast cancer, teen pregnancy and other contemporary epidemics. Female medical students go through an ordeal, but at least it ends with graduation. It is the patients who ultimately suffer the effects of sexist medical education.

Ω

Is Medical School the right choice for *you*?
A SELF-EVALUATION TEST FOR THE PRE-MEDICAL STUDENT

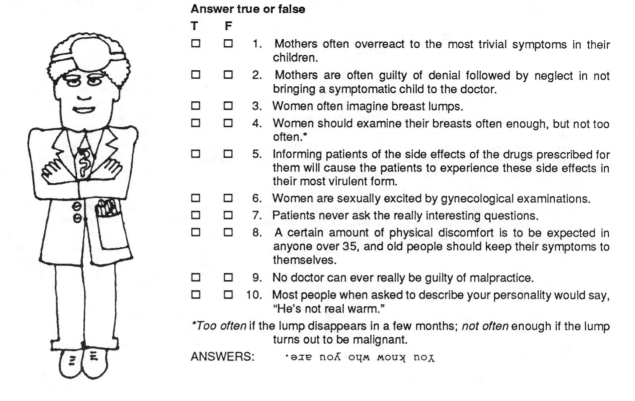

Answer true or false

T   F

- □ □ 1. Mothers often overreact to the most trivial symptoms in their children.
- □ □ 2. Mothers are often guilty of denial followed by neglect in not bringing a symptomatic child to the doctor.
- □ □ 3. Women often imagine breast lumps.
- □ □ 4. Women should examine their breasts often enough, but not too often.*
- □ □ 5. Informing patients of the side effects of the drugs prescribed for them will cause the patients to experience these side effects in their most virulent form.
- □ □ 6. Women are sexually excited by gynecological examinations.
- □ □ 7. Patients never ask the really interesting questions.
- □ □ 8. A certain amount of physical discomfort is to be expected in anyone over 35, and old people should keep their symptoms to themselves.
- □ □ 9. No doctor can ever really be guilty of malpractice.
- □ □ 10. Most people when asked to describe your personality would say, "He's not real warm."

Too often if the lump disappears in a few months; *not often* enough if the lump turns out to be malignant.

ANSWERS: You know who you are.

The Gynecologic Exam and the Training of Medical Students: An Opportunity for Health Education

by Judith Schmidt

This article is a personal account written by a senior health education major about her experience as a teaching associate (TA) in training medical students for the gynecological examination. This method of using teaching associates who "teach on their own bodies" has evolved in medical schools across the country in recent years. It is an attempt to counter inadequate medical school preparation in this important area of women's health and to improve the physician-patient relationship in gynecological medicine. Lack of sensitivity to female patients has taken the form of high rates of malpractice litigation in gynecology, a situation which might well be reversed given the improved communication between physician and patient. Medical school teaching staff across the country have now widely accepted the use of teaching associates as the most effective teaching method for this part of the complete physical examination.

One of the ideas emphasized in this approach is that of the "activated patient." An activated patient is one who is fully and equally involved as a participant in the examination process. One projected outcome of this approach is greater personal responsibility for one's health such as doing self-breast exams. But the potential of using this approach goes beyond mere "disease prevention" of traditional medical care. It gives female patients a sense of control over what happens to them—both inside and out of a gynecologist's office—and enters a psychological and social health dimension that makes the concept known as "high-level wellness" accessible. In the context of medical intervention by physicians during the gynecological exam, the potential exists to take steps toward the goal of optimal wellness. This article attempts to explore that potential.

"What's it like doing that sort of thing?" curious and sometimes incredulous friends ask. I have just told them about my job. I am a teaching associate (TA) for the instruction of the gynecological examination to first and second-year medical students. As such, I am a "professional patient." I give feedback to these students about their technique and attitude, and most important, about the way they communicate with me as a patient during the gynecological exam.

I respond to my friends' questions by telling them my job is demanding. I experience the same feelings that any woman facing a breast and pelvic exam does, including anxiety and nervousness. But overall, I feel good about doing it. I feel that what I am doing is important.

The next question, "Does it pay well?" The implication is that the only reason for my engaging in such an occupation must be money. "Yes, it does," is my answer. "And well it should! My job takes a good deal of knowledge and ability." Not only does it require knowledge of female sexual and reproductive anatomy, but it means that I must be comfortable discussing my own anatomy with others. It requires good teaching and interpersonal skills, plus a lot of sensitivity about a topic that is emotionally loaded for students and patient alike.

"But money isn't the main reason I do it," I explain. My own experiences with gynecologists have for the most part not been satisfactory. The opportunity to improve this area of women's health through my input into the training of medical students appeals to me. Also, as a student majoring in health education at the same university, I see the potential for patient education and the role physicians

might play in this process. As a TA, I feel I have some influence in this direction.

"Does your job take training?"

"Yes it does," I respond, as I visualize our initial training sessions. In these first sessions, we learn right along with the medical students. We all become part of a "learning team" which I can now see is beneficial for reducing anxiety and developing a comfortable working relationship with the students prior to the actual examination.

Just as the medical students do, we watch the Bates videotape, "Female Pelvic Examination." And just as they do, we practice inserting the speculum and examining internal anatomy manually on the plastic Gynny model. As I practice using the speculum on the Gynny model, the idea then seems less scary to me. I wonder, as a health educator, whether offering other women this experience on a Gynny model prior to a pelvic exam might lessen their anxiety, as it has mine.

In these initial training sessions my actual teaching role begins. I am called upon to recall my own feelings during the gynecological exam. The medical students are also encouraged to explore the kinds of feelings that they, as physicians, might experience. How should the physician, for example, handle a situation in the best interests of the patient and him or herself if sexually attracted to the patient prior to the examination? Issues such as these are dealt with in these sessions.

Emphasis in these training sessions is put on the importance of involving the patient during the process of the exam itself. An activated patient who is involved in such a way has some sense of control over what is happening to her during her exam. Again, as a teaching associate I am called upon to describe how being "activated" in this way as a patient allows me to feel less victimized during the gynecological exam.

From HEALTH VALUES, Vol. 10, No. 2, March/April 1986, pp. 33–36. Copyright © 1986 by Judith Schmidt. Reprinted by permission of the author.

Part of this initial discussion focuses on empathy. To learn to empathize with female patients, all the students are required to disrobe, drape, and get into the lithotomy position—or into the stirrups, as it is commonly called. Through this first-hand experience, medical students can vividly relate to the feelings of vulnerability shared by their female patients as they lie naked, legs suspended, waiting to be examined—covered only by a thin piece of paper that fails to intercept the cool flow of air over one's usually concealed private anatomy.

After these preliminary training sessions, my difficult work begins. I find that my anxiety soon disappears as I get actively involved in teaching. The students are much more nervous than I am so that relating to them in a calm and confident way has the effect of putting us both at ease.

The nature of the suggestions that I give during the actual examination stresses technique. I might suggest that a student flatten his or her hand while palpating my abdomen. I might help a student identify that fleeting moment when my ovaries roll past. But I do not emphasize the mechanics, as I know these will improve with practice.

The general feedback I give each student in turn afterward about how well he or she communicated with me and attended to my emotional needs is far more important. I begin by reinforcing those things which I like. This might include confirming that the student maintained eye contact with me and watched my face for non-verbal signals indicating discomfort. Or it might mean commending a student's effective use of firm and reassuring touch. Then, I follow with a suggestion for improvement. This might include suggesting to the student that he or she replace specialized medical jargon with common conversational language that the patient can more easily understand.

Occasionally, my job demands that I be assertive. For example, I had to tell a male student that I was uneasy having his groin against my knee, while having my breast examined—under ordinary circumstances a female patient might interpret this in a sexual way. We were both embarrassed, but he expressed appreciation for telling him this.

Only once did I find it necessary to tell a student about poor attitude. "I am uncomfortable with the way you treated me—as if I were a plastic model," I had to say. Fortunately, this is rare as most students are respectful and caring to the extreme.

I am proud of the student who is able to include me actively and equally as a participant. I keep a mental check-list during the exam of the various ways the student might accomplish this. Does the student remember to offer me a mirror? Does he or she offer it in such a way that is *not* just an off-hand question? ("Do you want a mirror?") But rather in a way so that *I*, as patient, understand that it is important and acceptable to know about my own female anatomy. "Would you like to hold a mirror while I examine your pelvic area? That way I can better explain to you what *I* see, and *you* can see everything for yourself?"

There are other check-offs on my mental list. Does the student offer me the option of having my head raised during the pelvic part of the examination to facilitate communication between us? Does the student actively solicit my verbal input; not just telling and explaining, but questioning and encouraging any questions *I*, as patient, might have regarding my anatomy or sexual functioning?

Finally, I consider certain non-verbal aspects of our communication exchange. I consider the student's attitude. Is it flippant or overbearing in any way? Does the student display appropriate respect and a willingness to share power in the interaction that goes on between us? What clues do I get from facial expression, body position and movement that support my assessment?

By assessing the answers to all these questions, I am able to evaluate how well I was activated as an involved and equal participant during the examination. When done effectively, this process allows me to feel in control—not as a passive bystander whose body is "being done to."

At this point, relating the notion of the activated patient to the idea of wellness begins. By actively engaging female patients in the gynecological exam itself, the physician can play an important role in aiding the female patient in knowing and being comfortable with her body. Not only might this have a spin-off effect of encouraging women to practice self-examination and prevention at home, (I am an example of one who only began doing regular self-breast exams since beginning this job even though I had long known the appalling statistics about breast cancer) but it might help overcome those culturally programmed negative feelings that many women still have about their bodies and lead to a greater degree of sexual satisfaction.

At the end of the teaching session, it is my time for reinforcement. The students all express their gratitude. They are relieved that doing a procedure that had worried them has turned into a positive learning experience; they give me credit. I accept their thanks and express my hope that they will use what they have learned here to make the experience of the gynecological exam a better one for their patients.

One of my fears when I took this job was how the students would react when we would meet in public after the training sessions. I knew this was inevitable as I am a student on the same campus in a small city. Contrary to my worries, I have not felt the slightest embarrassment. Rather I sense a mutual respect between us resulting from the difficult task we shared together.

This feeling of mutual respect might not be something peculiar to my own particular experience. Perhaps it is a reflection of this kind of interaction between a patient-oriented physician and an activated, involved patient. It is an interaction that is designed to allow the patient to feel more in control and, in so doing, to enhance her self-esteem.

The positive effect of this interaction for the patient and its contribution to her overall health status should not be minimized. Replacing negative feelings that many women still have regarding their sexual-reproductive anatomy with positive ones can enhance a woman's sense of well-being and personal fulfillment. Satisfying such a psychological health need represents a step on that continuum toward that elusive concept known as high level wellness.

Entering this psychological and social health dimension goes beyond the purely physical realm of traditional medical care.

Medical intervention by a physician which attempts to accomplish such a task is a concrete way to lessen the gap between disease prevention and that lofty goal of optimal wellness. It is an intervention mutually rewarding to patient and physician alike.

Bibliography

1. DiMatteo RM, Friedman HS: *Social Psychology and Medicine*. Oelgeschlager, West Germany, Gum and Hain, Publishers, Inc., 1982.
2. Miller GD: They gynecological examination as a learning experience. *Journal of the American College Health Association* 1974; 23(2).

Ω

PRO

Women's Health: Developing a New Interdisciplinary Specialty
by Karen Johnson, M.D.

Abstract. This paper argues that medicine is based on a male paradigm that does not permit high-quality comprehensive care for women within existing medical specialties. Suggestions are made to alleviate the shortcomings of the current paradigm by including women. A call for the development of a specialty in women's health is made. Types of resistance to this proposal, stemming from sexism, economics, and alliances to existing specialties, are also discussed. Finally, it is argued that bringing the study and practice of women's health to parity with the understanding and treatment of men must be achieved rapidly and comprehensively using an active and multifaceted approach.

Introduction

No existing medical specialty is devoted exclusively to the comprehensive care of women. Many of us providing health care for women in a variety of existing specialties believe that the absence of such a comprehensively trained specialist is a significant problem in the health care services offered to women.[1] This problem could be solved through the development of an interdisciplinary specialty in women's health.

Medicine as a Paradigm Based upon Experiences with Men

With the exception of physicians in one surgical specialty, obstetrics-gynecology, physicians caring for women base the majority of their diagnoses and interventions on clinical trials and studies with men, often unknowingly.[2] However benevolent the original intentions in excluding women from drug trials and clinical studies, their absence has led to unnecessary morbidity and premature mortality. For example, the Baltimore Longitudinal Study on Aging started in 1958 did not include women for the first 20 years. This omission delayed the discovery of the link among osteoporosis, calcium, estrogen, and progesterone, resulting in the needless suffering and death of hundreds of thousands of women.

More recently the AIDS epidemic has highlighted the serious consequences of assuming that diseases in women manifest with exactly the same signs and symptoms as diseases in men. Until 1991 the Center for Disease Control (CDC) criteria for AIDS was based on men. HIV positive women presenting with cervical cancer, pelvic inflammatory disease, and vaginal thrush were diagnosed much later in the disease process. Not only did these uniquely female diagnoses delay treatment and thus shorten life expectancy compared with men, they often caused undue economic hardship because meeting the CDC criteria was a prerequisite to receiving public assistance available to patients with AIDS.

Other problems are created by the assumption that our experience with men is transferable to women. Although cardiovascular disease is the leading cause of death in women, we would hardly know it based on most of the research in this field.[3] The initial study affirming that aspirin could be used as preventive therapy for coronary disease included more than 22,000 subjects, all male. The Mr. FIT study (Multiple Risk Factor Intervention Trials) identified coronary disease risk factors in 15,000 subjects, again all men. Even when women's risk of cardiovascular disease is assessed, clinical experience and interventions with men may not be applicable to women. Women may present with different symptoms in the office; they often arrive further in the progression of a myocardial infarction in the emergency room; they are more likely to die in the operating room.

Many diseases common in both men and women have a substantially higher incidence in women. It is not entirely clear why. Diseases of the gastrointestinal tract are just one example. Gallstones occur earlier in women and women continue to have a greater prevalence of them throughout their lives. Biliary dyskinesia occurs more often in women. Irritable bowel syndrome and gastroparesis are three times more common in women than men. Women are more susceptible to the hepatotoxic effects of alcohol than men. However, as is often the case in diseases that occur in both genders, clinical investigations have been carried out mostly in men. As a result in caring for women we cannot be confident that our diagnostic techniques and medical interventions are sound.

Health matters that occur exclusively (or primarily) in women such as menstruation, premenstrual symptoms, uterine fibroids, menopause, and breast cancer have received less attention than the patient population (52% of adults) would warrant. This has hindered our ability to offer advice with confidence.

Sometimes relying on the male paradigm is nothing short of ludicrous. Consider the study at Rockefeller University in which researchers were analyzing the effects of obesity on estrogen activity and the tendency to develop breast and uterine cancer. All the subjects were male.[4] Although it is finally a widely held belief that women and men are equal they are not the same—physiologically or psychologically.[5,6] Using men as the medical standard from which women diverge is unpardonable.[7]

Crossing Boundaries

Now that the consciousness of medicine has been raised, it has been suggested that improving women's health care can be achieved by making adjustments in the education of physicians within existing specialties.[8] This plan on its own would not address the numerous health concerns experienced by women that do not easily fit into any existing specialty. Consider the woman whose abdominal pain is finally diagnosed as endometriosis. Lacking an interdisciplinary-trained women's health specialist, the recommended interventions are likely to be biased by the specialty training of her provider. A primary care physician may be inclined to prescribe analgesics for pain, whereas a gynecologist leans more toward hormonal or surgical interventions. A psychiatrist or other mental health provider may need to be included to assist with corollary emotional distress or sexual dysfunction. Two or more physicians are required to provide complete care, an inefficient and expensive process.

Many medical problems experienced by women present similar dilemmas. Two additional examples are pre-

menstrual symptoms and domestic violence. Premenstrual symptoms are inadequately defined within the existing paradigm, but they are certainly experienced by many women. Lacking agreement about diagnosis and treatment, specialists tend to interpret symptoms through their own frame of reference. Domestic violence is a major health hazard for American women, but it is overlooked by many physicians.[9] Untrained in a broader understanding of women's health, physicians' impressions are biased by the perspective of their own specialty. When presented with only a small part of the clinical problem, they often fail to piece together the larger diagnostic picture. A women complaining of insomnia or suffering with a fracture may be treated in an emergency room or family practice center, but never asked directly about physical abuse. Although the lack of a unified approach to premenstrual symptoms can lead to discomfort and distress, the failure to accurately diagnose domestic violence can be life threatening. What is called for in these and many other situations experienced by women is an interdisciplinary approach.

Correcting the Paradigm

Most physicians until recently have been unaware that the practice of medicine is based on a male paradigm.[10] Many of the problems that have arisen because of this have been identified. There is now relative agreement within the medical profession that these problems must be addressed, but we are by no means in agreement as to the method.

Some believe that we have crossed the barriers to the full inclusion of women's health care needs and that we can correct the existing medical paradigm by alterations within current specialties. This belief is at odds with the limited achievements women have made in other areas when analogous omissions were brought to light, as noted in Faludi's *Backlash*.[11]

Representatives from at least three specialties—internal medicine, obstetrics-gynecology, and family practice—have argued that these specialties can adequately meet the comprehensive needs of women patients. I question their assertions. Unless practitioners of these specialties have taken it upon themselves to round out their standard residency training, few are qualified to call themselves women's health specialists in the manner I am arguing is required.

At present most internists have inadequate knowledge of women's reproductive health, extremely limited experience with the psychosocial aspects of women's health care, and a discipline that is built entirely on a male paradigm. Although obstetrics-gynecology training is based upon experiences with women, it is arguable whether it can genuinely be considered a primary care specialty. The training is fundamentally surgical, and the inclusion of a psychosocial perspective is also limited.

Family physicians argue that they are in the best position to offer high-quality comprehensive care for women. This is true within the context of the current medical

15

paradigm. Their interdisciplinary training serves them well in approaching the multiplicity of women's health care concerns. However, the training and practice of family medicine require these physicians to divide their attention among women, men, and children.

Certainly family physicians treat the young as well as the elderly and more than other specialists gain a psychosocial perspective in their training. Nevertheless, this has not negated the need for the specialty of pediatrics or the subspecialty of geriatrics. Pediatricians' focused attention on children and geriatricians' focused attention on the elderly have led to improved health care for the youngest and the oldest of patients. Specialists in women's health will bring similar benefits to all our woman patients—no matter what specialty we practice.

I do agree with colleagues who caution that a specialty in women's health must not be viewed as alleviating the imperative that every existing medical specialty revise its content to include the accurate and respectful treatment of women.[12] However, I do not believe that these efforts will be adequate. Nor do I think that these improvements and the development of a new interdisciplinary specialty are mutually exclusive. They would be complementary.

Placing Women's Health in the Larger Context

The idea of a specialty in women's health is a logical extension of the women's health movement that began in the 1960s.[13] Physicians influenced by this movement began to articulate the need for a specialty in women's health by the 1980s.[14,15] The recent increased interest in women's health at all levels is gratifying; however, attention to the concerns of women has been inconsistent during this century. It would be a mistake to assume the current flurry of activity in women's health will continue without formalizing the specialty.

Having a medical specialty in women's health could be viewed much like having a room of one's own.[16] Just as departments of women's studies have been instrumental in assuring that women's experiences are accurately represented in the academic community, a specialty in women's health would serve a similar purpose in medicine.

Those who believe it will be sufficient to simply add women's health to existing specialties would be wise to study the history of science, the sociology of knowledge, and the role of values in science if the missed opportunities of other pioneers are to be avoided. Nineteenth century scientists argued that the rigors of a university education would drain energy from women's reproductive organs. These and other socially expedient biases were used to justify the exclusion of women from positions of authority and decision making. Unless health issues are approached from a solid interdisciplinary, pro-woman perspective, I am not confident that current or future physicians will serve women significantly better than their earlier counterparts. We have already seen a great deal of the money targeted for new research in women's health funneled into the existing "old boys'" research network.[17] This is wor-

risome and disappointing to those of us who had hoped for more adventuresome funding and innovative projects. Rest assured, the age-old debate of autonomy versus integration will wage on as we struggle with how to include women's health in medical training. Common sense and experience suggest that we must do both. It is from the power base of a residency in women's health that efforts to mainstream are most likely to be successful. Furthermore, women's health is a separate body of knowledge and deserves to be treated as a legitimate area of inquiry.

Positioning a Women's Health Specialty

There are several possible routes to specialization. Women's health could be a primary care specialty like pediatrics or subspeciality like geriatrics. Alternatively, much like toxicology, it could be a field of study. Entry from any number of specialties would be possible. The positioning of the specialty is less critical than its content. Women's health must be based on research and experience with women, not men.

Those of us interested in fostering the development of an interdisciplinary specialty in women's health have many resources to turn for valuable advice and information. Nursing, a female-dominated profession, has had training programs in women's health for over a decade. Feminist scholars in health psychology and women's studies also have much to offer.

There are already many interesting and active steps being taken within medicine to assure a better response to women's health care needs. Since 1982, hospital-affiliated multidisciplinary women's health centers have offered a closer approximation of an interdisciplinary approach than more conventional group practices.[18] This summer Harvard Medical School held their fifth annual conference on women's health, combining internal medicine, obstetrics-gynecology, and psychiatry. The American Medical Women's Association is preparing a multidisciplinary postgraduate course on the health care needs of women. Fellowships in women's medicine have started to appear at several institutions, and a number of medical schools offer electives in women's health.[19] Nevertheless, a growing number of medical students longing to specialize in women's health express frustration at the lack of a residency program anywhere in the United States. For now, highly motivated trainees are left to customize existing residencies to achieve their goal of specializing in women's health (D. Moran, personal communication).

Resistance

The resistance to this proposal has been intense and is no doubt determined by many factors. Change is almost always anxiety provoking. In this case the anxiety is fueled by forces as divergent as sexism, economics, and alliances to existing specialties.

Treating women with knowledge drawn from research on men is enough of a problem without being compounded by pervasive sexism.[20] This is an issue in patient care that we have hardly begun to address.[21] Sexist behavior ranges from simple patronizing[22] to explicit harassment and abuse.[23] One male obstetrician has suggested that unless male physicians correct their sexist attitudes and behavior, they should not be allowed to provide health care for women.[2,24]

Unfortunately sexism is not unique to male physicians. It is embedded in the professionalization of almost every medical student. How else can we interpret the disturbing revelation this year of a graduating medical student that in the anatomy lab female breasts were designated as "waste" and tossed in the trash without careful dissection and examination?[25] This behavior is unconscionable when one in nine American women can expect to develop breast cancer within her lifetime.

Arguments that a specialty in women's health will lead to costly fragmentation and overspecialization do not make sense. It is the current arrangement that causes these problems. Divisions in medicine are arbitrary and based on any number of factors including physician interest, expanding scientific knowledge, and political agendas. Siphoning funds from other critical areas such as AIDS and cancer research will undoubtedly be used as economic scarecrows. At a less conscious level some will be concerned that specialists in women's health will compete more favorably for women patients. Women are the greatest users of health care. Yet another potential financial loss is hard to swallow when physicians are already feeling under siege.

Those of us specializing in the care of women have been cautioned against proposing the development of a new specialty just as medicine is being forced to tighten its belt. The proposal of a new specialty at this time may seem to burden a crumbling system. But it is in this climate that attending to the health care needs of women is even more urgent. Unless we are vigilant about the quality and availability of care for women, it is likely with any of the insurance reforms currently under consideration that health care services for women will be the first to suffer.[26]

Even many well-meaning physicians are unconvinced that a specialty is needed. They believe that theirs is either providing perfectly adequate care for women or that with only modest efforts the quality of care can be raised to acceptable levels. Their identification with their own training interferes with an accurate understanding of the problem.

ʾraming the Solution

What most opponents fail to appreciate is that women's ʾh is a unique body of knowledge and skills based upon ε ʾence with women that cross the boundaries of existing sp ʾes. Women's health care needs are not being met, and can. ʾ met, within the existing medical paradigm.

T. ʾterion of the American Board of Medical Specialist. a new specialty is that it must "represent a distinct vell-defined field of medical practice" such as "special concerns with problems of patients according to age, sex, organ systems or interaction between patients and their environment." With practice specialties ranging from addiction medicine to undersea medicine,[27] I am hard pressed to understand why a specialty embracing 52% of the adult population is unreasonable or unnecessary.

Conclusion

When it comes to women's health, there are far more questions than answers. Specialists devoted to women's health care in a number of fields are beginning to provide some answers, but the information is fragmented and unknown to physicians who have no particular interest in the field.

It is not only discriminatory, but truly dangerous to fail to bring the study and practice of women's medicine to parity with the understanding and treatment of men rapidly and comprehensively. This can and must be achieved through an active and multifaceted approach. This includes physicians examining their practices and attitudes for social or cultural biases that affect medical care, funding medical research in women's health, and increasing the number of women in positions of authority in teaching, research, and the practice of medicine.[28] The Women's Health Initiative,[29] a multidisciplinary, multiinstitute intervention study to address the major causes of death, disability, and frailty among middle-aged and older women, is an important step, as is the creation of the Office of Research on Women's Health. However, as valuable as these efforts are, they are insufficient. Women deserve no less than children who have specialists in pediatrics and the elderly who have specialists in geriatrics. A new interdisciplinary specialty in women's health is required.

References

1. Johnson K, Dawson L. Women's health as a multidisciplinary specialty: An exploratory proposal. J Am Med Wom Assoc 1990;45:222–224.
2. Rodin J, Ickovics J. Women's health: Review and research agenda as we approach the 21st century. Am Psychol 1990;45:1018—1034.
3. National Women's Health Resource Center. Cardiovascular disease. In: Forging a women's health research agenda, 1990;1–20.
4. Flynn T. Female trouble: Imagine a study about uterine cancer that only examines men. Chicago Tribune 1986 Oct 29; Sec 7:26
5. Miller JB. Toward a new psychology of women (2nd ed.) Boston: Beacon Press, 1986.
6. Johnson K. Trusting ourselves. New York: Atlantic Monthly Press, 1991.
7. Toward a women's health research agenda: Findings of the scientific advisory meeting. Society for the Advancement of Women's Health Research. Washington, DC: Bass and Howes, Inc. 1991:1–16.
8. Your opinion: Women's health specialty. Internal Medicine World Report 1990; Sept 15–30:30
9. Novello A. Cited in: Fore J. Doctors urged to ask about abuse. San Francisco Examiner 1992 June 17:A–10.
10. Liebert MA. From the publisher. J Wom Health 1992;1:xix.

11. Faludi S. Backlash. New York: Crown, 1990.
12. Harrison M. Women as other: The premise of medicine. J Am Med Wom Assoc 1990;45:225–226.
13. Ruzek S. The women's health movement: Feminist alternatives to medical control. New York: Praeger, 1979.
14. Johnson K. Seminar presented at the Center for Educational Development, University of Illinois, Chicago, April 1982.
15. Wallis L. Presentation to the National Association of Women Health Professionals, Chicago, Oct 1989.
16. Woolf V. A room of one's own. New York: Harcourt Brace Jovanovich, 1929.
17. Hamilton JA. Women's health research: Public policy issues. Presented at Second Annual Syntex Women's Health Roundtable, Washington, DC, Feb 1992.
18. Johnson K. Women's health care: An innovative model. Wom Ther 1987;6:305–311.
19. Montgomery K, Moulton A. Undergraduate medical education in women's health. Wom Health Forum. 1992;1:1–2.
20. Novello A. Cited in: Surgeon general says sexism is a problem. San Francisco Examiner 1992 May 13: A–15.
21. Eichler M, Reisman A, Borins E. Gender bias in medical research. Paper presented at Conference on Gender, Science an Medicine, Toronto, November 1988.
22. Wallis LA, Klass P. Toward improving women's health care. J Am Med Wom Assoc 1990;45:219–221.
23. Gartrell N, Milliken N, Goodson W. Thiemann S. Physician patient sexual contact: Prevalence and problems. Western J Med. In Press.
24. Smith, JH. Women and doctors. New York: Atlantic Monthly Press, 1992.
25. Fugh-Berman A. Tales out of medical school. The Nation 1992 January 20; 1:54–56.
26. Jecker NS. Age-based rationing and women JAMA. 1991;266:3012–3015.
27. List of self-designated practice specialty codes. Chicago: American Medical Association, 1992.
28. Council on Ethical and Judicial Affairs. Gender disparities in clinical decision making. JAMA 1991;266:559–562.
29. Healy B. The Yentl syndrome. N Engl J Med 1991: 325:274–275.

CON

Women's Health As a Specialty: A Deceptive Solution
by Michelle Harrison, M.D.

Abstract. A proposed call for a new specialty in women's health is an attempt to rectify current inadequacies in the care of women. This paper discusses ninteenth century origins of the current organization of medical specialties in which the male body is the norm and woman becomes "other." Nineteenth century attitudes toward women, with the belief in the biological inferiority of women due to their sexual organs, and the replacement of midwives by physicians, became the basis of this bifurcated system of care in which women require two physicians for their ongoing care. A reorganization of medical specialties is proposed in which: (1) Internal medicine incorporates the primary care aspect of gynecology, as does family medicine; (2) Obstetrics and gynecology remains the surgical and referral specialty that it is; (3) Interdisciplinary research addresses gaps in understanding the role of reproductive events, hormones, and cycles to normal and pathological functioning; (4) Medical students are taught to identify across gender lines; (5) All specialties are examined for the pupose of making them "user friendly" to women; and (6) The medical profession addresses and rectifies past inequities in the conceptual framework about women and their subsequent denial of leadership opportunities. The need for education in women's health is acknowledged, but with the goal of making that need obsolete. A new specialty has the potential to further isolate women's issues from mainstream medicine and to marginalize its practioners.

The proposition that women's health become a separate specialty derives from the failure of the established medical system to address adequately the health care needs of women. These inadequacies exist in the social, medical, educational, and research aspects of women's health. Even though women consume proportionally more medical services than do men, the basic organization of medical specialization has been based upon a male standard to which woman is the eternal exception. Although the establishment of a separate specialty of women's health may initially seem appealing, it has the potential of further isolating the women's perspective in delivery of health care, while simultaneously marginalizing those practitioners who commit themselves to its practice.

This paper discusses the history of the development of the current system of medicine with its adaptation toward the male body and psyche. A model of health care in which women's bodies are the norm, not the exception, is developed.

Nineteenth Century Attitudes

The current treatment of women has its roots in the history of medicine in America, which in turn reflected the

From JOURNAL OF WOMEN'S HEALTH, Vol. 1, No.2, 1992. Copyright © 1992 by Mary Ann Liebert, Inc. Reprinted by permission.

prevailing cultural attitudes toward women. Dr. Charles D. Meigs, Professor of Midwifery and the Diseases of Women and Children at Jefferson Medical College in Philadelphia, in 1838 translated the following from the French physician Velpeau:

Puberty, or the marriageable age, is announced in girls, as it is in boys, by numerous changes. . . . The young girl becomes more timid and reserved; her form becomes more rounded. . . . Her eyes, which are at once brilliant and languishing, express commingled desires, fears, and tenderness; the sensations she experiences and the sense of her own weakness, are the causes why she no longer dares to approach the companions of her childhood but with a downcast look.[1]

The biological transition from girl to young woman was seen as the causative factor in her change in personality. Biology was deemed destiny, and hers was to be one of fear and weakness.

The nineteenth century saw the development of a sizable population of women who, because of industrialization and urbanization, became part of a middle class in which women's employment outside the home was unnecessary. So, while the vast majority of women throughout the world toiled in fields and factories, bore child after child, then aged and died early, Western Europe and America were creating a new version of woman expressive of new political and economic times. The new version conveniently placed women out of competition with men and created a biological basis for that exclusion. Meigs, in an 1859 collection of his own lectures, wrote, "The sexuality of the woman does in its essence consist in the possession of that peculiar structure called ovarian stroma—her heart, brain, lungs, all her viscera, all indeed that she is, would not make her a female without the primordial central essence—stroma."[2] He continues, "She demands a treatment adapted to the very specialties of her own constitution, as a moral, a sexual, germiferous, gestative, or parturient creature."[2] Women's sexuality then became the heart of the justification of difference, and difference invariably meant lesser.

Laqueur, in *Making Sex: Body and Gender from the Greeks to Freud,* describes the Greek model in which the genders were measured by metaphysical perfection in hierarchical relation to each other. This early model of "one sex" in various states of perfection and imperfection was replaced in the nineteenth century with a model of biological divergence based upon anatomical and physiological incommensurability.[3] What had previously been a variation on a single human body became two distinct sexes, believed to be different in every aspect. The shift had been one of changing from comparing grades of apples to comparing apples and oranges, male and female.

Laqueur argues that the polarities of gender can be understood as polarities of power and that "the competition for power generates new ways of constituting the subject and the social realities within which humans dwell."[3] As if to illustrate Laqueur's point, Dr. Alfred Stille in his presidential address to the American Medical Association in 1871 stated, "If, then, woman is unfitted by nature to

become a physician, we should, when we oppose her pretensions, be acquitted of any malicious or even unkindly spirit."[4] Woman had been discovered to be a new species, one conveniently unsuited to compete with men in the profession of medicine.

Nineteenth century medicine developed along two lines simultaneously. The body of medicine treated men and the nonreproductive aspects of women's health. Childbirth and common gynecologic problems were usually left to midwives, in part because of prohibitions against male physicians examining female sexual organs. Women's genitals began to be "observed" by physicians in the mid nineteenth century.[5] With the development of gynecologic surgery, which established gynecology as a recognized field, and the successful effort on the part of medicine to define childbirth as a surgical procedure, female midwives were replaced by male obstetricians and gynecologists.

The lifting of cultural prohibitions against the gynecologic examination of women by men opened the way for increasing male knowledge about female reproductive anatomy and physiology. If not for the pursuit of economic and professional power on the part of physicians, there might have been a partnership with the midwives, with benefit to both professions and especially to women as patients. Instead there was the destruction of midwifery and a loss of the ways in which women had for centuries attended to the needs of other women. The midwives' care of women exclusively meant that for midwifery, the female body was the standard, the normal, the regular. With the transfer of care to a male medical profession, in which the standard was the male body, the body without female parts, woman's body became "other."[6] With the destruction of midwifery and the paucity of women physicians, the woman's body with its sexual organs was now a foreign body to the overwhelmingly male medical profession and the exclusively male gynecologic surgeons.

The stage was thus set for the current organization of medicine in which internal medicine attends to the nonreproductive aspects of women's health and the generative-related conditions are relegated to the obstetrician-gynecologist. The woman's body with its sexual and generative functions had been medicalized, even in those processes that can be viewed as normal functions. Because medicine was organized around a male body and because physicians were male, nothing about a woman's menstrual cycle or reproduction was "normal." It was all new. She had to be "managed," an approach to women that has not significantly changed.[7]

Nineteenth century medicine attributed the state of women's mental health to the health of their ovaries. Mental illness (at times defined as the inability to accept culturally defined roles, with symptoms including a desire to run away from home, dislike of a husband, or a refusal to sleep with him[8]) was attributed to the dysfunction of sexual organs. The reproductive organs became the seat of not just sexual passions but were seen as the cause of insanity. Clitoridectomy was the first operation performed to check woman's mental disorder.[9] Proponents of castration described the benefits of removal of the ovaries: "the moral sense of the patient is elevated . . . she becomes tractable, orderly, industrious, and cleanly."[9] There was apparently some recognition that castration could lead to postoperative insanity, in which case further surgery was recommended, namely removal of the uterus and Fallopian tubes. Clitoridectomy, castration, and hysterectomy were the nineteenth century treatment of uncontrolled female emotions.[9] The operation was successful if the woman "was restored to a placid contentment with her domestic functions."[10]

Normality was defined as male, with sanity therefore being closer to male function than to female function. Barker-Benfield suggests that the identification of female sexuality with madness was a result of the assumption that "man's madness" was the norm within the society and therefore woman's was easier to cure.[11] Female "madness" was also easier to see because to the extent it expressed resistance to stereotypic roles, it stood in sharp contrast to the social and political prohibitions of the society.

Such practices as the nineteenth century surgical treatments to return women to their acceptable "passivity" may seem shocking by contemporary standards. Less obvious are the current ways in which society accommodates male behavior and male "madness." For example, although the current diagnosis of postraumatic stress disorder describes the woman's reaction to rape, an adequate framework to describe the causative behavior on the part of the male aggressor is lacking. The psychological effects of sexual harassment on the part of the victim can be described, but the language and understanding of perpetrators is wanting.

The long delay in recognizing wife battering and marital rape may be traced to the nineteenth century when, "throughout much of the bourgeois century, all across the Western world, women remained virtual chattels in the hands of their fathers, and later, of their husbands."[12] For the last two centuries it was the women victims of battering and marital rape who were brought for mental health services. Society's acceptance of, and possibly hopelessness about, male violence may prevent perception of these acts as deviant and destructive.

Sex role stereotyping within the mental health field was aptly described by Broverman et al., who described sex biases in interpretation of behavior by clinicians. In their 1970 study, a healthy adult (nonspecified sex) had attributes more like a healthy male than a healthy woman. They found that "clinicians are more likely to suggest that healthy women differ from healthy men by being more submissive, less independent, less adventurous, more easily influenced, less aggressive, less competitive, more excitable in minor crises. . . ."[13]

These findings from 1970 are not unlike the descriptions of Velpeau (quoted above) in 1838 or those describing results of castration. In those intervening 130 years, a civil war was fought, women organized and fought for the right to vote, they organized against alcohol, they entered the professions of medicine and law against great odds,

they joined the military for two world wars, and yet the stereotypes prove more resilient than reality. Women's sex and sexuality continued to be perceived as the basis for her inferiority. Physicians had, "turned the stereotype of feminine frailty into a medical principle."[14]

The diagnosis of late luteal phrase dysphoric disorder was added to the *Diagnostic and Statistical Manual* of the American Psychiatric Association in 1987.[15] This diagnosis describes a mental disorder whose etiology is the menstrual cycle and whose language includes anger as a symptom of mental illness. Although few would dispute that the menstrual cycle may affect how some women feel, including anger, there is an important distinction between influencing and causing symptoms and behavior.

Men and women are influenced in mood by weather, light, diet, general health, and day of the week, but few would designate those as the determinants of mental illness. However, old beliefs persist, in practitioners and in women. When a contemporary woman visits her gynecologist because she is irritable with her children premenstrually, she is the "medical" expression of the nineteenth century view of women's mental state being controlled by her ovaries. Likewise, her gynecologist is supporting this premise when ovariectomy is the treatment recommended for the woman's mood or behavioral problems. Chemical and surgical castration remain accepted treatments for disorders of mood.[16-18]

Educating for Women's Health

The establishment of training programs in women's health is a separate issue from the creation of a new specialty. There is an enormous job to be done in educating the medical profession and institutions. Ideally, this would be a task undertaken with the aim of eventual obsolescence. Fellowships are needed in order to teach and to create meaningful research. However, to create a new specialty, to certify those physicians trained to take care of women, would allow the rest of those in medicine to feel absolved of responsibility for addressing the needs of women, and more inclined to leave the sensitive care of women to those few practitioners who are now the "experts." In reality, only a very small percentage of women (and of a given social class) would have access to this care, and the vast majority of women would continue as they do now with their bifurcated care.

The Call for a Specialty

The problems in contemporary medicine that have brought forth the call for a new specialty in women's health are related to: (1) unexplored and unanswered questions in research and education related to women's health; (2) the ways in which women's health needs are not met; and (3) the bifurcation of routine medical care of women.

Given the shortcomings of the present medical system, the call for a separate specialty is understandable. It comes out of frustration, disappointment, and mistrust. The presence of increasing numbers of women physicians has led to a reassessment as to whether medicine could do a better job in addressing needs of women patients. However, there is no aspect of this new proposed specialty that should not be an integral part of the education and practice of every physician, male or female. Rather, the solutions lie in a reorganization of current medical specialization and a demand for the provision of services that more adequately address the needs of women patients.

Questions for Research and Education

Major gaps exist in the understanding of differences in female physiology and pathology, related, but not restricted, to the menstrual cycle. Because of the "foreign nature" of female bodies to a male medical profession, the menstrual cycle and its effects were for a long time ignored, stigmatized, or left strictly to gynecology. Were all males to menstruate, the interrelated effects of the menstrual cycle on other aspects of a person's health would have been considered essential, even fascinating, areas of study, worthy of the best research and funding. In fact, the vast majority of physicians have never experienced menstruation, looked at sanitary pads, handled tampons, or had cramps. Though it may not be necessary to experience illnesses in order to understand or treat them, the lack of understanding or familiarity with what is normal may result in a tendency to pathologize the entire process. That deficiency in personal experience may limit one's ability to be comfortable with integrating menstruation into a "normal" body.

On the other side, the fact that women are not defined by their menstrual cycles does not mean that this process is irrelevant. It is clear that many medications react differently over the course of the menstrual cycle, yet this area remains largely unexplored. Pharmacologic research has been done on males in part because the menstrual cycle becomes a confounding factor in analysis of results. However, the drugs are then used on women and those confounding effects become clinical effects—poorly understood because of a paucity of research. The research that is needed is not necessarily on the menstrual cycle itself, but rather interdisciplinary research that looks at the menstrual cycle in relation to heart disease, asthma, seizures, and lupus, areas where it is already clear that gender is relevant.[19-25] Interdisciplinary and gender-conscious research is needed to look at osteoporosis in relation to nutrition, exercise, vitamins, *and* the menstrual cycle. Current research and understanding of substance abuse lacks any systematic or "systems" study of the effects of the menstrual cycle or of menopause.

The designation of obstetrics and gynecology as *the* woman's specialty may have actually isolated the understanding of interrelations between menstruation, pregnancy, and other metabolic processes. And, because of the bifurcation in treatment and approach to women's health, the rest of medicine has tended to leave these questions to obstetrics and gynecology.

There is a consistency to the problems identified in the care of women. The common thread is the lack of integration of women's physiologic and metabolic processes into the body of medicine. As a result, the female body remains somewhat "foreign," something a bit more alien to (primarily male) physicians than a regular (male) body.

The Problem of Shortcomings in the System

The differential attention paid to male versus female patients has been documented. Armitage, Schneiderman and Bass, in a study of physician response to complaints in men and women, speculate that "they might be responding to current stereotypes that regard the male as typically stoic and the female as typically 'hypochondriacal.'"[26] Recent literature has addressed differences in referral patterns for male and female cardiac patients[27] and in their selection for coronary angiography and coronary revascularization.[28] This research attempts to discriminate between bias in the care of women and their different needs because of different courses of specific illness. If there is bias in the care of women cardiac patients, it must be addressed, but it does not warrant the development of separate surgery based upon the "female" heart as opposed to a "male" heart. Whatever differences exist in severity of illness, circulation of coronary arteries, or innervation of conducting muscle, they are all within overlapping variations of both male and female hearts. With the exception of those organs involved in reproduction, the vast majority of human organs are truly androgynous.

The Bifurcation of Medical Care of Women

Internal medicine is founded on the model of a male body, with women as "other."[29] That specialty attends to the medical illnesses of the entire male body and part of the female body, whereas obstetrics and gynecology treats those parts of the body related to reproductive health. The result is that most women during their reproductive years must go to two physicians to get their whole body attended to, or use one and forgo the services of the other.

The archaic nature of this arrangement is nowhere more evident than in the assessment of abdominal disorders. The partitioning of the abdominal cavity into the domain of two specialties reflects the dual origins of internists descending from the regular physicians and ob-gyns replacing midwives. No clear anatomical distinction exists, however, between abdomen and pelvis in a female. The area is a continuous cavity divided by imaginary lines that delineate the boundaries of the specialist's territory rather than anatomical structures. The gastrointestinal tract passes through the pelvis and may adhere to the ovaries; endometrial tissue may migrate to the diaphragm, and yet the woman with abdominal pain must visit two doctors, each of whom only partially examines her and then communicates findings with the other by phone or written report, or though the patient. In a male it would be akin to having initial chest pain evaluated by two different doctors, one for the heart and one for the lungs. One doctor would only listen to heartbeats, the other only to breath sounds. Each would then write reports back to the other as to whether the shortness of breath and pain on deep inspiration were of cardiac or pulmonary origin. The need for two physicians to evaluate abdominal pain in a woman is equally absurd.

It is the organization of medical knowledge and practice that are the problem, not the female body. Whereas internal medicine and ob-gyn fall short of addressing the whole woman, family medicine takes care of the whole woman, but in the context of her family, a social role not a medical condition. The one specialty that teaches care of the whole woman also includes children and men. In other words, either a specialty treats only parts of the woman, or it treats all of her and her family.

Rather than the establishment of a new specialty based upon the care of more than half of all adult patients, the current system, in both its structure and content, must address the needs of women as an integral and legitimate aspect of the practice of medicine within every specialty. There simply is no special training for an orthopedist treating women or a radiologist reading women's films or a cardiologist listening to a woman's heart. There is rather the necessity for all orthopedists, all radiologists, and all cardiologists—indeed, all physicians—to look beyond bias and sex stereotyping, and to view being female as only one aspect of the biological, social, and psychological person.

If all human bodies were female and social structure was based upon some other factor than gender, the thorough knowledge of the body would be the medical standard. For instance, anatomically, the physician would examine the whole body because vaginas would not be alien anatomical parts but rather within the norm. If men had large breasts, they would be included in the routine examination of a person. The same physician who examines for spleens and prostrates would be expected to feel for breast lumps. The internist examining for abdominal pain would also do a pelvic exam as part of the assessment, and at the same time, would also do a Pap if needed. In other words, the female reproductive and sexual parts would be part of the everyday practice of an everyday physician.

Even though childbirth has become a surgical procedure,[30] pregnancy remains a metabolic process with the major risk factors being related to the medical health of the woman. Hypertension and diabetes, normally the domain of internists, in pregnancy becomes the domain of the obstetrician-gynecologist, a highly trained surgeon. The major difficulties of the postpartum period are likewise not surgical. Bleeding may occasionally be a problem, but the physician is more likely to encounter thyroid disease, depression, and questions about medications that might pass into breast milk. These are areas more appropriately addressed by an internist or family physician than by a surgeon.

Marginalization of "Women's Health" Specialists

The entrance of women and minorities into male-dominated fields has more commonly led to what the anthropologists term "ritual contamination" of a field than to an increase in the prestige of the women who enter the profession. A field created for the nonsurgical routine care of women, whose practitioners would invariably be mostly female, would likely become a relatively low-paid, low-status field with little or no opportunities for advancement or access to power within universities or specialty societies. Just recently in this century women have entered into medicine in significant numbers. However, their continued inability to achieve positions of power makes it likely that "women's health" would become a marginalized area for a few dedicated (probably most female) physicians. Meanwhile, the rest of medicine would continue as it is, with both the male body and male psyche the standard of normality and health. And, as long as the standard is male, "other" invariably will mean less.

Women do not need special practitioners. Except for diseases of the male reproductive tract and some rare genetic diseases, there are no illnesses restricted to men only. The basic diseases of man are the diseases of woman. The surgical care of women's reproductive organs would rightfully remain the domain of the obstetrician/gynecologist. Although ob-gyns would like to be designated as the primary care physicians of women, it is more likely that internists or family physicians will retain expertise in pelvis exams rather than ob-gyns adding to their training the routine management of diabetes, hypertension, heart disease, gastric ulcers, pneumonia, and all the other diseases encountered in the routine primary care of women.

Necessary Changes

The changes needed to rectify current shortcomings are broad in scope but necessary if anything except cosmetic changes are to be made. Hospital facilities can be dressed up in pink colors and new labeling, but unless the need for fundamental changes in the structure of medicine are acknowledged and implemented, health for the vast majority of women will go unaltered. The basic deficiencies and biases that exist in the conceptual framework of woman—as a biological, psychological, and social person—will continue to undermine any attempt to put women on an equal medical and professional footing with men. The changes needed are as follows.

1. The current specialty of internal medicine must incorporate the menstrual cycle and reproduction into its conceptual framework. The routine gynecologic care of women must be a part of the practice of internal medicine. Family medicine, while continuing to provide primary care for a woman, must recognize her individual existence separate from the family.

2. Obstetrics and gynecology should remain the specialty for referral of obstetric and gynecologic difficulties.

3. Interdisciplinary research must address gaps in the understanding of female functions and their relationship to normal and pathological conditions.

4. Medical students must be taught to identify with patients across gender lines.

5. All medical specialties must be examined for ways in which they are or are not "user friendly" to women.

6. Organized medicine, including medical schools and professional societies, must begin to actively address and rectify those unfounded assumptions about the biological inferiority of women that have been the basis for exclusion of women from medicine and from positions of leadership and power within medicine.

It is not clear what medicine would look like without the standard of the male body and the concomitant underlying assumptions of a biological basis for female passivity and weakness. However, we have the opportunity to find out. Women as patients and as professionals should not settle for a small corner of medicine as a women's health specialty, however appealing that might be. Women instead need to establish their rightful place and perspective within the body of medicine, a body that has been entirely too male in its conceptual framework as well as its membership. There is no medical imperative for a new specialty. Instead, there is an urgent social and economic imperative to restructure medical specialization and to create a nonadversarial body of knowledge and code of practice, in which gender may represent difference but not "other," and certainly not less.

References

1. Velpeau ALM. An elementary treatise on midwifery (CD Meigs, trans.; 2nd Am. ed). Philadelphia: Grigg & Elliot, 1838:83.
2. Meigs CD. Woman: Her diseases and remedies. Philadelphia: Blanchard and Lea, 1859:51, 55.
3. Laqueur T. Making sex: Body and gender from the Greeks to Freud. Cambridge, MA: Harvard University Press, 1990:5–8, 11.
4. Fishbein M. A history of the American Medical Association 1847 to 1947. Philadelphia: WB. Saunders, 1947:83.
5. Barker-Benfield GJ. The horrors of the half-known life. New York: Harper Colophon Books, 1976:85.
6. Harrison M. Woman as other: The premise of medicine. J Am Med Wom Assoc 1990;45:225–226.
7. Harrison M. A woman in residence. New York: Random House, 1982:199.
8. Corea G. The hidden malpractice (updated ed.). New York: Harper Colophon Books, 1985:102–103.
9. Barker-Benfield GJ. The horrors of the half-known life. New York: Harper Colophon Books, 1976:120–126.
10. Ehrenreich B, English D. For her own good. Garden City NY: Anchor Books, 1979:124.
11. Barker-Benfield GJ. The horrors of the half-known life. New York: Harper Colophon Books, 1976:84.
12. Gay P. The bourgeois experience. Vol. 1: Education of the senses. New York: Oxford University Press, 1984:174.
13. Broverman IK, Broverman DM, Clarkson FE, Rosenkrantz PS, Vogel SR. Sex-role stereotypes and clinical judgments of mental health. J Consult Clin Psychol 1970;34:1–7.
14. Corea G. The hidden malpractice (updated ed.). New York: Harper Colophon Books, 1985:96.
15. American Psychiatric Association. Diagnostic and statistical manual of mental disorders (3rd ed., rev.). Washington, DC: American Psychiatric Press, 1987.
16. Casper RF, Heart MT. The effect of hysterectomy and bilateral oophorectomy in women with severe premenstrual syndrome. Am J Obstet Gynecol 1990:162:105–109.
17. Casson P, Hahn PM, Van Vugt DA, Reid RL, Lasting response to ovariectomy in severe intractable premenstrual syndrome. Am J Obstet Gynecol 1990;162:99–105.
18. Muse KN, Cetel NS, Futterman LA, Yen SSC. The premenstrual syndrome: Effects of a "medical ovariectomy." N Engl J Med 1984; 311:1345–1349.
19. Stampfer MJ, Willett WC, Colditz GA, Rosner B, Speizer FE, Hennekens CH. A prospective study of postmenopausal estrogen therapy and coronary heart disease. N Engl J Med 1985;313:1044–1049.
20. Wilson PWF, Garrison RJ, Castelli WP. Postmenopausal estrogen use, cigarette smoking, and cardiovascular morbidity in women over 50. N Engl J Med 1985;313:1038–1043,
21. Wolf PW, Madans JH, Finucane FF, Higgins M, Kleinman JC. Reduction of cardiovascular disease-related mortality among post-menopausal women who use hormones: Evidence from a national cohort. Am J Obstet Gynecol 1991;164:489–494.
22. Eliasson OK, Scherzer HH, DeGraff Jr. AC. Morbidity in asthma in relation to the menstrual cycle. J Allergy Clin Immunol 1986;77:87–94.
23. Lenoir RJ. Severe acute asthma and the menstrual cycle. Anesthesia 1987;42:1287–1290.
24. Price TRP. Temporal lobe epilepsy as a premenstrual behavioral syndrome. Biol Psychiatry 1980;15:957–963.
25. Steinberg AD, Steinberg BJ. Lupus disease activity associated with the menstrual cycle. J Rheumatol 1985;12:816–817.
26. Armitage KJ, Schneiderman LJ, Bass RA. Response of physicians to medical complaints in men and women. JAMA, 1979;241:2186–2187.
27. Bickell NA, Pieper KS, Lee KL, et al. Referral patterns for coronary artery disease treatment: Gender bias or good clinical judgment? Ann Int Med 1992;116:791–797.
28. Krumholz HM, Douglass PS, Lauer MS, Pasternak RC. Selection of patients for coronary angiography and coronary revascularization early after myocardial infarction: Is there evidence for a gender bias? Ann Int Med 1992;116:785–790.
29. Harrison M. Woman as other: The premise of medicine. J Am Med Wom Assoc 1990;4:225–226.
30. Harrison M. A woman in residence. New York: Random House, 1982:93.

Ω

♀

The Health Insurance Conspiracy

by Peg Byron

When Jackie Winnow found she had breast cancer, she figured that her hospital treatments would be covered by her comprehensive insurance policy, obtained through her job as the Lesbian/Gay Liaison for San Francisco's Human Rights Commission.

But almost a year after Winnow's death in September 1991, her lover, Teya Schaffer, is still settling hospital bills and insurance claims. Instead of Winnow's spending her final, pain-filled days comforting her 11-year-old son, Asher, whom she was raising with Schaffer, she was forced to write letters in triplicate to convince the insurance company that it had to cover her hospital bills. The company, faced with the mounting medical claims, told her she was no longer insured. It was a mistake, the company eventually admitted, but the computer kept rejecting payment requests from hospital bill collectors.

"When you're no longer financially independent, the worry of those bills gets magnified. It was very emotionally distressing for her," Schaffer says. Winnow founded the acclaimed Women's Cancer Resource Center in Berkeley, California, after a lump in her breast was diagnosed as malignant. Near the end, however, Schaffer says, "She just wanted some peaceful last months. The insurance hassle made it much harder for her."

■ In the 1970s, Cosby Totten of Tazewell, Virginia, went to work in Appalachia's coal mines after her divorce left her as the sole support of six children. She needed the job—and the insurance for her family that came with it.

"That was one of the reasons I went into the mines," she says, dismissing the broken fingers, ribs, and chipped elbow she suffered below ground as "not serious," while she earned $49 a day to start. Recently, the former coal miner found herself unemployed and uninsured again. "Well, I don't know what I'd do if I got sick. It would depend on how sick," she says. "It might be better, cheaper, and easier to just stay home and die. You could at least do it your way."

■ At a nonprofit New York City clinic, cuts in public funding have led to requirements for payment from destitute but non-Medicaid-eligible clients. The payments demanded are modest by New York standards but they cause the poor to forgo follow-up visits or stay away altogether, sometimes with terrible consequences.

"Even the least amount is hard for a lot of people," says Dr. Vicki Alexander, the medical director. "A patient comes wanting just birth control pills and complaining of a little abdominal pain. We treat her for a pelvic infection before we get the results of the cultures. She goes out thinking she's probably been taken care of. But the cultures show something else and she ends up having something that can sit inside her for a long time. By the time she comes back, she needs seven days in the hospital with intravenous treatment, and we have to remove her uterus, tubes, ovaries, everything," says Alexander.

Then there are the self-employed, and workers whose employers provide no insurance at all. If they can afford it, they may buy policies as individuals or as part of a group. But insurers offering such policies often drastically raise rates or even refuse to renew a policy if, for example, a serious health problem develops. Insurance rates for a family can start at about $4,000 a year and escalate to triple that amount if one member discovers a chronic condition. And anyone who has what insurers call a "preexisting condition" most likely cannot buy any policy at all.

Insurance is the key to U.S. health care. Yet an estimated 36 million U.S. residents, or 15 percent of the population, lack health insurance. (The Bush administration's figures are the lowest of expert estimates, putting the number of uninsured at 32 million.) Only one other country in the industrialized world is without a national health insurance program—South Africa.

As a result of these disparities, a revolution in the economics of the U.S. health care system is looming. The question is not whether the system will be changed, but by how much. Three basic types of change are being debated among more than a hundred proposals. The two least adequate ones are supported by the most powerful Republican and Democratic factions. The third proposal calls for health services available to everyone, paid for through the government.

The results of the presidential election and the maneuverings of congressional forces will influence the outcome, but the public's fears and anger about the current system may prove to be the determining force in the drive for change. A 1991 *Wall Street Journal* poll found about 70 percent of U.S. citizens want a program of universal health care like Canada's, which guarantees care for all residents through a centrally paid system. None of the tons of paperwork that is routine in this country is required in Canada, where everyone, rich or poor, expects the same treatment.

The Crisis in Costs

Annual health care costs of $2,700 per person in the United States are the highest in the world, though statistical measures like life expectancy and infant mortality show the population is far from the healthiest. With costs

From *MS. Magazine*, Sept./Oct. 1992, pp. 40–45. Copyright © 1992 by Ms. Magazine. Reprinted by permission.

increasing at double the rate of inflation, health care spending will total about $817 billion this year, far outpacing the military budget and making up 14 percent of the gross domestic product, according to Commerce Department estimates.

The epidemics of AIDS, unemployment, homelessness, and drug abuse are adding to the U.S. health care bill, even while many thousands go without help. Hospitals, the most expensive providers of care, report being swamped with poor patients who would be better off getting help earlier as outpatients but who wait to go to emergency rooms because they can't afford to visit a doctor or clinic.

Women pay an extra high price for the current U.S. system. Uninsured women are likely to forgo vital screening tests for breast and cervical cancer, or skip prenatal care while pregnant. And, although 51 percent of people with insurance are women, 5 million of those insured women between the ages of 15 and 44 are not covered for reproductive care, according to a study in *Consumer Reports*. In addition, most publicly funded programs (and, often, private insurance plans) fail to cover simple preventive care like Pap smears and mammograms, yet those same programs do pay for expensive procedures once cancer is diagnosed.

In the U.S., health care is mostly provided through a system where fees are tied to services ordered; the medical services performed reflect the fear of malpractice lawsuits. Greed is also a factor: a study in the *Journal of the American Medical Association* found that women with more comprehensive coverage were more likely to have repeat cesarean sections than uninsured women, even though vaginal deliveries are recommended as safer for most women who have previously given birth via C-section. Indeed, the Washington, D.C.-based National Women's Health Network suggests the only way to reduce unnecessary C-sections may be to raise physician compensation rates for vaginal deliveries.

The annual bill will top $2 trillion by the year 2000—just a decade before baby boomers begin to reach their sixties and expect their health care to be covered by Medicare. This sizable elderly group will include a majority of women, given women's longer life span. The government will be forced to pick up the tab, but that will add to the pressure for a system that covers everyone—which, once implemented, would eliminate the need for Medicare and Medicaid.

The Big-Money Interests

The U.S. system, pieced together during this century, is shaped around the payment structure, which has been controlled by hospital, physician, and insurance interest groups. In the past, those groups resisted proposals for change with cries of "socialized medicine" and "rationing" sure to hurt the middle-class consumer. In fact, profits make the health business the fastest growing sector of the economy and the male-dominated levels of its work force are among the highest paid of U.S. professionals. Cost

control in any form means income control for doctors, hospitals, insurers, and their ancillaries. Herein lies the controversy.

Debate about the health care system is not new. It began before World War I when doctors were struggling to get established at the expense of other health care providers such as midwives. During the Depression and after World War II, reform efforts resumed, with one national health care proposal even introduced by then Representative Richard Nixon. The attempt failed.

Only since the 1940s has health insurance become a benefit of employment—most commonly as hospital insurance. This further tilted health care toward hospitals, high-cost technologies, and surgeries. In 1965, even Lyndon Johnson couldn't get a national health insurance program passed. After heavy lobbying by organized medical interest groups like the American Medical Association (AMA), only Medicare and Medicaid emerged—in forms that also heavily supported hospital and fee-for-service care.

Many providers now cry that regulation and bureaucratic demands, especially through malpractice lawyers and bloated insurance companies, have carved into their profits. Nonetheless, in 1990 hospitals accounted for $256 billion in health expenditures; doctors, $125.7 billion. The top 20 health insurers received $26.7 billion in premiums, scraping by with $759.6 million in profits.

These are formidable lobbyists. The AMA, during a recent election year, ranked second in size among the Federal Election Commission's top 50 PACs.

A sore point in trying to reform insurance companies is their practice of skimming the healthy from the sick and those at risk of being sick. Many companies have switched from the traditional "community rating" method, which spread cost risks among all those insured, to the "experience rating" method that bases policy price, or premium, on the claims made from the individual or group insured. As a result, people insured through small groups or on their own may see premiums rise to well over $10,000 per year.

Employers who pay premiums for more than 139 million workers have their own methods of skimming to contain their costs and save profits under the current system, through devices like higher deductibles and "managed care" plans, as well as by rejecting those who are or might become sick.

The Horror of Getting Covered

A $350 annual deductible kept Betty Geralds of Freeport, Long Island, from using her company's health insurance plan. Working as a loan processor for less than $20,000 a year and caring for her granddaughter, she just couldn't afford the deductible. So to get treated for high blood pressure, she would either go to a county clinic or, in spite of the risks, go without care altogether.

Worried about her health, she switched this year to HIP, her company's health maintenance organization (HMO), a form of managed care coverage that is increasingly popular for controlling costs. HMOs charge members low rates, which can range from $2 to $10 per office visit, and a similar nominal amount for prescriptions, with no deductible or insurance claims to file. In exchange, the user must choose only plan-approved doctors, have procedures authorized in advance, and use only program-approved hospitals.

But the nearest hospital Geralds could use was in the next county, almost an hour away, and although the HIP doctors seemed capable, she had not been able to see the same doctor in three different visits since enrolling. "With HIP, it has to be within their guidelines," she says. "If I could afford to have it my way, I would not be involved with HIP."

Other forms of managed care can take the form of utilization review within more traditional insurance policies (whereby all non-emergency treatment must be pre-approved or the insurer will not pay) and "preferred provider" networks, which offer discounts for using doctors who have agreed to hold down fees and treatment costs. But insurers are finding the higher administrative costs eat much of the savings. Self-insurance by companies is an increasingly popular attempt at cost control, where the employer takes on the risk and pays medical bills through an administrator. For the user, this can slow reimbursements, depending on the company's cash flow interests; if the company goes out of business, all benefits are lost, without the otherwise required insurance extension protections.

"Eighty percent of U.S. labor conflicts in the last few years have been over medical benefits," said Leni-Anne Zibor, assistant to the president of District Three of the International Union of Electronic, Electrical, Salaried Machine and Furniture Workers for New York and New Jersey. "Health care happens to be one issue people are willing to go out on the street for. They know they could be destroyed financially, and they want to be able to take care of their families," Zibor says.

But people with no insurance commonly find the price of an individual policy way beyond their means. Brooklyn artist Nisa Rauschenberg, who works as an illustrator and photo editor to support her painting, says, "I'm not on welfare. I'm taxed to death, and I just can't do it," referring to insurance. While Rauschenberg, 32, is fortunate in her good health, she says, "I want to have children at some point and I've got to have health insurance for that." One policy premium jumped 10 percent in the time it took for her just to receive the application. "I thought, For crying out loud, I might have to get married to get insurance. It's the most ridiculous reason I can think of to get married."

Three Prescriptions for Change

Dozens of health system reform proposals are before Congress, but they boil down to three basic cures.

▪ President Bush announced his version less than a week before he declared his campaign for reelection, no doubt aware of Democrat Harris Wofford's decisive Sen-

ate victory, using the health care issue, to beat Bush's ex-attorney general Dick Thornburgh in Pennsylvania.

Bush's plan is based on tax breaks and insurance vouchers. The government would provide vouchers to the poor and tax credits to the middle class for health care purchases, with $1,250 a year allocated for individuals, $2,500 for couples, and up to $3,750 for families of three or more. Tax deductions would be capped according to income. The self-employed would be able to deduct all health insurance premiums. Changes mandated for the insurance industry would allow small businesses to pool employee health plans and require insurers to cover people with preexisting conditions without delay when they change jobs. Managed care plans for Medicaid and Medicare would be promoted. States would be pressured to limit malpractice awards.

The Bush program is estimated to cost about $35 billion a year, and part of that would be paid for with caps on Medicaid costs. The plan would slash Medicaid increases (federal payments in 1990 were generally about $800 per child and $1,400 per adult). But outside of restricting options for the poor, the plan lacks cost controls. The Bush plan would benefit insurers, hospitals, and doctors; it would cost businesses nothing. It offers nothing to the uninsured or the underinsured.

▪ Powerful Democrats like Senate Majority Leader George Mitchell and Senator Edward Kennedy are promoting a compromise plan called AmeriCare, known as the "pay or play" approach. This requires employers either to provide insurance to workers or pay a tax to fund a new government insurance plan to replace Medicaid and cover the unemployed; Medicare would be untouched. This approach is often described as "popular," but it is most popular with special interest groups such as the AMA, which supports a version of the plan.

AmeriCare would leave the health insurance industry in place with some reforms. Cost controls still would not be placed on doctors or hospital providers. AmeriCare would try to reduce costs by developing treatment guidelines to limit reimbursement and to encourage doctors to cut down on "defensive medicine" aimed mainly at avoiding malpractice lawsuits. Copayments of up to 20 percent would be set for those living above the poverty level, with deductibles of up to $500 per family. The uninsured and medically uninsurable would benefit from ending discrimination in the insurance system.

▪ The single-payer plan. One of the most comprehensive versions of this proposal, similar to the Canadian system, was sponsored by Representative Marty Russo, who lost his Illinois Democratic primary this spring. Senator Wofford and Senator Paul Wellstone (D.-Minn.) have each offered his own version. This approach breaks the link between insurance and employment, using federal and state taxes for financing; payments would be administered from one central agency, with the same insurance card provided to everyone. The government is the payer and, hence, the negotiator of rates. Fifteen hundred complicated insurance plans, as well as Medicaid and Medicare, would be eliminated. Under Wofford's proposal, states could devise their own approaches to provide every person with guaranteed coverage.

Opponents claim the single-payer plan would not allow people to choose their own doctors and there would be long waits or rationing of care. Sponsors emphatically deny both threats. Several women's groups are backing the single-payer system, including the Asian Immigrant Women's Association and the National Latina Health Project in conjunction with MADRE, the National Black Women's Health Project, the Boston Women's Health Book Collective, the National Women's Health Network, and the Older Women's League. Democratic presidential candidate Bill Clinton is advocating a plan that falls between the AmeriCare and single-payer plans.

It will take women's participation in this national debate to ensure coverage for all reproductive health care services, as well as the many chronic health problems like high blood pressure and diabetes that tend to require primary more than tertiary care. Women, more often than men, both need and provide long-term care and that also must be factored into health insurance reforms, as it is in Wofford's but not in Russo's version.

Health care as it stands now is a business. It involves massive financial interests, from the concrete contractors who build the hospitals to the entrepreneurial physician in private practice. Such interests have distorted the debate as well as driven up the price. Now the high costs may be the system's downfall.

Things are so bad in health care that U.S. citizens will have to overcome their disgust with government to support universal health care through a national program. But no plan should be supported uncritically. Accountability of hospitals, doctors, and other providers must be improved. The power of a single-payer system should be wielded against unethical or incompetent providers.

The centralized, national funding of a universal health care system is preferable because it would ensure equal access and uniform quality. It also creates needed leverage in cost controls and would reduce administrative costs— estimates range from $40 billion to $270 billion—enough to pay for health care even for the currently uninsured. Real change also should address access to experimental and alternative treatments, some of which are cheaper than available licensed treatments that have been dismal failures for diseases like breast cancer.

Once universal health coverage is a reality, women like Betty Geralds, Nisa Rauschenberg, Cosby Totten, and Jackie Winnow will be able to focus more on the joy of living than on the fear of illness.

Ω

Health Care Rationing
by Adriane Fugh-Berman, M.D.

Although health care rationing already exists in this country, it is more subtle, more convoluted, and more pathological rationing than that which exists in any other country. Poor people get less health care and the relatively rich get more health care. Ironically, neither group gets optimal health care. We tend to confuse high-tech diagnostics and therapeutics with good health care (as in the statement "The United States has the best health care in the world . . ."), but health itself is in short supply even in our well-insured populations.

We already have rationing—in the best light, it is random rationing; at worst, it is rationing only for the poor because it is based on the ability to pay. Emergency rooms (ERs) have become the primary care provider for many of the uninsured and underinsured. They are not very good places to get primary care: one rarely sees the same

provider twice; ER personnel are so overworked that they are irritable with those they don't consider to be bonafide emergencies; preventive health care is not possible; and follow-up is rarely adequate. Emergency rooms have become a nightmare because once the wards fill up, there is no place to put new patients until an inpatient dies, is discharged, or is transferred. Meanwhile the patients stay in the emergency room, with more coming in all the time. At some point, the ER may close and is said to be "on diversion", meaning that ambulances are not to deliver patients there. There are occasions when every hospital in New York City is on diversion and ambulances must drive around until one of the ERs opens up. There is regular meal service in New York City ERs, a necessity because the average waiting period between the time a patient is officially admitted and the time he or she actually gets a bed is 24 hours. Some patients wait days, psychiatric patients may wait a week. Many of the doctors who work in the ER are excellent; care is compromised not because doctors aren't conscientious, but because they are overwhelmed.

From The Network News, March/April/May 1991. Copyright © 1991 by National Women's Health Network. Reprinted by permission.

Patients are sent home before they are ready to leave the hospital because DRGs (diagnostic-related groups) limit how long people can stay on the basis of their diagnosis, not their actual condition. Doctors learn tricks: I have kept a patient on intravenous medication when I could have switched him to oral medication because this would allow the patient to stay in the hospital longer. Patients are transferred from public to private hospitals if they can pay and, more commonly, from private to public hospitals if they cannot. It is not so very different from the days of segregated hospitals; these days we separate by ability to pay instead of by race.

Other public hospitals stagger and sway under the weight of the chronically ill, the acutely ill, the casualties of the drug wars, the boarder babies, the mental patients, the dysfunctional adults who cannot be discharged because they have no place to go. In New Jersey each hospital bill carries a 13% surcharge to help make up for uncollected bills (nationally, uncompensated care totaled more than $8 billion in 1988). Hospitals try to make up the money elsewhere, through such mechanisms as government subsidies. Private hospitals court well-off patients with carpeted floors, gourmet meals in private rooms, grooming services—or establish high-profit services such as open heart surgery.

Prince George's Hospital Center in Maryland was recently fined for its mini-version of an equitable health plan; they were charging patients who could pay more in order to subsidize patients who couldn't pay.

The Montefiore-associated Family Health Center is a model of excellent health care in the South Bronx. Because it is in an underserved area, it received Federal funds until some bureaucrat decided that because the clinic was now in the underserved area, the area was no longer underserved and therefore not entitled to more funds . . .

Public hospitals provide less than optimal care because they are overloaded. This results in a diffusion of attention to patients, a survivalist mentality among health care practitioners, and discouraging mortality statistics. Washington, D.C. General Hospital, for instance, has been disparaged unfairly. This hospital takes care of the poorest and the sickest patients, so the death rate is higher because patients arrive sicker. Some of the patients who don't do well have been transferred from private hospitals, which are blatantly allergic to patients without insurance. One study found that 87% of patient transfers to Cook County Hospital in Chicago were the result of lack of medical insurance. Almost a quarter of the patients were medically unstable before being transferred and were transferred anyway (Schiff, et al., *New England Journal of Medicine* Vol. 314, no.9, Feb. 27, 1986, "Transfers to a public hospital").

Medicaid covers less than half of the nation's poor. It was not meant to do otherwise. One must be not only poor, but often far below the poverty level in order to qualify—in Alabama a family of three is ineligible for Medicaid if its annual income exceeds $1,416 (*Washington Post*, Jan. 6, 1991).

Many people who are not poor have no health insurance, including people working for small businesses, part-time workers, the self-employed, and those taking early retirement. Uninsured women are much less likely to undergo screening for breast cancer, cervical cancer, or glaucoma (diseases in which screening is worthwhile and where early intervention is crucial). Five million women of childbearing age (15–44 years) are covered by private health insurance—but it often doesn't even pay for prenatal care! (*Consumer Reports*, August 1990).

Employers are reluctant to hire older workers because their health insurance premiums are so high. Many insurance companies now require a negative HIV test result before granting coverage.

Insurance for Whitman-Walker Clinic health workers more than quadrupled in a year and a half, nearly driving the primary provider of service to HIV-positive patients in Washington D.C. bankrupt. Although HIV-positive patients are in the most dire need of insurance, they are the least likely to get it. We have accepted that the sickest patients should bear the greatest financial burden. Isn't that health care rationing?

In 1989 the American Medical Association took out a series of Canada-bashing ads which accused our northern neighbors of rationing health care. A picture shows a young girl with the caption: "In some countries she could wait months for her surgery." Another reads "Elective surgery: should it be up to you or up to a committee?" It is interesting that when the most powerful lobby for the medical profession in the U.S. takes aim at Canada, all it could come up with was diversionary whining. Yes, you may wait months for ELECTIVE surgery in Canada. It's called elective for a reason; it means it is not an emergency. If it's an emergency, you get faster service. There are far too many "elective" procedures done in the United States.

Canadians are very happy with their system; and a majority of Americans would prefer it too. So what if you have to wait for elective surgery—Canada has us beat on life expectancy (longer), infant mortality (lower), and spending percentage of GNP (lower).

Although England's National Health Service is having problems of its own because of intentional dismantling by Conservative governments, it's kind of fun to bring it up to those who oppose a National Health Plan. It always provokes the same response: "Did you know that you can't get kidney dialysis there if you're over 55?!" And in this single example it's true that it is relatively easy to obtain dialysis here (because of a rider attached to a Congressional bill). You're not entitled to preventive medicine, prenatal care, routine medical care, dental care, hospital care, prescriptions, home health care, or anything else— but if your kidneys fail, rest easy! It's the one medical condition that we actually take care of in this country.

While poor patients don't get enough health care, patients who can pay suffer excess procedures and tests. Good insurance, in fact, is a reliable risk factor for Caesarean-sections.

A study published in *JAMA* (Jan. 2, 1991) found that women with good insurance were much more likely to have repeat C-sections than were uninsured women. Despite recommendations that it is safer for women who have undergone a previous C-section to have vaginal births, 87% of women in this California study who had C-sections undergo repeat C-sections for later births. In private, for-profit hospitals, the rate was more than 95% (*Washington Post* 1/2/91). It has been said that the only way to reduce C-section rates is to raise the physician compensation rate for vaginal deliveries above that for C-sections!

Some firms use telemarketers to contact patients and offer them free physicals. The offer is only made to well-insured patients whose insurance carriers are later billed for as much as $30,000. Patients may receive an 18-panel urinalysis, a 26-panel blood workup, an EKG, echo-cardiography, sonograms of vital organs and the vascular system, and pulmonary function tests. None of these tests are valuable for routine screening although telemarketers are instructed to tell the clients that these tests are good preventive medicine! (*Medical Economics*, July 23, 1990, "Is this the ultimate health care fraud?").

The answer to these problems is a national health plan. The answer is not to pour more money into Medicaid. It's not to pass a bill on long-term care. It's not to pass a catastrophic health bill. It's not to pass a women's health bill. The problems are all related to the fact that we have no minimum standard of care to which every person is entitled. As a society, we would rather complain about the inequity of rationing high-tech care while people are dying from lack of access to simple, boring, but essential, low-tech care. We have chosen to ration primary care and preventive medicine on the basis of ability to pay. We have chosen not to ration the resources to keep permanently comatose patients alive, to try to save babies who weigh less than a pound, to do organ transplants and other high-tech procedures. We can ration by choice or we can ration by chance. These are our only options. Isn't it time we made better choices?

Ω

Women in Prison, Women in Danger:
Reproductive Health Care Denied
by Brenda V. Smith

While much has been written over the past months about the increasing prison population in this country, little attention has been paid to the fastest growing group among the incarcerated population, women, and in particular women of color. With the number of women prisoners growing and prison health care, particularly reproductive health care, existing at a substandard level, we are on the verge of a crisis—depriving prisoners of their rights and endangering their very lives. The examples illustrated below suggest the potential of this crisis.

In the last decade, female prison population growth has significantly outstripped that of the male prison population. In 1980, there were approximately 13,000 women serving sentences in state and federal prisons. By the end of 1989, that number had risen to over 41,000. In 1989 alone, the female prison population grew by 24% compared to a 13% growth in the male prison population.

Preliminary figures from 1990 suggest that this trend has abated somewhat and that for the first time since 1981, the male growth rate in the prison population exceeded the growth rate in the female population (8.3% and 7.8% respectively).

The primary reason for the increase in both the male and female prison population has been this country's war on drugs. By primarily focussing the war on interdiction, not on treatment and prevention, the prison population has witnessed an astronomical increase. While the male prison population has increased by 112% since 1980, the female prison population increased by over 200%.

A larger percentage of women than men are serving sentences for drug offenses. The most current information from the Bureau of Justice Statistics, collected in 1986, reveal that 22% of all women prisoners compared to 16% of men prisoners were serving sentences for drug offenses.

Recent figures suggest that figure has only increased. For example, the Federal Bureau of Prisons reports that while 55.1% of all federal prisoners are serving sentences for drug offenses, 62% of women prisoners are serving sentences for drug offenses. Though disturbing, this statistic is not surprising since women are overwhelmingly convicted of non-violent crimes with an economic motive such as drug sales, theft, forgery and prostitution.

From *Common Ground—Different Planes,* Summer 1991, pp. 4–6. Copyright © 1991 by The Women of Color Partnership Program of the Religious Coalition for Reproductive Choice. Reprinted by permission.

Women prisoners are disproportionately women of color. African-American women comprise over 50% of the total female prison population. In the District of Columbia, 99% of women prisoners are African-American.

The majority of these women are between 21 and 35, in their prime childbearing years. About 80% of women prisoners have children. Almost 90% of those who reported having children indicated that at least one of their children was under the age of eighteen. About 25% of women prisoners are pregnant or postpartum (8-10% are pregnant). The District of Columbia Department of Corrections estimates that 20% of women prisoners are pregnant at intake.

Typically, women enter prisons and jails with a host of medical problems including HIV infection and other sexually transmitted diseases, diseases associated with poor nutrition such as obesity, diabetes, hypertension, and alcohol and other drug addictions. A conservative estimate suggests that 70% of women prisoners have alcohol and other drug problems. These women are clearly in need of comprehensive health care services.

While the system of medical care for all prisoners is poor, the situation is far worse for women prisoners. Prison medical care systems were created for men. Essentially, women must "fit in" to the existing inadequate framework. Though the situations of individual women outlined below may appear extreme, they are unfortunately all too common.

Routine gynecological care, such as pap smears, breast exams and mammograms, is very rare in state or federal prison systems. The care that exists is generally administered only when the medical situation becomes an emergency. As demonstrated, the emergency often becomes a disaster, with women dying or becoming severely injured.

Quality prenatal care has become another pressing need, given the increasing numbers of pregnant women entering prison. Many pregnant prisoners suffer from alcohol and drug problems. Most prisons, however, offer these women little or no assistance in detoxing, despite clear medical data which shows the serious harm both women and their fetuses can suffer when allowed to detoxify without appropriate medical supervision. Prenatal care for these women is even more vital given the increased chances of complications with the pregnancy or the newborn due to prior drug and alcohol use.

Pregnant women also have increased nutritional needs which are not met in jails and prisons. Though Congress passed legislation last year allowing states, at their option, to provide the Women, Infant and Children ("WIC") food program to pregnant prisoners, only Alabama and Arizona have chosen to do so. The WIC program provides additional food such as cheese, milk, cereal, infant formula, eggs, peanut butter and juice for pregnant women, new mothers, infants and children under age five with family incomes below 185% of the poverty level.

In addition to food supplements, WIC provides health and nutritional counseling—including smoking cessation, and alcohol and drug abuse prevention—to foster comprehensive long-term improvement in the health status of WIC program participants and their families.

These WIC programs are core services pregnant prisoners need in order to ensure the healthiest pregnancies and outcomes for them and their children. Practically speaking, the WIC program could be used to expand services to pregnant prison population and provide services which prisons and jails cannot fund through their own budgets.

Women prisoners also desperately need access to reproductive counseling. There is little health care counseling within prisons and even less related to women's reproductive health. Male and female prisoners engage in sexual practices both before and after their incarceration that put them at high risk for unplanned pregnancies and for sexually transmitted diseases, including HIV infection.

Though abortion is technically available for prisoners, depending on the laws of the particular state, it is difficult and practically impossible for most women to obtain. In the District of Columbia a pregnant prisoner who wishes to obtain an abortion has a number of seemingly insurmountable obstacles.

A District of Columbia prisoner must be able to pay for the abortion. While government funds can be used for almost any type approved medical procedure for prisoners, District of Columbia funds cannot be used to pay for elective abortions for women prisoners (or any other low-income woman for that matter). Because most women prisoners were unemployed prior to their incarceration, they have little personal or family resources to pay for the procedure.

Even if a D.C. prisoner can pay for an abortion, she must make her own arrangements to have the abortion performed at a private clinic. D.C. General which provides routine medical care for prisoners no longer performs abortions. Generally, women prisoners get ten minutes per day to make phone calls. If she is able to make the arrangements, she must then secure approval to have a guard transport her to the facility to have the abortion performed.

Approval could take weeks because of the shortage of guards or because of prison overcrowding. If all these obstacles are surmounted, she will be transported by a guard, often male, who is required by prison regulations to be present at all times during the procedure.

Comprehensive counseling on reproductive health is essential to the health of prisoners. Additionally, they must have meaningful access to abortion and contraception. As noted, sex continues even during incarceration. Though prison administrators have in the past turned a blind eye to sexual practices within prisons, they can no longer afford to ignore the consequences of such activity. Contraception, both barrier and oral methods, must be made available to women prisoners.

Women prisoners are a forgotten and undeserved population. Both prison officials and the public justify their neglect of women prisoners because they are law violators, drug addicts, "bad" mothers or all of the above. These women reflect the end product of what happens when we ignore the needs of low-income women, in particular the need for economic and family support and good health care including reproductive services and counseling.

The need for these services does not halt when women are incarcerated. These women have needs which are just as critical, if not more critical, than the needs of women in the free world. We must press prison officials, public health officials, and the public to respond to the concerns of these women in a comprehensive and caring manner. Services to these women will benefit not just them but their children and the communities to which they will ultimately return.

Ω

♀

How to Tell Your Doctor a Thing or Two

by Morton Hunt

If you're like most Americans, you've lost a lot of faith in doctors in recent years. In 1966 the Louis Harris survey organization reported that 73 per cent of Americans had a great deal of confidence in the medical profession: by 1977 the figure had dropped to 43 per cent.

As a result a new kind of patient has appeared—a patient who is questioning and even argumentative, sometimes mistrustful, often balky. This patient goes doctor-shopping, files complaints with medical societies, sues for malpractice. She may join one of the hundreds of new medical-consumer (patient) organizations that defend patients against their own docrtors. She—or he—no longer silently listens to the doctor with awe but speaks up, wants to be told everything and to be convinced, and reserves the right to reject the doctor's advice or to ask for a second opinion.

I've been talking to leaders of the medical profession and of medical-consumer groups, and both sides agree on one thing: Doctors throughout America are seeing the new kind of patient increasingly often in their offices. Although some doctors—including my own—look approvingly on patients of this new breed, the majority view them with disapproval and even hostility. By training, position and tradition, doctors tend to play the role of Wise Patriarch Whose Word is Law, and they expect their patients to be Good Children Who Obey Without Argument. They consider the new breed "difficult," "troublemakers" and—above all—"bad" patients.

But there is growing evidence that nowadays the "bad" patient is a better one, in terms of medical results, than the "good" patient. According to a number of recent research studies, the passive, uncomplaining, unquestioning patient is less likely to get well quickly than the new kind. Or as Eli Glogow, director of the graduate program in health administration at the University of Southern California, succinctly puts it, "the 'bad patient' gets better quicker."

Why? Not because the "bad" patient—whom I'll call the "active" patient—refuses to follow instructions. Indeed, medical journals report that the independent patient is apt to carry out doctors' orders faithfully, once he or she accepts them, while the passive patient is more likely to forget or quietly disobey.

But following instructions is only part of it. What gives the active patient better odds at regaining health quickly or staying healthy is a whole new concept of the patient's role. Essentially it consists of taking responsibility for one's own health care—becoming an adult rather than a child in the doctor-patient relationship. That means finding the best doctor available but getting another opinion if doubtful about a major recommendation; defending oneself against overmedication and unnecessary surgery; and in general acting as the doctor's partner, collaborator and equal.

It is out of necessity that such patients are becoming ever more numerous for there has been a revolution in the nature of medical practice. In recent years the doctor-patient relationship has become coldly impersonal, and not very reassuring to the patient. Here are some of the reasons:

• The number of drugs, tests and special technological procedures has vastly increased. As a result, patients spend more time with nurses and technicians, less time with the doctor himself. Diseases get treated but treatment becomes an assembly-line affair.

• The new technology makes for greater specialization. Specialization makes for higher fees—and so more doctors want to specialize (more than four out of five now do so). In consequence there are fewer general practitioners, and the patient has to wait longer and settle for less time with a G.P. than ever before.

• Specialization also means that the patient is subdivided and parceled out among doctors—the gynecologist, the allergist, and so on—and is to each not a person but a symptom in some part of the body. Many patients get medical care from several doctors but have no one doctor who cares. There's the rub. Dr. W. Walter Menninger of

Reprinted with permission from Bread & Roses, Women's Health Center, Milwaukee, Wisconsin.

the Menninger Foundation, a center of psychiatric research, says that most of the grievances patients have against doctors involve breakdown in the *caring* aspect of the physician-patient relationship, not in the quality of technical care.

One young woman I know worried about menstrual spotting and went to a busy gynecologist who, with little explanation, did a suction extraction of the endometrium (the mucus lining of the uterus). Unprepared for the invasive and painful procedure, she left the office shaken and burst into tears on the sidewalk. Months later she said to him as casually as she could, "Doctor, that last visit was so unpleasant I thought I might never come back"—to which he replied just as casually, "If you ever feel that way again, I think you *shouldn't* come back." Caring? He'd sneer at the word.

- We Americans move about more than ever. We become separated from the doctor who knows us best, and what he or she knows about us is, in most cases, lost or forgotten. Yet you, the patient, have no legal right in most states to make the doctor turn over his records to you. (If you ask, he'll send them to another doctor—but few patients ask.)

- Group practice, growing by leaps and bounds, gives the busy doctor much-needed relief and free time and assures you that someone will be on hand when needed. But the substitute doctor rarely knows your medical history or has time to read through your folder. Unless you can fill in the gaps in this stranger's knowledge of you-and have the courage to do so—you may get indifferent or even hurtful treatment.

One 30-year-old woman went to her medical group when a rash spread over her arms and chest. An overworked doctor who had never seen her before asked her a few questions and concluded—correctly—that it was an allergic reaction; summer sunshine and an antibiotic she'd been taking didn't go well together. He prescribed a form of cortisone to be taken by mouth, and a week later she was in the hospital with a bleeding ulcer. Buried in her folder and unread by the doctor had been notes about a tendency on her part toward ulcers: cortisone treatment brought the condition to an acute state.

- The profit motive has altered the patient-doctor relationship. Profitmaking is an old, respectable incentive to businessmen and professionals alike, but it can easily lead to exploitative and unfair practices. That's why watchdog agencies protect consumers from impersonal big business. But medicine, though it too is now impersonal and big business—doctor's fees total over $26 billion a year—remains virtually unregulated except by itself.

Exploitation by doctors takes many forms. In a study of one group of internists, researchers found that some of the doctors ordered patients to come back for follow-up visits twice as often as others did, even though all were treating the same kinds of patients. Three of four doctors polled by the American Medical Association this year admit that they now order anywhere from one to several extra tests

per patient—not for the patient's benefit but for their own, as protection from potential malpractice suits. But it is the patient who pays—and who is exposed to extra risks.

The most serious conflict between the patient's best interest and the profit motive occurs when the doctor stands to gain the most. A surgeon who will earn many hundreds of dollars from performing an operation is likely to be less objective, when deciding whether to recommend it, than a surgeon who is not involved and therefore impartial. A recent Congressional study indicates that one of every six operations is unnecessary: that's more than 3 million needless operations per year, costing $4 billion and leading to nearly 12,000 postoperative deaths. In some specialties the figures are even higher; various research teams have termed anywhere from a quarter to a half of the 800,000 hysterectomies performed each year "unjustified" or "unnecessary."

Reaction to all this was inevitable. Liberal doctors and medical administrators drafted "bills of rights" for patients, and a few legislators tried to get some of them enacted into state law. Labor unions and veterans' organizations began to fight for "patients' advocates" in clinics and hospitals, to listen to patients' grievances and take their complaints to the authorities. Everywhere the new breed of patient began to appear.

And perhaps most important, medical-consumer organizations sprang up, most of them offshoots of the 1960s consumer movement. Public Citizen, the national organization headed by Ralph Nader, set up the Health Research Group in Washington, D.C. Headed by Sidney M. Wolfe, a dynamic young doctor, it gathers research data and uses them to lobby for stronger Government controls over drug advertising, prescription writing, the use of x-rays; for the patient's right to obtain personal medical records; and for controls over cost and quality of health care in general.

In recent years other medical-consumer groups have been started in many cities by churches, by campus organizations and by women's groups. Some of them, chiefly educational, publish pamphlets, newsletters or books on medical matters, or operate Tel-Med libraries. (You phone, ask to hear a tape on a medical matter that concerns you and get plugged in to a four-to-seven minute cassette at no charge.) Others also offer counseling and advice and make referrals to doctors or clinics. Still others, like Nader's health group, are interested chiefly in bringing pressure to bear on city and state officials to control medical costs and practices and in getting consumer-minded representatives onto the governing boards of hospitals, medical-insurance plans and relevant state agencies.

In the long run it will be these collective efforts that will rebuild the patient-doctor relationship in a new, democratic form. Meanwhile what can you, the individual, do for yourself? A good deal. From my conversations with medical-consumer leaders I have put together a seven-point program for the new-style patient:

1. *Care for yourself as far as possible.* Save the doctor's time and your own—and your money—by doing at home certain things you can learn through community-

health projects and self-care courses taught by medical-consumer groups. You can learn to take and record your own blood pressure and that of your husband and children (these days *everyone's* blood pressure is considered important information; the equipment costs as little as $20). You can learn to adjust the dosage of your own or your children's medication, within limits set by the doctor. You can give yourself or others in your family regular injections (allergy shots, for instance), when needed. Professor Lowell S. Levin, of the Yale University School of Medicine, a specialist in public health, says that the time has come for the "rediscovery of the lay function in health," and maintains that the informed patient can become the most important practitioner in the medical-care system.

2. *Keep your own medical records.* Since in most states you can't gain access to doctors' records, ask your doctor for his findings every time you visit him—your pulse, blood pressure, hemoglobin and white-cell count—whatever he checks; and don't settle for "It's fine." You have a moral if not a legal right to precise information. So start a notebook. Keep track of whatever the doctor tells you, plus the dates of illnesses, their symptoms and duration, diagnoses, medications taken and their effects.

Also ask your doctor for the results of all tests and lab reports. A few doctors already provide such information; others do not but will if you ask; and many others will refuse. If your doctor refuses, you can either accept defeat or look for another doctor. You also can ask any medical-consumer group what the law is in your state; it may support your claims, and if it does, tell the doctor so.

3. *Come to the doctor prepared.* Before your visit, jot down everything you want to tell the doctor. Include the questions you want to ask. It's amazing how things will slip your mind when you're talking to a hurried doctor or when you're spraddled out on an examination table with some unseen gadget making its way into you. Many feminist groups urge patients to take along a friend to hold the list of questions and remind you of things you forget. Most doctors will ask a third party to leave before an examination, but this is only custom: A.M.A. spokesmen and consumer-group leaders agree that doctors should, and for the most part will, allow a third party to remain if the patient asks them to.

4. *Exercise your right to choose and refuse.* Even with a doctor you believe in—and all the more with one who is new to you—you should take an active part in decisions affecting you. Ask for a detailed explanation of the possible side effects of any recommended drug or procedure. Ask if there are alternate ways to treat your problem. Give due weight to the doctor's preference, but also to your own. It's your body and your life.

If the doctor calls for tests, ask how necessary they are; it's quite in order for you to say you'd like to keep costs down. And ask about risks; it's quite proper for you to say you'd like to avoid any x-rays that are of only marginal value, since it's not the individual exposure that endangers you but an excessive lifetime total of exposures. And it's also your right to say that you prefer to live with your medical problem—or even die of it—rather than submit to a painful, risky treatment if the outcome is highly uncertain.

But if you question the doctor's advice or decline to follow any of his recommendations, won't he be angered? It depends in part on how you put it—and on what kind of person he is. Says Dr. Wolfe, of the Health Research Group, "The doctor who gets huffy when you ask questions or express preferences is a doctor to stay away from. The doctor you should look for is the one who realizes that you have a right to ask questions and to decide what you want to do with your life."

Do you really have a right to refuse any of the doctor's orders? Medical-consumer leaders and A.M.A. officials agree that unless your disease endangers the public welfare, you do have such a right—but that if you exercise it, the doctor may exercise a corresponding right to stop treating you. If you're pregnant or seriously ill or worried, you may be afraid to risk it; you may choke back your questions or objections and play the part of the "good" patient.

But speaking up needn't mean confrontation. Denise Fuge, coordinator of the Women and Health Committee of the New York Chapter of NOW, says patients shouldn't *confront* the doctor, but should seek to *communicate* their fears, wishes and personal values openly and honestly. "Most doctors," she says, "don't know what women are thinking, and they'd like to. They'd respond to the patient much more sensitively if they did."

5. *Get a second opinion.* Before you agree to surgery or any other major procedure, or when some ailment isn't getting better under your doctor's management, tell him that you'd like a second opinion and that you feel sure he wouldn't mind your getting one. He probably will mind, but won't say so or threaten to stop treating you; publicly, most doctors are opposed only to mandatory (legally required) second opinions. Privately, though, many of them feel like Dr. James Sammons, executive vice-president of the A.M.A., who is against them in general.

"I'm opposed to them," he told me, "because the patient's right of choice is lost—he tends to assume the second opinion is more intelligent than the first one." What Dr. Sammons ignores is that the second opinion, though not necessarily more intelligent than the first, is disinterested and hence less subject to unconscious bias. Not all doctors, incidentally, are against second opinions; one quarter of a sample of doctors polled by the magazine Medical World News favored them, and the trend is in that direction.

6. *Ask for enough time.* Don't let yourself be rushed. "You're paying for an expensive service," says Maryann Napoli, of New York's Center for Medical Consumers and Health Care Information, "and consultation is part of it. It's important for your mental health as well as your physical health to have your questions fully answered and your doubts resolved."

Denise Fuge, of NOW, recommends that you say something like, "Doctor, I came to you because I've been worried, and I need more time to talk to you. If you're too busy today, please tell me when you can spend more time with me and I'll come back." A women's medical-consumer group in New York, HealthRight, also suggests that you ask the nurse some of your unanswered questions; nurses are often sympathetic and less rushed than the doctor.

But if your doctor regularly allows less time than normal—15 minutes is the national average duration of routine office visits—and doesn't respond to your request for more time, he may be the wrong doctor for you.

7. *Don't let yourself be treated as an inferior.* This is one of the trickiest points, and perhaps one of the most important. Many doctors treat you in ways that put you at a psychological disadvantage. Some gynecologists in particular address patients by their first names even when they scarcely know them; it makes the patient feel a little like a child. Many women resent this; a few fight back. When a gynecologist greeted one woman, whom he had seen only once before, with "What brings you here today, Lillian?" she said sweetly, "I've got galloping vaginitis again, Bernard." Bernard took the hint. Generally, though, a more formal way of setting the matter straight will work better. For instance: "Doctor, I would much prefer to be called Ms. So-and-so," or, "I really don't like being addressed by my first name."

Similarly, it may make you feel inferior to be undressed and in a gown when you first meet the doctor. If so, tell the nurse you want to speak to him before you undress. This is a delicate matter; the doctor may have set office rules. But Dr. Menninger points out that when you come to exhibit some disease to the doctor, you are apt to feel shame and humiliation, and since such feelings tend to make you a docile patient rather than an active one, it is important to resist anything that intensifies them.

Things will never be what they once were. But the new doctor-patient relationship need not be one of antagonism; it can be one of equality and co-operation. This is what most of the medical-consumer groups, and most active patients are really seeking.

And within the ranks of doctors there are signs of evolution toward a new image of the good doctor—no longer the wise patriarch whose word is law, but a dedicated expert who is ready to give you the help you need and the kind of help you choose. Increasingly, medical journals carry articles advocating democratic ways of dealing with patients and favoring patient participation in the making of medical decisions.

Professor Julia Frank, of the Yale University School of Medicine, writing in the New England Journal of Medicine, urges doctors everywhere to make the patient "an equal member of the team." An editorial in a recent issue of the Journal of the American Medical Association, noting the spread of "participatory democracy" in our society, says, "It is simply no longer possible for the physician to make moral and value decisions for his patients." And Professor Levin, writing in Public Health Reports, sounds a call for massive self-reform by the health professions: "The high value placed on the compliant patient must be transferred to the active, even resistant, patient." He predicts the creation of a "new social contract between professionals and lay persons"—a contract from which the doctor will benefit, by sharing responsibility with those he treats.

And it is a contract from which the patient will benefit by gaining self-respect and a sense of control over her own life—and by getting better quicker.

Ω

♀

More Than One Womb

by Louise Marsden

For the first 31 years of my life, I thought I had a fairly good idea of what my body was like; it functioned 'normally', and since I had a paramedical education, having trained as a pharmacist, I thought that I was informed. Then for various reasons I decided to have a child. I am a woman, I can bear children, so it should be straightforward, I thought. (It couldn't be quite straightforward, I am a lesbian.) I was trying for a year, towards the end of which I began to think I was infertile. I suspect that friends wondered at my continued attempts to become pregnant, as infertility seemed more and more of a possibility. Then one month just when my period was due, I became sick with what seemed incredibly like German measles. It *was* German measles, and my period did not come that month, and I was pregnant. There was no question of whether or not to have an abortion: the effects of German measles on a foetus are usually ghastly. It was not too difficult to get an NHS abortion, although there was some delay, of course! In my anaesthetic haze after the abortion (or termination as they say), the doctor came around and told me that there had been 'scanty products' from the abortion. He looked skeptical and told me to come back in ten days. By then

From Women's Health: A Spare Rib Reader (England) edited by Sue O'Sullivan. Copyright © 1987 by Louise Marsden. Reprinted by permission of the author.

the results of the histology tests — the examination of the embryonic tissue — would be ready. He did not stay to explain. The ward sister assured me that at least one woman every week has scanty products from an abortion.

During the next ten days I tried to find out why there would be 'scanty products'. Perhaps the embryo had already died. This sometimes happens and if it is in the first three months our bodies can reabsorb the 'products'. Perhaps with the German measles it had not grown much anyway. Perhaps the whole pregnancy had been hysterical. I had been trying hard to get pregnant, and maybe I'd forced my body to pretend that it was. Confidence in my own judgment seeped away a little. Were these symptoms psychological?

Anyway, I waited, searching for information as usual. On the appointed day I went, they did not have the histology results, of course. However, I was examined and my uterus was still swollen. It was a different doctor and he decided to have a look around, or rather a feel around. Finally he found something: 'a vaginal septum perhaps', yes, a vaginal septum. Did I mind a student doctor having a look? No, but what are you looking at? He explained that I had a piece of flesh dividing my vagina into two, nothing else. He asked for another sample of urine and I was asked to return to see the consultant in two days and dismissed.

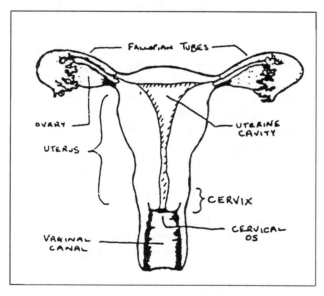

Figure 3. Average female reproductive organs: here is a diagram of what are called 'the female reproductive organs', but we'll call them average female reproductive organs' *Teresa Savage (SR 88 October 1979)*

I immediately did a pregnancy test at home, it was still positive. Great! The consultant was very apologetic, another abortion immediately. But it may not be simple; he may have to cut the septum; he may not be able to remove the foetus without doing a caesarian type abortion, which means cutting me open. He didn't quite know, but it seemed that I had a double uterus. Well, the abortion was quite straightforward fortunately (we have to be thankful

for small mercies); my uterus is completely divided into two, it's a uterus didelphys. From the outside I look like any woman does, there is one entrance to my vagina, but once inside a little, there is this tissue — septum — which divides the pathway into two, going up to two cervixes, then into the two uteruses. The pathway on the left is much narrower and until this abortion business, had never been discovered, although I had had countless internal examinations by doctors for one thing or another. What follows is what I've learned since. I want as many women as possible to know that these anomalies exist.

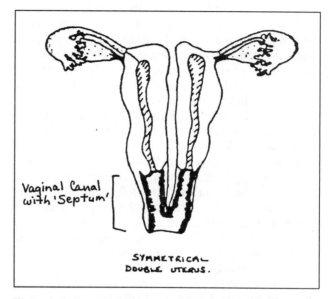

Figure 4. Symmetrical double uterus: here you get two uteruses, two cervixes. There is a fallopian tube attached to each uterus, so the usual number of fallopian tubes and ovaries. The duplication can continue down to the vagina. This is called a Uterus Didelphys *Teresa Savage (SR 88 October 1979)*

In the first 12 weeks when the egg is dividing into different cells (when it is called an embryo), two tubes form and they are called Mullerian ducts. There is one on either side, and they come together to form one tube or vessel, and eventually, the uterus, cervix and upper vagina. If they do not join together completely, and fuse, then these variations on the theme of the female reproductive system develop. The urinary tracts, the kidneys, urethras (tubes going down to the bladder) and bladder also form during this fusion of the Mullerian ducts. So if you get incomplete joining of those ducts, it is possible to have variations in that area too. I have a double lot of kidneys and urethras, but the urethras join together before getting to the bladder. Again they have never caused me any trouble, although some variations can.

It is not known why these things happen, they just do. These things are not passed on from mother to child, so they are not hereditary.

There are a number of possible variations in the uterus and vagina in the female reproductive system. You can have extra ovaries, but that seems to be extremely rare.

You can be born without the top part of the vagina or with a very strong division across it.

The Problems Caused by the Different Variations

Infertility: there is complete infertility if the path to the cervix and vagina is blocked and there is relative infertility if the pathways are narrowed and there are divisions or septa in any of the paths. So with a Unicornuate uterus, one side is completely missing, including one ovary: this means fertility will be considerably reduced.

Miscarriage: miscarriage is more common because implantation of the fertilized egg can happen on a septum, and the septum is likely to have a weaker blood supply and will not be strong enough to support the growing egg (embryo). Also the space inside the uterus may be irregular, and this will prevent growth.

Premature labour and premature rupture of the membranes (waters): both of these happen for the same reasons as miscarriage happens. The foetus may not be able to position itself properly for birth, because of the shape of the uterus. So 'malpresentation' is more common. The baby may lie across the uterus, or upside down (breech).

Dystocia (abnormal labour): the uterine contractions may not be co-ordinated, also the non-pregnant side of the uterus can block the way of the baby. Placenta can remain in the uterus, again because of the uncoordinated contractions, so it has to be removed by hand.

All of the above problems are to do with childbirth, but with a uterus which has a blind side, you can get a build up of menstrual blood because there is no way for it to come out. So periods can be very painful and eventually after some years, you can get a big lump which is made up of old menstrual blood and it falls down into the vagina. Its removal would have to be by surgery.

It is hard to find very much written on how often these variations occur; they are often not discovered at all because they are not always problematic. Ian Donald in *Practical Obstetric Problems* says that two out of every thousand women have a 'congenital deformity' that is bad enough to interfere with pregnancy. This is 0.2% and presumably he means that 0.2% of women have problems conceiving because of one of these variations. Belscher and Mackay in *Obstetrics and the Newborn* say, however, that the incidence of variation is approximately 1%, but if minor forms of duplication like a septate uterus are included, it could be close to 5%. So five women in every 100 have some variation, and this knowledge is kept in weighty medical tomes, hidden from us.

The gynecology consultant whom I saw for the abortion said that he sees about one woman a year with some variation. I have spoken to midwives who have been practicing for years, and who have seen only two or three — not surprising, really, as midwives deal with women who have successfully conceived, and not with women who are having problems.

Until I decided to get pregnant, my double uterus caused me no difficulties at all; most of the problems do seem to happen in pregnancy. If a lot go unnoticed, it's possible that they are trouble free. Ian Donald quotes that from 42 pregnancies where there were uterine variations, 19 ended in miscarriage, five in premature labour, eight with unstable presentation, that is breech or sideways, and in five the placenta had to be removed by hand. Out of the 23 pregnancies reaching labour, four babies died. He also says that the more minor the variation, then the more treacherous; for example, in some variations the growing foetus could lie with its head in one side, and body in the other, and this would be very dangerous. Since mine is completely separate, the problems are minimized.

That is all the technical information I have been able to find; there is not a lot written, just two or three pages in gynaecology books in chapter headed 'Congenital Anomalies/Abnormalities'. Are we not told much about the abnormalities of the female reproductive system because these women are not normal, possibly not reproductive, or is it a continuation of the mystification that prevents us from having control over our bodies and our lives?

In the past few months I have heard of other women with such variations, but as yet I have not met any others. It would be good to hear of other women's experience. I have not had a lot to do with doctors since the discovery. My GP was mildly amused and the consultant at the hospital objectively curious.

I am pregnant again now; it happened the first time I tried after the second abortion, clever body, so I have been to an antenatal clinic. I suspect that I am a curiosity there. I don't mind people learning from my parts; the more who know the better. But I think that I will have to undergo more examinations than usual for the sake of medical science and I also think that I will not be told what they are seeing or what they are thinking. I object to being seen as a medical specimen and not just as a variation. I am not sick. I do not feel any different from how I felt for the first 31 years of my life.

My present lover noticed ages ago that there were 'two ways that she could go' inside my vagina, and she often felt worried about it. Why don't we trust our own discoveries? The 'experts' have made us totally dependent. Now that I am pregnant, I feel less in control than I might overwise have felt. I keep thinking that perhaps I should be doing things that other pregnant women don't need to do, I don't know quite what. I suppose I am feeling that I do have some deformity for which I am responsible. The feeling is not strong and I resist it, but it's there. I feel angry that some of my confidence has been taken from me. We should know that these variations are possible, but of course there is so much that we should know and we don't.

Neither the woman I am involved with nor I were shocked or horrified by the knowledge, only curious and we sought out as much information as we could, as quickly as we could. Other women have been shocked and thought it peculiar, but I think that reflects a standard acceptance of what is 'normal'. We're fighting the 'norms' of this society.

They say that these variations often go undetected, that is until they present a problem. But if we knew about them, some we could easily discover ourselves like double vaginas. We would not be taken by surprise and the possibility of thinking it 'odd' would at least be reduced.

Ω

Self-Help Health Education:
Models from Diverse Communities
from National Women's Health Network's *Network News*

The National Women's Health Network sponsored an exciting panel discussion at the recent annual meeting of the American Public Health Association. Presenters from six groups shared strategies about integrating the self help approach into programs and services provided to women in their communities. Common themes seen in self help projects were highlighted by Carol Downer, in her introduction, "Self help starts with women's own experience as its base, and validates women. This leads to trying to change the world outside women, not women themselves. Self help can't be used to control others, rather it gives them knowledge to make them independent." The communities using self-help techniques were incredibly diverse: homeless women, Spanish-speaking women in California and New Mexico, African American women in Atlanta, women interested in menstrual extraction, and Native American women dealing with diabetes, violence, and fetal alcohol syndrome. Each group had found that their programs were popular with women in their communities.

For more information about the projects conducted by each group contact:

Judith Costlow, **Santa Fe Health Education Project,** PO Box 577, Santa Fe, New Mexico 87504-0577. The Project publishes the *Health Letter,* a bilingual newsletter covering women's and family health topics. They have recently revised *Menopause:A Self Care Manual* which is available for $5.

Carol Downer, **Federation of Feminist Women's Health Centers,** 1680 N. Vine Street, Suite 1005, Los Angeles, CA 90028, (213) 957-4062. The Federation has published books and pamphlets on gynecologic self-help,

and is currently sponsoring a speakers bureau and self-help tours to work with groups interested in learning menstrual extraction.

Paulita Ortiz, **National Latina Health Organization,** PO Box 7567, 1900 Fruitvale Ave., Oakland, CA 94601, (510) 534-1362. The organization conducts a Spanish-language class series, Better Health Through Self Empowerment in the East Bay area of Northern California. The Organization also coordinates the Latinas for Reproductive Health Rights project and distributes a newsletter.

Charon Asetoyer, **Native American Women's Health Education Resource Center,** PO Box 572, Lake Andes, SD 57356, (605) 487-7072. The Center is run by women who live and work on the Yankton Sioux reservation in South Dakota. The Center concentrates on confronting the root of so many health problems in the Native American community, alcohol. The Center has developed health education resources for women on HIV disease, fetal alcohol syndrome, Norplant, and diabetes.

Terry Boykins, **Calvert Workers Cooperative,** 9 Gammon Avenue, SE, Atlanta, GA 30312. The cooperative is a community development center for a public housing project. In addition to supporting other projects, the cooperative also sponsors self-help groups for teens and women living in public housing.

Stephanie Stevens, **Women's Health Education Project,** PO Box 20284, Tompkins Square Station, New York, NY 10009. The project conducts women's health workshops in homeless shelters in New York City. They have produced a pamphlet, "Having a Baby: A Guide to Resources in New York City" and are working on a guide to other reproductive health services.

Ω

Women and the Health Care System

1. The list below mentions a few of the issues women's health activists have organized around:

   - more women doctors
   - women's health centers run *by* women *for* women
   - self-help groups
   - better information for personal informed decision-making
   - excellent health services equally available for rich & poor
   - consent forms which must be read and signed by a woman before she has birth control inserted/injected or before any surgical process

   a. If you were to identify the priorities for the activities for a women's health organization, list the rank that you would give to each of the above. (Are there different issues you would add to your six priorities?)

issue	b	c
1.		
2.		
3.		
4.		
5.		
6.		

   b. In the column b, for each of the issues above, identify whether that issue can (yes) be taken care of within the present system or (no) whether such a "demand" calls for fundamental changes in the health care system.

   c. In column c, for each of the issues, identify whether you think the last 20+ years of activism have improved this issue.

   - − = there have been set-backs
   - 0 = little change
   - + = situation improved
   - ++ = situation very much improved

2. Identify five things which every woman should be able to expect as a part of a good gynecological examination:

   a.

   b.

   c.

   d.

   e.

3. Describe your "best" and "worst" health care experiences. Briefly, identify the behaviors (or other characteristics) which were different for the health providers in the two situations. Referring to "How to Tell Your Doctor a Thing or Two," can you identify ways that you were or were not an "active patient" in the two situations?

4. Outline *both* sides of the debate on the question, "Will increasing the number of women doctors increase the quality of care which women receive as health care consumers?"

    yes

    no

5. Go through several medical journals and look at the images of women as health care consumers. What patterns emerge?

6. After doing question 5, compare present day images of women as consumers in medical journals to what was presented in the same journal five, ten, or twenty years ago. In what ways are the representations of women changing or not changing?

Chapter

2

Diversity and Health Issues

A core part of developing an analysis of women's health issues is working towards an understanding of why "some women have a better chance of being healthy than other women." This involves learning how racism, anti-semitism, poverty, homophobia, ageism, attitudes towards disabilities, fatphobia, and other forms of oppression multiply the effects of sexism, impact on women's mental and physical health, affect access to the determinants of health (nutrition, environment, housing, education, and rewards for employment), and influence or determine one's access and/or relationship with the health care system. Articles in this chapter are chosen to stimulate dialogue on this and help us work towards a better understanding of how oppressions impact on health so that working against oppressions and our own ways of perpetuating oppressions can be an on-going part of our work towards a health care system more appropriate for *all* women (and men.)

The reader is reminded that this book is planned to complement, rather than overlap with, *The Black Women's Health Book.* As African-American women, and the National Black Women's Health Project specifically, have played a leadership role in the documentation and expression of how racism is a major health issue, much of the most ground-breaking work on this topic is covered or reflected in *The Black Women's Health Book.*

The first three articles set the tone for how this book and its editors try to work on diversity issues. Audre Lorde's classics, "Age, Race, Class and Sex: Women Redefining Difference" and "There Is No Hierarchy of Oppressions" look at the interactions of *all* forms of oppression and how a basic understanding of power and control issues (who benefits from the inequalities in society and what weapons are used to keep the status quo/the inequalities in place) is fundamental to understanding any and all forms of oppression. (It is important to note that while Audre Lorde's life was devoted to educating us about the widest range of oppressions and begging us to look at their intersections rather than looking at a hierarchy of oppressions, Lorde also emphasized that in a racist society, racism plays a dominating role in maintaining power differentials.)

Ricky Sherover-Marcuse, a Jewish feminist, also devoted her life to anti-oppression work. Her "Unlearning Racism" article captures some of the essence of the powerful, life changing Unlearning Racism Workshops which she facilitated around the country, encouraging each of us to take responsibility for starting to unlearn oppressive misinformation which we have learned as a part of our socialization in a racist society. Perhaps her most inspiring work was to stimulate everyone committed to anti-oppression work to look at how we could consciously work at being *allies* for each other and for "each other's issues."

"Infant Mortality in the US" and "The Class Gap" provide rare discussions on the intersection of race and class as health determinants in the US and provide a feel for the complexity of these issues which too often get left out of our debates when we simply try to look at race or class issues. Internationally, infant mortality rate (IMR) is considered the key figure to use for comparing health determinants in different populations. When IMRs are used for looking internally at what is happening in the US, we see a drastic difference between the IMR for wealthy white populations and the IMR for poor Black communities. As Paul Wise says, "infant mortality represents a stark if not ultimate expression of social and economic injustice in our society." "The Class Gap" provides an unusual glimpse at what we could learn about the influence of class on health *if* we had access to such information. Class analysis, building on officially published figures (always open to criticism, such as, why does a woman's class get defined by her husband's occupation?), is core to women's health writing in many other countries, but "the U.S., unlike most industrialized nations, does not regularly collect and publish mortality statistics (or other health information) by class." Is that a reason for, or a reflection of, Americans' confusion about the role of class in our lives? "Strained Class Windows" is one of a series of articles in the special class issue of *Sojourner* (January 1994) looking at the role of class in women's lives. Class differs from other forms of oppression in a very fundamental way. For other issues, a goal is to celebrate and value our differences and to eliminate *the oppression* related to the issue. With class (poverty), the goal is to *eliminate that form of difference.* As Judith K. Witherow says at the end of her article, "I would like to see the problems caused by classism worked on continually until all women share equally in the benefits of society."

In order to recognize the ways that racism and other forms of oppression impact on every health issue, we have tried to include articles by a diverse group of women in many chapters of this book. The next articles in this chapter are intended to highlight, rather than isolate, a few of the many special issues which are related to racism, anti-semitism and disability issues. "Angry Women Are Building: Issues and Struggle Facing American Indian Women Today" and "The Health of Native People in the US" summarize, from very different perspectives, many of the key issues which Native American women live with daily when literal survival is the central issue in their lives. "Blazes of Truth" and "JAP: The New AntiSemitic Code Word" discuss the oppression and meanings of using the term "Jewish American Princess." Irene Klepfisz's "Consciousness-Raising Questions on Anti-Semitism" is a set of questions (discussion starters) designed to help us discover the degree to which we (as Jews or as allies) have internalized or tolerate anti-semitic oppression. "Disability and the Medical System", "On Being an Outreach Group: Women with Disabilities" and "Simply . . . Friend or Foe?" give us an overview of some of the health and medical abuse issues for women with disabilities, provide specific ideas for how women's organizations can make more meaningful connections with women with disabilities, and through illustrations, offers the able-bodied ideas for how to be allies to people with disabilities.

This chapter closes with two very different papers which address what happens or can happen in the classroom when diversity becomes an issue. "Gender and Race in the Classroom: Teaching Way Out of Line" looks at how easily the material is seen to be "volatile" and the classroom can become "explosive" when someone other than a white male teaches the class or becomes the center of attention. As the title states, "Ideas for Anti-Racism and Pro-Diversity Work and Discussion in a Women's Health Class" brings together a number of ideas and exercises which have been used successfully in trying to make diversity issues core to the teaching and learning about women's health.

Age, Race, Class, and Sex:
Women Redefining Difference*

by Audre Lorde

Much of western European history conditions us to see human differences in simplistic opposition to each other: dominant/subordinate, good/bad, up/down, superior/inferior. In a society where the good is defined in terms of profit rather than in terms of human need, there must always be some group of people who, through systematized oppression, can be made to feel surplus, to occupy the place of the dehumanized inferior. Within this society, that group is made up of Black and Third World people, working-class people, older people, and women.

As a forty-nine-year-old Black lesbian feminist socialist mother of two, including one boy, and a member of an interracial couple, I usually find myself a part of some group defined as other, deviant, inferior, or just plain wrong. Traditionally, in american society, it is the members of oppressed, objectified groups who are expected to stretch out and bridge the gap between the actualities of our lives and the consciousness of our oppressor. For in order to survive, those of us for whom oppression is as American as apple pie have always had to be watchers, to become familiar with the language and manners of the oppressor, even sometimes adopting them for some illusion of protection. Whenever the need for some pretense of communication arises, those who profit from our oppression call upon us to share our knowledge with them. In other words, it is the responsibility of the oppressed to teach the oppressors their mistakes. I am responsible for educating teachers who dismiss my children's culture in school. Black and Third World people are expected to educate white people as to our humanity. Women are expected to educate men. Lesbians and gay men are expected to educate the heterosexual world. The oppressors maintain their position and evade responsibility for their own actions. There is a constant drain of energy which might be better used in redefining ourselves and devising realistic scenarios for altering the present and constructing the future.

Institutionalized rejection of difference is an absolute necessity in a profit economy which needs outsiders as surplus people. As members of such an economy, we have *all* been programmed to respond to the human differences between us with fear and loathing and to handle that difference in one of three ways: ignore it, and if that is not possible, copy it if we think it is dominant, or destroy it if we think it is subordinate. But we have no patterns for relating across our human differences as equals. As a result, those differences have been misnamed and misused in the service of separation and confusion.

Certainly there are very real differences between us of race, age, and sex. But it is not those differences between us that are separating us. It is rather our refusal to recognize those differences, and to examine the distortions which result from our misnaming them and their effects upon human behavior and expectation.

Racism, the belief in the inherent superiority of one race over all others and thereby the right to dominance. Sexism, the belief in the inherent superiority of one sex over the other and thereby the right to dominance. Ageism. Heterosexism. Elitism, Classism.

It is a lifetime pursuit for each one of us to extract these distortions from our living at the same time as we recognize, reclaim, and define those differences upon which they are imposed. For we have all been raised in a society where those distortions were endemic within our living. Too often, we pour the energy needed for recognizing and exploring difference into pretending those differences are insurmountable barriers, or that they do not exist at all. This results in a voluntary isolation, or false and treacherous connections. Either way, we do not develop tools for using human difference as a springboard for creative change within our lives. We speak not of human difference, but of human deviance.

Somewhere, on the edge of consciousness, there is what I call a *mythical norm*, which each one of us within our hearts knows "that is not me." In america, this norm is usually defined as white, thin, male, young, heterosexual, christian, and financially secure. It is with this mythical norm that the trappings of power reside within this society. Those of us who stand outside that power often identify one way in which we are different, and we assume that to be the primary cause of all oppression, forgetting other distortions around difference, some of which we ourselves may be practicing. By and large within the women's movement today, white women focus upon their oppression as women and ignore differences of race, sexual preference, class, and age. There is a pretense to a homogeneity of experience covered by the word *sisterhood* that does not in fact exist.

Unacknowledged class differences rob women of each others' energy and creative insight. Recently a women's magazine collective made the decision for one issue to

*Paper delivered at the Copeland Colloquium, Amherst College, April 1980.

print only prose, saying poetry was a less "rigorous" or "serious" art form. Yet even the form our creativity takes is often a class issue. Of all the art forms, poetry is the most economical. It is the one which is the most secret, which requires the least physical labor, the least material, and the one which can be done between shifts, in the hospital pantry, on the subway, and on scraps of surplus paper. Over the last few years, writing a novel on tight finances, I came to appreciate the enormous differences in the material demands between poetry and prose. As we reclaim our literature, poetry has been the major voice of poor, working class, and Colored women. A room of one's own may be a necessity for writing prose, but so are reams of paper, a typewriter, and plenty of time. The actual requirements to produce the visual arts also help determine, along class lines, whose art is whose. In this day of inflated prices for material, who are our sculptors, our painters, our photographers? When we speak of a broadly based women's culture, we need to be aware of the effect of class and economic differences on the supplies available for producing art.

As we move toward creating a society within which we can each flourish, ageism is another distortion of relationship which interferes without vision. By ignoring the past, we are encouraged to repeat its mistakes. The "generation gap" is an important social tool for any repressive society. If the younger members of a community view the older members as contemptible or suspect or excess, they will never be able to join hands and examine the living memories of the community, nor ask the all important question, "Why?" This gives rise to a historical amnesia that keeps us working to invent the wheel every time we have to go to the store for bread.

We find ourselves having to repeat and relearn the same old lessons over and over that our mothers did because we do not pass on what we have learned, or because we are unable to listen. For instance, how many times has this all been said before? For another, who would have believed that once again our daughters are allowing their bodies to be hampered and purgatoried by girdles and high heels and hobble skirts?

Ignoring the differences of race between women and the implications of those differences presents the most serious threat to the mobilization of women's joint power.

As white women ignore their built-in privilege of whiteness and define *woman* in terms of their own experience alone, then women of Color become "other," the outsider whose experience and tradition is too "alien" to comprehend. An example of this is the signal absence of the experience of women of Color as a resource for women's studies courses. The literature of women of Color is seldom included in women's literature courses and almost never in other literature courses, nor in women's studies as a whole. All too often, the excuse given is that the literatures of women of Color can only be taught by Colored women, or that they are too difficult to understand, or that classes cannot "get into" them because they come out of experiences that are "too different." I have heard this argument presented by white women of otherwise quite clear intelligence, women who seem to have no trouble at all teaching and reviewing work that comes out of the vastly different experiences of Shakespeare, Molière, Dostoyefsky, and Aristophanes. Surely there must be some other explanation.

This is a very complex question, but I believe one of the reasons white women have such difficulty reading Black women's work is because of their reluctance to see Black women as women and different from themselves. To examine Black women's literature effectively requires that we be seen as whole people in our actual complexities—as individuals, as women, as human—rather than as one of those problematic but familiar stereotypes provided in this society in place of genuine images of Black women. And I believe this holds true for the literatures of other women of Color who are not Black.

The literatures of all women of Color recreate the textures of our lives, and many white women are heavily invested in ignoring the real differences. For as long as any difference between us means one of us must be inferior, then the recognition of any difference must be fraught with guilt. To allow women of Color to step out of stereotypes is too guilt provoking, for it threatens the complacency of those women who view oppression only in terms of sex.

Refusing to recognize difference makes it impossible to see the different problems and pitfalls facing us as women.

Thus, in a patriarchal power system where white-skin privilege is a major prop, the entrapments used to neutralize Black women and white women are not the same. For example, it is easy for Black women to be used by the power structure against Black men, not because they are men, but because they are Black. Therefore, for Black women, it is necessary at all times to separate the needs of the oppressor from our own legitimate conflicts within our communities. This same problem does not exist for white women. Black women and men have shared racist oppression and still share it, although in different ways. Out of that shared oppression we have developed joint defenses and joint vulnerabilities to each other that are not duplicated in the white community, with the exception of the relationship between Jewish women and Jewish men.

On the other hand, white women face the pitfall of being seduced into joining the oppressor under the pretense of sharing power. This possibility does not exist in the same way for women of Color. The tokenism that is sometimes extended to us is not an invitation to join power; our racial "otherness" is a visible reality that makes that quite clear. For white women there is a wider range of pretended choices and rewards for identifying with patriarchal power and its tools.

Today, with the defeat of ERA, the tightening economy, and increased conservatism, it is easier once again for white women to believe the dangerous fantasy that if you are good enough, pretty enough, sweet enough, quiet enough, teach the children to behave, hate the right people, and marry the right men, then you will be allowed to co-exist with patriarchy in relative peace, at least until a man needs your job or the neighborhood rapist happens along. And true, unless one lives and loves in the trenches it is difficult to remember that the war against dehumanization is ceaseless.

But Black women and our children know the fabric of our lives is stitched with violence and with hatred, that there is no rest. We do not deal with it only on the picket lines, or in dark midnight alleys, or in the places where we dare to verbalize our resistance. For us, increasingly, violence weaves through the daily tissues of our living—in the supermarket, in the classroom, in the elevator, in the clinic and the schoolyard, from the plumber, the baker, the saleswoman, the bus driver, the bank teller, the waitress who does not serve us.

Some problems we share as women, some we do not. You fear your children will grow up to join the patriarchy and testify against you, we fear our children will be dragged from a car and shot down in the street, and you will turn your backs upon the reasons they are dying.

The threat of difference has been no less blinding to people of Color. Those of us who are Black must see that the reality of our lives and our struggle does not make us immune to the errors of ignoring and misnaming difference. Within Black communities where racism is a living reality, differences among us often seem dangerous and suspect. The need for unity is often misnamed as a need for homogeneity, and a Black feminist vision mistaken for betrayal of our common interests as a people. Because of the continuous battle against racial erasure that Black women and Black men share, some Black women still refuse to recognize that we are also oppressed as women, and that sexual hostility against Black women is practiced not only by the white racist society, but implemented within our Black communities as well. It is a disease striking the heart of Black nationhood, and silence will not make it disappear. Exacerbated by racism and the pressures of powerlessness, violence against Black women and children often becomes a standard within our communities, one by which manliness can be measured. But these women-hating acts are rarely discussed as crimes against Black women.

As a group, women of Color are the lowest paid wage earners in america. We are the primary targets of abortion and sterilization abuse, here and abroad. In certain parts of Africa, small girls are still being sewed shut between their legs to keep them docile and for men's pleasure. This is known as female circumcision, and it is not a cultural affair as the late Jomo Kenyatta insisted, it is a crime against Black women.

Black women's literature is full of the pain of frequent assault, not only by a racist patriarchy, but also by Black men. Yet the necessity for and history of shared battle have made us, Black women, particularly vulnerable to the false accusation that anti-sexist is anti-Black. Meanwhile, womanhating as a recourse of the powerless is sapping strength from Black communities, and our very lives. Rape is on the increase, reported and unreported, and rape is not aggressive sexuality, it is sexualized aggression. As

Kalamu ya Salaam, a Black male writer points out, "As long as male domination exists, rape will exist. Only women revolting and men made conscious of their responsibility to fight sexism can collectively stop rape."*

Differences between ourselves as Black women are also being misnamed and used to separate us from one another. As a Black lesbian feminist comfortable with the many different ingredients of my identity, and a woman committed to racial and sexual freedom from oppression, I find I am constantly being encouraged to pluck out some one aspect of myself and present this as the meaningful whole, eclipsing or denying the other parts of self. But this is a destructive and fragmenting way to live. My fullest concentration of energy is available to me only when I integrate all the parts of who I am, openly, allowing power from particular sources of my living to flow back and forth freely through all my different selves, without the restrictions of externally imposed definition. Only then can I bring myself and my energies as a whole to the service of those struggles which I embrace as part of my living.

A fear of lesbians, or of being accused of being a lesbian, has led many Black women into testifying against themselves. It has led some of us into destructive alliances, and others into despair and isolation. In the white women's communities, heterosexism is sometimes a result of identifying with the white patriarchy, a rejection of that interdependence between women-identified women which allows the self to be, rather than to be used in the service of men. Sometimes it reflects a die-hard belief in the protective coloration of heterosexual relationships, sometimes a self-hate which all women have to fight against, taught us from birth.

Although elements of these attitudes exist for all women, there are particular resonances of heterosexism and homophobia among Black women. Despite the fact that woman-bonding has a long and honorable history in the African and African-American communities, and despite the knowledge and accomplishments of many strong and creative women-identified Black women in the political, social and cultural fields, heterosexual Black women often tend to ignore or discount the existence and work of Black lesbians. Part of this attitude has come from an understandable terror of Black male attack within the close confines of Black society, where the punishment for any female self-assertion is still to be accused of being a lesbian and therefore unworthy of the attention or support of the scarce Black male. But part of this need to misname and ignore Black lesbians comes from a very real fear that openly women-identified Black women who are no longer dependent upon men for their self-definition may well reorder our whole concept of social relationships.

Black women who once insisted that lesbianism was a white woman's problem now insist that Black lesbians are a threat to Black nationhood, are consorting with the

*From "Rape: A Radical Analysis, An African-American Perspective" by Kalamu ya Salaam in *Black Books Bulletin,* vol. 6, no. 4 (1980).

enemy, are basically un-Black. These accusations, coming from the very women to whom we look for deep and real understanding, have served to keep many Black lesbians in hiding, caught between the racism of white women and the homophobia of their sisters. Often, their work has been ignored, trivialized, or misnamed, as with the work of Angelina Grimke, Alice Dunbar-Nelson, Lorraine Hansberry. Yet women-bonded women have always been some part of the power of Black communities, from our unmarried aunts to the amazons of Dahomey.

And it is certainly not Black lesbians who are assaulting women and raping children and grandmothers on the streets of our communities.

Across this country, as in Boston during the spring of 1979 following the unsolved murders of twelve Black women, Black lesbians are spearheading movements against violence against Black women.

What are the particular details within each of our lives that can be scrutinized and altered to help bring about change? How do we redefine difference for all women? It is not our differences which separate women, but our reluctance to recognize those differences and to deal effectively with the distortions which have resulted from the ignoring and misnaming of those differences.

As a tool of social control, women have been encouraged to recognize only one area of human difference as legitimate, those differences which exist between women and men. And we have learned to deal across those differences with the urgency of all oppressed subordinates. All of us have had to learn to live or work or coexist with men, from our fathers on. We have recognized and negotiated these differences, even when this recognition only continued the old dominant/subordinate mode of human relationship, where the oppressed must recognize the masters' difference in order to survive.

But our future survival is predicated upon our ability to relate within equality. As women, we must root out internalized patterns of oppression within ourselves if we are to move beyond the most superficial aspects of social change. Now we must recognize differences among women who are our equals, neither inferior nor superior, and devise ways to use each others' difference to enrich our visions and our joint struggles.

The future of our earth may depend upon the ability of all women to identify and develop new definitions of power and new patterns of relating across difference. The old definitions have not served us, nor the earth that supports us. The old patterns, no matter how cleverly rearranged to imitate progress, still condemn us to cosmetically altered repetitions of the same old exchanges, the same old guilt, hatred, recrimination, lamentation, and suspicion.

For we have, built into all of us, old blueprints of expectation and response, old structures of oppression, and these must be altered at the same time as we alter the living conditions which are a result of those structures. For the master's tools will never dismantle the master's house.

As Paulo Freire shows so well in *The Pedagogy of the Oppressed,** the true focus of revolutionary change is never merely the oppressive situations which we seek to escape, but that piece of the oppressor which is planted deep within each of us, and which knows only the oppressors' tactics, the oppressors' relationships.

Change means growth, and growth can be painful. But we sharpen self-definition by exposing the self in work and struggle together with those whom we define as different from ourselves, although sharing the same goals. For Black and white, old and young, lesbian and heterosexual women alike, this can mean new paths to our survival.

> *We have chosen each other*
> *and the edge of each other battles*
> *the war is the same*
> *if we lose*
> *someday women's blood will congeal*
> *upon a dead planet*
> *if we win*
> *there is no telling*
> *we seek beyond history*
> *for a new and more possible meeting.* **

Ω

---

*Seabury Press, New York, 1970
**From "Outlines," unpublished poem.

There Is No Hierarchy of Oppressions

by Audre Lorde

I was born Black, and a woman. I am trying to become the strongest person I can become to live the life I have been given and to help effect change toward a liveable future for this earth and for my children. As a Black, lesbian, feminist, socialist, poet, mother of two including one boy and a member of an interracial couple, I usually find myself part of some group in which the majority defines me as deviant, difficult, inferior, or just plain "wrong."

From my membership in all of these groups I have learned that oppression and the intolerance of difference come in all shapes and sizes and colors and sexualities; and that among those of us who share the goals of liberation and a workable future for our children, there can be no hierarchies of oppression. I have learned that sexism (a belief in the inherent superiority of one sex over all others and thereby its right to dominance) and heterosexism (a belief in the inherent superiority of one pattern of loving over all others and thereby its right to dominance) both arise from the same source as racism—a belief in the inherent superiority of one race over all others and thereby its right to dominance.

"Oh," says a voice from the Black community, "but being Black is NORMAL!" Well, I and many Black people of my age can remember grimly the days when it didn't used to be!

I simply do not believe that one aspect of myself can possibly profit from the oppression of any other part of my identity. I know that my people cannot possibly profit from the oppression of any other group which seeks the right to peaceful existence. Rather, we diminish ourselves by denying to others what we have shed blood to obtain for our children. And those children need to learn that they do not have to become like each other in order to work together for a future they will all share.

The increasing attacks upon lesbians and gay men are only an introduction to the increasing attacks upon all Black people, for wherever oppression manifests itself in this country, Black people are potential victims. And it is a standard of right-wing cynicism to encourage members of oppressed groups to act against each other, and so long as we are divided because of our particular identities we cannot join together in effective political action.

Within the lesbian community I am Black, and within the Black community I am a lesbian. Any attack against Black people is a lesbian and gay issue, because I and thousands of other Black women are part of the lesbian community. Any attack against lesbians and gays is a Black issue, because thousands of lesbians and gay men are Black. There is no hierarchy of oppression.

It is not accidental that the Family Protection Act, which is virulently anti-woman and anti-Black, is also anti-gay. As a Black person, I know who my enemies are, and when the Ku Klux Klan goes to court in Detroit to try and force the Board of Education to remove books the Klan believes "hint at homosexuality," then I know I cannot afford the luxury of fighting one form of oppression only. I cannot afford to believe that freedom from intolerance is the right of only one particular group. And I cannot afford to choose between the fronts upon which I must battle these forces of discrimination, wherever they appear to destroy me. And when they appear to destroy me, it will not be long before they appear to destroy you.

Ω

Reprinted with permission from *Council on Interracial Books for Children Bulletin*. vol. 14, No. 3-4, 1983. (1841 Broadway, Rm. 500, New York, N.Y. 10023)

Unlearning Racism
by Ricky Sherover-Marcuse

Because racism is both institutional and attitudinal, effective strategies against it must recognize this dual character. The *undoing* of institutionalized racism must be accompanied by the *unlearning* of racist attitudes and beliefs, and the *unlearning* of racist patterns of thought and action must guide the practice of political and social change.

Institutionalized racism can be defined as the systematic mistreatment of people of color (Third World people). Defining racism in this way highlights the fact that racism is not a genetic disease which is inherent in white people, but that it is a form of social oppression which is the result of the institutionalized inequalities in the structure of a given society.

Attitudinal racism can be defined as the set of assumptions, feelings, beliefs, and attitudes about people of color and their cultures which are a mixture of *misinformation* and ignorance. By "misinformation" I mean any assumption or attitude which in any way implies that people of color are less than fully human. Defining attitudinal racism as misinformation about people of color which has been imposed upon white people means that racism is not a moral defect which some (bad) white individuals have, but a social poison which has been given to all of us, albeit in many different forms.

Attitudinal racism and institutional racism feed off each other. The systematic mistreatment of any group of people generates misinformation about them which in turn becomes "explanation" of or justification for their continued mistreatment. As a result, misinformation about the victims of social oppression becomes socially empowered or *socially sanctioned misinformation*. This is what differentiates this sort of misinformation from prejudice. Socially sanctioned misinformation gets recycled through the society as a form of conditioning which becomes part of our "ordinary" assumptions, and as a result social oppression is viewed either as "natural" or as the fault of the victims themselves.

For example, the misinformation that people of color are stupid or indifferent to the value of human life becomes the "explanation" as to why there is a higher rate of infant mortality among certain groups in the populations. This "explanation" then justifies the attitude that there is really nothing one can do about infant mortality since this problem is basically due to the character or personality structure of the ethnic group involved.

For the past five years I have been doing workshops with groups of white people on "Unlearning Racism". The purpose of these workshops is to help whites to become aware that we have a personal stake in overcoming and unlearning the racist conditioning that was imposed upon us. Having racist beliefs and attitudes is like have a clamp on one's mind. *Unlearning* racism is partly a process of *relearning* how to get accurate information from and about people of color. This involves *relearning* how to really listen to people of color without making judgments or assumptions about what we think they are going to tell us.

When white people become aware of the ways in which *our lives* have been limited and restricted by racism, we become aware of *our interest* in ending this oppression. The most effective action that white people can take against racism will be action which springs not from a sense of guilt or pity, but from our own *knowledge* that in working against racism we are moving towards our own human liberation.

Ω

Reprinted with permission from the Coalition for the Medical Rights of Women.

Infant Mortality in the U.S.

by Paul Wise

Infant mortality has a long history as a sensitive indicator of the general well being of a population in that it is closely related to the nutritional, sanitary, and medical conditions of a society. Early in 1983 a series of reports pointed to rising infant mortality rates in areas of high unemployment.[1] In response, the Senate committee charged with the oversight of childhood nutrition programs, the Committee on Agriculture, Nutrition and Forestry, chaired by Jesse Helms, held hearings on this issue.

The reaction of government officials and many academicians was to fault these reports on the unreliability of their statistics. They pointed to the "randomness" inherent in annual mortality data from a small geographic area (e.g., city or state) whereby increases in rates my occur by chance alone. Their advice was not to view these increases as real, and further that the declines in infant mortality over the past decade would indeed continue. The committee's dismissal of the short-term rise in mortality precluded, however, the very real possibility that the mortality reflected transitory but very real change in social conditions. A related issue underlying much of the debate was the notion that cities or states with large black populations should not be compared to others with primarily white populations or to a national average. Helms stated it best when he noted as part of a question:

Some observers have noted that the comparative use of inner city statistics—where black populations are often higher— with the national average is inappropriate because black infant mortality is historically close to double the national rate.[2]

The implication is that rates for blacks and whites must be viewed separately, as black rates have been "historically" so much higher than those of whites. This discussion highlighted two fundamental observations. First, that racial differentials in infant mortality are enormous and persistent. Second, and far more subtle, was the unspoken attitude that high mortality was both tolerable and somehow related to inherent racial differences. The "history" of high black infant mortality implied some form of natural order, not particularly responsive to public policies, and a source of statistical error if not controlled for in comparative studies. The true implications of these differentials were rarely approached, and only in the written testimony of Dr. Peter Budetti, a respected public health researcher and child advocate, did their devastating presence receive the attention they deserved. The concentration of infant mortality in the black community has become so marked that the ranking of states by infant mortality generally corresponds to the percent of their population that is black. The precise causes of this high black infant mortality remain unclear. However, recent efforts to better understand the nature of infant mortality trends have shed light on some areas of special concern.

Neonatal Mortality: Disparity Between Blacks and Whites

Infant mortality is defined as the number of deaths experienced in children from birth to one year of age, and is usually expressed per 1000 live births. In 1982, the infant mortality rate for the United States was 11.2. This implies that for every 1000 children born alive in the United States, an average of 11.2 of them will die before their first birthday. It has been known for some time that the majority of infant deaths occur shortly after birth from causes significantly different from those which kill infants later in the first year. In the United States approximately 70% of all infant deaths occur during the newborn, or "neonatal" period, defined as the first 28 days of life. Therefore, discussions of infant mortality must primarily address trends in neonatal mortality.

The neonatal mortality rate (NMR) in the U.S. has been falling for more than a century. However, despite the considerable variation in NMR over the years, there has been one constant observation: for any given year, the NMR for black newborns is substantially higher than that for whites. The long history of high black mortality rates has provided the basis for a widespread acceptance of unequal mortality and the accompanying view that it is in large part due to innate characteristics of black women and infants. A closer look at these data, however, suggests that black rates ultimately assume the level of white rates; it is just that it takes more than ten years to occur. The white rate was 17.2 in 1960, but it took until 1974 for the black rate to reach that level. The white rate reached 15 in 1967, while the black NMR did not fall below 15 until 1977.

Also intertwined with the issue of racial differentials is the larger question of class. In this society racial patterns of mortality are heavily influenced by social and economic forces. When one compares the neonatal mortality experience of wealthy whites with that of poor whites, poor whites reveal much higher rates of death. The same inverse relationship with income has been documented for black neonates. Therefore, poverty is associated with poor birth outcome for infants of both races. However, when neonatal mortality is analyzed for each race and income level, black

From SCIENCE FOR THE PEOPLE, March/April 1984, pp. 23–26. Copyright © 1984. Reprinted by permission of the author.

Paul Wise teaches pediatrics at Children's Hospital in Boston, and is in the Division of Health Policy Research and Education at Harvard University.

mortality has been shown to be higher than that of whites even within the same income groups. This suggests that in the U.S., black neonatal mortality is associated not only with income effects but also residual social influences more closely related to race than to income.

Birth Weight as a Crucial Factor

An important insight into the nature of these patterns in neonatal mortality can be gained by partitioning neonatal mortality into its component parts. It has been well documented that the risk of death in a newborn is closely related to its weight at birth. In general the lower the birth weight the higher the risk of death. This is due to the fact the birth weight is a relatively good proxy measure of the maturity and intrauterine growth of the child. Neonates can then be categorized into various birth weight groupings each associated with its respective mortality risk. Commonly newborns under 1500 gm (3.3 lbs.) are termed very low birth weight (VLBW), below 2500 gm (5.6 lbs.) low birth weight (LBW) and above 2500 gm normal or high birth weight. The group with the highest mortality is the VLBW group. The smallest risk is in those newborns with birth weights above 2500 gm. This general framework of risk stratification allows neonatal mortality in a population to be broken down into two parts: 1) the distribution of birth weights in that population and 2) the relative survival of newborns in that population that are born at a given birth weight. The first component is usually labeled the "birth-weight distribution", and the second the "birth-weight-specific mortality." Therefore, to analyze differences in mortality one must establish whether one group had a higher proportion of births born with weights associated with high risk (VLBW and LBW groups) and subsequently any differences in survival once they are born at a given birth weight.

This partitioning has helped explain why newborns in the United States experience higher mortality than in 16 other industrialized countries. Comparisons between the U.S., Norway[3] and Sweden[4] reveal that the cause of relatively high NMR's in the U.S. are due to unfavorable birth weight distribution. The U.S. experiences much higher rates of VLBW and LBW births. Birth-weight-specific mortality rates were in fact significantly better for these newborns in the U.S. Once an infant is born in the U.S., its chances of survival are somewhat better than that of newborns of the same birth weight born in Norway and Sweden. The problem in the U.S. is that due in large part to poor nutrition particularly prevalent among black and low income mothers, a far higher percentage of infants are born at low birth weights.

When racial and income differentials are analyzed in this manner a similar pattern emerges. For the most part, black birthweight-specific mortality rates for LBW babies are better than those of white neonates. Once born at a given birth weight, black newborns' survival is even better than white survival. Then why are black NMR's so much higher than those of whites? The answer is that blacks have much higher rates of low birth weight births. In fact, blacks experience approximately twice the low birth weight rate of whites.

The Issue of Low Birth Weight

Unlike birth-weight-specific-mortality, declines in low birth-weight rates have not been similar for both races. Reports from diverse locations including North Carolina,[5] California,[6] and Boston,[7] have shown that white LBW rates fell more steeply than did those of blacks. National estimates have echoed these findings. This divergence has helped to widen the gap between white and black NMR's.

Attempts are often made to explain these observed racial and income differentials in NMR's based on differences in the demographic characteristics of the compared populations. Most notably has been the argument that the different rates are due to a higher portion of births to young women among blacks. It has been known for some time that newborns of women under 16 years are at significantly higher risk of death. It has also been well documented that the number of births for black and poor white teen-age women is almost double that for wealthy whites. This has led some to the conclusion that by preventing teen-age births much of this racial differential in NMR could be extinguished. This proves false, however, when one considers that less than 5% of black or low income white births occur to women under 16. If all births to women under 16 were prevented, less than 10% of the racial and income differential would be reduced. The mortality risk associated with births to women 17 to 20 years is not appreciably higher than that of women 20 to 35 years. Therefore, teenage pregnancy cannot be held responsible for the mortality differentials. Programs dealing with pregnant teenagers and young parents are important because these births are associated with high medical and social risk and require special resources to help improve their outcome. However, they should not be viewed as a means of significantly reducing inequalities in overall neonatal mortality. Rather the focus must be on preventing the relatively high rates of low and very low birthweight births. Until this is accomplished the racial and income gaps in neonatal mortality rates will not be reduced, and indeed may widen.

The major recent declines in NMR's in the U.S. may have even exacerbated racial differences. Both national[8] and state-specific analyses[9, 10] have suggested that both blacks and whites have experienced remarkable reductions in birthweight-specific-mortality rates over the past decade. Once born at a given birthweight, newborns today are much more likely to survive than they were ten years ago. However, the birthweight distribution component has not fared as well. The percentages of all births which are of low birthweight has fallen much more slowly than birth-weight-specific mortality rates. Continued efforts to improve the quality and access to intensive neonatal care when needed will remain an important aspect of neonatal care for all infants in the years to come. However, the concentration of mortality into the very low birthweight category of newborns makes it unlikely that differentials can be reduced through greater reliance on neonatal intensive care. What is needed is greater emphasis on preventive strategies.

Preventive Strategies

Nutrition supplementation programs have generally proved effective in increasing the birthweight of newborns. The most important of these has been the Women, Infant and Child (WIC) supplementation program. A federal program administered through state agencies, WIC provides coupons for nutritious foods for eligible pregnant and lactating women and children under five years of age. Eligibility is based on nutritional and income criteria. In conjunction with coupon distribution, nutritional and medical consultation is an ongoing requirement. While controversy over its impact persists, the WIC program has been shown to increase the birthweight of neonates born to enrolled women. The Reagan administration has made recent efforts to significantly reduce funding for WIC and lighten eligibility requirements despite the fact that less than half of all eligible women and children in the U.S. are presently served by WIC.[11]

Caring and conscientious monitoring of the woman, fetus, and family from the first trimester until delivery are directly associated with an improved rate of infant survival.[12] However, numerous studies has shown that poor black women are much less likely to receive prenatal care than are whites. In some cities as many as one half of all black women will receive no prenatal care or begin care just weeks before their scheduled due date.

Improvements in the quality of and access to comprehensive prenatal services, therefore, would seem to be more important than ever. The critical importance of LBW birth rates to overall racial differentials in NMR's has never been greater. However, all indications are that prenatal services for poor women in the U.S. are beginning to erode due to constriction of federal programs in this area. Cutbacks in the WIC program and funds supporting the delivery of general prenatal services have already occurred. Further efforts by the Reagan administration to curtail funding for these and related programs can only reduce the already inadequate resources dedicated to this area of preventive care.

While understanding the patterns of neonatal mortality is useful in assessing the need and nature of medical and social initiatives, it also helps focus attention on the presence and the scope of social disparity in the United States. That poor, black neonates experience almost four times the mortality of wealthy white neonates provides insight into the human toll of continued structural inequalities, and helps explain why the issue of infant mortality becomes so heavily contested in the political arena. It is in this sense that infant mortality represents a stark if not ultimate expression of social and economic injustice in our society, and at some level, reminds all of the brutal cost this disparity exacts from its youngest and most vulnerable citizens.

References

1. For instance see Food Research and Action Center, "Infant Deaths Go Up, While WIC Program Funds Stay Low," presented in Hearings, Committee on Agriculture, Nutrition and Forestry, U.S. Senate, March 14, 1983
2. Hearings, Committee on Agriculture, Nutrition and Forestry, U.S. Senate, March 14, 1983
3. Erickson, J.D., F.B Bjerkedal, Fetal and infant mortality in Norway and the United States. JAMA 1982; 247:987-991.
4. Guyer, B., L.A. Waklack, S.L. Rosen. "Birth-weight standardized neonatal mortality rate and the prevention of low birth weight: how does Massachusetts compare with Sweden?" N. Engl. J. Med. 1982, 306:1230-1233.
5. David, R.J., E. Siegel. "Decline in neonatal mortality, 1968 to 1977: better babies or better care?" Pediatrics 1983; 17-531-540.
6. Williams, R., P.M. Chen. "Identifying the sources of the recent decline in perinatal mortality rates in California." N. Engl. J. Med. 1982; 306:207-214.
7. Wise, P.H., M. Wilson, M. Wills, M. Kotelchuck. *Childhood mortality in the City of Boston*. Part I: Neonatal Mortality. (In Press).
8. Lee, K, et al. "Neonatal mortality: an analysis of the recent improvements in the United States." Am. J. Public Health 1980; 70:15-21.
9. David, R.J., E. Siegel, 17-531-540.
10. Galdenberg, R.I., J.I. Humphrey, C.B. Hale. "Neonatal death in Alabama, 1970-1980: an analysis of birth weight and race specific neonatal mortality rates." Am. J. Obstet. Gynecol. 1983; 145:545-552.
11. Hearings, Committee on Agriculture, Nutrition and Forestry, U.S. Senate, March 14, 1983.
12. Ibid.

Ω

The Class Gap

by Vicente Navarro

Much attention has recently been paid to the growing disparity in the mortality rates of blacks and whites. There is a moral imperative to mobilize social resources to reverse this trend. But there is another mortality gap, one that is not talked about: the social class gap. Because the United States, unlike most industrialized nations, does not regularly collect and publish mortality statistics by class, we do not know how many more years a corporate lawyer lives than an unskilled blue-collar or service worker.

On one of the few occasions that the government did gather such information, however, in 1986 (and measuring only deaths from heart and cerebrovascular diseases), the results were stunning. People of any race with less formal education, with lower incomes and belonging to the working class (those whom the Census classifies under the terms "operator" and "services") die at higher rates than people belonging to the upper classes (those designated "managers" and "professionals"). The death rate from heart disease, for example, was 2.3 times higher among unskilled blue-collar operators than among managers and professionals. By contrast, the mortality rate from heart disease in 1986 for blacks was 1.3 times higher than for whites.

Did these enormous gaps close or widen during the 1980s? We have no means of knowing. But we do know that class differentials in the rates at which people get sick have been growing. From 1983 to 1988 the percentage of individuals with an annual income over $60,000 who had limited activity due to a chronic condition declined, while for those with incomes less than $10,000, it increased. It is fair to assume that the class differentials in mortality have been increasing as well. And the rise in the black death rate offers further grounding for this assumption, since blacks, because of racism, are disproportionately concentrated in the low-income groups.

In the 1980s the U.S. population underwent severe class polarization, with a reduction of the middle class, a slow growth of the upper and upper-middle classes, and a rapid growth of the low-paid, unskilled working class. The low earners are a heterogeneous group—blacks, Latinos, whites, men and women—whose standard of living is fast deteriorating. They belong to the 40 percent of the population that received only 15.7 percent of the total income in 1984, the lowest amount since such figures were first kept, in 1947. On the other hand, the wealthiest 20 percent received 42.9 percent of the total income, the highest ever. This growing disparity of wealth and income is the main, if not exclusive, reason for the growing differentials in morbidity and mortality between whites and blacks. The deteriorating working and living conditions of the low-wage working class are reflected in the statistics on death and disease. Within each class, minorities are even worse off. This is why the life expectancy of blacks has been declining, and that of whites is improving at an unprecedentedly slow rate. It is also the reason that the publication of health statistics in racial terms is insufficient.

We as a nation need to do much more to eliminate racism, but we also need to eliminate the fatal consequences of classism. The growing mortality differentials between whites and blacks are part of larger mortality differentials—class differentials. The publication of health statistics in racial terms assumes that white unskilled workers have more in common with white lawyers, for example, than with black unskilled workers. They do not. White workers have far more in common, in the way they live, get sick and die, with black workers than with white lawyers. And the same may be said of black workers and black lawyers. Yet the way in which statistics are kept does not help to make white and black workers aware of the commonality of their predicament. The collection and publication of mortality statistics by race *and* class would help to unite rather than separate black and white laborers.

Class differentials in mortality rates are not unique to the United States. In other industrialized nations not only do they exist but they are on the rise, and great national and international debates on the reasons for this have begun. Meanwhile, in the United States the silence persists.

Vicente Navarro is a professor of health policy and sociology at Johns Hopkins University.

Ω

♀

Strained Class Windows

by Judith K. Witherow

You People. Every time I hear those ignoble words used, I know it isn't going to be good. They will always make me mentally and physically cringe.

When you hear those words from birth on, as part of your name, you know which rung of the ladder you're standing on.

"You People should have indoor plumbing. How can you stand that outhouse?" "You People need to have electricity and running water." "Your house looks so small. How many of You People sleep in one bed?" (I shared a bed with two sisters, and, in the winter, our body heat was probably the only thing that kept us from freezing to death.) "Why don't You People paint your house?"

Gee, poverty makes you so damned dumb that none of these things ever occur to you. Someone pointing them out is like a giant wake-up slap on the forehead.

We could have painted any bare wood shack we ever lived in seven different colors, and it wouldn't have changed a thing. Oh, people would have said, "You People are so gaudy," but that is how much tangible difference it would have made. There would have been less money for food and other survival necessities, but what the hell, it might have made us easier to look at. That's what it is all about, isn't it? Looks?

Not the kind of looks where someone is rolling their eyes while they are "trying" to talk to you. This habit is the twin of "You People," and you just want to haul out a piece of tape and hold their eyes still so they can clearly see what you are saying.

I'm 49 years old, and I still don't have this class thing figured out. For that matter, I don't know for sure whether classism or racism is worse. Most times I can't even figure out why I'm being treated the way I am.

I honestly thought I could be objective writing this article, but the deeper I dig into old buried familial grief graves, the more angry and sad I become. If this weren't so God awful important, I'd throw the dirt back on, but how are we ever going to change anything unless all sides are totally truthful?

As a poor, mixed blood Native American, raised in the northern Appalachians, I invite you into my life and reveal to you the sights, tastes, smells, and life-limiting experiences that you might not have been privy to.

I keep wanting to say I know all the big words I'm using. It's very important to me that you know I'm not being

From *Sojourner: The Women's Forum,* January 1994, Vol. 19, No. 5, pages 1, 34, 35. Copyright © 1994 by Sojourner: The Women's Forum. Reprinted by permission.

Judith Witherow is a Native American, Lesbian author and artist.

pretentious, that these are no one else's words but mine. If that is classism in reverse, I will readily say I am sorry. My partner, Sue, helps me proofread but that is the extent of the input. Sometimes people assume someone of my background could not be literate. I can't tell you how many times someone has asked me if I actually wrote a particular article.

I hear the same thing from many family members, but for a different reason. The first time I showed my mother a poem I had written, she asked if I really knew all those words, or did I find them in a dictionary? Often I get quizzed about an article I've written. Someone will say, "Did that really happen?" It's like, "Judith, you'll be in deep, deep trouble if you put a lie in print." Right. The nonfiction police will bust my butt.

The printed word has always been cause for heated discussion in my family. They don't believe anyone would print something that isn't true. This includes *The National Enquirer.* I've learned that the older generation can survive easier without the ugly truths at this late date, so I concentrate on working with the younger ones. The truth doesn't always set you free. It bruises and bleeds like no other injury ever could, but pain can open the gates to gain.

I graduated from high school and made my family very proud. Looking back, I can see I was purposely kept at lower class levels even though I had good grades. No one ever mentioned scholarships or college to me. (As a result, I earned a living as a textile factory worker, waitress, and housekeeper.) I believe you get weeded out of the further education track at an early age. It's not the grades that count. It's your family's potential that is measured by the class yardstick. (You People would just take up a space that could be used by someone really serious.) Some very fine minds get lost this way. Yes, you could go to college at a later date, but by then life has had so many whacks at you that it rarely leaves you with the time or confidence to try it. Survival often means feeding the belly before the brain. The deprivation of either causes lifelong pain. There is only so much humiliation you can cram into a child before you effectively crowd her out of the system.

My father quit school in third grade to help raise his brothers and sisters. He was self-educated and gave me an abiding love of the written word. My mother made it to the eighth grade. Her one clothing outfit for school was the top of a dress for a blouse and the bottom of a man's overcoat for a skirt. She never stopped grieving for her lost chance. She often spoke of her proudest moment as winning a poetry recital before she had to quit school.

When my father was in his seventies and dying of cancer, he asked me to cover for him because he had told the nurse a lie. I thought she must have asked him about smoking or drinking. He said, "She asked me how far I had went in school. I thought fifth grade sounded much better so I told her that. You back me up, kid." I asked him why he didn't just say he had graduated? He looked like someone had pulled a gun on him. "Jesus, girl, you can't say anything like that." I tried to explain to him it was a bullshit question, but he was having none of it.

You see, after many years of subjugation, you become your own overseer. To this day, I see my nieces and nephews trash each other before the rest of society gets a chance. I understand the dynamic perfectly. If you make fun of or hurt each other, then the second time around it doesn't hurt as much. You have already been prepared. When you depersonalize pain and suffering, you can ignore it. Only when a human face is superimposed on poverty will this barbaric practice end.

The first house I remember us living in contained three small rooms. (The next tenants used it as a chicken coop.) My father had to walk stooped over because the ceilings were about five feet high. He was six foot tall. There was no water or electricity, of course. The creek out back served as a washing machine, a refrigerator, and a bathtub.

We never lived in a place that had screen doors or screens in the windows. This allowed everything, including snakes, to come and go at will.

We learned at an early age to pound on the floor before getting out of bed. This was so you didn't accidentally step on a rat and get bitten. Why the hell do rats always overrun the poor? I can tell you it is not for the food. Maybe it's just easier access.

When it snowed in the mountains, it would drift in through all the cracks that weren't full of paper or rags. We had very few blankets, so coats, rugs, or clothes helped to keep us warm. The roof had so many holes that we didn't have enough pots or cans to catch all the rain that trickled through. Too bad we didn't have one of those glass ceilings I hear so much about. I'll bet those suckers could keep you dry, warm, and in your place.

This basically describes all the houses we grew up in. Each move was a little better than the last. When I was five, we moved to a house that had electricity. At age 14, we moved to a house that had both water and electricity. We never acquired a place with screens or one that wasn't overrun with rats. Yes, we set traps. Yes, we put out poison. Many times my brother and I would sit in the basement with a .22 rifle and pick them off when they popped their heads out.

People many times equate poverty with laziness. We always worked. Dad worked at a sawmill and as a lumberjack. Later on, he became a carpenter. He never missed work, and he never received any benefits.

My dad, a good-looking, proud man, came from a long line of alcoholics, as did my mother, but only he succumbed to it. It still follows the male lineage on both sides of the family. Twice while growing up, I heard people use my dad's name as a synonym for drunk. If the alcohol colored and clouded the ugliness and made it bearable, I can understand and forgive that. Yes, I'm sure the cheap wine he drank took material and mental tolls on all of us, but it was an illness he fought all of his life.

One time Dad committed himself to an alcohol rehabilitation institution. Mom had to apply for welfare and sign a non-support order that she was told would never be served. It was protocol. (It was the only time she applied for benefits.) On the day of Dad's release after two months of treatment, the police came and took him away in handcuffs because of the nonsupport warrant. On the way home from jail, he stopped and bought a bottle of wine. It caused a breach in my parents' relationship that never healed. None of us had ever been in any trouble with the law. The law was something you feared with all of your being. It still is for us older ones.

Mom worked as a housekeeper for several families. I was ashamed of her for doing that. When high school girls whose homes Mom cleaned would tell me in a loud voice at school what a wonderful job Mom did, I wanted to die. On the other hand, to Mom's dying day, she would brag about what a good job she had done and how pleased her employers were.

She also did waitress and factory work and thought it was a great honor that she had never been fired from any job. Me, I just wanted to shake her when she would start these raps and say, "Of course, they didn't fire you. You were every shit-working boss's dream. You never complained, and you left a piece of your heart and health everywhere you worked." Of course, I never said it out loud to her.

She looked at me in total amazement whenever I tried to say that perhaps things weren't as cut and dried as they appeared. She was the dearest, kindest woman I have ever known. I will never stop missing her truly honest compassion. May she rest in peace. I doubt I ever will.

Work. That's all we ever knew from childhood up. You name it, and we sold it or did it. We picked and sold strawberries, blackberries, elderberries, and blueberries. We sold Rosebud salve by the gross. Remember those tacky cardboard mottos that said "HOME SWEET HOME?" Sold them. Countless packs of seeds also sold door to door. Lawnmowing, gardening, babysitting, etc.

One of the hardest jobs was picking princess pine. It's used to make funeral and Christmas wreaths, etc. You find it growing wild in the wintertime. It looks like wispy little pine trees. You get paid six cents a pound for it. Believe me, it takes more back-breaking work than you can ever imagine to fill a burlap sack with it. Digging through the snow in search of it without the benefit of gloves or boots is something you wouldn't wish on anyone. We would miss school to help with this. Whoever was the youngest at the time would be placed in a hurriedly fashioned lean-to for shelter from the elements. Another young one would stay nearby and keep the fire going while the rest of us picked.

Our favorite spot, one where you weren't walking forever to find the pine, was on a state game reserve. One time, after picking all day, we dragged our sacks up to the dirt road where Dad was to meet us. Instead of Dad, we were met by a game warden. He made us dump out all of our piney. He said he had been watching us work all day long, and he wanted to teach us a lesson. Granddad and the rest of us were scared, but Mom told us it would be all right.

Later that night we went back and picked it all up by the light of the moon. Mom said that it was too much work picking something growing wild—that should be yours for free—only to have it wasted by someone who didn't know the first thing about nature.

Because of background and lifestyle, our family is riddled with disease and disability. The water we drank wherever we lived came out of mountains that had been strip-mined for coal. This same water would flow down the river and kill all of the fish and other living organisms.

The little town of 400 where we were raised is now full of cancer, multiple sclerosis, and many other diseases. I had cancer and had a section of my right foot removed. I have multiple sclerosis as do other members of my family. It is uncommon to have so many cases in such a small region. It's not contagious, so what is the common denominator?

We moved from the mountains in 1964, but apparently not in time. All of us have arthritis. Most have several of the following: high blood pressure, diabetes, emphysema, vitiligo, learning disabilities, heart and lung disease, sarcoidosis, eczema, kidney or liver disease or alcoholism.

I wish there had been free lunch programs back then. I know our health problems due to malnutrition could have been avoided. When I hear anyone go into a diatribe about all You People wanting handouts, I go a bit crazy. My main memory of my childhood is always being hungry. Oh sure, we gardened, hunted, and fished, but it was never enough to feed eight or more people at one time.

Does society still not get it? An unhealthy child will be an even more unhealthy adult. A sick, uneducated adult will not be able to work and contribute like a healthy educated one can. This dynamic will cost from the cradle to the coffin if it is not interrupted. Unlimited resources that are now being spent to make war all over the globe could be redirected to save the same amount of people.

My hope is that after all of the articles on class are printed in this issue, they will not just be read and then forgotten. If more people aren't willing to work to help us change our destiny, the loss will soon be insurmountable. I would like to see the problems caused by classism worked on continually until all women share equally the benefits of society.

Ω

♀

Angry Women Are Building:
Issues and Struggles Facing American Indian Women Today
by Paula Gunn Allen

The central issue that confronts American Indian women throughout the hemisphere is survival, *literal survival,* both on a cultural and biological level. According to the 1980 census, the population of American Indians is just over one million. This figure, which is disputed by some American Indians, is probably a fair estimate, and it carries certain implications.

Some researchers put our pre-contact population at more than 45 million, while others put it at around 20 million. The U.S. government long put it at 450,000—a comforting if imaginary figure, though at one point it was put at around 270,000. If our current population is around one million; if, as some researchers estimate, around 25 percent of Indian women and 10 percent of Indian men in the United States have been sterilized without informed consent; if our average life expectancy is, as the best-

informed research presently says, 55 years; if our infant mortality rate continues at well above national standards; if our average unemployment for all segments of our population—male, female, young, adult, and middle-aged is between 60 and 90 percent; if the U.S. government continues its policy of termination, relocation, removal, and assimilation along with the destruction of wilderness, reservation land, and its resources, and severe curtailment of hunting, fishing, timber harvesting and water-use rights—then existing tribes are facing the threat of extinction which for several hundred tribal groups has already become fact in the past five hundred years.

In this nation of more than 200 million, the Indian people constitute less than one-half of one percent of the population. In a nation that offers refuge, sympathy, and billions of dollars in aid from federal and private sources in the form of food to the hungry, medicine to the sick, and comfort to the dying, the indigenous subject population goes hungry, homeless, impoverished, cut out of the American deal, new, old, and in between. Americans are daily made aware of the worldwide slaughter of native peoples such as the Cambodians, the Palestinians, the Armenians, the Jews—who constitute only a few groups faced with genocide in this century. We are horrified by South African apartheid and the removal of millions of indigenous African black natives to what is there called "homelands"—but this is simply a replay of nineteenth-century U.S. government removal of American Indians to reservations. Nor do many even notice the parallel or fight South African apartheid by demanding an end to its counterpart within the borders of the United States. The American Indian people are in a situation comparable to the imminent genocide in many parts of the world today. The plight of our people north and south of us is no better; to the south it is considerably worse. Consciously or unconsciously, deliberately, as a matter of national policy, or accidentally as a matter of "fate," *every single government,* right, left, or centrist in the western hemisphere is consciously or subconsciously dedicated to the extinction of those tribal people who live within its borders.

Within this geopolitical charnel house, American Indian women struggle on every front for the survival of our children, our people, our self-respect, our value systems, and our way of life. The past five hundred years testify to our skill at waging this struggle: for all the varied weapons of extinction pointed at our heads, we endure.

We survive war and conquest; we survive colonization, acculturation, assimilation; we survive beating, rape, starvation, mutilation, sterilization, abandonment, neglect, death of our children, our loved ones, destruction of our land, our homes, our past, and our future. We survive, and we do more than just survive. We bond, we care, we fight, we teach, we nurse, we bear, we feed, we earn, we laugh, we love, we hang in there, no matter what.

Of course, some, many of us, just give up. Many are alcoholics, many are addicts. Many abandon the children, the old ones. Many commit suicide. Many become violent, go insane. Many go "white" and are never seen or heard from again. But enough hold on to their traditions and their ways so that even after almost five hundred brutal years, we endure. And we even write songs and poems, make paintings and drawings that say "We walk in beauty. Let us continue."

Currently our struggles are on two fronts: physical survival and cultural survival. For women this means fighting alcoholism and drug abuse (our own and that of our husbands, lovers, parents, children);[1] poverty; affluence—a destroyer of people who are not traditionally socialized to deal with large sums of money; rape, incest, battering by Indian men; assaults on fertility and other health matters by the Indian Health Service and the Public Health Service; high infant mortality due to substandard medical care, nutrition, and health information; poor educational opportunities or education that takes us away from our traditions, language, and communities; suicide, homicide, or similar expressions of self-hatred; lack of economic opportunities; substandard housing; sometimes violent and always virulent racist attitudes and behaviors directed against us by an entertainment and educational system that wants only one thing from Indians: our silence, our invisibility, and our collective death.

A headline in the *Navajo Times* in the fall of 1979 reported that rape was the number one crime on the Navajo reservation. In a professional mental health journal of the Indian Health Services, Phyllis Old Dog Cross reported that incest and rape are common among Indian women seeking services and that their incidence is increasing. "It is believed that at least 80 percent of the Native Women seen at the regional psychiatric service center (5 state area) have experienced some sort of sexual assault."[2] Among the forms of abuse being suffered by Native American women, Old Dog Cross cites a recent phenomenon, something called "training." This form of gang rape is "a punitive act of a group of males who band together and get even or take revenge on a selected woman."[3]

These and other cases of violence against women are powerful evidence that the status of women within the tribes has suffered grievous decline since contact, and the decline has increased in intensity in recent years. The amount of violence against women, alcoholism, and violence, abuse, and neglect by women against their children and their aged relatives have all increased. These social ills were virtually unheard of among most tribes fifty years ago, popular American opinion to the contrary. As Old Dog Cross remarks:

Rapid, unstable and irrational change was required of the Indian people if they were to survive. Incredible loss of all that had meaning was the norm. Inhuman treatment, murder, death, and punishment was a typical experience for all the tribal groups and some didn't survive.

The dominant society devoted its efforts to the attempt to change the Indian into a white-Indian. No inhuman pressure to effect this change was overlooked. These pressures included starvation, incarceration and enforced education. Religious and healing customs were banished.

In spite of the years of oppression, the Indian and the Indian spirit survived. Not, however, without adverse effect. One of the major effects was the loss of cultured values and the concomitant loss of personal identity. . . . the Indian was taught to be ashamed of being Indian and to emulate the non-Indian. In short, "white was right." For the Indian male, the only route to be successful, to be good, to be right, and to have an identity was to be as much like the white man as he could.[4]

Often it is said that the increase of violence against women is a result of various sociological factors such as oppression, racism, poverty, hopelessness, emasculation of men, and loss of male self-esteem as their own place within traditional society has been systematically destroyed by increasing urbanization, industrialization, and institutionalization, but seldom do we notice that for the past forty to fifty years, American popular media have depicted American Indian men as bloodthirsty savages devoted to treating women cruelly. While traditional Indian men seldom did any such thing—and in fact among most tribes abuse of women was simply unthinkable, as was abuse of children or the aged—the lie about "usual" male Indian behavior seems to have taken root and now bears its brutal and bitter fruit.

Image casting and image control constitute the central process that American Indian women must come to terms with, for on that control rests our sense of self, our claim to a past and to a future that we define and that we build. Images of Indians in media and educational materials profoundly influence how we act, how we relate to the world and to each other, and how we value ourselves. They also determine to a large extent how our men act toward us, toward our children, and toward each other. The popular American media image of Indian people as savages with no conscience, no compassion, and no sense of the value of human life and human dignity was hardly true of the tribes—however true it was of the invaders. But as Adolf Hitler noted a little over fifty years ago, if you tell a lie big enough and often enough, it will be believed. Evidently, while Americans and people all over the world have been led into a deep and unquestioned belief that American Indians are cruel savages, a number of American Indian men have been equally deluded into internalizing that image and acting on it. Media images, literary images, and artistic images, particularly those embedded in popular culture, must be changed before Indian women will see much relief from the violence that destroys so many lives.

To survive culturally, American Indian women must often fight the United States government, the tribal governments, women and men of their tribe or their urban community who are virulently misogynist or who are threatened by attempts to change the images foisted on us over the centuries by whites. The colonizers' revisions of our lives, values, and histories have devastated us at the most critical level of all—that of our own minds, our own sense of who we are.

Many women express strong opposition to those who would alter our life supports, steal our tribal lands, colonize our cultures and cultural expressions, and revise our very identities. We must strive to maintain tribal status; we must make certain that the tribes continue to be legally recognized entities, sovereign nations within the larger United States, and we must wage this struggle in many ways—political, educational, literary, artistic, individual, and communal. We are doing all we can: as mothers and grandmothers; as family members and tribal members; as professionals, workers, artists, shamans, leaders, chiefs, speakers, writers, and organizers, we daily demonstrate that we have no intention of disappearing, of being silent, or of quietly acquiescing in our extinction.

Notes

1. It is likely, say some researchers, that fetal alcohol syndrome, which is serious among many Indian groups, will be so serious among the White Mountain Apache and the Pine Ridge Sioux that if present trends continue, by the year 2000 some people estimate that almost one half of all children born on those reservations will in some way be affected by FAS. (Michael Dorris, Native American Studies, Dartmouth College, private conversation. Dorris has done extensive research into the syndrome as it affects native populations in the United states as well as in New Zealand.)
2. Phyllis Old Dog cross, "Sexual Abuse, a New Threat to the Native American woman: An Overview," *Listening Post: A Periodical of the Mental Health Programs of Indian Health Services.* vol. 6, no. 2 (April 1982), p. 18.
3. Old Dog cross, p. 18.
4. Old Dog cross, p. 20.

Ω

The Health of Native People in the U.S.
by Amy Markus

When I was a child growing up in the suburbs, t.v. westerns were popular. As a consequence I watched countless white settler families attacked by the inevitable, paint-streaked Apaches (always a favorite tribe of Hollywood). Usually the cavalry came to the rescue, but if they weren't around the family was somehow always able to fight off two or three hundred whooping Apache braves. For years this was the basis of my information about native

By Amy Markus from *WomenWise*, Vol. 8, No. 1, 1985. Copyright © 1985 by the Concord Feminist Health Centers. Reprinted by permission.

people in this country. I learned more as a teenager when, in 1973, the American Indian Movement (AIM) and the occupation of Wounded Knee, S.D. filled the evening news night after night. That's when I began to read books like *Bury My Heart at Wounded Knee*. And that's when I began to realize the horrors that Native Americans endured at the hands of the white man. The Indians, historically, were treated brutally and this treatment has culminated in generations of poverty-stricken life on the reservation. While some non-Native Americans feel great sorrow for the repression of the rich cultures of Native American peoples, and others even have a sentimental yearning for a return to a time of the "Noble Savage," there seems to be no realistic or urgent commitment by non-Native people to the survival of Indian peoples or their culture. Further, there seems to be little understanding of the "new" Indian war that threatens the survival of native people in this country.

I was only vaguely aware of this threat when I went to work with the Northwest Indian Women's Circle in the state of Washington last summer. There I learned that the health of native people—spiritually, psychologically, and physically—faces the menace of this "new" Indian war sponsored by the U.S. government and large corporations. Some of the grim statistics include the mortality rate from all causes associated with alcoholism which is 22 times the national average; suicide is twice the average of the general American public; death from chronic diseases such as diabetes mellitus is 15 times the national average; and the rates of cancer and birth-defects are high among native populations, especially in the western United States. But there are committed groups and individuals fighting for a healthier, more traditional, way of life, among them many native women. Some fight the siting of the MX missile in Nevada, others study the effects of toxic chemicals on breastfed infants, still others provide traditional birthing care for native women, believing in the connection between the health of the earth and the perpetuation of human life. This concern for their people and the strength and power needed to struggle for their survival is not a new phenomenon for Indian women. They have always had more status and authority than was perceived by the white culture. There is a Cheyenne proverb which says, "A nation is not conquered until the hearts of its women are on the ground. Then it is done, no matter how brave its warriors or how strong its weapons." The heart of Indian women today are heavy but they are not on the ground. The struggle continues.

One of the most profoundly damaging phenomenon for Native Americans has been the psychological results of hundreds of years of domination and oppression by a foreign culture. I have learned that the Indian way values harmony and balance between the material and spiritual sides of life. One respects the earth and takes only what one needs in order to leave the earth as bountiful for the seven generations to come as it was for you. There is an understanding that human beings are only a very small part of a larger universe and as such, have no right to dominate others who share the earth. The Europeans came along, to whom domination, over the earth, over other people, was (is) the means to material ends, the accumulation of which was the ultimate achievement. Through spreading of disease and physical violence the white man was able to force what was left of Indian nations onto the least desirable lands in this country. The old ways of life were interrupted and with it language, religion and traditions were forcibly replaced by those of the dominant society. For years, we have forced negative cultural images onto the Indian people. This has been particularly true for Indian women, who have struggled against images that were drawn and defined by a white culture unfamiliar with the cultures in which Native American women lived.

In truth, Indian women play(ed) important roles in their tribes, many of which were matriarchal. As one Sioux woman, an anthropologist, wrote, "Of course, we did walk ten paces behind—that's documented—and the reason we did it was to tell you where to go." Women were the keepers of the culture, they provided continuity and stability to the community and were highly valued for their role in healing, growing food, and giving life. These were qualities held in high esteem by their society. It is part of the tragedy of American society that we do not place a truly high value on such roles in life. If we did, then no sickness would go untreated, no child would go hungry, and the women would, as among the Iroquois, "decide when the people will go to war, because when the war is done, it is the women who weep."

Physically, Native Americans were extremely healthy before contact with Europeans. There was no experience with diseases such as smallpox, scarlet fever, measles, cholera or yellow fever. Without immunity to these contagious diseases entire villages were often wiped out; sometimes this was a calculated act on the part of white people who would give disease-laden blankets to the Indians. Other conditions such as obesity, tuberculosis, heart disease, and diabetes, now prevalent among Indian populations, were also unknown. Their diet of wild game, fish, plants and berries was high in protein and rich in vitamins without high levels of fat. As the Indian way of life was destroyed, so too was the physical health of the people. Farley Mowat eloquently relates the disruption of the lives of the Idthen Eldeli of northern Canada in *People of the Deer*, published 35 years ago. In it, he tells what is an archetypal story for native people. The Idthen Eldeli needed to eat the red meat and fat of the deer in order to survive in the harsh, arctic climate. White traders came and encouraged the people to stay South in the summers, not to follow the great herds of deer. The traders sold the Idthen Eldeli white flour, sugar, guns and shells on credit. In order to pay off debts the people were encouraged to kill the deer for trade, not solely for survival. Farley Mowat writes,

"It has been nearly 100 years now since the Idthen Eldeli began to starve. Starvation first came to them when they began to exist on a winter diet which now consists of 80% white flour, with a very little lard and baking powder, and in summer almost nothing but straight fish. The Idthen people now get little of the red meat and white fat of the deer, once their sole food. Three generations have been born and lived—or died—upon a diet of flour bannocks and fish eaten three times a day and washed down with tea. Each of these generations has been weaker and had less 'immunity' to disease than the last."

Today, foods high in fats and sugar are the norm among Indian populations. Over half of all nutrition for Indian populations comes from governmental sources which consist of foods low in nutritional value—white bread and dyed American cheese to name two. Native people are dependent on the U.S. government for many of the material things which sustain them precisely because that is how the government designed things. It is imperialism at home, at its most debilitating, with the intention of making all Indian children dependent on the state for nurturing. Such "nurturing" may well destroy the Indians as a people.

The ability to continue the cycle of life is a cherished and sacred element of Native American life. To a Native American population of only 1.4 million people (according to the 1980 census) the ability to bear strong, healthy children is of the utmost importance. But this process of healthy reproduction is being threatened in many ways. In the 1970s, Dr. Connie Uri, a Native American doctor, made an official inquiry into the sterilization of native people in the United States. In 1975 she found that 25,000 native women had been sterilized within Indian Health Service facilities (a federal program). It is thought that as many as 42 percent of native women and 10 percent of native men have been sterilized, many of whom were coerced or given inadequate information about the permanent effects of the operation. For instance, on the Rosebud Reservation in South Dakota a 16 year old delivered her first child, emerged from the anesthesia and was told she was "fixed" so she couldn't have children until she was 18. At 21 she was married and unable to conceive. As Dr. Uri wrote, "Zero population growth may be all right for the white man . . . But for the Indian, it's genocidal."

What is perhaps even more dangerous and threatening to native people is the fact that the U.S. government and various corporations want to further exploit the land, once thought to be worthless, and thus appropriated to Indians. Here are some reasons: in the United States, 80 percent of the uranium reserves, 33 percent of strippable coal, and unknown amounts of oil, copper, timber and other raw materials are on Indian land. In many areas of the west, especially in South Dakota and the southwest, intense energy development has been going on for years. The consequences of such development are reflected in the health, or rather ill-health, of the people—mostly Native Americans—living in these areas. The National Cancer Institute cites significantly high cancer mortality of Indians in the west. People of the Dine nation in the southwest, particularly near Shiprock and Oaksprings where uranium mining has been going on for decades, experience an abnormally high rate of birth defects. On the Pine Ridge Reservation in South Dakota, where the poorest people in America live, a health study was undertaken in 1980 by W.A.R.N. (Women of All Red Nations). Serious health problems were documented, among them:

- in one month in 1979, 38 percent of pregnant women on Pine Ridge had spontaneous abortions
- since 1962, an elder in 10 out of 12 families died of cancer

- 60 percent to 80 percent of newborns on the Pine Ridge Reservation suffer breathing complications because of undeveloped lungs and/or jaundice
- breast and uterine cancer, leukemia and sterility among Lakota women are of epidemic proportion.

Not content to merely recite these appalling statistics, W.A.R.N. went on to investigate why these conditions run rampant on Pine Ridge. What they found is that the source of water for Pine Ridge residents, the Lakota Aquifer, is contaminated at the source with herbicides, insecticides and radioactive particles. Tests done on the aquifer by a Rapid City, SD biochemist showed that the water on Pine Ridge contained lethal does of radioactive particles—19 picocuries per liter. Above 5 picocuries is considered dangerous by the U.S. Public Health Service. Pine Ridge is located 80 miles south of a mining town and energy development is big business in this area of South Dakota. But what W.A.R.N. discovered isn't an isolated case. The Indian Health Service and the EPA have discovered radioactive contaminants in 19 out of 150 wells tested on reservations in Arizona, New Mexico, and California.

It is this kind of unbridled greed at the expense of the environment and people, that is threatening the survival of Native Americans as a people. In the Four Corners region of the southwest, an area rich in uranium, the U.S. government is trying to relocate thousands of Hopi and Dine people who have lived there for centuries. The government is willing to disrupt 10,000 individual lives and an ancient culture for 30 years of uranium for nuclear power plants, the waste of which can kill us all. What is happening to native people in this country—the cancer and birth defects from pollutants produced by man, and the high rate of diabetes and heart disease from diets high in sugar and fats—is only a distillation, a more concentrated form, of what is happening to all of us. If Americans do not begin to see the wisdom of the traditional Indian ways of respect and care for the earth and all of its creatures, then 30 years of energy scraped from the soil will be of no value. We must work for a fundamental restructuring of what we, as humans, value most; choices for the future must take into account the fact that if we take, we must give, and that there *are* limits to be faced if human beings are to survive on this planet. Americans still have much to learn from the native peoples of this land, if only we will ask and listen. Then perhaps there will come a day when the words of a holy woman from the Wintu tribe do not ring so true:

The white people never cared for the land or deer or bear. When we Indians kill meat, we eat it all up. When we dig roots, we make little holes . . . When we burn grass for grasshoppers we don't ruin things. We shake down acorns and pine nuts. We don't chop down trees. But the white people plow up the ground, pull down the trees, kill everything . . . how can the spirit of the earth like the white man? . . . Everywhere the white man has touched it, it is sore.

Bibliography

Akwesasne Notes. May 1980, Late Summer 1982, Late Fall 1982, Winter 1983, Spring 1984.

Calif. Urban Indian Health Council, Inc. *California Indian Maternal and Child Health.* Oakland, CA, 1981.

Hammerschlag, Carl, M.D. *Excerpts from a Workshop on Mental Health.* March 12, 1983.

Katz, Jane B., e.d. *I Am the Fire of Time—The Voices of Native American Women.* New York: EP Dutton, 1977.

LaDuke, Winona. *Infant Formula in Native America.* Cambridge, MA: Harvard Univ., 1982.

MATRIX. Dec. 1980, Jan. 1981.

Matthiessen, Peter. *In the Spirit of Crazy Horse.* New York: Viking Press, 1980.

Mowat, Farley. *People of the Deer.* Boston: Little, Brown & Co., 1951.

Prout Bulletin. October 1978.

Thorpe, Dagmar. *A Context for Grantmaking to Native Women: A Discussion Paper Developed for the National Network of Grantmakers.* Forestville, CA, 1984.

Ω

Blazes of Truth

by Susan Schnur

When I was 12 years old, my parents sent me off to Camp Ramah in the Poconos. That June, I was a dull kid in an undershirt from Trenton, New Jersey, outfitted in lime-green, mix-and-match irregulars from E.J. Korvette's. By the end of August, though—exposed as I was, for two months, to suburban Philadelphia's finest pre-adolescent fashion cognoscenti—I had contracted that dread disease: "*JAP*itis."*

Symptoms included not only the perfection of an elaborate, all-day, triple-sink procedure for dyeing white wool bobby socks to the requisite shade of dirty white (we called it oyster), but also my sudden, ignominious realization that the discount "Beatlemania" record my mother had bought for me the previous spring was not, after all, sung by the real group.

I'm not even sure that the term *JAP* existed yet back then (I don't think it did), but, in any case, by October I was—more or less—cured. I put the general themes of entitlement, of materialism, of canonized motifs (in those days, Lord and Taylor was the label of choice rather than Bloomingdale's) at the back of my mental medicine chest for the next two decades.

It wasn't until six months ago, actually—while teaching a course at Colgate University called "Contemporary Issues of Jewish Existence"—that I again gave the subject of *JAPs* a moment's pause.

This article was originally published in LILITH, the independent Jewish women's quarterly; subscriptions are $16.00 per year, from LILITH, 250 West 57th Street, New York, NY 10107. It is being reprinted here by permission.

Susan Schnur is a rabbi and a writer and has been a Visiting Professor in the Philosophy of Religion Department at Colgate University.

*The term JAP refers to Jewish American Princess.

A unit of *JAPs* was decidedly *not* on my course syllabus (I taught the standards: Holocaust—Faith—Immigration—Assimilation—Varieties of Religious Experience—Humor—Israel—Women). But my students, as it turned out, were obsessed with *JAPs*.

Week after week, in personal journals that they were keeping for me, they talked *JAPs*: the stereotypes, dating them, hating them, not *being* them, *JAP* graffiti, *JAP* competitiveness, *JAPs* who gave them the willies back home in Scarsdale over spring break.

I had been raised on moron jokes; *they* had been raised on *JAP* jokes. ("What does a *JAP* do with her asshole in the morning? Dresses him up and sends him to work.")

Little by little, I came to realize that the *JAP* theme was by no means a one-note samba. It was kaleidoscopic and self- revealing; the students plugged it into a whole range of Jewish issues. I began to encourage them to look at their throwaway *JAP* comments with a measure of scrutiny.

The first, and most striking, ostinato in the students' journals was the dissociative one. As one Jewish student framed it, "There are so many *JAPs* in this class, it makes me sick." (An astonishing number of students were desperate to let me know this.)

Since over one-third of the class was not Jewish (the enrollment was 30), and since there was no one in the class that I would have identified sartorially as a *JAP*, this was an interesting fillip.

"That's funny," I started commenting back in these students' journals. "The other students think *you're* a *JAP*."

Eventually, one Jewish student wrote, "Maybe when I talk about *JAPs* and that whole negative thing, it's a way for me to get 'permission' to assimilate."

Another wondered why he feels "like every *JAP* on campus somehow implicates me. That's a very 'minority culture' reflex, isn't it? Why am I so hung up on how everyone else perceives Jews?"

Some students perceived the *JAP* phenomenon, interestingly, as a developmental phase in American Judaism—a phase in which one parades both one's success and one's entitlement. "When my best girlfriend from childhood was bat mitzvahed," wrote one student after reading *A Bintel Brief* and *World of Our Fathers*, "her grandmother gave her a '*JAP*-in- training' diamond-chip necklace. It's like the grandmother was saying, 'When I was your age, I had to sew plackets in a Lower East Side sweatshop. So you girls be *JAPs*. Take whatever you can and be proud of it."

A Black student mentioned—during a talk about the socialization of Jewish women—that Jewish women, like their Black counterparts, are encouraged to be extremely competent, but then are double-bound with the message that their competence must *only* be used for frivolous purposes. (Like Goldie Hawn, in *Private Benjamin*, scolding her upholsterer with impressive assertiveness: "I specifically said—the ottoman in mushroom!", or informing her superior officer that she refused to go to Guam because "my hair will frizz.") "Minority women are warned not to be a real threat to anyone," the student explained, "That's how *JAPs* evolve."

Another theme of the students touched on their perception that Jews are sometimes discriminated against not because they are *less* endowed than others, but because they are more endowed (smarter, richer, more "connected"). *JAPs*, then, become, in the words of an Irish Catholic student who was doing reading on theology and the theme of chosenness, "the 'chosen of the chosen'. Unlike Irish Catholics who have been discriminated against because we seem 'un-chosen'," she mused, "people hate *JAPs* because they seem to have everything: money, confidence, style."

Of course, it's probably unnecessary for me to point out that the most prolific *JAP* references had to do with the venerable old feud—the Jewish War-Between-The-Sexes.

One pre-law Jewish male in the class (who was under a lot of pressure and had developed colitis during that semester) stated point-blank that he did not date Jewish women. I was shocked by the number of 20-year-old, seemingly fully-assimilated Jewish males who were right up there with Alexander Portnoy on this subject.

Several students responded to his comment in their journals. "He's angry at *JAPs*," one woman wrote, "because they get to be needy and dependent, whereas the expectations on him are really high."

Another student related the experience of two friends of hers at SUNY Binghamton: "Someone spray-painted the word *JAP* on their dormitory door," she recounted.

"But now I wonder—which one of the girls was being called a *JAP*? The one with the dozen Benetton sweaters, or the one who'd gotten 750 on her L-SATs?" The question being, of course, which is ultimately more threatening . . . the demanding woman or the self-sufficient one?

An Hispanic woman in the class talked about what she called "the dialectic of prejudice"—that is, the contradictory nature of racist or sexist slurs as being, in itself, a diagnostic of irrational bias. "A *JAP* is portrayed as both frigid and nymphomaniacal," she wrote. "She's put down both because of her haughty strut that says, 'I'm independent', and because of her *kvetching* that says, 'I'm dependent'."

A twist on this theme was provided by a Jewish woman who commented, "Whatever Jewish men call us—cold, hot, leech, bitch—it's all the same thing: They're afraid they can't live up to our standards."

A psych major in the class took a different tack. "It's not that the Jewish male really believes Jewish women are terrible, rather that he simply wants majority culture males to believe it. It's like when territorial animals urinate on a tree," she explained. "It's a minority male's possessive instinct. Like a sign that says, 'Robert Redfords—stay away!'"

Finally, several Jewish students framed their relations with one another in the context of Jewish family systems. "Lashing out at Jewish women—calling them all *JAPs* or refusing to marry them—is a way to get back at the entire high-expectation, high-pressure Jewish family," stated one student in response to a film I showed in class called "Parenting and Ethnicity." "You can lash out by becoming an academic failure," he went on, "or you can become a doctor—which is less self-destructive—and then simply refuse to marry a Jewish woman."

Towards the end of the term, a feminist friend pointed out to me something I had not considered: that the characterizations of *JAPs* and Yuppies are often identical—the difference being, of course, that a Yuppie designation is still generally taken as neutral or even positive, whereas there is hardly one of us left—I don't think—who would compete for the label of *JAP*.

All in all, I trust that the larger lessons in all of these *JAP* ruminations have not been lost on my students. For example: Why has it become socially sanctioned to use a *Jewish* designation (*JAP*) for a description that fits as many Christians as Jews? Or why—along the same lines—is it okay to use a *female* designation (again, *JAP*) for a description that fits as many men as women? Or sensing what we now sense, shouldn't we refuse any truck altogether with the term *JAP*?

Ω

JAP: The New Antisemitic Code Word

by Francine Klagsbrun

Isn't it odd that the term *JAP*, referring to a spoiled, self-indulgent woman, should be so widely used at a time when women are working outside their homes in unprecedented numbers, struggling to balance their home lives and their work lives to give as much of themselves as they can to everybody—their husbands, their kids, their bosses?

Jewish women, like women throughout society, are trying to find their own paths, their own voices. And, along with other changes that have taken place, they have been finding themselves Jewishly. And yet we hear the term *JAP* being used, perhaps almost more now than ever before. Why?

The new found, or rather newly accepted, drive of women for achievement in many arenas threatens many men. What better put-down of the strong woman than to label her a "Princess"? She is not being attacked as a competitor—that would be too close to home. No—she's called a princess, and that label diminishes her, negating her ambition and her success.

One may note, and rightly so, that there are materialistic Jewish women—and men too. But are Jews the only people guilty of excesses in spending? Why should the word "Jewish" be used pejoratively to describe behavior we don't approve of?

I think the answer is that there is an underlying antisemitic message in that label. Loudness is somehow "Jewish." Vulgarity is somehow "Jewish." All the old stereotypes of Jews come into play in the use of the term *JAP*. In this day, polite Christian society would not *openly* make anti-Jewish slurs. But *JAP* is O.K. *JAP* is a kind of code word. It's a way of symbolically winking, poking with an elbow, and saying, "well you know how Jews are—so materialistic and pushy."

What is interesting is that this code word can be used in connection with *women*—the Jewish American *Princess*— and nobody protests its intrinsic antisemitism.

This article was originally published in LILITH, the independent Jewish women's quarterly; subscriptions are $16.00 per year, from LILITH, 250 West 57th Street, New York, NY, 10107. It is being reprinted here by permission.

Francine Klagsbrun is the author of *Married People: Staying Together in the Age of Divorce* (New York: Bantum, 1985) and of *Voices of Wisdom: Jewish Ideals and Ethics for Everyday* (New York: Pantheon Books, 1980). These excerpts are from a speech delivered by Klagsbrun recently at Temple Israel of Great Neck NY

Consciousness-Raising Questions on Anti-Semitism

by Irena Klepfisz

The following are some questions that both Jews and non-Jews might consider asking in trying to identify in themselves sources of shame, conflict, doubt and anti-Semitism. The questions are designed to reveal the degree to which they have internalized the anti-Semitism around them. By examining their own anti-Semitism, Jews will conclude that anti-Semitism, like any other ideology of oppression, must never be tolerated, must never be hushed up, must never be ignored, and that, instead, it must always be exposed and resisted.

1. Do I have to check with other Jews in order to verify whether something is anti-Semitic? Do I distrust my own judgment on this issue?

2. When I am certain, am I afraid to speak out?

3. Am I afraid that by focusing on anti-Semitism I am being divisive?

4. Do I feel that by asking other progressives to deal with anti-Semitism I am draining the movement of precious energy that would be better used elsewhere?

5. Do I feel that anti-Semitism has been discussed too much already and feel embarrassed to bring it up?

6. Do I feel that the commercial presses and the media are covering the issue of anti-Semitism adequately and that it is unnecessary to bring it up? Am I embarrassed by the way anti-Semitism/the Holocaust is presented in the media? Why?

7. Do I have strong disagreements with and/or am ashamed of Israeli policies and as a result, feel I can't defend Jews wholeheartedly against anti-Semitism? Is it possible for me to disagree with Israeli policy and still oppose anti-Semitism?

8. Do I feel guilty and/or ashamed of Jewish racism in this country and, as a result, feel I can't defend Jews wholeheartedly against anti-Semitism? Is it possible for me to acknowledge Jewish racism, struggle against it, and still feel Jewish pride? And still oppose anti-Semitism?

9. Do I feel that Jews have done well in this country and, therefore, should not complain?

10. Do I feel that historically, sociologically and/or psychologically, anti-Semitism is "justified" or "understandable," and that I am, therefore, willing to tolerate it?

11. Do I feel that anti-Semitism exists but it is "not so bad" or "not so important"? Why?

12. Do I believe that by focusing on the problem of anti-Semitism I will make it worse? Why?

13. Do I feel that Jews draw too much attention to themselves? How?

14. Do I associate the struggle against anti-Semitism with conservativism? Why?

15. What Jewish stereotypes am I afraid of being identified with? What do I repress in myself in order to prevent such identification?

Ω

Disability and the Medical System
by The Boston Women's Health Book Collective

Women with disabilities constantly struggle to find health care workers who are sensitive to their needs. For nondisabled women, experiences such as childbirth tend to raise awareness of abuses in the medical system. But women with disabilities, particularly those raised with a disability or with very severe medical difficulties, constantly encounter patronizing attitudes and ignorance by health care practitioners, damaging their sense of independence and well-being, and seriously reducing the quality of care.

The overlap of sexism with discrimination against people with disabilities restricts employment, education, and participation in the community for the approximately 30 million U.S. women with disabilities, who are among the most frequent consumers of medical services. While not all disabled people need medical treatment, such nonmedical services as Social Security benefits, wheelchair transportation, and personal care attendant benefits require "certification as disabled" by a doctor.

Yet physicians get little, if any, training about or exposure to people with disabilities. A woman with cerebral palsy reported going to the doctor for an ear infection; he

---

PREVENTING DOCTOR ABUSE

1. Remember: you are in charge of your care; regard the doctor and other health workers as consultants who are employed by you.

2. Don't accept inappropriate or hurtful interaction. If confronting your doctor is hard, role playing first with friends may help you assert yourself.

3. Take a friend with you to take notes and provide support. Make sure the doctor knows that the friend or interpreter, if you use one, is not your guardian and that all communication should be directed to you.

4. To find a good doctor, ask women you trust; avoid the phone book or other listings. Call first to ask if the doctor has experience with your disability; ask about wheelchair or other accessibility.

5. Ask your general practitioner to find out about a specialist's experience with disabled people before referring you for an appointment.

6. Get a new doctor if you feel frightened, threatened, abused, or not respected as a capable adult; if your friend isn't allowed in the examination room without an acceptable reason; if the doctor isn't understandable and willing to learn from you about disabled people.

7. If you like your physician, tell her or him why. Refer others to that doctor.— M.S.

Marsha Saxton, a disability rights and women's health activist, herself disabled with spina bifida, is director of the Project on Women and Disability, a program sponsored by the Boston Women's Health Book Collective.

told her he'd never met a person with CP and spent 20 minutes asking her probing questions unrelated to her ear. When another woman visited a dermatologist because of a blister from her brace, he became visibly alarmed to find a woman in a wheelchair in the examining room. On the other hand, some doctors only meet disabled people who are in medical crisis, and disability is viewed solely as a dysfunction; medical schools offer virtually no training in the social and political issues of disability, let alone the impact of sexism, racism, or homophobia on women with disabilities.

The recent passage of the Americans with Disabilities Act of 1990, which has sweeping provisions for accessibility of facilities and services, signals the growing political strength of disabled people. But the medical system lags behind in recognizing disabled women as adults, capable of independent, self-directed lives. For example, if a disabled woman questions a doctor's recommendation, the response is often brutal; a blind diabetic woman who questioned her doctor's prescription was told, "You are hardly in a position to decide. If you'd followed your doctor's advice, you probably wouldn't be blind."

Disabled women, often displayed with little or no clothing in front of groups of medical students, are beginning to communicate their feelings of violation and humiliation. Doctors justify this kind of objectification—bordering on abuse—as necessary to teach students; they are baffled that disabled women have begun to protest.

One of the most pervasive myths is that disabled women are not sexual beings capable of sexual relationships and motherhood. A woman with spina bifida asked her gynecologist for birth control and was asked, "What for? What would you do with it?" The medical system has lagged in addressing the reproductive health needs of women with various kinds of disabilities. By far, most of the medical research on the topic focuses on male reproduction and sexual function.

Medical benefits are another quagmire of inequity. Women with disabilities must fight harder than men to justify their need for benefits since women may not have "worked" in the Social Security system enough to qualify for Medicare. Often only the most sophisticated self-advo-

cates who have access to legal advice can obtain their rights in the system. Others become discouraged by the vast bureaucratic requirements and give up.

With the increasing competition and privatization in the health care industry, hospitals are under pressure to be profitable. Screening technologies such as genetic testing, and extensive investigation into family medical histories, are being used increasingly to identify patients who may be poor financial risks. This strategy, called "skimming," often used by insurance companies to disqualify policyholders, hits women the hardest.

Another area of concern is personal care attendant services, which would allow severely disabled people to live in the community outside of institutions; obtaining such services is the new priority of the Denver-based activist organization Americans with Disabilities for Attendant Programs Today (ADAPT), which led the successful fight for wheelchair-accessible transportation.

Women with disabilities have few resources to challenge abuses; many are just now gaining the confidence to speak out, and their organizations have only begun to identify the nature of the mistreatment. As a group, disabled women tend to be poor, unemployed, and unlikely to pursue malpractice litigation; pro bono legal services are needed to support the legal rights of this emerging constituency.

We must assist disabled women in becoming more assertive, understanding their legal rights, and exploring medical alternatives, so that all of us can function as informed consumers of medical services.

For more information contact: ADAPT, (303) 733–9324; Disability Rights Education and Defense Fund, (202) 986-0375; Project on Women and Disability, (617) 277-5617. Also, the following books are available: *Past Due: A Story of Disability, Pregnancy and Birth,* by Anne Finger (Seal Press, $10.95); *Women with Disabilities: Essays in Psychology, Culture and Politics,* edited by Michelle Fine and Adrienne Asch (Temple University Press, $35); and *With Wings: An Anthology of Literature by and About Women with Disabilities,* edited by Marsha Saxton and Florence Howe (The Feminist Press, $12.95)
—Marsha Saxton

Ω

♀

On Being an Outreach Group: Women with Disabilities

by Marsha Saxton

Americans with Disabilities Act

The Americans with Disabilities Act (ADA), signed into law on July 26, 1990, will significantly expand civil rights protection for people with physical and mental disabilities, in several key areas. They include:

•**Employment.** Private companies with more than 25 employees (and eventually those with more than 15 employees) cannot discriminate in hiring practices and must make their facilities accessible to disabled employees (unless the cost to do so is prohibitively expensive).

•**Public Access.** Public facilities, such as restaurants, stores and services, that are constructed after the bill was signed must be made accessible to persons with disabilities. Existing buildings, unless they are substantially rehabilitated, are not affected, except those for whom modifications are "readily achievable," i.e., not of excessive cost.

•**Transportation**. Newly purchased trains and buses with Amtrack, commuter rail systems, and local and intercity lines must be accessible to wheelchair users through lift devices or ramps. Station terminals must eventually be made accessible, though in some cases, with up to a 30-year time frame.

•**Communications.** Telephone companies are required to offer communication relay systems, to enable hearing- or speech-impaired people who have teletype devices to communicate with hearing people via phone lines.

•**State and Local Governments** must make their facilities and services accessible to people with disabilities.

Regulations for enforcement of the ADA will be developed by various federal agencies and phased in over the next few months or up to several years, depending on the scope of changes required.

For more information on the Americans with Disabilities Act, contact Disability Rights Education and Defense Fund, 1616 P Street, N.W., Suite 100, Washington, D.C. 20036, (202) 328-5185, or the President's Committee on Employment of People with Disabilities, Suite 636, 1111 20th Street, N.W., Washington, DC. 20036-3470, (202) 653-5044.

A woman called me at my office recently, seeking a consultant on disability. She works for a women's organization which had gotten a grant that required her group to include people with disabilities. She asked me, "How do you get *them* to come to our events?" I guess she didn't realize that I am one of "them." Once again, I wondered, "Why is reaching out to people with disabilities so difficult?" After several years of doing consulting and training in disability awareness, I'm just starting to fathom how hard it is for people to think about access for people with disabilities. I've thought about disability all my life because of frequent hospitalizations and surgery at Shriner's Hospital to treat the weakness in my legs from my birth condition, spina bifida. I've been familiar with other disabled people, in wheelchairs, with speech differences, vision and hearing impairments, and with needs for various medical treatments. Disability doesn't seem like such a big deal for me. But it's clearly a big deal for people who are not familiar with it.

There have been many positive changes in the past few years, including the recent passage of the Americans with Disabilities Act, as well as a shift in women's organizations toward remembering to include disabled people in their "list" of outreach groups. Even so, it's not easy being an "outreach group." While everyone else is focusing on the topic of the event, "outreach groups" must field all the comments and behaviors that arise out of people's discomfort. We deal with feeling like one of "them," feeling objectified for being asked to join just because we're one of the target groups. We are the ones responsible for putting you at ease about our differences—differences which you may find distressing.

As disabled women, we must push through feeling like a bother if we need assistance, especially if the environment has not been made accessible so that we can function relatively independently. We are often expected to be a representative of our group in ways that are unreasonable: "Well Sarah, what do handicapped people feel about this issue?"

One of the most common assumptions that disabled women face is that efforts to include us are altruistic: we are being included through the generosity of others or we should be included so we won't have to feel so bad about ourselves. Other assumptions are made about us. Nearly everyone has had the flu or an injury, where daily activity and responsibilities are temporarily suspended and we need the help of others. But nondisabled people assume that a person with a chronic illness or disability must suspend their activities permanently. They express amazement at a disabled person's ability to adapt to physical limitations and proceed with life.

People are not relaxed around us. Some people are overly helpful: grabbing a blind person's arm to "assist" them or pushing a person's wheelchair without asking or introducing themselves. Some people show their fear by actually leaning backwards, as if to avoid physical contact. Some people attempt to ignore the disability entirely, assuming or pretending that the person's disability is not a factor in their life. I've had people tell me, "I've known

From *Sojourner: The Women's Forum,* Nov. 1990.

Marsha Saxton is the director of the Project on Women and Disability, and a board member of the Boston Women's Health Book Collective. She coedited, with Florence Howe, *With Wings, An Anthology of Literature by and about Women with Disabilities* (The Feminist Press, 1987).

someone for five years who uses a wheelchair, but I've never asked her why she doesn't walk."

What has made it so hard to include us? When I've asked people this question, the most common response initially is, "We don't know what to do about ramps or sign-language interpreters, or how to get materials done in Braille." While there are some key pieces of information that can help organizations with the logistics of accessibility, the real issue seems to be discomfort with the issue of disability.

About one-sixth of the population, or 43 million people, has some sort of disability or illness that restricts daily life in some way and requires accommodation. Multiply that number by the family, friends, and coworkers of disabled people, and nearly everyone is currently directly or indirectly affected by disability. We rarely regard disability as the commonplace experience it actually is. Disability is a cultural taboo, like death or sex. When we were children, our natural and sometimes unabashed curiosity in encountering a disabled person was often met with our parents' embarrassed "Hush, don't ask and don't stare." Simple curiosity was replaced with embarrassment, fear, and mistrust.

Our culture's poor treatment of disabled people is evidence of our inability to think generally about all of our physical differences and physical needs. As a society, we tolerate poor quality air, water, and food, in exchange for convenience. We accept and wear uncomfortable fashions and even use harmful products to alter and disguise our bodies. Although we seem to value athletic prowess and reduced cholesterol, ironically, we place low value on the physical well-being of workers in the workplace. By choosing high-stress lifestyles, productivity and profit over our physical well-being, we are literally disabling ourselves.

Just as the fundamental behaviors and attitudes of racism and sexism are communicated to children from their earliest learning, disability oppression starts with child-rearing practices: we've all been babies and have had the experience of total dependence on others for feeding, dressing, bathing, mobility, communication, and so have, in a sense, experienced being "disabled" by cultural standards. The way our dependence and bodily needs were regarded by our caretakers, whether as a bothersome, disgusting burden or as a natural part of being human, affects our ability to think and function in a relaxed and thoughtful manner around someone else's physical needs.

We are entering a transition period where the taboo against acknowledging disability is lifting. The once common behaviors of shouting at a deaf person or of assuming that someone with another kind of disability can't hear, or even think, are declining. My friends who use wheelchairs report that waiters are somewhat less likely to ask the person accompanying them, "What would *she* like to eat?"

Because of this gradually increasing awareness, unasked questions are emerging. In disability awareness presentations I and friends of mine give to school children, we hear such honest and unabashed questions as, "What do blind people eat?" "How do you drive your wheelchair up onto the bed at night?" Adults never got a chance to ask all those questions, although they harbor the same kinds of confusions.

Go ahead and help us lift the taboo! Take the risk that you might make a mistake. In fact, if you are serious about moving through this oppression, you probably will. The worst that will happen is that you may feel embarrassed. The best will be that you will learn something about disability, and get to know us better. You might even learn something important about yourself.

Leaving out people with disabilities is a great loss to any movement for justice and equality. Despite the stereotypes, we have a full range of skills, and may have been forced, because of our disabilities, to sharpen our sense of setting priorities, organizing our time, asking for help and delegating, skills essential to any organization. Women with disabilities who have dealt with the oppression and have moved beyond the physical or emotional struggles of a disability are pretty tough characters and will be an asset to your organization.

When colleges in the '70s and '80s began reaching out to Black students, administrators couldn't comprehend the criticism that the traditional curricula, based on white culture, didn't address the educational needs of African-American students. By the same token, making an event logistically accessible to wheelchair users, for example, is just the beginning. In events such as lectures or concerts, accessibility is an adequate welcome to people with disabilities. But in events where the nature of the interaction requires thoughtfulness, attention, communication, and close physical proximity, there is need for sensitivity and openness to disability.

While the group "people with disabilities" do not share a common cultural background, the pervasive discrimination for disabled people means we do have common experiences. The way to make a program accessible and relevant to disabled people is to include us in the planning and leadership of your organization. In approaching disabled individuals or disability organizations that may be interested in your programs ask, "How can we include a broader group of people with disabilities? What would make our event welcoming and relevant?"

In the women's movement, we're slowly realizing that we can reach beyond our own groups to include other people with very different experiences, perspectives, and needs. Those of us from more mainstream groups are starting to realize that reaching out to people of various differences is for our own benefit, not just for the benefit of those typically left out.

But how easy it is to lose sight of the reasons for reaching out to underrepresented groups, and to proceed with the effort out of a sense of obligation. We sometimes forget that the goal of "diversity" is not improved percentages, or political correctness, but learning, pushing though fear, getting close to new friends and meeting and working with very different leaders in our many struggles for liberation. We benefit from the increased strength of a broad-based movement with diverse perspectives and sources of insight and power. Here are some guidelines in beginning to think about outreach:

(1) If this group is not your priority to learn about and include, don't pretend it is. Just adding disability organizations to your mailing list doesn't mean you or your organization can really reach out in a manner that works.

(2) If your organization is serious about reaching out to people with disabilities, get a group together for discussion about disability. Try reading, as a group, a good book on disability, such as one of the books listed below, and discuss what issues come up for members. Focus on such questions as: What have you been told about disabled people, by your family, your early schooling? What are common stereotypes? When was the first time you met, or saw, a disabled person? How did that encounter influence your feelings about disabled people? Do you know disabled people now? What do you imagine their lives to be like? Are you shy, awkward, or "not yourself" around disabled people? This kind of discussion and exploring of feelings helps defuse the discomfort and helps people be willing to risk making mistakes and move toward making friends with disabled people.

(3) A good place to start with any effort to reach out to people with diverse backgrounds and experiences is to begin to explore and appreciate the diversity in your own group. Spend some time talking about ancestry, class backgrounds, lifestyle choices.

(4) Encourage the members of your organization to talk about their own disabilities. When the taboo around disability is broken, often people will begin to reveal their previously unmentioned physical conditions: back problems, hearing losses, allergies, chronic illness and so forth. Discuss accommodations for the people already in your organization who have hidden disabilities.

(5) Be honest. Don't advertise "wheelchair accessible" if your site doesn't comply with architectural standards, including the bathrooms. If your building has a level or ramped entrance, but no accessible bathrooms, state that on your flyers.

(6) Publicize the accessibility you do have! Put "wheelchair accessible" or the universal access symbol if that's the case.

(7) Plan ahead. If your organization doesn't have money for sign-language interpreters in your budget (which can cost up to $50 an hour depending on how long events are and how many interpreters are required) then reaching out to deaf people is not feasible for you now. Plan on including interpreters in next year's budget.

(8) Set outreach goals that make logical sense for your organization's goals. You don't have to reach out to everybody all at once. (Unless your agency or business *is* covered by the Americans with Disabilities Act, in which case you must comply with the new law for public accommodation.) "Disabled people" is a diverse group of people. There may be subgroups of disabled people who find your services or activities relevant. For example, a literary group may decide to put materials on tape for blind people

and publicize events within the blind community. A labor activist group may seek people disabled on the job.

(9) Don't act on your guilt! Disabled people can sniff pity or guilt a mile away! If you are an activist organization, reach out to us because you want our input and involvement, not because you feel bad for having left us out. If you offer services, include us because you can competently serve this population.

(10) Be flexible. Even if your building is not wheelchair accessible, you can consider holding events or services at other locations.

(11) Be communicative and patient about accessibility with your membership. If you are reaching out to women with environmental illness (severe allergies) regularly mention to your members *why* wearing scented products make the environment inaccessible to some people. Keep remembering how hard it is for people to understand this issue, even after *you* catch on!

(12) Remember to focus on what you're doing well. Change is slow, and less than instant results doesn't mean you're doing it wrong. If you or your group focus only on failures, frustration and self-blame will actually slow you down. It takes a long time for any new group to trust that you're earnest.

As social institutions recognize the legitimate needs of people with disabilities for access and accommodation, and as individuals become more familiar with disability issues, we can move beyond emotional reactions to disability and beyond the logistical issues of accessibility, and begin to ask questions that can move us all forward. For example: How does the economic system perpetuate the oppression of disabled people? How do racism, sexism, or other types of prejudice operate together with disability oppression? How does disability oppression hurt all people, disabled or not? How can women's peace, labor, or environmental groups take on the fight against disability oppression, and how can disabled people and disability organizations effectively participate and take leadership in these other movements? These are the exciting questions.

People with disabilities are a significant part of the population of every other constituency. Just as sexism hinders the effectiveness of any other movement—for economic justice, racial equality, or peace—the oppression of people with disabilities limits these movements. All other liberation movements must come to include people with disabilities. Your personal commitment to people with disabilities is a critical step in ending oppression of all people. Even more important, you can take the lead in your organizations, workplaces, families, and communities in joining us to end this oppression.

Resources and Readings:

The Project on Women and Disability offers leadership training and resources for women interested in disability issues, and provides consultation and training on how to involve people with disabilities, and create programs and events which address the needs of women with disabilities. Call (617) 727-7440. Ask for our bibliography of readings on women and disability.

The Information Center for Individuals with Disabilities has extensive listings on disability organizations and resources in Massachusetts. They publish a monthly newsletter, *Together,* on local and national disability news. Call (617) 727-5540.

The Massachusetts Rehabilitation Commission Library is a good place to browse in the disability literature, at Fort Point Place, 27-43 Wormwood St., Boston.

With the Power of Each Breath: A Disabled Women's Anthology, edited by Susan Browne, Debra Connors, and Nanci Stern. Cleis Press, 19185.

Building Community: A Manual Exploring Issues of Women and Disability, by the Women and Disability Awareness Project. Educational Equity Concepts, Inc. 1985.

Past Due: A Story of Disability, Pregnancy and Birth, by Anne Finger. Seal Press, 1990.

With Wings: An Anthology of Literature by and about Women with Disabilities, edited by Marsha Saxton and Florence Howe. The Feminist Press, 1987.

Women with Disabilities: Essays in Psychology, Culture, and Politics, edited by Michelle Fine and Adrienne Asch. Temple University Press, 1988.

Disabled, Female, and Proud: Stories of Ten Women with Disabilities, by Harilyn Russo. Exceptional Parent Press, 1988.

Why Can't Sharon Kowalski Come Home? by Karen Thompson and Julie Andrzejewski. Spinsters/Aunt Lute, 1988.

Escape: A Handbook for Battered Women Who Have Disabilities. Finex House, 1988. Jamaica Plain, MA.

Dykes, Disability, and Stuff. Quarterly Journal, Catherine Lohr, Publisher, PO Box 6194, Boston, MA 02114.

Ω

Simply . . . Friend or Foe?

from New Internationalist

The able-bodied can be allies of disabled people—or they can be patronizing oppressors. Here are a few ways in which non-disabled readers can be friends instead of foes.

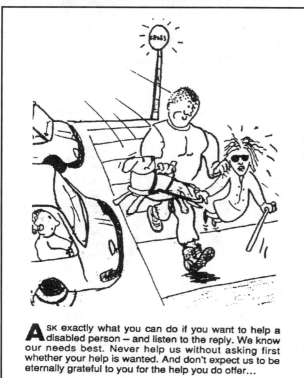

ASK exactly what you can do if you want to help a disabled person – and listen to the reply. We know our needs best. Never help us without asking first whether your help is wanted. And don't expect us to be eternally grateful to you for the help you do offer...

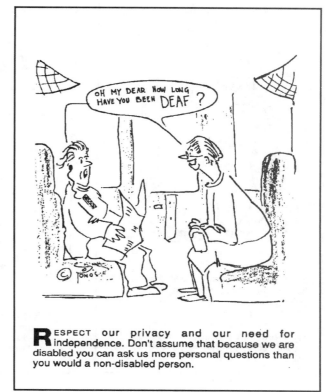

RESPECT our privacy and our need for independence. Don't assume that because we are disabled you can ask us more personal questions than you would a non-disabled person.

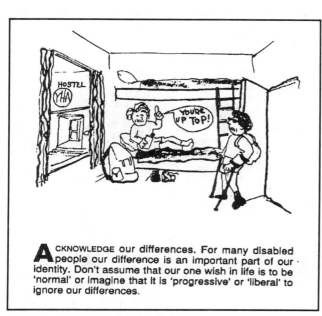

ACKNOWLEDGE our differences. For many disabled people our difference is an important part of our identity. Don't assume that our one wish in life is to be 'normal' or imagine that it is 'progressive' or 'liberal' to ignore our differences.

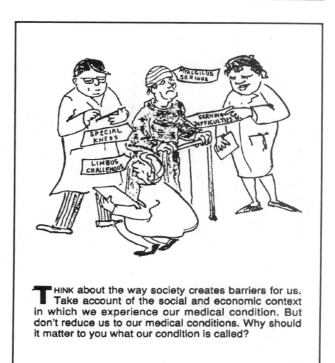

THINK about the way society creates barriers for us. Take account of the social and economic context in which we experience our medical condition. But don't reduce us to our medical conditions. Why should it matter to you what our condition is called?

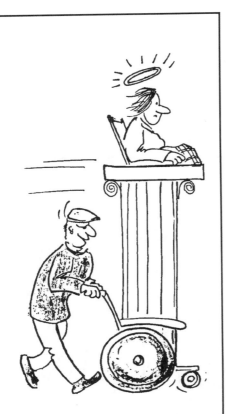

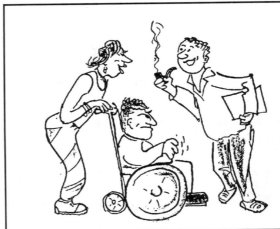

RECOGNIZE our existence. A gaze can express recognition and warmth. Talk to us directly. Neither stare at us — nor immediately look away either. And never talk about us as if we weren't there.

Challenge patronizing attitudes towards us. We want your empathy not your pity. Putting us on a pedestal or telling us how 'wonderful' and 'heroic' we are does not help. This attitude often conceals the judgment that having an impairment is intolerabale — which is very undermining for us.

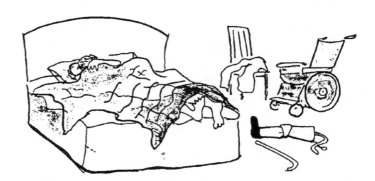

REALIZE that we are sexual beings, with the same wishes, needs and desire for fulfilling relationships as non-disabled people. Don't assume that we will never have children. And if a disabled person has a non-disabled lover don't jump to the conclusion that the latter is either a saint or has an ulterior motive.

APPRECIATE the contribution that we make to society in the fields of work, politics and culture. We engage in these activities for the same reasons as you do — but we may have some different insights to offer. Don't assume that we are passive — or that our activities are a form of 'therapy' to take our mind off our disability. Most disabled people are financially hard up and so we may have a greater need to earn a living than you.

This section is inspired by *Pride Against Prejudice* by Jenny Morris and produced in conjunction with Claire King and Beverly Ashton. The cartoons are by Tony Meredith.

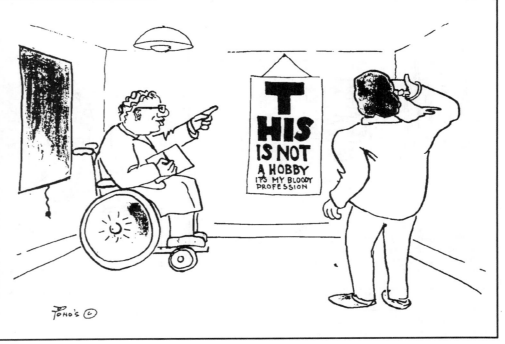

Gender and Race in the Classroom:
Teaching Way Out of Line

by Lana F. Rakow

Both students and teachers have experienced and participated in relationships of domination, submission, oppression, and privilege which have helped to shape who they are and how they interpret the world. This recognition of students and teachers as historically situated subjects with conflicting gender, race, and class interests is vital to understanding the possibilities and limits of the classroom (Weiler 1988,125).

Kathleen Weiler is among a growing number of scholars interested in feminist and critical pedagogy who call our attention to the fact that classrooms are not and can never be neutral sites for the production or reproduction of knowledge. Those of us who step into classrooms as professors and as students do not shed our identities at the door with our coats. We enter those rooms as humans situated as subjects and as objects of discourses that give us the identities we claim for ourselves and that are assigned by others. We cannot set aside the social relationships of the larger world—a world in which classifications of gender, race and class are among the most paramount—as we take up the more temporary relationship of professor and students.

In the traditional classroom, these identities are hidden or may be viewed as irrelevant. In fact, the traditional academic definition of a good teacher and of a successful classroom could be described as this: a generic professor, with sufficient knowledge of and enthusiasm for his subject matter, using appropriate pedagogical techniques, incites his generic students to the impassioned mastery of the material he brings to them. But scholars using feminist, ethnic studies and other critical perspectives have debunked the myth of the generic—in the English language and in the classroom (for a good example, see Bisseret Moreau 1984). This generic professor is, as the language indicates, presumed to be a white male, and the students who successfully master his content will probably be those most like him. Because the white male who enters the classroom simply adds the compatible identity of professor to his other identities, his own subject position may appear to be and may feel unproblematic. While gender, race and class identities may seem irrelevant as a consequence, they are actually the foundational structure upon which the traditional classroom—and the academy as a whole—is built.

When women and men of color and white women enter the classroom, "there's sure to be trouble" (Schuster and Van Dyne 1985, 162). The identity of professor is almost certainly incompatible with their gender and racial identities, since, as we have seen, the "generic" professor is white and male. They stand out as a member of a group or groups, their gender and race visible where the gender and race of the "norm" fades away. They disrupt old certainties and civilities (Schuster and Van Dyne's words, 163), because the normal discourse of the academic classroom becomes problematic. How will students position and "read" the professor and the text of the classroom and vice versa?

Even in a classroom with a traditional format and content, the professor who is the Inappropriate Other (see Ellsworth 1989, 321) must struggle for the authority and respect that is granted automatically to a white man (see Friedman 1985,206). Thus, this professor must engage in tiring "identity work" (McDermott and Church 1976) in a constant relational negotiation with colleagues and students. When the professor cannot or will not take up an expected identity, conflict ensues. Susan Friedman explains that even where authority and respect are accorded, they may be granted with great resentment and even hostility. Citing Norma Wikler, she points out that students may pressure women to take up the identity of an all-forgiving, nurturing mother who gives unconditional approval, perhaps one of the few identities women can successfully meld with that of professor. However, hostile challenges to their authority may come at grading time or other times when women are perceived as punitive, since this violates the expectations of the mother identity, though not of professor (Friedman 1985, 206; also, see Martin 1984).

When the professor who is the Inappropriate Other, however, self-consciously chooses to bring a different text to the classroom, a text that challenges the traditional curriculum because it centers the theories and experiences of people of color and white women, she or he has committed a further transgression and heightens the salience of personal gender and racial identities in the classroom. The material is "volatile" (Anderson and Grubman 1985, 221), and the classroom can become "explosive" (Culley 1985, 209). Because gender and race are such inseparable parts of the identities of *all* of us, students find it difficult to acknowledge their existence. Hence, the content, as well as the instructor, may be resisted for this and other reasons,

From *Teaching Forum*, Vol. 12, No. 1, December 1990. Copyright © 1990 by the Undergraduate Teaching Improvement Council, Madison WI. Reprinted by permission.

Lana Rakow is Associate Professor and chair of the Communications Dept. at UW-Parkside, where she specializes in gender and communication. This paper was presented at the annual conference of the International Communication Association in Dublin, Ireland, in June, 1990.

not the least of which is that, as Elizabeth Spelman puts it, "For the most part, educational institutions do not know how to reward students for learning about themselves or about others unless the others are (1) male, (2) white and (3) dead" (Spelman 1985, 243). In addition, white women and racial minority women and men may have little interest in or appreciation for their own histories and for understanding their own experiences, particularly since this material seems to have so little relevance for their own upward mobility.

Not surprisingly, however, it is white males who most object to being de-centered in the classroom. The introduction of discourses that place women and racial minorities as subjects and that permit women and racial minorities in the classroom to speak in their own discourses is both a new experience and a threatening one for many white males. A number of feminist teachers (see Mumford 1985 and Rothenberg 1985) have reported aggressive and disruptive attempts on the part of white male students to bring the classroom back to the dominant sexist, racist and homophobic discourse. While it is true that others in the classroom may also be more comfortable with a dominant discourse, it is generally white males who are accorded the powerful subject position in that discourse to act on it aggressively. If the teacher is a woman, the attempt may be made to relocate her as the sexist object of this discourse, thereby negating her authority as a professor in academic discourse. Several examples illustrate how this occurs.

In one example, Margo Culley describes an incident that happened to her on the first day of class for the Women's Studies section of a course, "Man and Woman in Literature." Upon hearing which section he was in, a male student walked past her in the front of the room, made noises as if to vomit, and stopped at the door to wave to the class and say, "See you later, girls," to the nervous laughter of the rest of the class (Culley 1985, 214). Despite any other terms on which Culley wished to present herself or the course, the dominant patriarchal discourse and this student's position of power within it could negate them.

Another example illustrates how individuals' expectations of gender can be established and played out at quite young ages. Valerie Walkerdine (1981) reports an interaction between four-year-old British nursery school boys and their teacher, who is a woman about 30 years old. The boys make explicit sexual commands to the teacher ("show your knickers"), delighting in their use of obscenities as well as in the power they command over her as a sexual object. As Walkerdine explains, in the classroom the boys exist simultaneously as objects of powerlessness in the institutional discourse where the teacher has power and as subjects of patriarchal discourse, where they can render the teacher the object of their sexist discourse, where she signifies not as "teacher" but as "woman."

A third example is closer to home. One semester, when I introduced a section on gender in a communication class, I began with a presentation summarizing scholarly research that questions the "generic" masculine in English,

thinking it would be a non-threatening introduction to the topic of gender identity. Before I had gone far, a white male student burst out with an angry, "You are way out of line shoving this dogma down our throats!"

The student had successfully placed me in a double-bind situation. If I responded punitively, as my professor subjectivity permitted, I was indeed "out of line" for a woman, and I would have confirmed his and probably other students' reading of me, exacerbating their antagonism. If I capitulated to his complaint and appeared apologetic or "weak," he would have successfully drawn me back as the object of sexist discourse, in which I would signify as "woman" but not as "professor." His use of male sexual imagery ("shoving this dogma down our throats") illustrates how he had collapsed the dominant academic and sexual discourse so that only a male could "rightfully" take up the subject position in either. My example illustrates that the resistance we face is as much to the material we bring to the classroom as it is to the discursive subject position we wish to take up, a position that can be taken up only if granted by the students with whom we interact. The combination of material about gender and race with the subordinate subject position of the instructor as woman and/or racial minority can mean both are dismissed by students because the instructor is seen to have a personal bone to pick with the world.

Despite such attempts to re-center themselves through the assertion of the dominant discourse, white male students are more likely to feel themselves silenced because they learn their discourse will not pass uncritiqued (as it did not in the above case). They may report on student course evaluation forms that the professor does not let students disagree or that she does not like men (or in the case of a professor of color, does not like whites or treats them unfairly), while other students may report they have felt encouraged to speak for the first time. One Hispanic woman reported in a workshop that she conducted on teaching material on women of color that a student had written on her course evaluation form, "The problem with this course is that there is no tolerance for racism and sexism." Students may feel there is too much emphasis on race and gender because it stands out in such marked contrast to the supposed neutrality of the rest of the material they encounter in their undergraduate careers (see Miner 1987). They may see lecture materials and readings as "biased" or "one-sided" because the politics of writers and researchers are generally made explicit. One of my students (white and male) reported to me in my office that he did not like a reading by a white feminist, because "it sounds like she wrote it on the 28th day of her month." Margo Culley offers the somewhat reassuring reminder that, "If she [the feminist instructor] initiates a process challenging the world view and the view of self of her students, she will surely—if she is doing her job—become the object of some students' unexamined anger" (Culley 1985, 213).

Of course, not all students resist the material and the instructor, and some students respond with enthusiasm, particularly those typically marginalized in the classroom. However, the presence of other, resistant discourses can present its own struggle. Despite the good intentions expressed by feminist, ethnic studies and critical scholars, the classroom cannot become an egalitarian place where all those who are silenced and marginalized by the dominant discourse can find equal opportunity speaking rights. Elizabeth Ellsworth (1989) examines the complexity in relation to one of her own teaching experiences at the UW-Madison. Even in a course of students representing a wide diversity of "differences" and all committed to challenging racism, conflicting discourses and the shifting subjectivities of students and professor made the classroom a site of struggle. The injustices of race, class and gender outside the classroom cannot be overcome in the classroom, she explains, no matter how committed the teacher and students (316). For example, ". . . a Chicana student had to define her voice in part through opposition to—and rejection of—definitions of 'Chicana' assumed and taken for granted by other student/professor voices in the classroom" (311). Ellsworth and her students found they had to struggle against oppressive ways of being known by others, even when those others were articulating their own experiences and self-definitions.

Ellsworth's experience teaches us the lesson that despite what might be our own sensitivity to the marginalized positions of others, we cannot hope to achieve equality *in* the classroom since it does not exist *outside* the classroom. Weiler's analysis of an incident in a public school classroom (Weiler 1985, 140-141) illustrates the problem. In a classroom discussion about Malcolm X's autobiography, a black male student attempted to interpret a passage in a discourse out of his lived experience of racism. The white feminist teacher, though she was sensitive to black experience and on other occasions encouraged such discourse, persisted in reading the passage from the interpretive framework of an academic discourse about socialization. The student dropped the course.

Weiler does not criticize this teacher for her actions, but rather points out that "the classroom is always a site of conflict" whether the teacher is a traditional one or a feminist or critical one. Students and instructors "read" texts and the classroom according to their gendered, raced and classed subjectivities (Weiler 1985, 137).

The discourse of the classroom is not completely controlled by teachers, but teachers can open the possibility that other discourses besides the dominant sexist and racist discourse can be heard. Elizabeth Spelman (1985, 241) suggests that to combat marginalization we use material that has some chance of speaking to the lives of all members of the class, if not everyone all of the time, then everyone some of the time. What happens in this kind of classroom cannot be predicted, nor can the pedagogical approach that is appropriate be learned through any kind of "cookbook" approach to teaching methods. Each classroom will be different, depending upon the constellation of subjectivities that come together and are invoked in the course of the semester (Ellsworth 1989, 323).

While those of us who enter such classrooms as teachers will no doubt continue to think of strategies and assignments and frameworks to try, hoping to derive better ways to deal with the conflicts and resistance and to come out the other side of the semester less bruised, our identities more intact, these are only individual and limited solutions. We need institutional support. The colleges and universities in which we teach generally express their approval of teachers who do not take risks in the classroom, who do not re-think the content and format of their courses, who do not address the potentially explosive social relations of their classrooms, who speak and encourage the dominant discourse that silences and explains away most people of the world, including many of those represented in their own classrooms.

The UW System, for one, is advocating the value of "diversity" in hiring, student enrollment and the curriculum. But an attention to diversity cannot be advocated without attention to the teaching situations that will be produced and the differential impact such teaching has on racial minorities and white women. We will ultimately have to convince not only administrators, but our colleagues, that we are up to something different in the classroom that cannot be assessed in the way that classroom teaching has traditionally been assessed. We will have to convince them that what goes on in our classrooms should be going on in their classrooms as well. They will have to learn to acknowledge and account for their own subjectivities and those of their students, a process that will unmask the "objective" curriculum and the neutral classroom.

References

Anderson, J., and S. Grubman. "Communicating Difference: Forms of Resistance." In *Women's Place in the Academy: Transforming the Liberal Arts Curriculum*, ed. M.R. Schuster and S.R. Van Dyne, 221-231. Totowa, NJ: Rowman & Allanheld, 1985.

Bisseret Moreau, N. "Education Ideology, and Class/Sex Identity," In *Language and Power*, ed. C. Kramarae, M. Schulz, and W.M. O'Barr, 43-61. Beverly Hills: Sage, 1984.

Bromley, H. "Identity Politics and Critical Pedagogy," *Educational Theory* 39, no.3 (1989):207-223.

Butler, J.E. "Toward a Pedagogy of Everywoman's Studies." In *Gendered Subjects: The Dynamics of Feminist Teaching*, ed. M. Culley and C. Portuges, 230-239. Boston: Routledge & Kegan Paul, 1985.

Culley, M. "Anger and Authority in the Introductory Women's Studies Classroom." In *Gendered Subjects: The Dynamics of Feminist Teaching*, ed. M. Culley and C. Portuges, 209-218. Boston: Routledge & Kegan Paul, 1985.

Ellsworth, E. "Why Doesn't This Feel Empowering? Working Through the Repressive Myths of Critical Pedagogy." *Harvard Educational Review* 59, no. 3 (August 1989):297-324.

Friedman, S.S., "Authority in the Feminist Classroom: A Contradiction in Terms?" In *Gendered Subjects: The Dynamics of Feminist Teaching*, ed. M. Culley and C. Portuges, 203-208. Boston: Routledgte & Kegan Paul, 1985.

Martin, E. "Power and Authority in the Classroom: Sexist Stereotypes in Teaching Evaluations." *Signs* 9, no. 3 (1984):482-492.

McDermott, R.P. and J. Church. "Making Sense and Feeling Good: An Ethnography of Communication and Identity Work." *Communication*, vol. 2 (1976):120-142.

Miner, M. "Another Women's Play? Doesn't That Make Like Number 6?" *Radical Teacher* (April 1987):1-4.

Mumford, L.S. "'Why Do We Have to Read All This Old Stuff?' Conflict in the Feminist Theory Classroom." *Journal of Thought* 20, no. 3 (Fall 1985):88-96.

Rothenberg, P. "Integrating the Study of Race, Gender and Class: Some Preliminary Observations." Paper presented to the National Women's Studies Association Conference, Atlanta, June 1987.

—. "Teaching About Racism and Sexism: A Case History." *Journal of Thought* 20, no. 23 (Fall 1985):122-136.

Schuster, M.R. and S.R. Van Dyne. "The Changing Classroom." In *Women's Place in the Academy: Transforming the Liberal Arts Curriculum*, ed. M.R. Schuster and S.R. Van Dyne, 161-171. Totowa, NJ: Rowman & Allanheld, 1985.

Spelman, E.V. "Combating the Marginalization of Black Women in the Classroom," In *Gendered Subjects: The Dynamics of Feminist Teaching*, ed. M. Culley and C. Portuges, 240-244. Boston: Routledge & Kegan Paul, 1985.

Walkerdine, V. "Sex, Power and Pedagogy," *Screen Education* (1981):38-51.

Weiler, K. *Women Teaching for Change: Gender, Class & Power*. South Hadley, MA: Bergin & Garvey, 1988.

Ω

♀

Ideas for Anti-Racism and Pro-Diversity Work and Discussion in a Women's Health Class

by Nancy Worcester[1]

A core part of developing an analysis of women's health issues is examining why "some women have a better chance of being healthy than other women" and learning how racism, anti-semitism, poverty, homophobia, ageism, attitudes towards disabilities, and fatphobia affect women's mental and physical health, affect access to basic resources (housing, rewards for employment, nutrition, environment and education) which can be primary determinants of health, and influence or determine one's access or relationship with the health care system.

While my goal in teaching women's health is to try to teach every topic from an openly anti-oppression/pro-diversity viewpoint and to include readings and perspectives of many different women, I have found there are limitations to this approach. First, as a white woman struggling to unlearn my own racism (and other oppressive attitudes), I cannot always provide the leadership I strive for! Equally important, in a course where both the subject matter and the effort to build a pro-diversity classroom environment may be new to students[2], too often students (and teachers) find it challenging to deal with the already controversial topics and feel it is "too complicated" ("there isn't enough time" or "we don't have the tools/information to adequately deal with other issues") to look at the impact of racism and other oppressions on each topic. Even successfully managing to do exactly that can feel equally unsatisfactory if at the end of a class, there is the feeling that we have done a superficial "laundry list," mentioning a wide range of groups but never adequately reaching an understanding of the impact and perpetuation of institutional and attitudinal oppressions.

For these reasons, I try to plan at least one session, approximately a quarter of the way into the course (after we have started on the materials so it should be apparent why anti-oppression work is central to the course and we still have the rest of the semester to build on work done in this session) which concentrates on pro-diversity/unlearning racism exercises and discussions. The teaching team constantly experiments with different approaches, always evaluating (and debating) the most effective strategies. I believe that learning about racism must be the core of this work. However, at this stage, I have found it most effective (with groups where the majority of students are white and mostly new, but open, to unlearning racism) to do this as a part of workshops on diversity awareness rather than starting with specific unlearning racism workshops. The advantage of this approach is that people new to working against racism may be able to build on their experiences of working against other oppressions or their experiences of being a part of an oppressed group to see the similarities with racism. The disadvantages of this approach are that the facilitator and the group have to be careful that the racism component does not get "diluted", that attention is paid to ways that racism is unique and destructive in ways different from other oppressions, and that institutional as well as attitudinal oppression is addressed.

I. SETTING THE SCENE FOR UNLEARNING RACISM PRO-DIVERSITY WORK

A. It is useful to establish ground rules, such as the following:

- It will be hard work.
- We need to listen and think.
- We need to share and be honest when we do.
- We may not always feel comfortable
- We may make mistakes. But it is a bigger mistake not to work on this.
- Guilt will only keep us stuck.
- Information shared in this session should not go out of this room.

Many people feel these two ground rules also help an introduction to racism:

- Our emphasis will not be on violent racism. We will concentrate on more subtle forms which are a part of everyday life for all people of color.
- We will not talk about reverse discrimination. In a society where one group has power over another, "reverse discrimination" is, in fact, a complex and inaccurate concept.

B. Working definitions of racism need to be clarified. Ricky Sherover-Marcuse's "Unlearning Racism" is a key article for this work (p. 48). She uses these basic definitions:

INSTITUTIONALIZED RACISM = Systematic mistreatment of people of color.

ATTITUDINAL RACISM = set of assumptions, feelings, beliefs and attitudes about people of color and their culture which are a mixture of misinformation and ignorance.[3]

C. It can also be useful at this stage to introduce the issues of internalized oppression and affirmative action. The paper by Thompson and Disch has excellent ideas for how to talk about affirmative action. These are issues which students often want to discuss, but they can side track the class from the more central topics unless they are planned to be a part of the other topics.

II. IDEAS/EXERCISES FOR PRO-DIVERSITY AWARENESS.

Introduce Audre Lorde's concept of "mythical norm" (see p. 43) and Ricky Sherover-Marcuse's use of terms "target and non-target" (see IV. Target Group Exercise below.) Introduce the inter-relationships of power and control, attitudinal and institutional oppressions, and the perpetuation of "social order".

Mythical Norm[1] (non-targets)[2]	Oppressions	Targets[2]
White people	Racism	People of Color
Men	Sexism	Women
Young (not too young)	Ageism	Old/Very Young
Heterosexual	Heterosexism/ Homophobia	Gays/Lesbians/ Bisexuals
Able-Bodied (mentally & physically)	Abelism	People with Disabilities
Christian	Anti-Semitism (Religious Narrowness)	Jews (Other Religious Groups)
Thin	Fatphobia	Fat People
Middle Class (access to resources)	Classism	Poor People

[1]The term "Mythical Norm" comes from Audre Lorde's writings, particularly in *Sister Outsider*.
[2]Ricky Sherover-Marcuse used the terms "non-target" and "target" groups in her Unlearning Racism Workshops.

Exercises:

In setting up exercises, the challenge is to make sure that no one feels invisible, conspicuous, or is put in the position where they try to speak for everyone in a group.

A. Similarities and Differences

(This works well as a large group activity)

Have participants identify similarities between all forms of oppression and what is unique about different forms of oppression. (i.e. We want to work towards "celebrating" most differences but what is the one form of difference we want to eliminate? [class, poverty]. What is the one "difference" we all hope to grow into? [Age] What is the role of invisibility with some oppressions? Are we better or worse at understanding the "differences" which could affect us [ageism, classism, disability, body size, sexual identity] than those we know will never be personal issues [a change of sex or race]? In what ways is the impact of racism different than other forms of oppression?)

B. Target vs. Non-Target

(This works well as small group follow-up to the target exercise described below).

Have each person identify a *non-target* group they are in, list benefits and privileges they have simply because they are a part of this group, and at what age/in what situation they first remember recognizing this phenomena.

Have each person identify a *target* group they are in. How does the experience of being in a target group help them see ways that they can use their *non*-target group situation(s) to actively work against oppression?

Have each person identify a *target* group they are in and think of a time when *internalized oppression* has made them, as a member of the target group act in an oppressive way (jokes, comments, not hiring) towards someone of the same target group. Describe how effective internalized oppression is and why it is very confusing to people outside the target group who do not understand internalized oppression.

C. Sexism and Racism

For people who have actively worked against sexism, it is sometimes useful to look specifically at similarities between sexism and racism (In what ways is being a white woman in this society similar to being a Black man? As men have power, men must be involved in working against sexism, and as whites have power, white people must be involved in working against racism) before looking at ways in which racism and sexism are different.

Questions for Discussion

Have people work in groups of 2 or 3 to discuss questions. If there is time, larger groups can discuss what came up in small groups.

    a. (For women) Describe the first time you remember being at a disadvantage because you were female. How did you feel about that? Did you do anything to resist? Now, looking back on that stage, what do you wish you had done or what would you want a daughter or sister to do in that same situation today? (For men) Describe the first time you remember being at an advantage because you were male. How did you feel about that?

    b. Think of some things you do now in your daily life to work towards equality for women.

    c. Concerned men often want to know what they can do about sexism. What do you say to a man who asks "What can I do about sexism?"

    d. Identify ways in which men working against sexism is similar to white women working against racism. List specific ways white people can do anti-racism work

D. Power and Control

The power & control wheel (p. 347) was put together by battered women to describe the many ways their abusers controlled them in their relationships. Using that wheel, identify similar ways institutional structures and different forms of oppression work to perpetuate inequalities.

E. Vision of a Diverse Society

Throughout the next week, every time you are in a group situation, observe the diversity or lack of diversity of the group. Identify who is making the decisions, who benefits from the present power dynamics, what are the visible and invisible barriers which keep others from participating in the group. Create a vision for yourself of a diverse group/community in which you *benefit* from working/playing with people different than you. Identify ways in which you can work toward making this diversity vision a reality for your life.

III. IDEAS FOR BEGINNING DISCUSSIONS ON RACISM

An introduction to racism needs to look at how all white people in a racist society are taught to be racist. (This helps to remove guilt and moves us on to more positive attitudes. It may help change the useless theme of "But I'm not racist" into "How can I work to not be racist?")

Some Questions to Work on in Small Groups

Do you remember when you were first aware of there being people of color or that you were a person of color? What did you learn from this experience?

(For white people) How did you learn to be racist? How did your family or your home environment treat people of color? Did you learn that people of color (or a specific group) were "bad"? Do you remember early racist jokes/actions you witnessed? Did you learn to pretend that you didn't notice differences and to act like "we're all just alike"? Did you learn to be artificially nice to/to feel sorry for people of color? In what ways do white people benefit from being white? Why is racism a white person's issue?

(For people of color) Identify ways in which you observed racism affecting family members, friends, or people you didn't even know. Identify several different ways (overt, subtle, being ignored, or being treated as if someone didn't notice your race) racism has had an impact on your life as a child, as a teenager, and presently. Identify ways you have worked against racism. If you could say several things to white people about racism, what would you say?

IV. RICKY SHEROVER-MARCUSE'S TARGET GROUP EXERCISE

This exercise is adapted from an exercise used by Ricky Sherover-Marcuse in Unlearning Racism Workshops I attended in Madison, WI and at the Iowa City Women Against Racism conferences. Ricky's workshops and this exercise in particular, were powerful and inspirational in helping me have the courage to play more of a leadership role in anti-racism work "even though I didn't feel ready." (The more I work on anti-racism, the more questions I have and the fewer answers, so I now realize I will never feel "ready"!) Writing up my version of this exercise (which I have now used successfully in various ways, in many settings) is one way I am keeping the promise I made to myself at the time of Ricky's death that I would do what I could to keep her work alive and inspiring to others.

Ricky Sherover-Marcuse suggested that by looking at groups as "targets" and "non-targets", rather than as "oppressed" and "oppressors", we can better:

- Avoid feeling guilty! None of us want to think of ourselves as oppressors.
- See that we benefit from being in a non-target group even if we do not actively engage in targeting the other group.

Purposes of this exercise:

- To help everyone see the wide range of target groups which are a part of our lives.
- To help individuals see for themselves that they probably belong to both target and non-target groups. We benefit whenever we are in a non-target group. We are at a disadvantage whenever we are a part of a target group.
- To help individuals have some sense of what it feels like to be in one group or another. (Does it feel worse to be in some target groups than others? Does it feel better to be a part of a target group if there are many people in that group? How does it feel to be the only person in a target group? What does it feel like to be separated from a friend or potential friends because of the group identified?)
- To help set the scene for looking at people of color as a target group and white people as a non-target group.

Exercise

A room with space for everyone to move around in is required for this exercise.

Everyone is in the middle of the room while the exercise is introduced.

The workshop leader will call out a target group/non-target group combination. Each person in the target group moves to one side of the room. Each person in the non-target group moves to the other side of the room. Each person defines their own identity. People can stay in the middle of the room if they cannot decide which side they should be on or prefer not to identify with either group.

There should be a moment or two after everyone is in the appropriate place for everyone to quietly think about what it feels like to be a part of this particular target or non-target group. (There is no group discussion until the exercise is completed).

The workshop leader then calls out the next target group non-target group combination. The exercise is repeated with everyone moving to the side of the room which represents their identity on this particular issue. The exercise is repeated a number of times until 10-12 target/non-target combinations have been called.

Target groups are always on the same side of the room. Nontarget groups are always on the opposite side of the room. If 10-12 combinations are used, many people will have had the experience of being on both the target and non-target sides of the room. (Warning! Often the non-target group is numerically small but they still have the power. This can be very confusing to someone new to the issues of power and control. A challenge of this exercise is to make sure that someone who is always on the non-target side [i.e. a white, middle class man] or who is the only non-target [i.e. the only man in a women's studies class] sees the difference between the numerical size of a group and who has power in society)

TARGET GROUP EXERCISE
Non-target/Target Combinations

Non-target Groups	Target Groups
men	women
under 50	over 50
under 40	over 40
over 20	under 20
did not grow up poor	grew up poor
one parent went to college	neither parent went to college
parents' native language = English	parent's lang = not English
not Jewish	Jewish
non-rural	rural
never called or felt fat	called or felt fat
physically/mentally abled	disabled

Do *not* use examples where people have to choose between identifying themselves in a way which could put them at risk or denying a part of their identity. For example, in many situations it will not be safe to ask women to identify themselves on the basis of whether they are lesbians or battered women. In these situations, have the workshop leader explain why people are not being asked to identify on certain issues and have everyone stand in the middle of the room and think of the ramifications of not being able to identify with a particular group. (Contrast this situation to racism where most people of color do not have the choice not to identify themselves.)

V. DEVELOPING DIVERSITY EXERCISES FOR SPECIFIC ORGANIZATIONS OR GROUPS

This exercise can be specifically designed to fit the needs of any organization or group committed to becoming more diverse. Having a group of people work together to think up "situations" which fit their group can be as important as actually doing the exercise!

This exercise helps people see the difference between merely learning to cope with/interrupt oppression, educating against oppression, and pro-actively working for social change.

The right range of "situations" will cover a wide range of issues from the very subtle to the less subtle. Each "situation" is described on a card and all cards are put in a hat.

Exercise:

Groups of two draw a "situation" from the hat and discuss it. The "situation" is discussed from three perspectives:

1. How do you handle this situation when you merely want to cope with it in a sensitive way?

2. How do you use the situation as an "teachable moment?"

3. How do you work on this issue if you see yourself as a social change activist?

Small groups report to the larger group (many issues can be covered in a short time.) The larger group discusses those situations where the small group got stuck or where the topic generates discussion.

Sample situations

A. A person you are working with tells you that she is thinking of quitting because she feels overwhelmed by all the poverty/sadness she sees.

B. A new woman is working on your shift. She is about 60 years old. You realize that for the last few days all your conversations have been about periods and premenstrual syndrome.

C. You are designing a new poster to recruit volunteers/new workers. You realize that all the images on the poster are of young, white, able-bodied women.

D. You meet an old friend and tell her about the work you are doing. She says "How can you do that? Isn't that work that just takes care of poor Black people all the time?"

E. There is a new woman on your shift who you think is Jewish. (You don't know for sure!) Other people have been talking about recent anti-semitic incidents in your community in a way you feel may be hurtful to this woman.

F. You have been working for your organization for more than one year. You realize you have never been aware of disabled women participating in your events.

G. A group of you are sitting around talking about what you hope to be doing in a couple of years. All the plans discussed depend on people having had a good education or access to money. You realize that some women (without money/without a college degree) are being left out of this conversation.

H. A large woman walks into the room. You realize that all the chairs in the room are quite small with arms on them so there is nowhere the woman can sit.

I. An African- American woman is waiting for your co-worker for help. You realize that your co-worker is purposefully not paying any attention to this woman.

J. You meet an old friend and tell her about the women's organization you are working/volunteering for. She says, "I didn't know you are a lesbian."

K. Your organization has been trying to work against racism, but you have noticed that all the information you have (all situations you have discussed) deals with only African-American vs. white issues. You feel issues for other people of color need to be discussed.

VI. DIVERSITY ISSUES AND WOMEN'S HEALTH

It is important to make the connections between anti-racism/pro-diversity exercises and the women's health course syllabus obvious to students. When articles from this book, readings from *The Black Women's Health Book,* newsletters from activist groups, etc. are assigned, it may be helpful if the discussions consciously refer back to and build on the issues covered in the exercises. For *every* women's health issue an effort can be made to work towards developing an over-all analysis of how the issues may be different, exaggerated, or multiply complex for women of color, Jewish women, lesbians, older women, poor women, fat women, or women with disabilities. The power and control exercise (IID) can be used as a basis for discussing many women's health topics. For example, with reproductive rights issues, how does institutional racism/oppression work (as the "using children" prong of the power and control wheel) to define who should and who should not have children? How does this affect access to infertility treatment, attitudes towards 'forced contraception or sterilization', and welfare and maternity leave policies?

Anti-oppression work can be very hard work: the issues can feel overwhelming. Without a clear vision of the long term goals of pro-diversity work, students can easily get "stuck" simply feeling that oppression is awful, only feeling sorry for their identified "victims" of oppression, and feeling that an individual can do little to change an oppressive system.

Just as easily, anti-oppression work can be the most rewarding work we do. My own commitment in teaching about oppressions is to thoroughly integrate identifying the problems and finding the solutions for each issue I teach. Positive images of women of color, Jews, lesbians, older women, fat women, and women with disabilities can be used as a central part of learning how oppression has affected these groups of women. Emphasizing the positive and influential work being done by activist groups can be a very empowering way to demonstrate that groups of women of all colors, sizes, ages, sexual identities, physical abilities, and classes, are already making huge changes in working for a society which values diversity and that a society which appreciates diversity will be a healthier society for all women.

The vision of a diverse society exercise (IIE) can be a powerful ending for a women's health course.

Notes

1. This paper draws together some of the exercises and activities which I have designed or adapted from many workshops I have attended in England and the USA in the last fifteen years. I thank the many people who have inspired and supported my unlearning oppressions work. I would welcome feed-back on this article and am always anxious to learn new ideas and resources for diversity work. Write Nancy Worcester, Women's Studies Program, University of Wisconsin, 209 N. Brooks St., Madison, WI. 53715.

2. "Feminist, Anti-Racist, Anti-Oppression Teaching: Two White Women's Experience" by Becky Thompson and Estelle Disch in *Radical Teacher,* number 41, 1992, pp. 4-10.

Ω

Diversity and Health Issues

1. Identify two ways that you think your sex, race, or family income have influenced your interactions with health care providers or your access to the health care system.

2. What is similar and what is different about the following?

    - men working against sexism
    - white people working against racism
    - middle class people working against class oppression

3. For this question, refer to the "Ideas for Anti-Racism and Pro-Diversity Work" article.

    a. Identify a *non*-target group you are in. Describe the age and situation in which you first became aware that you had certain privileges or power because of belonging to this group.

    b. Identify a target group to which you belong. Identify ways in which you think this is similar and different from belonging to another target group. (Be specific about which two target groups you are comparing.)

c. Having identified a target group you are in, describe ways in which you feel you may have internalized society's negative messages about this group.

4. List ways that in your daily life you could or do interrupt sexist, racist, anti-semitic, ageist, or homophobic incidents or behaviors.

5. You are helping to plan a women's health course. Choose two different women's health topics. Suggest specific ideas of how you could plan to make sure that diversity issues were central to the material covered for these topics.

3

Gender Roles, Images, and Stereotypes

Most introductory women studies courses devote some class time to a discussion of gender roles. Many of the inequalities in our society are reinforced through the perpetuation of gender roles and through the arguments that these roles are somehow biologically determined and inevitable. (We use the term *gender* roles to emphasize that these roles are socially and culturally determined, not biologically determined *sex* roles). Sex role stereotyping plays a part in every issue discussed in this book and has an impact on women's roles as health care consumers and providers. The first article, "Hazards of Health and Home," gives an excellent overview of women's health issues in the context of women's roles in society, exploring, among other issues, both the physical and psychological hazards of housework, the stress of caretaking and "emotional housework," and the impact of economic inequalities on women's health. The next article "Male and Female Hormones: Misinterpretations of Biology in School Health and Sex Education" critiques the presentation of information in textbooks in a way that makes gender roles seem biologically, rather than culturally or socially, determined. While trying to be nonsexist, the schools may actually be reinforcing sexist stereotyping in the guise of scientific material.

Examining the ways in which the media can reinforce these stereotypes is a useful way to raise consciousness on these issues. The film "Still Killing Us Softly," which focuses on images of women in advertising, is an excellent introduction to these issues which we use in our classes. The article "In Poor Health" specifically examines the images of women in advertising in medical journals, helping draw the connections between media stereotypes of women and the implications for health care. How health is represented in photographs in health textbooks is explored in "The Picture of Health." In images very similar to those seen in advertising, those portrayed as "healthy" exclude large segments of the population, leaving a group of young, white, thin, and physically abled to represent health. Health is presented in these images as a commodity that many will not be able to attain, in other words, a privilege, not a right. Finally, in "Super Women," Edward Dolnick counters the myths about women as "weaker," providing data and arguments to help us debate the interaction of biological and cultural issues in influencing health and longevity.

Hazards of Hearth and Home
by Lesley Doyal

Synopsis—Women's health cannot be understood simply in terms of their biological characteristics. Improved theoretical analysis and more effective political action both require an exploration of the causal links between women's daily lives and their experiences of health, illness and disability. Recent research relating to these issues is explored in two linked articles: "The Hazards of Hearth and Home" and "Waged Work and Women's Well Being" (Vol. 13 No. 6).

Domestic work varies around the world but it universally involves low status, lack of economic power, and extensive social and emotional responsibilities. The implications of this labour for women's health are explored in this first article through an examination of the physical and psychological hazards of housework, the impact of caring on women's well-being, the stresses of emotional housework, inequalities in the allocation of household resources, the social and economic context of the ageing process in women, and the effects of domestic violence. These issues are placed in the context of the feminisation of poverty and differences between women in the developed countries and the Third World are explored.

Introduction

Women's health has traditionally been understood in terms of their reproductive systems. Thus, doctors locate women's problems in the specialist areas of gynaecology and obstetrics and assume that this takes care of those health problems peculiar to the female sex. Even women's overrepresentation among those diagnosed as suffering from certain types of mental illness is frequently explained by reference to some ill-defined biological nature, related, however obscurely, to their reproductive characteristics.

The reductionist model of health and illness that lies behind these practices has come under increasing attack in recent years. Research has shown that social and economic factors such as class, race, and country of residence are crucially important in mediating the biological processes underlying disease, death, and disability in both sexes. People do not become sick or remain healthy simply because of their genetic inheritance and their accidental contact with disease causing agents. The causal processes involved are much broader, encompassing living and working conditions, access to basic necessities, power and autonomy, and the quality of human relationships.

Feminists have taken this analysis a step further, using these ideas to explore the particular health problems experienced by women. While most women have a longer life expectancy than men from the same social group as themselves, they report more ill health and distress than men, use primary care and hospital services more than men, and suffer more long-term disability. The nature and severity of women's health problems obviously vary according to race, class, and economic status, but this overall gender difference remains remarkably constant. Researchers are now beginning to explore the reasons for this, linking women's patterns of morbidity and mortality to the nature of gender divisions in society and particularly to the continuing inequalities between the sexes. Findings from this new research are used to explore the links between women's health and two main areas of activity in their lives—domestic labour and waged work.

Domestic Labour in a Global Context

Women have traditionally been responsible for most of the work done in the domestic sphere. However, very little is known officially about the nature of household work or the conditions under which it is performed. While there have been periodic panics about women's capacity to look after their families'—and therefore the nation's—health, the impact of their domestic work on women's own well-being has rarely been a cause for concern. Indeed the role(s) of housewife and mother have generally been seen as healthy, despite considerable evidence to the contrary. So what is the nature of this work that most women spend so much of their time performing?

Their domestic responsibilities involve women in a complex web of activities that are often difficult to disentangle. For most, the central threads consist of care of a husband (or male partner), care of children and other dependents, and housework. Although the balance of these responsibilities will vary during the life cycle, these basic jobs form the core of women's domestic work in most societies. Not surprisingly, the nature and volume of this labour and the circumstances under which it is carried out have profound effects on women's physical and mental health.

In the developed countries, the common stereotype of the housewife is of a consumer who does a relatively small amount of low status, unskilled work, much of which involves spending money earned by a man. The reality, however, is very different. In the first place, most domestic work is done not by full-time housewives, but by women who are also engaged in some combination of paid and unpaid work outside the home. This pattern now applies in the majority of countries around the world—rich and poor, socialist and capitalist. In the second place, domestic work involves many (often unrecognized) skills and much effort. Indeed, most women with children (with the exception of the very affluent) spend their lives in continuous activity, putting together what the Italian feminist Laura Balbo has called "survival strategies" for themselves and their families (Balbo, 1987, p. 45).

But despite its obvious social utility, women's domestic work is unpaid—a fact which demeans it, and sets it apart from most other work done by adults. This inevitably has psychological significance for women, lowering their self-esteem and minimizing their sense of their own worth. It also affects them in more material ways, by reinforcing their economic dependence on others. Although many mothers with young children are now in paid employment, few can earn enough to support themselves and their families while continuing to do unpaid domestic work. Hence, most are forced, along with full-time housewives, into economic dependence on a male wage earner. Others have to rely not on an individual man but on the state to provide for their basic needs. In either case, economic dependence seriously limits women's autonomy and inhibits their control over their own lives and their health.

At the same time, women also have to take responsibility for those who are dependent on them for emotional and physical sustenance. Most of their daily work involves women in the servicing of others (Kickbusch, 1981). Put in more romantic terms, women's work consists of care of their "loved ones." This care can range from washing a partner's clothes through cooking a child's dinner to comforting a teenager worried about spots or cleaning up after the dog has been sick. It is distinguished from the same work in a laundry, cafe, or health centre because it is done for love rather than money. That is to say, women are expected to care *about* other people as well as caring *for* them (Graham, 1984). Thus, many women bear the double burden of their own economic dependence on a man or the state along with the dependency of their families on them for physical and psychological survival.

So far we have been talking in general terms about the elements of domestic work as it is performed by women in most countries around the world. The recognition of these basic similarities is important in reminding us that whatever the circumstances, patriarchal societies give women ultimate responsibility for the well-being of their families, often at considerable cost to their own health. However, this responsibility will have different implications according to the socioeconomic circumstances in which it has to be fulfilled. This point is most clearly illustrated through contrasting the lot of the majority of women in the industrialized countries with those in the Third World.

Housework and childcare are not the same in Birmingham, England or Birmingham, Alabama, as they are in the slums of Sao Paolo or the rural wastes of the Sahel. The most obvious difference is the level of material resources to which a woman has access to meet her family's needs. As we shall see, poverty itself is a major factor influencing the impact that a woman's domestic work has on her health, and most Third World women are very poor by comparison with those in Britain or the United States. But

taking the analysis one stage further, we also need to recognize that the nature of domestic work itself is very different in the Third World.

Women in the rich countries work out their survival strategies through their own and often a partner's negotiations with the labour market and/or the state. This will often be difficult, time-consuming and exhausting, and the impact on the health of poor women should not be underestimated as they cobble together wages, benefits, subsidies, or rebates to underwrite the purchase of their necessities. However, even these options are not available to millions of women in the Third World. They have little or no money to spend in the cash economy and welfare services are not available to fill the gap. As a result, they have to weave their patchwork of survival through the direct production of their own and their family's needs. Many are engaged in subsistence agriculture, growing and then processing the food they are not rich enough to buy. Fuel is collected in the form of firewood rather than purchased from a gas or electricity supply company and water is collected from a local source rather than flowing to the house through pipes. Thus, the physical burdens of their domestic labour are very much greater and this is clearly reflected in their experiences of morbidity and mortality. These international variations will be explored in more detail as we look at the different aspects of women's domestic work and its impact on their health.

The Hazards of Housework

Throughout the world, women perform many millions of hours of housework every day—most of it unacknowledged and barely visible. In the developed countries it is widely assumed that technological innovation has led to a reduction in the hours spent on housework. However, there is little evidence to support this belief. The introduction of basic services, such as running water and gas and electricity, along with the later development of vacuum cleaners, washing machines, and other domestic appliances certainly ameliorated the hard physical labour that characterized the lives of so many workingclass women in the 19th and early 20th centuries (Oren, 1974; Pember Reeves, 1980; Llewellyn Davies, 1978; Spring Rice, 1981). However, there was little reduction in the number of hours worked (Vanek, 1974; Meissner et al., 1988). Nor is there evidence that women's greater participation in waged work has led to a more equal division of domestic labour. Instead, women have retained the moral responsibility for ensuring that all domestic work is done, whether they are employed outside the home or not. They must organize it and worry about it, even if they do not do everything themselves, with inevitable effects on their health.

Despite (or sometimes because of) the development of modern technology, housework can still be physically and mentally exhausting, especially when conditions are difficult. Domestic accidents are a common hazard, especially for older women, and are more likely to happen when the fabric of the home is substandard. An old and dilapidated house will be more difficult to keep clean and will often threaten the safety of women and children. Since they have to spend more time than men indoors, women are more affected by defects, such as condensation and dampness which can aggravate respiratory disorders, as well as increasing the physical burden of housework. Looking after a home and its inhabitants can also bring the worker into contact with a wide range of toxic chemicals that are largely unregulated and have often been inadequately tested (Dowie et al., 1982; Rosenberg, 1984). Most of these are domestic products of various kinds such as cleaning fluids, bleaches, detergents, insecticides, and pesticides that are commonly used in the home and garden. It has been estimated that the average household in the United States contains some 250 chemicals that could send a child to hospital (Rosenberg, 1984).

There is also growing evidence that in the course of their housework women may be put at risk by hazardous chemicals encountered by their partners at their place of work. Research has shown that they can be endangered by asbestos fibers and radiation brought home on their husband's clothes or on his person. It also seems likely that some cases of cervical cancer may be caused by substances to which the man is occupationally exposed, which are then passed on to the women during intercourse (Robinson, 1981). Thus, the domestic workplace is not necessarily free from the chemical hazards of the industrial setting. Toxic substances do not become safe simply because they cross the threshold of the home and more research is needed to identify these dangers, as well as more effective regulation to control them.

However, it is the psychological hazards of housework which have attracted most attention, at least in the developed countries. To understand the reasons for this we need to look more closely at the nature of the work itself, at its social and economic status, and at the conditions under which it is performed. We can then explore the effects these have on women's sense of themselves, their control over their lives, and their potential for growth.

In Ann Oakley's study of full-time British housewives, most saw the main advantage of their job as the negative one of freedom from the constraints of employment (Oakley 1974). Few were positively happy with their work, with 70% expressing themselves 'dissatisfied' overall (Oakley, 1974). The women described most of their household tasks as monotonous, boring, and repetitive. Interestingly, it is these very characteristics of unskilled labour that occupational psychologists have shown to be most stressful in the context of male waged work. Although they are not formally controlled by a boss, most women doing housework experience very powerful pressures, both from other people and from inside their own heads. Ann Oakley asked one of the women in her study whether she found housework monotonous. Sally Jordan replied:

Well, I suppose I do really, because it's the same thing every day. You can't sort of say, "I'm not going to do it," because you've got to do it. Take preparing a meal: it's got to be done, because if you didn't do it, the children wouldn't eat. I suppose you get so used to it, you do it automatically. When I'm doing housework, half the time I don't know what I'm thinking about. I'm sort of there, and I'm not there. Like when I'm doing the washing—I'm at the sink with my hands in water, and I drift off. I daydream when I'm doing anything really—I'm always going off in a trance, I don't hear people when they talk to me. (Oakley, 1976, p. 147)

Thus, women are able to get little job satisfaction from routine housework and this is exacerbated by their lack of social and economic status (Berk, 1980). Most adults are paid for their work, and lack of such rewards limits self-esteem and gives a sense of worthlessness. Moreover, housework tends to be noticed only when it has *not* been done, giving women little opportunity for positive reinforcement, even of a nonmaterial kind.

These negative feelings are reinforced by the circumstances under which domestic labour is carried out. Housework is paradoxical in that it is usually done at home in isolation from most other adults, but when combined with childcare it also offers little opportunity for solitude. Despite widespread social and economic change, women continue to do almost all their household tasks in individual nuclear family units, with modern architectural styles often reinforcing this separation. However, the housewife may also find that her time is not her own. She will have to respond to the needs of others, may find very little time or energy to do things for herself, and rarely has physical space of her own. Under these circumstances, the demands on women are often high, and the real possibilities for control are low—again a situation clearly identified as stressful in the context of waged work (Karasek, 1979).

An additional feature of domestic work which can pose a threat to women's health is its open-endedness. Just as there are no absolute goals or standards, so there is no obvious end to the working day. For men and older children, home is perceived as a place of rest and recovery from the stresses and strains of real work done in the world outside. However, for most women the home is also a workplace and remains so for most of their waking hours. Many find it difficult to separate work and leisure; indeed those with young children are never really off duty, and their working hours can even extend to periods of sleep.

Not surprisingly, surveys in the developed countries have shown that women indulge in fewer leisure activities than men. The hobbies and pastimes they do mention tend to be domestic or home-based (listening to records or tapes, watching TV, reading, needlework and knitting, crafts and cooking) and they are frequently combined with ironing or child care (Deem, 1986). Relatively few are able to have outside interests, and active participation in sport is rare indeed. The reasons for this are closely related to women's family situation: lack of material resources, reluctance of men to allow them out alone, and the difficulty of getting someone else to look after the children, as well as the male-domination of many leisure and sporting facilities. This lack of leisure in general, and sport in particular, has obvious implications for women's physical and mental health:

... the notion of "wellbeing" is closely tied up with opportunities for leisure. The fewer opportunities women have for leisure, the less the chance that they will see themselves as enjoying such wellbeing, which includes more than feeling healthy and/or fit and implies a sense of confidence about and enjoyment of life in general, which is difficult if that life consists mainly of being stressed, overworked, tense and continually feeling tired as well as having a poor body image. (Deem, 1986, p. 425)

Ultimately, the most damaging aspect of housework for women's mental health may be the lack of opportunity it offers for personal development. Some women do get a great deal of satisfaction from tasks done in and for their households, and develop considerable skills in the process. However, the structure of the job offers no opportunity for growth or advancement and few chances of wider social recognition for achievement. Of course, women do learn to deal creatively with challenges and crises throughout their lives. Indeed many individuals and families would not have survived without their tenacity, problem-solving abilities, and sheer hard work. However, those tasks are rarely of their own choosing and may offer little in the way of increased personal autonomy.

Why then do so many women go on doing housework under these conditions with so little complaint? One reason is their early socialisation which means that many have extreme difficulty in expressing any dissatisfaction they may have with housework. To do so may be to threaten their identity as a good wife and loving mother.

The power of this repression is reflected in what Jessie Bernard has called the "paradox of the happy marriage." During her classic investigation of male and female perceptions of marriage, men expressed a considerable degree of dissatisfaction, but appeared to have relatively good mental health as measured by a questionnaire. Women, on the other hand, were more likely to say they were happily married but exhibited much poorer mental health (Bernard, 1972). This contradiction was especially acute among full-time housewives, many of whom simultaneously expressed high levels of satisfaction with marriage, as well as serious psychiatric symptoms. Indeed Bernard describes what she calls the "housewife syndrome" consisting of nervousness, fainting, insomnia, trembling hands, nightmares, dizziness, heart palpitations, and other anxiety symptoms. She concluded that "the housewife syndrome is far from a figment of anyone's imagination" (p. 47) and that "being a housewife makes women sick" (p. 48).

But it is depression above all, that seems to be an occupational hazard among fulltime housewives, especially those with young children. Both clinical experience and community research have shown that many women staying at home experience intense frustration, which is usually expressed in feelings of emptiness, sadness and worthlessness (Brown & Harris, 1978; Nairne & Smith, 1984). Too often these feelings go unacknowledged; women are said to be "like that" and the front door closes on a great deal of misery and distress. George Brown and Tirril Harris working in South London found that one-third of a random sample of workingclass women with children under six who were full-time carers were suffering from what could be classified as "clinical depression." However, few had sought medical help. When women do take emotional problems to their doctors they are usually offered a chemical solution. In reality, however, it is the nature of women's domestic labour, their relationships with other people and their dependent status that makes them more likely than any other group to experience depression and anxiety, but less likely to confront the real reasons for their frustrations and dissatisfactions.

Who Cares for the Carers?

As well as doing the housework the majority of women also care for dependents. The intensity of this work varies over the lifecycle and some women never do it at all. However the vast majority become mothers at least once in their lives—in Britain the figure is now about 80%. This can be immensely rewarding and for many women motherhood is the most important and creative aspect of their lives. However, the reality of day to day childcare can also be both physically and emotionally demanding, especially under difficult circumstances (Graham & McKee, 1980; Richman, 1976; Boulton, 1983). For first-time mothers in particular, the responsibility of a tiny baby can be very onerous and nights without sleep exhausting and demoralizing.

Despite the lip service paid to motherhood as a social duty and a valued activity, few researchers have explored the reality of childcare from a woman's perspective. In an attempt to fill this gap, the British sociologist Mary Boulton recently carried out a series of in-depth interviews with young mothers (Boulton, 1983). Her intention was to disentangle women's feelings about the daily labour of childcare from their love for their children or their response to the status of motherhood itself. Almost two-thirds of women in the study experienced a strong sense of meaning, value, and significance in looking after their children. This is clearly important because a purpose in life is central to a feeling of well-being. However over one third did not feel this way (Boulton, 1983). Moreover, some 60% of her middle-class respondents and 44% of those who were working class found looking after children to be predominantly an irritating experience. Thus, the majority did not find childcare "naturally rewarding." Yet this was their fulltime work.

Many of the women referred to stress in their lives and identified a number of factors contributing to it. The lack of boundaries to their role meant that they were always trying to create structures and find themselves physical and mental space. They complained that childcare interfered with other activities, especially housework, and that children often undid what had just been achieved. For some women, childcare was isolating and limited them to relationships with other women in a similar position. Many also pointed out that children greatly curtailed their freedom of action because there was so much effort and anxiety involved in taking them out.

Overall, about 50% of Mary Boulton's sample said they were wholly content with their lives as mothers, about one-fifth were wholly discontented, while about one-quarter were in between. That is to say they accepted the situation, but wished it could be different. Significantly however, many of those who reported themselves satisfied also stated that their experiences of childcare were negative. This suggests that, as we saw in the context of housework, many women may simply accept situations over which they have no control, living much of their lives vicariously through others, with inevitable effects on their own well-being.

As well as caring for healthy children, women also look after dependent adults and chronically sick children. Again, precise information is difficult to obtain because this domesticated nursing is one of the most invisible of all forms of labour. In the British context, estimates suggest that at least 1.4 million people (out of a total population of just over 60 million) act as principal carers to adults and children with disabilities severe enough to warrant support in daily living tasks (Green, 1988). The vast majority of these are women. Some 15% of all British women of working age care for dependents over and above their normal family duties and many of them are also in paid employment (Martin & Roberts, 1984). Moreover, the need for such care is rising as the number of elderly and disabled people in the population increases. Indeed, the community care policies now fashionable in much of the industrialized world are based on the implicit assumption that women will continue with these unpaid labours (Osterbusch et al., 1987; Finch, 1984; Finch & Groves, 1983). Yet there is evidence that they may not be conducive to the promotion of women's own well-being.

The daily grind of caring has been well documented in a number of research studies (Equal Opportunities Commission, 1982; Finch & Groves, 1983; Briggs & Oliver, 1985). Caring for adults can be especially demanding both physically and psychologically. Much of the strain comes from the nature of the job itself—long hours, nightly disturbances and sometimes the trying behaviour of the person being cared for or the inability to hold a serious conversation. Stress is also caused by the conditions of caring, particularly the isolation that often results when the person cannot be taken out and no substitute care is available. Above all, caring for adults can cause emotional problems that do not arise in caring for normal children. The daughter who cares for a parent and the wife who cares for a husband may have to negotiate new relationships under difficult circumstances, often with very little support. One British woman looking after her husband has described her experiences in the following terms:

The tiredness associated with looking after someone disabled was the hardest thing for me to adjust to . . . the tiredness is, of course, due to different causes for each carer, but the exhaustive effect is the same—for me, the tiredness comes from the physical exertion of caring for someone with severe multiple sclerosis, and from the mental stress of seeing the person you love best in

the world suffering from such a disease. (Briggs & Oliver, 1985, p. 39)

Under these circumstances, women's own health will often suffer. This is especially true for women on what has been called the caring tricycle—the lifetime of responsibility which begins with care of children, continues into middle age with care of an aging parent, and ends with responsibility for a frail partner.

Doing Emotional Housework

Some of the more subtle aspects of women's domestic labour can be summarized as emotional housework. This is the least visible part of their work and consists of activities designed to ensure the happiness and emotional wellbeing of other family members—managing social relationships within the home to keep the old man happy and the kids quiet. While this labour is rarely perceived as such by women or their families, it is often a major burden. Arlie Hochschild has vividly described the processes involved:

The emotion work of enhancing the status and wellbeing of others is a form of what Ivan Illich has called "shadow labour": an unseen effort which, like housework, does not quite count as labour but is nevertheless crucial in getting things done. As with doing housework the trick is to erase any evidence of effort, to offer only the clean house and the welcoming smile. (Hochschild, 1983)

But who is looking after women's needs while they smile for others? Sadly, the answer for many is no one. The traditional division of labour in the family means that women frequently do not receive the emotional sustenance they might have expected from their nearest and dearest. While adult daughters may provide support, this is rarely true of grown-up sons and male partners.

Luise Eichenbaum and Susie Orbach have written extensively on this problem from their experiences as feminist psychotherapists (Orbach & Eichenbaum, 1984; Eichenbaum & Orbach, 1985). They make the important point that the social stereotype of the clinging, passive female leaning on a strong and independent man is usually the reverse of the truth. Most men, they say, are looked after by women all their lives, from their mothers and other female relatives through female teachers to their wives or female partners in adulthood. A girl, on the other hand, is brought up to assume that she will marry a man and provide nurturance, care, and emotional support for him and his children. While she is expected to *appear* "dependent, incompetent and somewhat fragile," the internal reality is rather different:

. . . behind this outward facade is someone who, whatever the inner state, will have to deal with the emotional problems met in family relationships, a person who knows that others will expect to rely and lean on her, a person who fears that she will never really be able to depend on others or never feels content about her dependency. (Eichenbaum & Orbach, 1985, p. 21)

Thus, many adult women cannot fulfill their own basic need for nurturance and emotional fulfillment, despite—or because of—their position at the hub of what is widely regarded as the most caring institution in modern society.

These insights derived from the psychoanalytic tradition are consonant with women's own accounts of their situation, as reported in a number of recent studies. Agnes Miles, a British sociologist, recently carried out in-depth interviews with some 65 women and men diagnosed as suffering from depression. About half of the women blamed their depression on an unhappy marriage, whereas most men referred to work and health problems (Miles, 1988). When asked about the support they had received, only 24 out of 65 women named their male partner as their main confidante and not all of these were satisfied with the quality of the relationship:

(Iris, 24, no children). "There is only my husband. I wish there was someone else. Mostly I keep my thoughts to myself. I hoard my thoughts, then I get upset and tell my husband because there is nobody else. I usually regret it afterwards. He is part of the trouble, but who else can I talk to?"

(Bridget, 29, two children 4 and 7). "I wish I had more people, I wish I had a woman friend. My husband is there but he doesn't want to talk, not like women talk to each other. He doesn't understand. He just says, don't bother me with nonsense." (Miles, 1988, pp. 94-95)

Many of the women in Miles' sample also expressed their fear of putting too much of a burden on other people. They were afraid that what little help was available would be withdrawn and, even more fundamentally, saw themselves as unworthy of support. Interestingly, the men in Miles' sample did not report the same problems in getting support from their wives. As Miles expressed it, "both took for granted that this was the natural order of things" (p. 113).

Susannah Ginsberg and George Brown uncovered a similar pattern in their study of women in the North London suburb of Islington. Again they were interviewing women who would be clinically diagnosed as a case of depression, in an attempt to see how relatives, friends, and doctors responded to their problems. This research repeated the now-common finding that signs of depression in women (such as inexplicable crying) are often given little attention since they are regarded as normal for women, especially when they are young mothers or menopausal (Ginsberg & Brown, 1982). Three quarters of those interviewed (27/37) who were living with their husbands felt that he had given little or no support. Mrs. Thomas, for instance, commented as follows:

"I told my husband how depressed I've been feeling. He just sits in silence. If he could just talk things out and suggest something—but he doesn't."

"Has he suggested you should go to the doctor?"

"No, he doesn't realize anything is wrong. He doesn't notice that I haven't been getting on with things." (Ginsberg & Brown, 1982, p. 93)

Three quarters of the women (34/45) also felt they received little or no support from their mother or other relatives such as sister, or friends. The majority (32/37)

who were living with their husbands said they did try to talk about their depression but most were unsuccessful. The majority of husbands apparently responded with such comments as "You're imagining it all," "Stop being silly," or "You mustn't talk like that, there's the baby" (Ginsberg & Brown, 1982, p. 95).

It seems, then, that women's domestic labour, especially their role in caring for others, is not always conducive to their own good health. Their mental well-being in particular will often be put at risk, and adequate support is not available when they are in need. As we shall see, this is especially true in the context of material poverty.

The Feminisation of Poverty

Women have always been overrepresented among the world's poor and recent years have seen a worsening of their situation (Scott, 1984). Although impoverished women are to be found in all countries, the majority live in underdeveloped parts of the world and it is here that the rigours of domestic work are at their most severe (Buvinic, Lycette, & McGreavey, 1983). Of course, men in the Third World are also poor, but it is women who must manage the consequences of poverty for the whole family. This often means performing physically heavier work and working longer hours than men (Dankelman & Davidson, 1988; Momsen & Townsend, 1987; Sen & Grown, 1988). In Tanzania, for instance, a recent study showed that women work an average of 3069 hours a year compared with 1829 hours for men (Taylor, 1985). Similarly, women in the Gambia spend 159 days a year on farmwork compared to men's 103 days (Mair, 1984). Moving to Asia, a study conducted in several rural villages in Kaunataka showed that the labour of women and children together contributed almost 70% of the total human energy expended on village work, even when strictly domestic tasks such as sweeping, washing clothes and childcare were excluded (Kishwar & Vanita, 1984).

Thus, women in the Third World bear a heavy weight of domestic responsibilities. Moreover, their material poverty and, for many, the exhaustion of frequent childbearing, add to their burdens. While climate, culture, and conditions vary between countries, these women are united by their poverty and the harshness of the social, economic, and physical environment in which they carry out their labours. As we shall see, this daily struggle is reflected in their general state of health and well-being.

In the richer parts of the world, most housewives can take for granted the existence of a constant supply of clean water. However, there are millions of women from rural areas of Bangladesh to the crowded barrios of Latin America who must face the daily task of acquiring enough water to meet the needs of their families. This is a physically demanding job which in rural areas will often mean a lengthy journey, but it is very rarely done by men.

Water is needed not just for drinking, but for sanitation and waste disposal, washing, childcare, vegetable growing, and food processing and also for economic uses such as keeping animals, irrigating crops, and brewing beer (Dankelman & Davidson, 1988). All this has to be fetched by women—usually on their heads because few have access to a vehicle of any kind or even a donkey (Wijk-Sijbesma, 1983). Many walk miles every day to a stream, well, or pond for a few pots of water. In urban areas, women depend on public taps which will usually mean long waits and no privacy for bathing. In many slums even public taps are not available, so that women face a long journey or the payment of a high price to a street vendor for water of dubious quality (Dankelman & Davidson, 1988).

Under these circumstances, water will have to be consumed sparingly, making other domestic tasks more difficult. Moreover, insufficient or polluted water will often result in illness, adding to the woman's burden. It is generally assumed that some 80% of all diseases in Third World countries are water-related. Diarrhoea, for instance, is a major cause of death among young children and is closely correlated with the absence of a clean water supply. Women themselves suffer additional problems caused by lack of adequate sanitation because religious and moral prohibitions mean they often have to wait until dark to avoid being seen in the act of defecation. This can lead to constipation and strain on the bladder and also exposes them to the risk of assault (Dietrich, 1986).

As well as supplying water, many Third World women are also responsible for ensuring an adequate amount of fuel for cooking, boiling water, and heating and lighting the house. Again, this very arduous task is rarely done by men and is a significant factor in the endemic exhaustion of many rural women. Throughout the world women are carrying loads of up to 35 kilograms, distances as much as 10 kilometers from home. This weight exceeds the legal allowance for women carrying heavy loads in an industrial setting in many countries. The distance women have to travel varies depending on where they live, and the time taken can be as much as three or four hours per day. In some areas including the Sahel, Gambia, and parts of India, the journeys can be even longer and deforestation means that they are increasing (Agarwal, 1986). As supplies of firewood diminish, women and children are having to spend even more time on collection. In parts of Bihar, for instance, where seven to eight years ago poor women could get enough wood at 1.5 to 2 kilometers, they now have to trek 8 to 10 kilometers every day (Agarwal, 1986).

This growing shortage of fuel has meant that cooking has now become more labour-intensive and traditional methods have to be adapted to conserve energy. In some places the traditional wood fuel has been replaced by substances, such as cattle dung and crop residues. These biomass fuels are less convenient for cooking; the fire has to be stoked continuously and the smoke is even more dangerous than woodsmoke (WHO, 1984). Emissions from biomass fuels are major sources of air pollution in the home, and studies have shown that cooks inhale more smoke and pollutants than the inhabitants of the dirtiest cities. In one study quoted by WHO, a female cook was said to inhale an amount of benzopyrene (a known carcinogen) equivalent to 20 packs of cigarettes a day. Chronic carbon monoxide poisoning has also been reported (Dankelman & Davidson, 1988). Pollution of this kind has been identified as a causal factor in the high level of respiratory and eye disease found among Third World women. It can also cause acute bronchitis and pneumonia, as well as nasopharyngeal cancer among those exposed from early infancy (WHO, 1984).

As well as ensuring supplies of water and fuel, many Third World women are also directly involved in the production of food for their families (Dixon-Mueller, 1985). They grow a variety of crops either for immediate consumption or to be sold or bartered in the village or local market, and raise poultry or small animals. When food is scarce or there is a drought, they may have to scour the countryside for edible matter such as the roots and leaves of plants. This raw food then has to be processed, often by laborious and lengthy methods. These processes will vary between cultures and climates, but Madhu Kishwar's account of Indian peasant women gives some indication of the quantity of work involved:

Grain or pulses to be consumed have to be hard-cleaned, little pebbles or pieces of dirt hand-sifted or painstakingly removed, one by one before the cooking of every meal. Many women have to hand-pound the paddy or grind the wheat two or three days a week in order to make it consumable. The paddy first has to be boiled and dried in the sun before it is husked. To husk 20 pounds of paddy, two women can easily spend two to three hours, and it takes much longer if a woman has to do it alone . . . Thus, cooking even the most simple and basic foods commonly used in the diet of ordinary families is very exhausting. (Kishwar & Vanita, 1984, p. 4)

These accounts make it clear that the domestic labour of most Third World women is extremely hard. The work is physically strenuous and the hours are long, leaving many millions exhausted, undernourished, and vulnerable to premature death. Moreover, most are involved in frequent childbearing, resulting in levels of debility which can only be guessed at, since morbidity data for rural women are rare, and mortality data crude and uninformative.

While some of the worst living and working conditions are suffered by women in the Third World, this should not blind us to the fact that there are also many women in the developed countries who suffer the ill effects of both absolute and relative poverty on their health (Gelpi, Hartsock, Novack, & Strober, 1983; Glendinning & Millar, 1987; Scott, 1984). In the United States, the richest country in the world, almost two-thirds of impoverished adults are women. This overrepresentation of women among the poor must be explained by reference to the sexual division of labour in the wider society. Women are confined to a secondary status in the labour market, yet their work in the home is not financially rewarded. State welfare benefits mirror this low earning capacity, thus perpetuating a lifetime of economic dependence and poverty for many working-class women. In Britain, for instance, working women make up over two-thirds of the 8 million people whose wages are below the poverty line. Similarly, some two-thirds of all elderly people live in poverty and six million of this nine million are women. Female-headed families, too, represent a significant group in poverty. Thus, many women in rich as well as poor countries suffer the ill-effects of poverty.

The ill health women experience as a result of deprivation is often compounded by the allocation of resources within the family. Research has shown that even in households where the aggregate income is above the poverty line, women may not have enough to meet their own needs. This is because the division of income and wealth between individuals is often unequal (Glendinning & Millar, 1987; Land, 1983; Pahl, 1980). Women tend to get (or take) less both because of their economic dependence and lack of power, but also because of their concern for other family members. Thus, women are more likely than men to be poor when living alone, they may be poor members in nonpoor households, or they may be the poorest in a poor household. In all cases, their health will be at risk.

Bread for the Breadwinner?

We can illustrate these inequalities in the allocation of household resources by looking at gender differences in nutrition. Although women are usually responsible for the purchase and preparation of food and often its production too, many do not have the power to determine distribution between family members, and their own health may suffer as a consequence. Adequate nutrition is a basic human need which cannot always be met for the entire household in conditions of poverty. Research in many countries around the world has shown that when the family income is too low, it is women who are especially prone to nutritional deficiency. Under these circumstances, food is often the only item of expenditure that can be manipulated to make ends meet and it is usually women who go short to ensure that the needs of the children and the breadwinner are met (Oren, 1974).

Yet women themselves have particular nutritional needs, which often go unrecognized or ignored. Menstruation, pregnancy, and lactation all increase women's need for protein and iron. This is difficult to measure precisely, but it has been estimated that pregnant women need 350 extra calories per day, while those feeding their babies need another 550 calories, as well as three times the normal intake of calcium and double the amount of vitamin A (Protein-Calorie Advisory Group, 1977). Research in both the developed countries and the Third World has shown that many women do not get enough of the right food to meet these needs.

A study carried out by the London-based Maternity Alliance in 1984 showed that despite the existence of the British welfare state some women are still not able to feed themselves adequately during pregnancy. The average cost of the diet recommended for pregnant women by the Department of Health in 1988 was £15.88. This repre-

sented nearly half the weekly benefit payable to a single person and a third of that for a couple (Durward, 1988). As a result, the many pregnant women on supplementary benefit could not afford to eat what was officially defined as necessary to sustain their own health and that of their unborn children.

In the Third World, the nutritional problems of poor women are, of course, much greater. The combination of lack of food and, in some countries, severe discrimination against women, results in serious undernutrition for many mothers and daughters (World Health Organization, 1986). According to the Protein-Calorie Advisory Group of the United Nations (PAG), there are definite indications of maldistribution of food at the family level in many parts of Africa with women getting the least even in pregnancy (Protein-Calorie Advisory Group, 1977). In some cultures, it is common for boys to be breastfed considerably longer than girls and for girl children to be fed less well than boys, thus reducing their chances of surviving infancy. Adult men often sit down to eat before their women and children, who get what remains (Leghorn & Roodkowsky, 1977; Carloni, 1981; Maher, 1981). Thus, food which is itself in scarce supply is distributed according to the prestige of family members rather than their nutritional needs. As a result, many women become anaemic, especially during pregnancy, due to a lack of basic nutrients. Estimates suggest that in the Third World as many as half of non-pregnant women and two-thirds of pregnant women are anaemic due to iron deficiency and folate and vitamin B_{12} deficiency combined with parasitic infections (WHO, 1979).

The authors of a recent study in Bangladesh set out to determine whether or not the very poor health record of women in that country could be explained by inequalities in the allocation of food and medical care (Chen, Huq, & d'Souza, 1981). The results were startling. Fourteen and four-tenths percent of female children in the sample were found to be severely malnourished, compared with 5.1 % of males. This appeared to be directly related to food intake because dietary surveys showed that per capita male food intake considerably exceeded that of females at all ages. Overall, males averaged 1,927 calories per capita compared with 1,599 calories for females. The male excess was as high as 29% during the childbearing years of 15 to 44. These differences remained even when the data were adjusted for body weight, pregnancy, lactation, and activity levels, indicating that they must be seen as a relevant factor in explaining women's excess mortality.

In concluding, the authors of the study make the important point that these gender inequalities in life and death should not be seen as merely the response to scarcity. Indeed, they were found in rich as well as poor families, reflecting the fundamental inferiority of women's position in a profoundly patriarchal society. Of course, the reasons for male preference are a complicated mixture of the material as well as the ideological—girls cannot earn as much to help the family budget, have to be given a dowry, and are not able to support their parents during old age. But all too often the end result is serious damage to the health of girls, with many of those who survive to adulthood passing on their debility to future generations.

Older Women: The Invisible Majority

So far we have talked mainly about the impact of domestic tasks on the health of women in their childbearing years. However, in the developed countries, at least, it is older women who are most often confined to the home and who form the largest single group living in poverty. Even those who are not materially deprived frequently face serious health problems, yet these go largely unnoticed in societies that prioritise youth, vitality, and innovation. A combination of ageism and sexism means that older women are all too often marginalised sexually, socially, and economically in ways that threaten their well-being.

Older women are now the fastest growing group in poverty in the United States and Britain. In the United States, one-fifth of women aged 65 and over are below the poverty line, and women are twice as likely as men to experience poverty in old age. The single elderly are poorest of all and are predominantly female—three-fifths of women over 65 are alone compared with only a quarter of men. This reflects both the age difference of most couples at marriage and women's longer life expectancy. Older women from ethnic minorities suffer disproportionately from the effects of poverty. Forty-two percent of aged black women are in absolute poverty and a staggering 82% in near poverty, according to the 1980 U.S. Census. A similar situation prevails in Britain, with two-fifths of elderly women (38%) living on or below the poverty line, compared with 25% of men; two-thirds of all older British women are on the margins of poverty (Walker, 1987).

The poverty of older women stems directly from their lifelong economic dependency on men, the nature of their domestic responsibilities, and the existence of a dual labour market. Those women who do not engage in waged work are never able to earn state benefit in their own right. Hence, dependency in their early and middle years is carried over into old age. Even those who do work outside the home are often unable to build up a reasonable income for themselves in retirement. Many worked in low paid jobs without pension provision. Moreover, their working lives are usually disrupted by childrearing and sometimes caring for elderly parents, giving them little opportunity to build up a reasonable contributions record. Most, therefore, remain dependent on men, who usually die first, leaving them with only a minimal state pension to rely on. As a result, many experience health problems either caused or exacerbated by inadequate living conditions, insufficient heating, and lack of a nutritionally balanced diet.

Of course, not all the health problems older women face can be related directly to poverty. Many also suffer the psychological problems associated with retirement from work. Almost no research has been carried out on this topic because it has generally been assumed either that women do not work outside the home or that they are not deeply attached to their jobs (Fennell, Phillipson, & Evers, 1988). Thus, women appear only as shadowy wives in studies of men's retirement problems. Yet the few accounts we have from older women themselves suggest that the tensions are very similar for both sexes, and are likely to result in similar health problems (Ford & Sinclair, 1987). Most older women also have to cope with the denial of their sexuality at the same time as the physical and psychological distancing of their children.

Very few studies have investigated the health problems of older women, and routine medical statistics tell us little about their well-being. However, we know that in both the United Kingdom and the United States, elderly women are much more likely than men to be disabled. Twice as many British women in the over-65 age group are severely or very severely disabled compared with men of the same age, while the figure is five times greater in the 75-plus age group (Harris, Cox, & Smith, 1971). Women suffer three times as much arthritis as men and osteoporosis is also a significant cause of reduced female mobility. Mental health problems are even more difficult to identify and measure, but older women appear to continue the excess identified in younger age groups, with higher rates of depression and dementia than their male counterparts. Alan Walker comments on the basis of British data that older women are "more likely than men to suffer from psychological problems such as loneliness or anxiety and to have lower levels of morale and life satisfaction" (Walker, 1987).

Overall, women seem to suffer longer periods of chronic ill health than men, but their deaths are rarely caused by the same disease(s) that disabled them in life. Men, on the other hand, tend to have shorter periods of disability and to die from the problems that have bothered them while they are alive (Verbrugge, 1985). Interestingly many older women seem to play down their ill health, either because of low expectations—"You can't expect much at my age"—or shame at being unable to manage any more (Fennell et al., 1988, p. 109). However, others seem to welcome illness as liberating them from a lifetime of caring for others, especially when their dependents are no longer alive (Herzlich, 1973). In any case, too many remain behind closed doors, struggling to look after themselves with little material or emotional support.

The situation of older women in underdeveloped countries is obviously different in several ways. In the first place, relatively few survive to old age at all, and those who do are often severely debilitated by frequent childbearing and hard physical labour. Second, they are more likely than women in the developed countries to be supported and looked after within the extended family. Indeed in many societies older women occupy important social roles—grandmother, mother, or mother in law, performer of religious or magical rites, senior wife—which offer more status than those of younger men. Those societies where women are required to be attached to a male adult usually have mechanisms to ensure that widows are not left alone. In India, for instance, remarriage is not encouraged among high-caste Hindu women and a son will be expected to support his mother while in some African societies, a widow is inherited by her husband's brother. Thus, older women in many parts of the Third World are less likely to suffer the isolation and invisibility of those in the developed countries, and in some cultures their status is even enhanced.

However, this is by no means always the case. Childless widows in particular often find themselves without social or financial security. Moreover, there is growing evidence that in many countries the breakdown of the traditional family-support system with industrialization and urbanization is increasing the vulnerability of divorced and widowed women (Youssef & Hetler, 1983). In parts of India, the expectation that a widowed daughter-in-law will be absorbed into her husband's family is no longer always adhered to. Instead, widows often return to their own families or set up (often very poor) households. Similar findings of lack of support for widows have been reported from Africa, from Upper Volta, Morocco, Zambia, and Swaziland (Youssef & Hetler, 1983). Thus, the problems of older women in the industrialized countries are increasingly being felt by those in the Third World as modernization removes their traditional sources of emotional and material sustenance, and therefore their access to reasonable health.

The Home as Haven?

Despite the dangers discussed above, it is a common myth that the home is a haven, offering protection from the dangers of the world outside. Indeed, many women are afraid to go out at night, staying behind closed doors to ensure their safety. The reality, however, is very different, as I explore in this final section.

It is clear that both the fear and the reality of domestic violence constitute a major threat to women's health. The use of physical force in the home is relatively common and most of it is inflicted on women by men (Dobash & Dobash, 1980). Precise estimates are difficult to achieve because so many victims are reluctant to reveal their private suffering. Indeed, the authors of a major British study suggest that only 2% of such assaults are reported to the police (Dobash & Dobash 1980). However, a number of studies designed to reveal the extent of this hidden violence have given broadly similar findings for the United States and Britain. A large-scale national study carried out by Murray Straus and his colleagues in the United States reported that over 12% of the married women interviewed had suffered severe violence at some point in their marriage, while a total of 28% had experienced physical violence of some kind (Straus et al., 1980). A British study involved interviews with all the women living in seven neighbouring streets in inner Leeds. About one-fifth of those interviewed had been the victims of violent attacks in their homes during the previous year (Hanmer & Saunders, 1984).

There is evidence of domestic violence in most countries around the world. In India, in particular, the uncovering of this abuse and its elimination has been a major focus of the new feminist movement (Mies, 1986). Urban and rural women, working class and middle class are all potential victims of domestic violence and Mies argues that their suffering has increased as the process of modernization gets under way. The most dramatic and widely publicized cases include the so-called dowry murders, in which women have been abused and eventually murdered because their husband and often his family are not satisfied with the money and goods she brought to the marriage. Many are deliberately burnt to death, but a cooking accident is blamed. Others commit suicide because the pressures on them are too great (Mies, 1986; Kishwar & Vanita, 1984).

Thus, the evidence demonstrates that a significant proportion of the women who live with men have the quality of their lives diminished by domestic violence. Moreover, this experience is shared by those in different social groups and societies, uniting women across class and racial divides. All women are potentially at risk from male violence, but paradoxically it is wives or cohabitees who get the worst treatment. Moreover, it is often their domestic work that provides the immediate excuse for a battering—a meal not ready on the table, a shirt not ironed, the house not clean enough, too much money spent on food, or a bout of "nagging." The physical damage caused is often severe, necessitating medical treatment or hospitalisation. In the Dobashes' study of the survivors of violence, nearly 80% reported visiting the doctor at least once during their marriage for injuries inflicted by their husbands. Nearly 40% said they had sought medical care on five or more occasions and many felt their husbands had prevented them from getting medical help when they needed it. Another study of women in British refuges found that 73% had put up with violence for three or more years. Thirty percent had suffered life threatening attacks or had been hospitalized for serious injuries such as fractured bones (Binney, Harkell, & Nixon, 1981).

As well as the physical damage, it is clear that domestic violence is a major cause of psychological stress and trauma. Sixty-eight percent of the British women in refuges said that mental cruelty was one of the reasons they left home (Binney et al., 1981). Many victims are emotionally debilitated by anxiety about the next attack and feel shocked, upset, angry, and bitter at what is happening to them. Sadly, many feel guilty and blame themselves:

I actually thought if I only learned to cook better or keep a cleaner house everything would be OK. . . It took me five years to get over the shame and embarrassment of being beaten. I figured there had to be something wrong with me. (Dobash & Dobash, 1980, p. 119)

The authors of a recent study in North London found that women who had been battered were twice as likely to be depressed and had lower self-esteem than those who had not received such treatment (Andrews & Brown,

1988). Years of violence often leave women in a situation where alternatives are difficult to visualize. The socially constructed dependencies that they already experience are exacerbated by physical intimidation and violence. Moreover, attempts to get help from social workers, police, and other authorities too often lead to further humiliation and rejection (Stark, Flitcraft, & Frazier, 1979).

Thus, women become double victims of the batterer and the social agencies who too often assign the blame to women and resist any intervention in the private lives of man and wife. Indeed, one American writer has used the term *learned helplessness* to describe the condition in which so many battered women find themselves (Walker, 1979). Constrained by lack of confidence, isolation, fear, and lack of money, too many are forced to remain for lengthy periods in relationships that threaten their health and sometimes even their lives.

Conclusion

Thus, research findings accord with some women's own subjective experience in associating many of their health problems with their domestic responsibilities. Women's traditional duties are not always good for their health, given the circumstances of inequality and sometimes deprivation under which they often have to be carried out. Not surprisingly perhaps, there is growing evidence that despite their subordination in the labour market, women sometimes improve their health by working outside the home. I explore the implications of this in Part Two.

References

Agarwal, Bina (1986). *Cold hearths and barren slopes: the woodfuel crisis in the Third World.* London: Zed Press.

Andrews, Bernice, & Brown, George. (1988). Violence in the community: A biographical approach. *British Journal of Psychiatry,* 153, 305–321.

Balbo, Laura (1987). Crazy quilts: Rethinking the welfare state debate from a woman's point of view. In Anne Showstack Sassoon (Ed.), *Woman and the state.* London: Hutchinson.

Berk, Sarah. (1980). *Women and household labor.* Beverly Hills: Sage.

Bernard, Jessie. (1972). *The future of marriage.* New York: World Publishing.

Binney, Val, Harkell, Gina, & Nixon, Judy. (1981). *Leaving violent men.* Leeds: National Womens Aid Federation.

Boulton, Mary. (1983). *On being a mother.* London: Tavistock

Briggs, Anna, & Oliver, Judith. (1985). Caring: *Experiences of looking after disabled relatives.* London: Routledge and Kegan Paul.

Brown, George, & Harris, Tirril. (1978). *Social origins of depression.* London: Tavistock.

Buvinic, Mayra, Lycette, Margaret, & McGreavey, William. (Eds.). (1983). *Women and poverty in the Third World.* Baltimore: Johns Hopkins Press.

Carloni, Alice. (1981). Sex disparities in the distribution of food in rural households. *Food and Nutrition,* 7, 3–12.

Chen, Lincoln, Huq, Emdadul, & d'Souza, Stan. (1981). Sex bias in the allocation of food and health care in rural Bangladesh. *Population and Development Review,* 7, 55–70.

Dankelman, Irene, & Davidson, Joan. (1988). *Women and environment in the Third World.* London: Earthscan.

Deem, Rosemary. (1986). *All work and no play.* Milton Keynes: Open University Press.

Dietrich, Gabriele. (1986). Our bodies, ourselves; organizing women on health issues. *Socialist Health Review,* March, 79–184.

Dixon-Mueller, Ruth. (1985). *Women's work in Third World agriculture.* Geneva: ILO.

Dobash, R. Emerson, & Dobash, Russell. (1980). *Violence against wives: A case against the patriarchy.* London: Open Books.

Dowie, Mark, et al. (1982). The illusion of safety. *Mother Jones,* June, 38–48.

Durward, Lyn. (1988). *Poverty in pregnancy* (with 1988 update). London: Maternity Alliance.

Eichenbaum, Luise, & Orbach, Susie. (1985). *Understanding women.* Harmondsworth: Penguin.

Equal Opportunities Commission. (1982). *Caring for the elderly and handicapped: Community care policies and women's lives.* Manchester: Author.

Fennell, Graham, Phillipson, Chris, & Evers, Helen. (1988). *The sociology of old age.* Milton Keynes: Open University Press.

Finch, Janet. (1984). Community care: Developing nonsexist alternatives. *Critical Social Policy* 9, 6–18.

Finch, Janet, & Groves, Dulcie. (1983). *A labour of love: Women work and caring.* London: Routledge and Kegan Paul.

Ford, Janet, & Sinclair, Ruth. (1987). *Sixty years on: Women talk about old age.* London: Women's Press.

Gelpi, Barbara, Hartsock, Nancy, Novack, Clare, & Strober, Myra. (1983). *Women and poverty.* Chicago: University of Chicago Press.

Ginsberg, Susannah, & Brown, George. (1982). No time for depression: A study of help seeking among mothers of preschool children. In David Mechanic (Ed.), *Symptoms, illness behaviour and help seeking.* New York: Prodist.

Glendinning, Caroline, & Millar, Jane. (1987). *Women and poverty in Britain.* Brighton: Harvester.

Graham, Hilary. (1984). *Women, health and the family.* Brighton: Harvester.

Graham, Hilary, & McKee, Lorna. (1980). *The first months of motherhood.* Research Monograph No. 3. London: Health Education Council.

Green, Hazel. (1988). *Informal careers (General Household Survey 1985—GHS no. 15 supplement A).* London: HMSO.

Hanmer, Jalna, & Saunders, Sheila. (1984). Well founded fear. London: Hutchinson.

Harris, Amelia, Cox, Elizabeth. & Smith, Christopher. (1971). *Handicapped and impaired in Great Britain, pt. 1.* London: HMSO.

Herzlich, Claudine. (1973). *Health and illness: A social psychological analysis.* London: Academic Press.

Hochschild, Arlie. (1983). *The managed heart: Commercialization of human feeling.* San Francisco: University of California Press.

Karasek, Robert. (1979). Job demands, job decision latitude and mental strain: implications for job redesign. *Administrative Science Quarterly* 24, 285–308.

Kickbusch, Ilona. (1981). A hard day's night—on women, reproduction and service society. In Margarita Rendel (Ed.), *Women, power and political systems*. London: Croom Helm.

Kishwar, Madhu, & Vanita, Ruth. (1984). *In search of answers: Indian women's voices from Manushi*. London: Zed Press.

Land, Hilary. (1983). Poverty and gender, the distribution of resources within families. In Muriel Brown (Ed.), *The structure of disadvantage*. London: Heinemann .

Leghorn, Lisa, & Roodkowsky, Mary. (1977). *Who really starves? Women and world hunger*. New York: Friendship Press.

Llewellyn Davies, Margaret. (1978). *Maternity: Letters from working women*. London: Virago.

Maher, Vanessa. (1981). Work, consumption and authority within the household: A Moroccan case. In Kate Young, Carol Wolkowitz, and Roslyn McCullagh (Eds.), *Of marriage and the market*. CSE books.

Mair, Lucy. (1984). *Anthropology and development*. London: Macmillan.

Martin, Jean, & Roberts, Ceridwen. (1984). *Women and employment: A lifetime perspective*. London: Department of Employment.

Meissner, Martin et al. (1988). No exit for wives: Sexual division of labour and the cumulation of household demands in Canada. In Ray Pahl (Ed.), *On work*. Polity Press.

Mies, Maria. (1986). *Patriarchy and accumulation on a world scale*. London: Zed Press.

Miles, Agnes. (1988). *Women and mental illness: The social context of female neurosis*. Brighton: Harvester Press.

Momsen, Janet, & Townsend, Janet. (1987). *Geography of gender in the Third World*. London: Hutchinson.

Nairne, Kathy, & Smith, Gerrilyn. (1984). *Dealing with depression*. London: Women's Press.

Oakley, Ann . (1974) . *The sociology of housework*. London: Martin Robertson.

Oakley, Ann. (1976). *Housewife*. Harmondsworth: Penguin.

Orbach, Susie, & Eichenbaum, Luise. (1984). *What do women want?* London: Fontana.

Oren, Laura. (1974). The welfare of women in labouring families in England 1860-1950. In Mary Hartman & Lois Banner (Eds.), *Clio's consciousness raised: new perspectives on the history of women*. London: Harper & Row.

Osterbusch, Suzanne, Keigher, Sharon, Miller, Baila, & Linsk, Nathan. (1987). Community care policies and gender justice. *International Journal of Health Services, 17*, 217–232.

Pahl, Jan. (1980). Patterns of money management within marriage. *Journal of Social Policy 9*, 313–335.

Pember Reeves, Maude. (1980). *Round about a pound a week*. London: Virago.

Protein-Calorie Advisory Group (PAC). (1977). *Women in food production, food handling and nutrition: With special emphasis on Africa*. Final report. New York: Author.

Richman, Naomi. (1976). Depression in mothers of preschool children. *Journal of Child Psychology and Psychiatry, 17*, 75–78.

Robinson, Jean. (1981). Cancer of the cervix: Occupational risks of husbands and wives and possible preventive strategies. In Joe Jordan, Frank Sharp, & Albert Singer (Eds.), *Preclinical neoplasia of the cervix*. London: Royal College of Obstetricians and Gynaecologists.

Rosenberg, Harriet. (1984). The home is the workplace: Hazards, stress and pollutants in the household. In Wendy Chavkin (Ed.), *Double exposure: women's health hazards on the job and at home*. New York: Monthly Review Press.

Scott, Hilda. (1984). *Working your way to the bottom: The feminisation of poverty*. London: Pandora Press.

Sen, Gita, & Grown, Caren. (1988). *Development, crises and alternative visions*. London: Earthscan.

Spring Rice, Margery. (1981). *Working class wives*. London: Virago. (Originally published in 1939.)

Stark, Evan, Flitcraft, Anne, & Frazier, William. (1979). Medicine and patriarchal violence. *International Journal of Health Services, 9*, 461–493.

Straus, Murray, Gelles, Richard, & Steinmetz, Suzanne. (1980). *Behind closed doors*. New York: Anchor Books.

Taylor, Debbie. (1985). Women: an analysis. *In Women: A world report*. London: Methuen and New Internationalist.

Vanek, Joann. (1974). Time spent on housework. *Scientific American, 231*, 116-120. (Reprinted in Amsden, Ann. (Ed.), *The economics of women and work*. Harmondsworth: Penguin.

Verbrugge, Lois. (1985). An epidemiological profile of older women. In Marie Haug, Amasa Ford, & Marian Sheator (Eds.), *The physical and mental health of aged women*. New York: Springer.

Walker, Lenore. (1979). The battered woman. New York: Harper & Row.

Walker, Alan. (1987). The poor relation: Poverty among older women. In Caroline Glendinning, & Jane Millar (Eds.), *Women and poverty in Britain*. Brighton: Harvester.

Wijk-Sijbesma, Christine van. (1983). *Participation of women in water supply and sanitation: Roles and realities*. Technical Paper 22. The Hague: International Reference Center for Water Supply and Sanitation.

World Health Organization. (1979). *The prevalence of nutritional anaemia in women in developing countries:* Country project. WHO Document FHE/79.3. Geneva: Author.

World Health Organization. (1984). *Biomass fuel combustion and health*. Geneva: Author.

World Health Organization. (1986). *Health implications of sex discrimination in childhood: Review and bibliography*. Geneva: WHO/UNICEF.

Youssef, Nadia, & Hetler, Carol. (1983). Establishing the economic condition of women headed households in the Third World: A new approach. In Mayra Buvinic, Margaret Lycette, & William McGreavey (Eds.), *Women and poverty in the Third World*. Baltimore: Johns Hopkins University Press.

Ω

Male and Female Hormones: Misinterpretations of Biology in School Health and Sex Education

by Mariamne H. Whatley

In identifying sexism in education and its impact on students, many educators have put a great deal of serious thought into identifying sex-biased language and examples in texts, as well as examining differential treatment of boys and girls in the classroom. However, one area that is left untouched because it is often considered not subject to bias is the presentation of biological or scientific "facts." Scientific research, far from being "pure" and unbiased, can be shaped by the social values of both the scientist and the surrounding society; the views of scientists (whatever their scholarly merits) can be used by the larger society for a variety of social purposes. This is particularly true in a society that claims to value "science" and "rationality."

Feminist scientists have, in recent years, been examining the ways biological research has been used to maintain the status quo in society, supporting racism and sexism by attributing biological causation to social behavior. The use of science to restrict women is by no means new, and the current backlash against feminism creates a climate in which the antifeminist implications of sociobiology and other biological determinist theories are readily accepted. In response to the growing body of literature in the field of sociobiology and the extensive work attempting to support biological determinism, feminist scientists have produced excellent critiques of biological research involving sex/gender issues (Bleier, this volume, Chapter 1; Bleier, 1984; Fee, 1983; Hubbard & Lowe, 1979; Sayers, 1982). However, these critiques have not filtered down to the textbooks and curricula in the schools, particularly in health and sex education, areas in which there are great possibilities for both bias and impact on students. Nor has any priority been given to consciously changing education in these areas in response to these critiques. Indeed, at the very suggestion that curricula be reviewed for sexism, conservative forces were activated to combat the possibility of change. The proposed "Family Protection Act" was intended in part to "preserve traditional family values" in the schools.

Health and sex educators in the schools are rarely trained in the evaluation of primary biological and physiological research. Therefore, they are likely to accept and teach a simplified and inaccurate version of biological findings. It is particularly important that the textbooks used to train future teachers and those used by teachers in the classroom be clear, accurate, and as free from bias as possible. Unfortunately, sexism in the fields of health and sex education is as common as it is in other areas.

An examination of health and sex education school curricular materials and teacher education texts reveals the often subtle misinterpretations of biology that can have a serious impact on both female and male students in terms of their perceptions of themselves and others. Often the implication is that the norm is biologically determined and that anything else is clearly deviation. The behaviors seen as part of a biologically determined natural path of development often reflect a sexist and heterosexist bias. From the scientifically incorrect use of the terms "male" and "female" hormones to the explanation of the roles of these hormones in growth and development to the implication of the inevitability of heterosexual dating, marriage, and childbearing, misinterpretation of biology helps teach teenagers to accept the status quo in sex roles. An educational policy at the level of schools of education in which teachers learn to view biological issues more critically and to identify sexism, as well as racism, in science is essential for combating sexism in the classroom, as well as influencing attitudes and patterns of behavior at a crucial stage of development.

In order to evaluate the materials teachers would be exposed to during their training, I examined 25 texts that were commonly used either in health and sex education classes at the college level or were education methods texts and curricular guides in these areas. These texts ranged in publishing dates from 1975 to 1984. In examining these texts, I was particularly looking for errors in facts, oversimplification to the point of inaccuracy, important information missing, and unwarranted social implications. In this chapter, I present several content areas in which flaws in texts have sexist implications.

"Male" and "Female" Hormones

The sex hormones that play a major role in changes occurring at puberty—estrogens and androgens, produced by the ovaries, testes, and adrenals—are present both in males and females. They can also be easily interconverted in different body tissues, often confounding experiments that look at the effects of hormones that are introduced into experimental animals. Though the average female tends to have higher levels of estrogens than androgens and the average male the reverse, there is a great deal of individual variation in the ratio of these hormones. As with most sex differences, there is significant overlap between the sexes

Mariamne H. Whatley, "Male and Female Hormones: Misinterpretations of Biology in School Health and Sex Education," pp. 67–88 in WOMEN, BIOLOGY AND PUBLIC POLICY, edited by Virginia Sapiro. Copyright © 1985 by Sage Publications, Inc. Reprinted by permission of Sage Publications, Inc.

in hormone levels. It is, therefore, not possible to determine biological sex based on hormone levels alone. In addition, these hormones are necessary for normal development in both sexes, and an increase in both hormones occurs in males and females at puberty.[1]

In most texts surveyed, there are discussions in which these hormones are consistently referred to as "male" (androgens) and "female" (estrogens) hormones. The majority of texts do not mention that both sexes produce these hormones and that their role is important in both sexes, though several of the most recent texts do point this out (Allgeier & Allgeier, 1984; Kilmann, 1984). It is rarely stated that androgens play a role in female development, though this has been presented occasionally (Sommer, 1978). Androgen plays an important role in the development of the female at puberty, in terms of growth, muscle and bone development, and hair distribution, yet it is called the "hormone of maleness" in one text (Hafen, Thygerson, & Rhodes, 1979, p. 259). The unstated implication is that such androgen-controlled aspects of development as muscle growth are essentially male. One of the texts illustrates this view in its explanation of the possible problems associated with a female having too much "male" hormone:

Too much androgen in a woman may enhance her sex drive and may cause her to become hirsute or abnormally hairy. (McCary & McCary, 1984, p. 31)

It is not clear whether hirsuteness is a price to pay for enhanced sex drive or whether they are both unhealthy and unfeminine effects of an overdose of the "hormone of maleness" in a female.

Science and science-based education are and should be based on precision and rigor. The imprecision of the preceding terminology is a serious problem because, by avoiding the subtleties of the roles of these hormones, the concepts of "male" and "female" and accompanying behavioral roles become fixed as if caused by the "male" and "female" hormones. After reading repeatedly that the androgens are male hormones and the estrogens are female hormones, one can easily forget that these terms are shorthand for hormones that are found predominantly but not exclusively in one sex or the other. From there it is easy to accept a rather broad role for these hormones in determining sex roles, though these are more likely to be culturally constructed than biologically determined.

The Role of Sex Hormones

All texts recognize that these hormones play an important role, either by themselves or interacting, in major pubertal changes, such as those in hair and fat distribution and the development and growth of breasts, genitals, muscles, and bones. Some texts expand beyond these well-established effects:

The onset of adolescence is triggered by the pituitary, which stimulates the secretion of the sex hormones that have important effects on various tissues of the body, including the brain. These hormonal changes are responsible not only for some of the physical changes that may greatly affect adolescent body image, but also changes in sexual, aggressive, and emotional behavior. (Hafen, Burgener, Hurley, & Peterson, 1978, p. 178)

Other texts support this idea of a biological basis for adolescent behavior. One text lists "Ten Basic Facts of Transescent Physical Development," which includes as a first fact, "Aggressive play and roughness among boys increase because of physiological changes at puberty" (George & Lawrence, 1982, p. 30).

The effects of hormones on the brain are simply not known. The arguments that claim a role for androgens in aggression are very weak, even in terms of the animal models that are generally much easier to study than humans. Biological research on aggression has serious problems relating to the nonrigorous definitions of that term that can range from rough-and-tumble play in nonhuman primates to competition in the business world to wars between nations. The loose definitions allow inappropriate extrapolation from results in animal studies to theories about human behavior. Currently, there is no proof for a causal relationship between physiological changes and aggressive behavior and much stronger arguments have been made for the role of socialization in aggression.[2] Considering the lack of scientific evidence connecting aggression and hormones, it might be wise for a teacher to look for nonbiological explanations of aggressive adolescent male behavior. The preceding passage set up a situation in which "normal" boys are expected to be rough and aggressive because of their hormones, whereas "normal" girls should not be. These expectations of gender-related behavior clearly can help create this socially accepted pattern of behavior without any aid from androgens.

Biology, Sex Roles, and Stereotypes

Educators have been making strong pleas to reduce sex role stereotypes and allow full development of the potential of all students, but the misunderstanding of the role of biology in determining sex roles can create confusion. For example, in an article originally published in Health Education, Dixie Crase (1978, p. 192) wrote the following:

In conclusion, whether sexual differences are due to biological and/or sociological factors, the sex of individuals continues to influence their development. It remains as important for a boy or girl to learn his or her sex role as ever. Educators and other adults must begin early to be aware of subtle, unconscious influences in early childhood which limit both boys and girls in terms of future self-concepts and interpersonal relationships. Individuals, families, and society can ill afford to limit the development of human potential.

Although she clearly wishes to avoid forcing constricting sex roles on girls or boys, she seems willing to accept a biological explanation. Earlier in the same article she wrote, "However, recently reported research suggests the newborn human infant is unequivocally a girl or a boy with feminine or masculine predispositions" (p. 187). Although the majority of newborns are unequivocally female or male in terms of external genitalia, the existence of feminine or masculine predispositions is hardly a given. On the contrary, several studies suggest that adults respond as if there were differences in predisposition though there is no objective basis for the described differences. Sex role stereotyping appears to begin at birth; gender "appropriate" descriptions of infants by parents appear not to reflect any real differences among infants (Rubin, Provenzano, & Luria, 1974). In fact, the concept of predispositions that Crase seems to accept serves to place limitations on the possibility of the full development of human potential that she seeks.

Often sex roles are covered as a separate topic in adolescent health and sex education. In texts, the presentation of these roles reflects some of the confusion expressed in the Crase article—that sex roles should not be limiting but that they are necessary, even, perhaps, biologically determined. A good example of these conflicting views can be found in the text, *Creative Teaching in Health* (Read & Greene, 1980, p. 216):

However, the long-term trend appears to be toward reducing the heretofore sharp distinctions in societal expectations for masculine and feminine patterns of interest and behavior.

Despite the vigorous actions of many feminist groups, certain underlying physiological differences will undoubtedly place limits on this effort and preserve the meaningfulness of sex roles.

It is not clear which underlying physiological differences are being referred to, whether simply to those few clear sex differences—potential to ovulate, gestate, lactate, versus the potential to inseminate—or differences such as those in aggression that are both vaguely defined and unproven as biologically determined. In any case, as with Crase, there is a hope expressed that the "meaningfulness" of sex roles will be preserved.

The lack of clarity about physiological givens versus cultural norms is expressed by Read and Greene (1980, p. 222) in a concept suggested for teaching sex roles:

8. Boys and girls develop typical differences in their personalities, interests, and modes of behavior as they mature. Physiological differences between men and women have traditionally led to different duties and responsibilities which in turn have produced general personality differences. Although based on physiological factors, this process of role definition is largely a cultural process.

The difference in duties and responsibilities that has a physiological basis is essentially that women can be the ones to give birth and breastfeed and that men cannot. Beyond that there are no roles that can be directly attributable to physiological differences. The token reference to the cultural process at the end of the sentence doesn't clarify at all what roles are attributable to what forces, so that the impression remains that physiology does play a large role in determination of personality differences. The use of the expression "typical differences" clearly indicates that there are specific patterns that are sex-related and, therefore, cannot or should not be altered. This lack

of precision leads to the implication that the norm is a biological given and all variations on these sex roles are deviance.

This view is stated much more directly in a list of concepts in a text called *Teaching Secondary Health Science* (Sorochan & Bender, 1978, p. 382):

12. Each person needs to accept his or her sexual-social role.

15. Sexual deviations often stem from unresolved emotional-social conflicts.

Here it is clearly stated that sex roles are given and unalterable; problems arise for individuals when they are unwilling to accept these givens.

The text also expresses the belief that in some cases biology itself might cause a "deviance" in behavior:

Adolescents often manifest extreme reactions to compensate for their size and other physical shortcomings. For instance, a tall girl in junior high may never go to dances because she is certain to be taller than most boys she dances with. Or a large girl may go in for athletics, masculine clothes, and a career because she cannot be "cute" and feminine. (p. 122)

Here what is defined as an "extreme reaction" is for a girl to stray from her sex role, pursuing athletics and a career because of a "physical shortcoming." In this paragraph, it has been clearly established that there is certain normal and healthy behavior for a girl. Instead of merely encouraging the educator to feel sympathetic for a "misfit," the authors could have introduced the idea of valuing individual differences and the possibilities of not fitting into a mold. It would also be an appropriate time to question some accepted standards of adolescent culture, such as girls having the option to dance only with boys who are taller or body size serving as a determinant of femininity. Educators should present athletics and a career as positive possibilities for all students.

Sorochan and Bender (1978, p. 384) even more clearly identify what they see as healthy behavior when they outline "exemplary informational behavioral objectives," some of which are listed below:

The student will be able to:

6. Date often

10. Accept sexual-social role

13. Demonstrate social dating skills

20. Describe how to select a marriage partner.

The clear core of these objectives is the acceptance of sexual-social roles, with dating and marriage as part of a normal continuum. The importance of dating as part of healthy development is emphasized in other texts as well, and an educator should question these statements. Texts could much better emphasize the importance of developing friendships with members of both sexes, learning to interact with other people in a number of different situations and at different levels of intimacy. Instead, only dating, which often puts extreme social and sexual pressure on an adolescent, becomes the important goal.

Although sex educators are always looking for ways to encourage adolescents to say no to unwanted sexual activity, they may be pushing them into the situation that can most easily trap them into saying yes. The impact in terms of self-esteem on those who are not considered datable, the pain of not being invited to a prom or party, the blow to the ego of an invitation rejection, have been well-documented in fiction and nonfiction. For health and sex educators to enforce subtly the status quo in teenage relationships, rather than calling them into question, is to place even more pressure on a group already facing emotional stress.

Male and Female Sexuality

In an effort to support continued "meaningful" sex roles, health educators often stress differences in sexuality as a basis for these roles:

Human sexuality refers to all of those qualities that distinguish between maleness and femaleness. The physiological differences are both obvious and important, but in addition there are the equally important differences in attitude, behavior, and responsibilities that define the male and female role in American society. (Read & Greene, 1980, p. 211)

First, it is crucial to note that in this passage human sexuality refers only to those differences and not to similarities between males and females, so that this reinforces the importance of difference between the sexes rather than the similarities of human beings. Sexuality becomes defined in terms of gonads, genitals, and culturally defined sex roles, rather than in any of those areas in which there might be overlap, such as affection, love, and nongenital response.

For example, this passage clearly ignores the fact that the basic physiological mechanisms of the sexual response, vasocongestion and myotonia, are actually the same in males and females. The well-known research of Masters and Johnson (1966) showed that what may seem to be very different responses, penile erection and vaginal lubrication, are actually controlled by the same mechanism, vasocongestion or buildup of blood in the genital area, and are indicators of similar levels of arousal. In addition, their classification of the phases of the sexual response, that is, arousal, plateau, orgasm, and resolution, apply to both males and females. After the pioneering research of Masters and Johnson, the overall message was clear that similarities are greater than differences in terms of the sexual response, so that according to the preceding passage, the sexual response would be eliminated from the definition of sexuality.

By maintaining the view of sexuality expressed in the previous passage, all sexually related behaviors become dichotomized into male and female behaviors and there is no longer an area of human sexuality. For example, there is the following discussion:

Within the male the sex drive is more specific and direct. It tends to be isolated from feelings of love and affection and directed more towards orgasm. Within the female the sex drive is more diffuse and is related to feelings of affection. Indirect stimuli such as sexual fantasies and provocative pictures have a much greater effect on the male than the female. (Read & Greene, 1980, p. 216)

Although it is never stated that the differences in sex drive are biological, it is implied because repeated references are made in the text to the role of physiological differences. (Because it has been shown that androgens play a role in libido, perhaps the suggestion is that the differences in sex drive are attributable to the different levels of androgens in males and females.) However, what makes this statement especially problematic is that it is not clear whether this is a description or prescription or both for "normal" sex drive for both sexes. Is a female who seeks orgasm or a male who seeks affection abnormal? Adolescents are worried and scared by issues of sexuality and want desperately to be "normal." The information from these texts serves to make life worse for them. By making this kind of statement in a book for educators, the authors, perhaps unconsciously, are supporting a common view of sexuality in our society. Texts should not reinforce the double standard. Without any attempt to show alternative approaches to adolescent sexual relations, sex education is often taught with the view that boys have a physiologically uncontrollable sex drive geared toward "doing it" and girls just want affection and a class ring. Therefore, adolescents learn what is "normal" in sexual behavior and try to follow those norms.

In addition to reinforcing certain societal views of sexuality, many health and sex education texts are strongly heterosexist, if not homophobic. A 1978 text (Hafen et al., 1978) reprinted an article from *Journal of School Health* that clearly expresses a negative view:

Homosexuality, as an enduring sexual pattern, is an illness, no different than any other illness and is a symptom of deep-seated emotional difficulty. Despite propaganda to the contrary, there is no such thing as a well-adjusted, happy homosexual. (Kriegman, 1978, p. 233)

The information provided is often biased and inaccurate, as in the following passage:

The practice of homosexual behavior leaves much to be desired if one wants to have children. This form of sexual behavior might prove unsatisfying for some, since mutual masturbation and oral-anal activity may amount to no more than impersonal encounters and are frowned upon by society. (Johns, Sutton, & Cooley, 1975, p. 209)

A number of criticisms of this passage can be made that also point out common omissions or misinterpretations in texts. For example, homosexuality does not preclude parenting. Many lesbians and gay men have had children while they were in heterosexual relationships and others choose to have children, often using artificial insemination, after they are in homosexual relationships. Another problem is that homosexuality is often used as synonymous with male homosexuality, so that descriptions given, accurate or stereotypical, often apply only to men, leaving lesbians invisible. A third point is that there is nothing inherently impersonal about homosexual behavior; it might be suggested that heterosexual intercourse can as easily lend itself to impersonal encounters as would mutual masturbation or oral-genital contact.

Returning to the previously discussed area of dating, the following statement appears as a concept to be taught under the topic of sex roles: "Adolescent dating activities and other heterosexual social activities serve important functions in the process of personality development" (Read & Greene, 1980, p. 240). Attention should be drawn to the use of the word "heterosexual" in the preceding passage. It is not clear whether the authors mean simply that both sexes are present or that the social activities are truly heterosexual. In the former case, social activities with both the same sex and opposite sex should be considered important for normal development. In the latter, the approximately 10 percent of the population that is homosexual is excluded by definition and those who are not interested in sexual activity at all are also precluded from the possibility of normal development.

From a simple misuse of the terms "male" and "female" hormones, it is easy to move step by step through the beliefs that certain feminine and masculine behaviors are biologically caused and, therefore, are normal. Deviance from sex roles, including deviance from heterosexuality, is seen as violation of biology. If instead it were clearly indicated that males and females are made up of a mixture of androgens and estrogens, in different proportions, it might be harder to fall into a trap of biological determinism. Flexibility in sex roles might be more easily viewed if it were recognized that there is similarity in hormonal constitution. What may seem a subtle distinction can have a major impact when viewed in terms of how sex roles are taught as part of health education.

"Facts" in Women's Health and Disease

Factual errors appear with surprising frequency in textbook descriptions of women's basic biology and of common diseases and disorders. Even worse than simply providing misinformation, these errors can greatly affect how women, especially adolescents, view their bodies. Providing good, accurate basic health information and demystifying the workings of the female body can help adolescents develop a much more positive view of their bodies and a stronger sense of control over what happens to their bodies at a time in development when changes may seem completely out of control. Through understanding basic physiological mechanisms and disease processes, they can become more active in maintaining their health. These changes can have a positive effect on other areas of their lives, such as enhancing self-esteem.

Textbook treatments of menstruation offer an important illustration of errors and misinterpretations of basic biology with sexist implications. Cramping during menstruation is generally caused by uterine spasms or contractions, which in turn can be caused by high levels of a substance called prostaglandins. Endogenous prostaglandins naturally cause smooth muscle contractions, including of the uterus, and are so powerful in their effect that they can be used as agents in the induction of second-trimester abortions. When it was recognized that high levels of prostaglandins could be causing dysmenorrhea, it was found that the use of inhibitors of prostaglandin synthesis could be potent relievers of menstrual pain. Both clinical and experimental evidence support the prostaglandin theory of causation of dysmenorrhea (Jones & Jones, 1982). Now the existence of such drugs as Motrin, Naprosyn, and Ponstel has eliminated what had been debilitating pain for a number of women.

Discussion of the cause and treatment of dysmenorrhea is particularly important in health education curricula because menstrual pain can be severe among adolescents, who need to understand what is happening to them and what can be done about it. Curiously, this topic leads many authors to minimize biological causation and to emphasize instead the problems of female psychology:

Painful menstruation or menstrual cramps, called dysmenorrhea, can be caused by a physical abnormality of the reproductive organs. But psychological causes (tense feelings about femininity, sexuality, and menstruation itself) are more common, especially in young women. (Eisenberg & Eisenberg, 1979, p. 428)

Another text agrees with the view that there is a chance that dysmenorrhea may be physiological in origin, but continues, "However, psychological problems, such as those related to tension or self-concept, appear to be the more prevalent cause" (Gay, Wantz, Slobof, Hooper, & Boskin, 1979, p. 117).

Hafen et al. (1979, p. 265) outline possible causes for dysmenorrhea:

1. an inflammation or infection,

2. constipation,

3. poor posture,

4. lack of regular physical activity,

5. psychological factors such as stress or lack of preparation for menstruation,

6. low pain threshold (some can tolerate pain better than others),

7. cysts or fibroid tumors, or

8. positioning of the uterus ("tipped uterus")

Some of these factors may increase the discomfort of dysmenorrhea, but there is no indication that poor posture, lack of preparation for menstruation, or lack of regular physical activity actually cause cramps. This approach is a classic case of blaming the victim. The adolescent girl who suffers severe cramps is seen as being at fault in any of a number of physical or psychological ways, except in extreme instances beyond her control such as having fibroid tumors. The pain of severe dysmenorrhea is stressful enough without also being held responsible for its cause. In addition, this approach helps perpetuate the stereotype of the hypochondriacal female who either imagines or causes her own ailments, a view prevalent in much of medical education.

Some more recent texts do mention the role of prostaglandins (Jones, 1984; Maier, 1984). Others mention no probable cause, which may be better than the blaming the victim policy, though a statement such as the following, while true, does not give much hope to an adolescent suffering cramps: "Cramping sensations, which are probably related to uterine spasms, seem to be less severe among women who have given birth" (Kilmann, 1984, p. 76). Other new texts ignore the subject of dysmenorrhea altogether (Allgeier & Allgeier, 1984), discussing only premenstrual syndrome (PMS), which is a distinct phenomenon, or confuse the two. One text (McCary & McCary, 1984, p. 31) says that high levels of progesterone cause dysmenorrhea, a theory that is held by a few people but never validated, whereas the prostaglandin theory of dysmenorrhea, which has been well-supported and documented, is not mentioned.

Textbooks should provide more thorough and accurate treatment of a problem that is so common among adolescent females. While nonmedical approaches to reducing cramps, such as exercise and salt reduction, should be discussed, it should also be pointed out that good treatments are available for debilitating cramps. There should never be an issue of a psychological component in dysmenorrhea unless people are willing to explore the subject in enough depth to prevent simplistic interpretations. An educator, especially a health educator who is involved with physical education as is often the case, must be aware that cramps are a real physiological phenomenon and not a rejection of femininity or simply an excuse for skipping gym class. Telling a girl that if she stood up straight, she probably wouldn't have cramps is hardly the answer, especially if she is doubled over from the pain.

It is also interesting to note that two texts that emphasize psychological origins for dysmenorrhea also subscribe to the notion that cystitis, a bladder infection caused by bacteria, may be psychological in origin (Gay et al., 1979, p. 118) and may respond to psychotherapy (Eisenberg & Eisenberg, 1979, p. 428). Cystitis is generally caused when *E. coli,* bacteria that are normal inhabitants of the large intestine, enter the urethra and move into the bladder. Though this infection can occur in males, it is much more common in females, largely due to the much shorter urethra in females. Contamination of the urethra can occur simply by wiping from back to front after defecation, but cystitis is certainly not necessarily the result of poor hygiene. In addition, vaginal intercourse can force bacteria up the urethra and the pressure of the penis can additionally irritate the urethra. However, cystitis can easily occur without any sexual activity.

Though many texts provide accurate medical information on the disease (e.g., Allgeier & Allgeier, 1984; Maier, 1984), another 1984 text describes cystitis as an inflammation of the bladder but never as a bacterial infection. It also adds, "sometimes cystitis is caused or aggravated by emotional factors, usually related to conflict over sexual matters" (McCary & McCary, 1984, p. 303). This view again places the burden of responsibility for causation on the sufferer. Because cystitis is often associated with heterosexual intercourse, it may be seen by a woman with the disease as being very much sexually related and, therefore, hard to discuss if she is also not comfortable discussing her sexual activity or if she is not sexually active at all. It is also important to recognize that it is a bacterial infection because many women suffer through it without seeking treatment and an untreated infection can spread, potentially causing kidney damage. Dysmenorrhea and cystitis are just two of the more obvious examples of the need for evaluating information in texts.

Conclusion

While educators who are eager to combat sexism may be carefully changing pronouns and making sure boys cook and girls do woodworking, they may be completely ignoring sexist information appearing in the texts that are used to train teachers. Many of these texts have serious flaws in the presentation of information on such common topics as changes during puberty and menstruation. These problems include oversimplification of information ("male" and "female" hormones), missing information (dysmenorrhea), incorrect information (emotional causes of cystitis and dysmenorrhea), and unwarranted attribution of human behavior to biological causes (aggression, sex roles). Some material carries the implication that, just as certain physical characteristics are biologically determined, so are sex roles. It is implied that variations on specific patterns of male/female behavior violate biological norms and are, therefore, unhealthy. What is stressed as normal and healthy includes a predictable pattern of heterosexual dating, followed inevitably by marriage. The status quo in society is enforced with little room for flexibility.

While stressing a biologically determinist view of sex roles, sexuality, and other behavior such as aggression, many texts offer a psychological explanation for some common problems experienced by females. Texts suggest that females suffering from such conditions as dysmenorrhea or cystitis are largely responsible for their problems due to their "tense feelings about femininity" or other emotional problems.

It is essential to be aware of overt or indirect implications of biological determination in male/female behavior. Sociobiology has become so popularized in its unexamined, simplified form that it can easily find its way into high school texts. Not only should authors of texts be more alert to their use of biology, but also in the training of teachers there must be a much stronger emphasis on a critical analysis of the texts they are using and the subtle ways in which biology can be distorted. In the training of health educators, much more emphasis must be placed on examining the actual biological and physiological information presented. Just as educators have learned to screen history texts for racial bias, we must screen for sexist and racist scientific information. Health and sex education texts must be carefully studied to identify this kind of biological error or misinterpretation. However, with the time delay involved in revising texts, it would certainly be unreasonable to wait for change to occur at that level. It is the health educators who must learn not to accept on faith so-called biological facts. This means that at the level of university schools of education, students must be taught not only content and methodology, but also critical reading of materials.

For those already teaching, workshops, inservices, and continuing education programs should be presenting and emphasizing these issues. Local departments of public instruction should take responsibility for providing revised curricular materials and for providing workshops in this area.

Alternative ways to teach these topics can be offered. For example, for an educator who is looking for a way to break out of the biological determinist approach to sex roles, it might be easiest to approach the issue cross-culturally. By examining variations in sex roles in other cultures, the biological argument can be called into question. It may also be easier for students to approach a discussion of sex roles in other cultures rather than to begin by questioning the assumptions and definitions they live with every day. An interesting example that could be used is drawn from Margaret Mead's (1935) *Sex and Temperament in Three Primitive Societies*. She examined a society in which the ideal adult of both sexes is gentle and nurturing, one in which both sexes are raised to be independent and hostile, and one in which the stereotypes of masculinity and femininity in our culture are reversed. Such examples can serve as a starting point to examine assumptions about sex roles in our own society. Biology cannot be viewed as pure unalterable fact by those who teach it, or we will be doing more to enforce sex role stereotypes than we can counter with the simple inclusion of s/he in the text.

Notes

1. For further reading on these hormones, I recommend Briscoe (1978), who has written a clear informative chapter, accessible to nonscientists.
2. A great deal has been written lately on theories of aggression and the relationship to hormones. Good discussions can be found in Bleier (1984, pp. 94–101) and Sayers (1982, pp. 66–83).

Resources

Allgeier, E. R. & Allgeier, A. R. (1984). *Sexual interactions*. Lexington: MA: D. C. Heath.

Bleier, R (1984). *Science and gender: A critique of biology and its theories on women*. New York: Pergamon.

Briscoe, A. M. (1978). Hormones and gender. In E.Tobach and B. Rosoff (Eds.), *Genes and gender*: I. New York: Gordian.

Crase, D.R (1978). Significance of masculinity and femininity. In B. Q. Hafen et al., *Adolescent health: For educators and health personnel*. Salt Lake City: Brighton.

Eisenberg, A., & Eisenberg, H. (1979). *Alive and well: Decisions in health*. New York: McGraw-Hill.

Fee, E. (1983). Women's nature and scientific objectivity. In M. Lowe and R. Hubbard (Eds.), *Woman's nature: Rationalization of inequality*. New York: Pergamon.

Gay, J., Wantz, M., Slobof, H., Hooper, C., & Boskin, W. (1979). *Current health problems*. Philadelphia: W. B. Saunders.

George, P., & Lawrence, G. (1982). *Handbook for middle school teaching*. Glenview IL: Scott, Foresman.

Hafen, B. Q., Burgener, R. O., Hurley, R. D., & Peterson, R. A. (1978). *Adolescent health: For educators and health personnel*. Salt Lake City: Brighton.

Hafen, B. Q., Thygerson, A. L., & Rhodes, R.L. (1979). *Health perspectives*. Provo, UT: Brigham Young University Press.

Hubbard, R. & Lowe, M. (Eds.) (1979). *Genes and gender II: Pitfalls in research on sex and gender*. New York: Gordian.

Johns, E. B., Sutton, W. C., & Cooley, B. A. (1975). *Health for effective living* (sixth ed.). New York: McGraw-Hill.

Jones, G. S., and Jones, H. W. (1982) *Gynecology* (3rd ed.). Baltimore, MD: Williams and Wilkins.

Jones, R E. (1984). *Human reproduction and sexual behavior*. Englewood Cliffs, NJ: Prentice-Hall.

Kilmann, P. R. (1984). *Human sexuality in contemporary life*. Boston: Allyn & Bacon.

Kriegman, G. (1978). Homosexuality and the educator. In B. Q. Hafen et al., *Adolescent health: For educators and health personnel*. Salt Lake City: Brighton.

Maier, R A. (1984). *Human sexuality in perspective*. Chicago: Nelson-Hall.

Masters, W. H., & Johnson, V. E. (1966). *Human sexual response*. Boston: Little, Brown.

McCary, S. P., & McCary, J. L. (1984). *Human sexuality: Third brief edition*. Belmont, CA: Wadsworth.

Mead, M. (1935) *Sex and temperament in three primitive societies*. New York: William Morrow.

Read, D. A., & Greene, W. H. (1980). *Creative teaching in health* (3rd ed.). New York: Macmillan.

Rubin, J. Z., Provenzano, F. J., & Luria, Z. (1974). The eye of the beholder: Parent's views on sex of newborns. *American Journal of Orthopsychiatry*, 44, 512-519.

Sayers, J. (1982). *Biological politics: Feminist and anti- feminist perspectives*. New York: Tavistock.

Shearin, R. B. (1978). Adolescent sexuality. In Hafen, et al., *Adolescent health: For educators and health personnel*. Salt Lake City: Brighton.

Sommer, B. B. (1978). *Puberty and adolescence*. New York: Oxford University Press.

Sorochan, W. D., & Bender, S. J. (1978). *Teaching secondary health science*. New York: John Wiley.

Ω

In Poor Health

by Anne Rochon Ford

"If she could cope she wouldn't have called."
"When women outlive their ovaries. . ."
"When compliance is an issue with your female patient . . ."

It's pretty hard to ignore advertising slogans like these. And yet most of us never see them. They appear in medical journals seen almost exclusively by doctors. They are the advertisements pharmaceutical companies use to advertise their products. They are not really available for the scrutiny of the lay public and understandably so, since the lay public are not the targets of these ads.

Many medical journals, from which doctors get a good deal of their updated medical information, are heavily supported by the pharmaceutical companies which advertise in them. While many of these journals are subscribed to by doctors, some are sent free and unsolicited to the doctors by the companies which subsidize them.

The advertisements placed in these journals by pharmaceutical companies are advertising products for one of the wealthiest industries in North America today. (Figures vary, but the pharmaceutical industry is consistently ranked in the top four most profitable industries.) Pharmaceutical companies have one aim—to sell their product. To achieve this, they invest millions of dollars annually in slick advertisements which sometimes run three or four pages an ad. These lace the journals doctors rely on for new information. Estimates of around $3,000 per doctor per year are spent by the pharmaceutical industry in Canada to convince doctors to buy their products.

In their glossy attempts to appeal to doctors, the advertisements frequently contain images of women which perpetuate long-standing negative stereotypes. Enough research has been done on the influence which advertising has on its viewers for us to know that doctors are affected by these negative images. The most well-intentioned doctors cannot help being influenced in whatever subtle way, by the myths and stereotypes portrayed in these ads.

Ivan Illich and Thomas Szasz are among a number of social thinkers who have stated that doctors serve as agents of social control or "social gatekeepers." If we accept this theory, we should then ask how much of what doctors learn or have reinforced about women in this advertising contributes to their "gatekeeper role"? Elissa Mosher, an observer of the pharmaceutical ads has noted:

"The suggestion is that women should be medically managed with mood-altering drugs when adapting to changes in their lives. . . . The "empty-nest syndrome" and

Reprinted with permission from *Healthsharing*, Spring 1986, Toronto.

the "irritable post-menopausal woman" are advertising creations developed in timely response to women's conflicts and search for identity and fulfillment in our society."

It is important to bear in mind who the pharmaceutical companies are trying to appeal to in these ads. It is not you or me, the potential consumers of these products; it is the doctor who will choose to write that prescription. This fact raises interesting questions about why doctors choose to prescribe drugs so readily for women. The late Ruth Copperstock of the Addiction Research Foundation found through a study of a Canadian population that women are more likely than men to receive a prescription for mood-altering drugs by a ratio of 2 to 1 and that that increases with age. She further found that symptoms presented by a woman—"My neck is always tense"—were more likely to elicit from a doctor the response of a drug prescription. The same symptoms presented by a man were more likely to result in the doctor sending him for lab tests or x-rays.

A few years ago, in some research I carried out for the federal Department of Health and Welfare, I looked at the image of women in the advertising pages of six Canadian and American medical journals between 1966 and 1983. The ads used women either to advertise a drug product specific to women (such as birth control pills or estrogen replacement therapy) or to highlight the use of a drug for women, even though the drug may have been indicated for both men and women (for example, tranquilizers.) I found that a series of images of women appeared consistently I have broken these down into a few themes:

Women Can't Cope

References to coping or the inability to cope are very prevalent in the ads dealing with women, often in highlighted copy, as in "If she could cope, she wouldn't have called." Emphasis is on the woman's powerlessness, an effective device in the promotion of drug products. It is a particularly popular theme in the advertisements dealing with drugs for menopausal symptoms. The menopause is referred to in one ad as a time when women simply "are beside themselves."

The inability-to-cope theme is one that we will likely be seeing more of in years to come as increasing numbers of women attempt to juggle both families and careers outside of the home. The theme has been used most flagrantly, however, in ads for drugs for the elderly. One ad speaks volumes: "She doesn't know if she's coming or going" is the type of comment one might overhear spoken by family members in semi-hushed tones, but the idea of using it in an advertisement, complete with trick photography, is in dubious taste. This ad, from a fairly recent medical journal, is, sadly, quite typical of ads for drugs for the elderly in which a figure (more often female than male) is portrayed as hopeless, pathetic and simply unable to cope anymore.

Doctor Knows Best

Again, we need to keep in mind that these ads are geared toward doctors, not toward the general public. Doubtlessly, pharmaceutical advertisers have recognized the increasing need to tell doctors that they're OK, in spite of increasing attacks on their profession. Positive reinforcement, seen in one ad for Premarin (a drug used for estrogen replacement therapy) shows a woman in distress. It reads, "When she can't manage, you can," reassuring doctors of their powerful and important role in society and of how much their patients truly need *them*. The tactic is simple: tell someone they're terrific often enough, and they'll probably buy your product!

Many ads are geared at appealing to "the expert" in the doctor, convincingly reinforced by short, clipped sentences, as in another ad for Premarin which reads: "You're the expert. . . . Think of all you know. . . . you know who should and who should not receive estrogens. . . . You're the only expert who can help. . . . You know your patient . . . her history . . . her family . . . her expectations . . . her concerns . . . her real needs." It's hard not to imagine that the positive reinforcement in the previous ad is not a direct response to a growing self-help movement within health care. The implication behind "You're the only expert who can help" seems to be, "So don't listen to what your patient heard from another health care giver, such as a chiropractor or naturopath, or what she might know herself about her needs for estrogen or not." This theme is also illustrated in an ad for birth control which states "The local high school expert on birth control says that the Pill makes you fat . . . She is often the primary source of information for her friends and her influence could lead to pill dropout. . . . Teenagers appear to be obtaining their information on oral contraceptives from the wrong sources."

Another ad for a medication for premenstrual and menstrual problems goes overboard in reassuring doctors that they are the experts in the business of women's health care. We learn in this ad that if a woman is not consulting the doctor because she has premenstrual tension it is because she is "indulging in a kind of conspiracy of silence, deliberately telling almost anyone but you (the doctor)." We are told that such patients are "cloaking" their "valid problems" behind a "feminine mystique" (exact words). In 1966, the year this ad appeared, premenstrual tension was quite routinely dismissed as "all in your head." The paranoia displayed in this ad copy is remarkable! In light of the text, the time at which the ad appeared is noteworthy—a few years after the appearance of Betty Friedan's *Feminine Mystique* and the gradual emergence of consciousness-raising groups.

Women Are Dumb

This theme in the ads doesn't appear to target a particular age group but, rather, crosses all of them. Often the graphic illustration accompanying the ad conveys the message that women are dumb more than the actual ad text. One of the most effective ways to illustrate that women are dumb is to treat them like children. "You're looking at a patient who needs an hematinic—chances are 1 out of 3 that she won't take it!" The smaller print reads "Many patients fail to comply with the prescribed hematinic dosage regimen. In pregnant women, non-compliance has been as high as 1 out of 3." Words like "comply" and "cooperation" appear in the text as easily as they might in a manual for training animals.

One ad for vitamin supplements refers to forgetful elderly patients, using an elderly woman in the ad. The text is worded in such a way—powerful, one-line statements spaced apart—as to elicit a nod of recognition from any doctor about how dumb and forgetful his female patients are (particularly the elderly). It causes one to wonder if ads making this kind of appeal might be creating a self-fulfilling prophecy and causing doctors to *look* for behaviour in patients which may or may not be there.

Women Can Be a Real Nuisance to Others

When we see how frequently ads with this theme appear, we can't help but wonder just who these drugs are for—the woman being prescribed them or her long-suffering family she has imposed her moods and crankiness upon? Another ad for Premarin, depicting an anxiety-ridden woman in the foreground and her family members looking puzzlingly at her from the background, reads: "Almost any tranquilizer might calm her down, but at her age, estrogen may be what she really needs." Again the idea is that she has been a bother to her family because of menopausal symptoms, but you can help her family by giving her *drugs*.

In the ads, she might not only be a nuisance to her family but to other members of the community. The language in this particular ad is clearly aimed at trying to make the doctor empathize not with the woman and her problem but with the poor, long-suffering bus driver who has put up with her. We're told in the ad text that "she makes life miserable for everyone she comes in contact with." Including, of course, the doctor.

Women are complainers, the advertising says, and the more that idea can be enhanced in the ads, the more convincing is the advertiser's argument for the drug which will, of course, help to silence them. About the mother who comes into the office with a colicky baby, one advertiser asks "How often will they be back with the same complaint?" In a study conducted by Cooperstock, the stereotype which doctors have of women as complainers revealed itself clearly. In her study, 68 physicians (general practitioners) were asked to describe a typical complaintive patient (to whom they had prescribed mood-modifying drugs). There was no reference to the gender of the person in the question. In their response, 4 per cent of the physicians spontaneously mentioned men as particularly complaintive, 24 per cent didn't mention either sex, and 72 per cent referred spontaneously to female patients.

One ad shows Cooperstock's observations in practice. The copy begins by referring to genderless "patients over 50," and before we know it, the hypothetical case has become a "her."

A Woman's Biology is Her Destiny

If we are to take pharmaceutical advertising as any kind of a reflection of reality, one of the worst things about aging for women is the menopause, signalling the end of the reproductive years. The implication here is that this is also the end of her useful years. Menopause is referred to as the time "when women outlive their ovaries" and as a simple state of "ovarian failure." Language packs a strong punch in this ad text. Failure has strong connotations and implies that they *should* be continuing to function but are not. In fact, it isn't a case of failure at all. The female human ovaries are *supposed* to stop functioning at a certain point in a woman's life cycle. It is tempting to imagine the outrage from the medical community if we were to suggest in advertising that "men outlive their testicles or their prostate" (which, eventually, they do, but this is not a fact given much attention).

So much are the reproductive years valued in our society that their end can trigger "depression with moderate anxiety" as one ad states, while another speaks of using estrogen replacement therapy "for the emotional symptoms of the menopause related to estrogen deficiency." In addition, heterosexuality, marriage and motherhood are assumed in the ads, and any disruption of those states is cause for alarm—and drugs.

Women Are a Homogeneous Group

It could be argued that this assumption is true in the depiction of women in most forms of advertising, not just pharmaceutical. It is a theme which is cleverly illustrated by a photograph of a woman and a reference to "her" in the text. In a 1981 ad for an oral contraceptive, the assumption of a universal experience with first sexual encounters is evident in the copy: "her comfort and appearance is particularly important to her." Again, the copy is really more concerned about the doctor than about the woman herself. The advertisers suggest that the pill "should not cause unnecessary problems such as break-through bleed-

ing, weight gain or acne which could jeopardize compliance." And again to reinforce the doctor's control over the patient they are reminded in the ad, "You want to be sure she stays on her pill. . . ."

Pharmaceutical company executives have also found it useful to adopt a language of pseudo-liberation by coopting the language of the women's movement. The "You've come a long way, baby" cigarette campaign was part of the same trend. One ad for an antibacterial drug, asks whether this particular drug "discriminates in favour of women." The full-page visual for this ad is of three long-haired jean-clad young women trying to convey to doctors that they (the advertisers) are with the times.

Another ad for Premarin tries to appeal to a sense of justice in doctors. It asks whether they don't think that it's a woman's "right" to be prescribed estrogen replacement therapy and thereby be entitled to "her own special quality of life." The ad copy tries to lead the doctor to believing that we have to accept that women have certain rights nowadays, and we owe it to them to be able to exercise their right to take this drug. In contrast with this attempt at showing women as having certain "rights," the copy writer relies on dated euphemisms like "the change of life" in referring to menopause.

When I have spoken with medical personnel about some of the images I have come across in pharmaceutical advertising, they reminded me that things really *are* improving—aren't they?—and that those horrible ads were from back in the sixties. It *is* true that the worst of the worst, the ads which provoke more of a laugh than a sense of anger, are found in journals from the sixties and seventies. The advertisers have had to clean up their acts to some extent, but in trying to do that, they have simply become slicker in their presentation. One notable improvement is that women doctors are appearing in the ads with greater frequency and women in nontraditional occupations are being portrayed. But there is still a need for improvement. The gratuitous use of attractive women to sell products is as prevalent today in pharmaceutical advertising as it is in most trade advertising. The depiction of elderly women is often questionable, but is probably as much a reflection of how our society feels about the elderly as of how it feels about women.

Perhaps a more important question is whether it is ethical at all to advertise drugs. In the late 1970s, the Consumer Association of Canada made valiant attempts to have all drug advertising to doctors banned. Although they were not successful in their attempts, a closer examination of how women are depicted in the advertising should provide enough incentive for some of us to pick up the torch.

Ω

The Picture of Health:
How Textbook Photographs Construct Health

by Mariamne H. Whatley

Photographs in textbooks may serve the roles of breaking up a long text, emphasizing or clarifying information in the text, attracting the buyer (the professor, teacher, or administrator who selects texts), and engaging the reader. But photographs cannot be dismissed merely as either decorative additions or straightforward illustrations of the text. Photographs are often far more memorable than the passages they illustrate and, because they are seen as objective representations of reality, rather than artists' constructions (Barthes, 1977), may have more impact than drawings or other forms of artwork. In textbooks, photographs can carry connotations, intentional or not, never stated in the text. The selection of photographs for a text is not a neutral process that simply involves being "realistic" or "objective"; selection must take into account issues such as audience expectations and dominant meanings in a given cultural/historical context (Whatley, 1988). In order to understand the ideological work of a textbook, a critique of the photographs is as crucial as a critique of the text itself.

Using ideological analysis to identify patterns of inclusion and exclusion, I examined photographs in the seven best-selling, college-level personal health textbooks. This chapter presents the results of that research. In the first part of the analysis, I examined the photographs that represent "health," describing who and what is "healthy," according to these representations. In the second part of the analysis, I determined where those excluded from the definition of health are represented in the approximately 1,100 remaining photographs in the texts.

Selling Health in Textbooks

Generally, textbook authors do not select specific photographs but may give publishers general descriptions of the type of photographs they wish to have included (for example, a scene showing urban crowding, a woman in a nontraditional job). Due to the great expense involved, new photographs are not usually taken specifically for texts. Instead publishers hire photo researchers to find appropriate photographs, drawing on already existing photographic collections. The result is that the choice of photographs depends on what is already available, and what is available depends to some extent on what has been requested in the past. In fact, because the same sources of photographs may be used by a number of different publishers, identical photographs may appear in competing books. Although authors may have visions of their books' "artwork," the reality may be limited by the selection already on the market. In addition, editors and publishers make decisions about what "artwork" will sell or is considered appropriate, sometimes overruling the authors' choices.

Photographs, especially cover-photos and special color sections, are considered features that sell textbooks, but they also can work as part of another selling process. Textbooks, in many cases, sell the reader a system of belief. An economics text, for example, may "sell" capitalism, and a science text may "sell" the scientific method, both of which help support dominant ideologies. Health textbooks may be even more invested in this selling process because, in addition to convincing readers to "believe" in health, their "success" depends on the readers' adoption of very specific personal behavioral programs to attain health. Health textbooks hold up the ideals of "total wellness" or "holistic fitness" as goals we can attain by exercising, eating right, reducing stress, and avoiding drugs. The readers' belief in health and their ability to attain it by specific behaviors is seen by many health educators as necessary to relevant educational goals; the belief in a clearly marked pathway to health is also part of a process of the commodification of health.

In North America and Western Europe, health is currently a very marketable commodity. This can be seen in its most exaggerated form in the United States in the proliferation of "health" clubs, in the trend among hospitals and clinics to attract a healthy clientele by advertising their abilities to make healthy people healthier (Worcester & Whatley, 1988), and in the advertisements that link a wide range of products, such as high fiber cereals and calcium rich antacids, to health. In a recent article in a medical journal, a physician examined this commercialization of health:

Health is industrialized and commercialized in a fashion that enhances many people's dissatisfaction with their health. Advertisers, manufacturers, advocacy groups, and proprietary health care corporations promote the myth that good health can be purchased; they market products and services that purport to deliver the consumer into the promised land of wellness. (Barsky, 1988, p. 415)

Reprinted by permission of the publisher from Ellsworth, Elizabeth and Whatley, Mariamne, THE IDEOLOGY OF IMAGES IN EDUCATIONAL MEDIA. (New York: Teachers College Press, © 1990 by Teachers College, Columbia University. All rights reserved.) "The Picture of Health: How Textbook Photographs Construct Health", pp. 121–140.

Photographs in health textbooks can play a role in this selling of health similar to that played by visual images in advertising a product in the popular media. According to Berger (1972), the role of advertising or publicity is to

make the spectator marginally dissatisfied with his present way of life. Not with the way of life of society, but with his own place within it. It suggests that if he buys what it is offering, his life will become better. It offers him an improved alternative to what he is. (p. 142)

The ideal of the healthy person and the healthy lifestyle can be seen as the "improved alternative" to what we are. It can be assumed that most of us will be dissatisfied with ourselves when measured against that ideal, just as most women are dissatisfied with their body shapes and sizes when compared with ideal media representations.

In effective advertising campaigns the visual image is designed to provoke powerful audience responses. In health textbooks the visual representation of "health" is calculated to sell, and it is likely to have a greater impact on the reader than discussions about lengthened life expectancy, reduction in chronic illness, or enhanced cardiovascular fitness. The image of health, not health itself, may be what most people strive for. In the attempt to look healthy, many sacrifice health. For example, people go through very unhealthy practices to lose "extra" weight that is in itself not unhealthy; being slim, however, is a basic component of the *appearance* of health. A recent survey found that people who eat healthy foods do so for their appearance and *not* for their health. "Tanning parlors" have become common features of health and fitness centers, though tanning in itself is unhealthy. As with being slim, having a good tan contributes to the appearance of what is currently defined as health.

The use of color photographs is particularly effective in selling the healthy image, for, as Berger (1972) points out, both oil painting and color photography "use similar highly tactile means to play upon the spectator's sense of acquiring the *real* thing which the image shows" (p. 141). The recent improvement in quality and the increase in number of color photographs in textbooks provide an opportunity to sell the image of health even more effectively than black and white photographs could.

Selection of Textbooks

Rather than trying to examine all college-level personal health (as opposed to community health) textbooks, I selected the best-selling ones, since those would have the widest impact. Based on the sales figures provided by the publisher of one popular text, I selected seven texts published from 1985 to 1988. Sales of these textbooks ranged from approximately 15,000 to 50,000 for each edition. (Complete bibliographic information on these textbooks is provided in the Appendix. Author-date information to these textbooks refer to the Appendix, rather than the chapter references.) Obviously, the sales figures depend on the number of years a specific edition has been in print.

For one text (Insel & Roth, 1988), I examined the newest edition (for which there could be no sales figures), based on the fact that its previous editions had high sales. A paper on the readability of personal health textbooks (Overman, Mimms, & Harris, 1987), using a similar selection process, examined the seven top-selling textbooks for the 1984–85 school year, plus three other random titles. Their list has an overlap with mine of only four texts, which may be due to a number of factors, including differences in editions and changing sales figures.

Analysis I: Healthy-Image Photographs

The first step in my analysis was a close examination of the photographs that I saw as representing "health," the images intended to show who is healthy and illustrate the healthy lifestyle. These included photographs used on covers, opposite title pages, and as openers to units or chapters on wellness or health (as opposed to specific topics such as nutrition, drugs, and mental health). While other pictures throughout the texts may represent healthy individuals, the ones selected, by their placement in conjunction with the book title or chapter title, can be seen as clearly connoting "health." I will refer to these as healthy-image photographs. I included in this analysis only photographs in which there were people. While an apple on a cover conveys a message about health, I was interested only in the question of who is healthy.

A total of 18 different photographs fit my criteria for representing health. I have eliminated three of these from discussion: the cover from Insel and Roth (1988) showing flowers and, from Dinitiman and Greenberg (1986), both the cover photograph of apples and the health unit opener of a movie still from the *Wizard of Oz*. (This textbook uses movie stills as openers for all chapters; this moves the photograph away from its perceived "objective" status toward that of an obvious construction.)

There are a number of points of similarity in the 15 remaining photographs. In several photographs (windsurfing, hang gliding), it is hard to determine race, but all individuals whose faces can clearly be seen are white. Except for those who cannot be seen clearly and for several of the eight skydivers in a health unit opener, all are young. No one in these photographs is fat or has any identifiable physical disability. Sports dominate the activities, which, with the exception of rhythmic gymnastics and volleyball played in a gym, are outdoor activities in nonurban settings. Five of these involve beaches or open water. All the activities are leisure activities, with no evidence of work. While it is impossible to say anything definitive about class from these photographs, several of the activities are expensive (hang gliding, skydiving, windsurfing), and others may take money and/or sufficient time off from work to get to places where they can be done (beaches, biking in countryside); these suggest middle-class activities, whether the actual individuals are middle class or not. In several photographs (windsurfing, hang gliding, swimming) it is hard to determine gender. However, excluding these and the large group of male runners in a cross-country race, the overall balance is 23 males to 18 females, so it does seem that there is an attempt to show women both as healthy individuals and in active roles.

How Health Is Portrayed

A detailed analysis of three photographs can provide insight into how these text photographs construct health. The first is a color photograph of a volleyball game on a beach from the back cover of *Understanding Your Health* (Payne & Hahn, 1986). As with most of these images of health, the setting is outdoors, clearly at a distance from urban life. The steep rock walls that serve as a backdrop to the volleyball game additionally isolate the natural beach setting from the invasion of cars[1] and other symbols of "man-made" environmental destruction and ill health. The volleyball players appear to have escaped into a protected idyllic setting of sun, sand, and, we assume, water. They also have clearly escaped from work, since they are engaged in a common leisure activity associated with picnics and holidays. None of them appears to be contemplating the beauty of the natural setting, but merely using it as a location for a game that could go on anywhere in which there is room to set up a net.

The photograph is framed in such a way that the whole net and area of the "court" are not included, so that some players may also not be visible. On one side of the net are three women and a man, on the other two women and a man. While this is not necessarily a representation of heterosexual interactions, it can be read that way. Two players are the focus of the picture, with the other five essentially out of the action. The woman who has just hit the ball, with her back toward the camera, has her arms outstretched, her legs slightly spread, and one foot partly off the ground. The man who is waiting for the ball is crouched slightly, looking expectantly upward. Her body is partially superimposed on his, her leg crossed over his. This is essentially an interaction between one man and one woman. It would not work the same way if the key players were both female or both male, since part of the "healthiness" of this image appears to be the heterosexual interaction. For heterosexual men, this scene might be viewed as ideal—a great male-female ratio on an isolated beach; perhaps this is their reward for having arrived at the end of this book—this photograph is on the *back* cover—attaining their goal of health.

All the volleyball players are white, young, and slim. The woman farthest left in the frame appears slightly heavier than the others; she is the only woman wearing a shirt, rather than a bikini top, and is also wearing shorts. Besides being an outsider in terms of weight, dress, and location in the frame, she is the only woman who clearly has short hair (three have long hair tied back in ponytails, one cannot be seen completely). Perhaps she can move "inside" by losing weight and changing her image. As viewers, we are just a few steps beyond the end of the court and are also outsiders. As with pick-up games, there is room for observers to enter the game—if they are deemed acceptable by the other players. By achieving health, perhaps the observer can step into the game, among the young, white, slim, heterosexual, and physically active. But if the definition of health includes young, white, slim, heterosexual, and physically active, many observers are relegated permanently to the outside.

If this photograph serves as an invitation to join in the lifestyle of the young and healthy, the second photograph, facing the title page of another book, serves the same function, with the additional written message provided by the title of the book—*An Invitation to Health* (Hales & Williams, 1986). The photograph is of six bicycle riders, three women and three men, resting astride their bicycles. This photograph is in black and white, so it is perhaps not as seductive as the sunny color of the first cover. However, the people in this photograph are all smiling directly at the viewer (rather than just leaving a space in back where the viewer could join in). Two of the women, in the middle and the right, have poses and smiles that could be described as flirtatious. They are taking a break from their riding, so it is an opportune moment to join the fun of being healthy.

As with the volleyball players, all the bicycle riders are young, slim, white, and apparently fit. Another similarity is the amount of skin that is exposed. Playing volleyball on the beach and riding bikes in warm weather are activities for which shorts and short-sleeved shirts are preferable to sweatpants and sweatshirts. The choice of these types of activities to represent health results in photographs in which legs and arms are not covered. Appearing healthy apparently involves no need to cover up unsightly flab, "cellulite," or stretch marks. A healthy body is a body that can be revealed.

The bikers are in a fairly isolated, rural setting. While they are clearly on the road, it appears to be a rural, relatively untraveled road. Two cars can be seen far in the distance, and there may also be a house in the distance on the right side of the frame. Otherwise, the landscape is dominated by hills, trees, and grass, the setting and the activity clearly distance the bike riders both from urban life and from work.

In a third photograph, a health unit chapter opener (Levy, Dignan, & Shirreffs, 1987), we can see a possible beginning to alternative images of health. The players in this volleyball game are still slim, young, and apparently white. However, the setting is a gym, which could be urban, suburban, or rural. While four players are wearing shorts, one woman is wearing sweatpants; there are T-shirts rather than bikini tops, and gym socks rather than bare legs. The impression is that they are there to play a hard game of volleyball rather than to bask in the sun and each other's gaze. Two men are going for the ball from opposite sides, while a woman facing the net is clearly ready to move. Compared with the other volleyball scene, this photograph gives more of a sense of action, of actual physical exertion, as well as a sense of real people, rather than models.

It is interesting to imagine how healthy the volleyball players and bike riders actually are, underneath the appearance of health. The outdoor groups, especially the beach group, are susceptible to skin cancer from overexposure to the sun. Cycling is a healthy aerobic sport, though it can be hard on the knees and back. It is particularly surprising, however, to find that the bikers represented in a health text are not wearing helmets, thus modeling behavior that is considered very risky. Compared with biking, volleyball is the kind of weekend activity that sends the enthusiastic untrained player home with pulled muscles, jammed fingers, and not much of a useful workout. The question also arises as to how the particularly thin women on the beach achieved their weight—by unhealthy weight-loss diets, by anorexia, by purging? The glowing image of health may have little to do with the reality.

Similarities to Advertising

Shortly after I began the research for this chapter, I was startled, while waiting for a movie to begin, to see a soft drink advertisement from which almost any still could have been substituted for a healthy-image photograph I had examined. There were the same thin, young, white men and women frolicking on the beach, playing volleyball, and windsurfing. They were clearly occupying the same territory: a never-never land of eternal sunshine, eternal youth, and eternal leisure. Given my argument that these textbook photographs are selling health, the similarities between soft drink advertising images and textbook healthy images are not surprising. They are appealing to the same groups of people, and they are both attempting to create an association between a desirable lifestyle and their product. You can enjoy this fun in the sun if you are part of the "Pepsi generation" or think "Coke is it" or follow the textbook's path to health. These can be considered one variant of the lifestyle format in advertising, as described by Leiss, Kline, and Jhally (1986).

Here the activity invoked in text or image becomes the central cue for relating the person, product, and setting codes. Lifestyle ads commonly depict a variety of leisure activities (entertaining, going out, holidaying, relaxing). Implicit in each of these activities, however, is the placing of the product within a consumption style by its link to an activity. (p.210)

Even a naive critic of advertising could point out that drinking a carbonated beverage could not possibly help anyone attain this lifestyle; on the other hand, it might be easier to accept that the same lifestyle is a result of achieving health. However, the association between health and this leisure lifestyle is as much a construction as that created in the soft drink ads. Following all the advice in these textbooks as to diet, exercise, coping with stress, and attaining a healthy sexuality will not help anyone achieve this sun-and-fun fantasy lifestyle any more than drinking Coke or Pepsi would.

These healthy-image photographs borrow directly from popular images of ideal lifestyles already very familiar to viewers through advertising[2] and clearly reflect the current marketing of health. The result is that health is being sold with as much connection to real life and real people's needs

as liquor ads that suggest major lifestyle changes associated with changing one's brand of scotch.

Analysis II: Where Are the Excluded?

For each textbook, the next step was to write brief descriptions of all other photographs in the books, totaling approximately 1,100. The results of the analysis of the healthy image photographs suggested a focus on specific aspects of the description of the individuals and activities in examining the remaining 1,100 photographs. The areas I selected for discussion are those in which "health" is linked to specific lifestyles or factors that determine social position/power in our society. I described the setting, the activity, and a number of observable points about the people, including gender, race, age, physical ability/disability, and weight. These photographs were all listed by chapter and when appropriate, by particular topic in that chapter. For example, a chapter on mental health might have images of positive mental health and also images representing problems such as severe depression or stress. These descriptions of photographs were used to establish whether there were images with characteristics not found in the healthy images and, if so, the context in which these characteristics were present. For example, finding no urban representations among the healthy images, I identified topic headings under which I did find photographs of urban settings.

White, young, thin, physically abled, middle-class people in the healthy images represent the mythical norm with whom the audience is supposed to identify. This not only creates difficulties in identification for whose who do not meet these criteria, but also creates a limiting and limited definition of health. I examined the photographs that did not fit the healthy-image definition to find the invisible—those absent from the healthy images: people of color, people with physical disabilities, fat people, and old people. I also attempted to identify two other absences—the urban setting and work environment. Because there were no obvious gender discrepancies in the healthy images, I did not examine gender as a separate category.

People of Color

After going through the remaining photographs, it was clear that there had been an attempt to include photographs of people of color in a variety of settings, but no obvious patterns emerged. In a previous paper, I examined representations of African-Americans in sexuality texts, finding that positive attempts at being nonracist could be undermined by the patterns of photographs in textbooks that, for example, draw on stereotypes and myths of "dangerous" black sexuality (Whatley, 1988). Rather than reviewing all the representations of people of color in these health textbooks, I will simply repeat what I pointed out earlier—that there is a strong and clear *absence* of photographs of people of color in the healthy-images category. People of color may appear as healthy people elsewhere in the text, but not on covers, title pages, and chapter openers. If publishers wanted to correct this situation, they could simply substitute group photographs that show some diversity for the current all-white covers and title pages.

People with Disabilities

From the healthy-image photographs, it is apparent that people with visible physical disabilities are excluded from the definition of healthy. Therefore, I examined the contexts in which people with disabilities appear in the other photographs. Out of the approximately 1,100 photos, only 9 show people with physical disabilities, with 2 of these showing isolated body parts only (arthritic hands and knees). One shows an old woman being pushed in a wheelchair, while the six remaining photographs all are "positive" images: a number of men playing wheelchair basketball, a man in a wheelchair doing carpentry, a woman walking with her arm around a man in a wheelchair, a man with an amputated leg walking across Canada, children with cancer (which can be seen both as a disease and a disability) at a camp (these last two both in a cancer chapter), and a wheelchair racer. However, three of these six are from one textbook (Payne & Hahn, 1986), and two are from another (Levy, Dignan, & Shirreffs, 1987), so the inclusion of these few positive images is over-shadowed by the fact that three books show absolutely none. In addition, none of these positive images are of women, and the only disabilities represented are those in which an individual uses a wheelchair or has cancer.

This absence of representation of disabled people, particularly women, clearly reflects the invisibility of the physically disabled in our society.

It would be easy to blame the media for creating and maintaining many of the stereotypes with which the disabled still have to live. But the media only reflect attitudes that already exist in a body-beautiful society that tends to either ignore or ostracize people who don't measure up to the norm. This state of "invisibility" is particularly true for disabled women. (Israel & McPherson, 1983, pp. 4–15)

In a society that values the constructed image of health over health itself, a person with a disability does not fit the definition of healthy. In addition, since the person with a disability may be seen as representing a "failure" of modern medicine and health care (Matthews, 1983), there is no place for her or him in a book that promises people that they can attain health. The common attitude that disability and health are incompatible was expressed in its extreme by a faculty member who questioned the affirmative action statement in a position description for a health education faculty member; he wanted to know if encouraging "handicapped" people to apply was appropriate for a *health* education position.

Looking at the issue of health education and disabilities, it should be clear that it is easier for able-bodied people to be healthy, so more energy should be put into helping people with disabilities maximize their health. Able-bodied people often have more access to exercise, to rewarding work (economically[3] as well as emotionally), to leisure activities, and to health care facilities. Health care practitioners receive very little training about health issues relating to disability (self-care, sexual health), though they may receive information about specific pathologies, such as multiple sclerosis or muscular dystrophy. The inability to see, hear, or walk need not be the impairments to health they often are considered in our society. Health education is an obvious place to begin to change the societal attitudes toward disability that can help lead to poor physical and emotional health for disabled people. Health textbooks could present possibilities for change by showing ways that both disabled and able-bodied people can maximize health, and this could be done in both the text and the photographs. For example, one of those color chapter openers could include people with disabilities as healthy people. This might mean changing some of the representative "healthy" activities, such as windsurfing. While there are people with disabilities who participate in challenging and risky physical activities, there is no need for pressure to achieve *beyond* what would be expected of the able-bodied.[4] Showing a range of healthy activities that might be more accessible to both the physically disabled and the less physically active able-bodied would be appropriate.

Fat People

There are no fat people in the healthy-image photographs. Some people who agree with the rest of my analysis may here respond, "Of course not!" because there is a common assumption in our society that being thin is healthy and that any weight gain reduces health. In fact, evidence shows that being overweight (but not obese) is *not unhealthy*. In many cases, being very fat is a lot healthier than the ways people are encouraged to attempt to reduce weight—from extreme low-calorie diets, some of which are fatal, to stomach stapling and other surgeries (Norsigian, 1986). In addition, dieting does not work for 99 percent of dieters, with 95 percent ending up heavier than before they started. Repeated dieting stresses the heart, as well as other organs (Norsigian, 1986). Our national obsession with thinness is certainly one factor leading to an unhealthy range of eating behaviors, including, but not limited to, bulimia and anorexia. While health textbooks warn against dangerous diets and "eating disorders," and encourage safe, sensible weight-loss diets, they do nothing to counter the image of thin as healthy.

Defining which people are "fat" in photographs is obviously problematic. In doing so, I am giving my subjective interpretation of what I see as society's definition of ideal weight. The photographs I have identified as "fat" are of people who by common societal definitions would be seen as "needing to lose weight." In the United States most women are dissatisfied with their own body weight, so are more likely to place themselves in the "need to lose weight" category than to give that label to someone else of the same size.

Not counting people who were part of a crowd scene, I found 14 photographs that clearly showed people who were fat. One appeared in a chapter on the health care system with a caption referring to "lack of preventive maintenance leading to medical problems" (Carroll & Miller, 1986, p. 471), one in a chapter on drinking, and one under cardiovascular problems. The remaining 11 appeared in chapters on weight control or diet and nutrition. Of the 11, one was the "before" of "before and after" weight-loss photographs. One showed a woman walking briskly as part of a "fat-management program" (Mullen, Gold, Belcastro, & McDermott, 1986, p. 125); that was the most positive of the images. Most of the photographs were of people doing nothing but being fat or adding to that fat (eating or cooking). Three of the photographs showed women with children, referring by caption or topic heading to causes of obesity, either genetic or environmental. Only 3 of the 11 photographs were of men. In these photographs, it seems we are not being shown a person or an activity, but a disease—a disease called obesity that we all might "catch" if we don't carefully follow the prescriptions for health. Fat people's excess weight is seen as their fault for not following these prescriptions. This failure results from a lack of either willpower or restraint, as implied by the photographs that show fat people eating and thus both draw on and lend support to the myth that fat people eat too much. The only health problem of fat people is seen as their weight; if that were changed, all other problems would presumably disappear. As pointed out earlier, the health problems of losing excess weight, particularly in the yo-yo pattern of weight loss/gain, may be greater than those created by the extra weight. In addition, the emotional and mental health problems caused by our society's fatphobia may be more serious than the physical problems (Worcester, 1988). These texts strongly reinforce fatphobia by validating it with health "science."

Health educators who consciously work against racism and sexism should carefully reevaluate how our attitudes help perpetuate discrimination against all groups. As Nancy Worcester (1988) points out,

The animosity towards fat people is such a fundamental part of our society, that people who have consciously worked on their other prejudices have not questioned their attitude towards body weight. People who would not think of laughing at a sexist or racist joke ridicule and make comments about fat people without recognizing that they are simply perpetuating another set of attitudes which negatively affect a whole group of people. (p.234)

An alternative approach would be to recognize that people would be healthier if less pressure were put on them to lose weight. Fat people can benefit from exercise, if it is accessible and appropriate (low impact aerobics, for example), without the goal needing to be weight loss (Sternhell, 1985). Photographs of "not thin" people, involved in a variety of activities, could be scattered throughout the text, and the pictures of those labeled obese could be eliminated completely. We all know what an obese person looks like; we do not need to have that person held up as a symbol of both unhealthiness and lack of moral character.

Old People

The healthy-image photographs show people who appeared to be predominantly in their teens and twenties, which is the age group toward which these college texts would be geared. Rather subjectively, as with the issue of weight, I will describe as old[5] those who appear to be about 65 or older. Obviously I probably judged incorrectly on some photographs, but since the representations seem to be skewed toward the young or the old, with the middle-aged not so prominent, my task was relatively easy. I identified 84 photographs that contained people I classified as old. Of these, 52 appeared in chapters specifically on aging or growing older, 10 appeared in chapters on death and dying, and the remaining 22 were distributed in a wide range of topics. Of these 22, several still focused on the issue of age. For example, a photograph of an old heterosexual couple in chapter entitled "Courtship and Marriage" is captioned, "While some people change partners repeatedly, many others spend their lifetime with a single spouse" (Carroll & Miller, 1986, p. 271). One text showed a similar photo and caption of a heterosexual couple, but also included an old gay male couple on the next page (Levy, Dignan, & Shirreffs, 1987). This represents an important step in terms of deghettoization of gay and lesbian images, and a broadening of views about sexuality and aging. Two photos showed old people as "non-traditional students"; another depicted a man running after recovering from a stroke; and yet another featured George Burns as a representative of someone who has lived a long life. In others of the 22, the age is incidental, as in a man painting (mental health), people shopping in an open market (nutrition), people walking (fitness), a man smoking.

As the societally stereotyped *appearance* of health diminishes, as occurs with aging, it is assumed that health unavoidably diminishes. In fact, while there is some inevitable biological decline with age, many health problems can be averted by good nutrition, exercise, and preventive health care. Many of the health problems of aging have economic, rather than biological, causes, such as lack of appropriate health insurance coverage (Sidel, 1986). In a society that is afraid to face aging, people may not be able to accept that they will experience the effects of aging that they so carefully avoid (if they are lucky enough to live that long). In addition, as with disability, the people who may need to do more to maintain health are those being most ignored.

It is significant that these texts have sections on aging, which contain many positive images, but it is also crucial that health be seen as something that can be attained and maintained by people of all ages. The attempt to include representations of aging in these books must be expanded so that people of all ages are seen to be able to be healthy—a state now seemingly, in those images of health, to be enjoyed only by the young.

Urban Setting

The healthy-image photographs showing outdoor scenes are situated at the beach or in other nonurban settings; it is possible some were set in city parks, but there are no urban markers in the photographs. Bike riding, running, kicking a soccer ball, playing volleyball can all be done in urban settings, though the hang gliding and sky diving would obviously be difficult. Considering the high percentage of the U.S. population that lives in cities (and the numbers of those that cannot easily get out), it seems that urban settings should be represented in the texts. Of the 28 other photographs I identified as clearly having urban settings, I could see only 4 as positive. Two of these showed outdoor vegetable/fruit markets, one showed bike riding as a way of both reducing pollution and getting exercise in the city, and one showed a family playing ball together. Of the rest, 9 appeared in chapters on the environment, with negative images of urban decay, smog, and crowded streets; 10 were in chapters on mental health or stress, showing scenes representing loneliness, stress, or anger, such as a crowded subway or a potential fight on a street corner. Drinking and drug chapters had two urban scenes: "skid row" alcoholics and an apparently drunk man unconscious on the street. There were also three urban scenes in sexuality chapters—two of streets with marquees for sex shows and one showing a "man 'flashing' Central Park" (Payne & Hahn, 1986, p. 348).

There is a clear message that it is unhealthy to live in the city. While this is partly true—that is, the city may have increased pollution of various kinds, specific stresses, less access to certain forms of exercise, and other problems— there are healthy ways to live in a city. One of the roles of health education should be to help us recognize healthier options within the limits imposed on us by economic or other factors. Rather than conveying the message that urban dwelling inevitably condemns people to ill health (unless they can afford to get away periodically to the beach or the mountains), scenes showing health within the city could be presented.

Options for positive images include scenes of outdoor activities in what are clearly city parks, people enjoying cultural events found more easily in cities, gardening in a vacant lot, or a neighborhood block party. Urban settings are excellent for representing walking as a healthy activity. City dwellers are more likely to walk to work, to shopping, and to social activities than are suburbanites, many of whom habitually drive. Urban walking can be presented as free, accessible, and healthy in terms of exercise, stress reduction, and reducing pollution. More indoor activities could be shown so that the external environment is not seen as a determinant of "healthy" activity. These might give a sense of the possibilities for health within what otherwise might appear to be a very dirty, dangerous, stressful place to be.

Work and Leisure

The healthy-image photographs I analyzed were all associated with leisure activities, so I tried to establish how these texts represent work in relationship to health. For this analysis, all photographs of health care workers were excluded, since these are used predominantly to illustrate health or medical issues. Of the 16 other photographs showing people at work, 4 were related to discussions of sex roles and women doing nontraditional work (phone "lineman," lawyer). This seems part of a positive trend in textbooks to reduce sexism. An obvious next step would be to show women in nontraditional work roles without commenting on them, as is done with a number of photographs of women as doctors. Six of the photographs of work accompany discussions of stress. Besides stress, there are no illustrations of health hazards at work except for one photograph of a farm worker being sprayed with pesticides. Three positive references to work show someone working at a computer (illustrating self-development), a man in a wheelchair doing carpentry, and an old man continuing to work.

Overall, the number of photographs representing work seems low, considering the amount of time we put into work during our lifetime. Blue-collar work is represented by trash collectors in an environmental health section, police officers in a weight control chapter, firefighters under stress, a construction worker in the opener for a stress chapter, the farm worker mentioned above, and women in nontraditional work. Blue-collar work is seen in terms of neither potential health hazards beyond stress nor the positive health aspects of working. The strongest connection between health and work presented involves the stress of white-collar jobs (symbolized by a man at a desk talking on the phone). The message seems to be that health is not affected by work, unless it is emotionally stressful.

The photographs in this book seem to be aimed at middle-class students who assume they will become white-collar workers or professionals who can afford leisure activities, both in terms of time and money. Those who work in obviously physically dangerous jobs, such as construction work, or in jobs that have stress as only one of many health hazards, are rarely portrayed. These people are also likely not to be able to afford recreation such as hang gliding (and also might not need the stimulus of physical risk taking if their job is physically risky in itself). These photographs serve to compartmentalize work as if it were not part of life and not relevant to health.

Rather than selecting photographs that reinforce the work-leisure split and the alienation of the worker from work, editors could include photographs that show the health rewards of work and the real health risks of a wide variety of work. For example, a photograph of a group of workers talking on a lunch break could be captioned, "Many people find strong support networks among their co-workers." Another photograph could be of a union meeting, illustrating that work-related stress is reduced when we have more control over the conditions of our work. In addition the mental health benefits of a rewarding job might be emphasized, perhaps in contrast with the stress of unemployment. Health risks, and ways to minimize them, could be illustrated with photographs ranging from typists using video display terminals to mine workers. A very important addition would be inclusion in the healthy-image photographs of some representation of work.

Conclusion

The definition of health that emerges from an examination of the healthy-image photographs is very narrow. The healthy person is young, slim, white, physically abled, physically active, and, apparently, comfortable financially. Since these books are trying to "sell" their image of health to college students, the photographs presumably can be seen as representing people whom the students would wish to become. Some students, however, cannot or may not wish to become part of this vision of the healthy person. For example, students of color may feel alienated by this all-white vision. What may be most problematic is that in defining the healthy person, these photographs also define *who can become healthy*. By this definition many are excluded from the potential for health: people who are physically disabled, no longer young, not slim (unless they can lose weight, even if in unhealthy ways), urban dwellers, poor people, and people of color. For various social, economic, and political reasons, these may be among the least healthy groups in the United States, but the potential for health is there if the health care and health education systems do not disenfranchise them.

The healthy-image photographs represent the healthy lifestyle, not in the sense of the lifestyle that will help someone attain health, but the white, middle-class, heterosexual, leisure, active lifestyle that is the reward of attaining health. These glowing images imitate common advertising representations. An ice chest of beer would not be out of place next to the volleyball players on the beach, and a soft drink slogan would fit well with the windsurfers or sky divers. It must be remembered, however, that while college students may be the market for beer, soft drinks, and "health," they are not the market for textbooks. Obviously, the biggest single factor affecting a student's purchase of a text is whether it is required. The decision may also be based on how much reading in the book is assigned, whether exam questions will be drawn from the text, its potential future usefulness, or its resale value.

The market for textbooks is the faculty who make text selections for courses (Coser, Kadushin, & Powell, 1982). While the photographs may be designed to create in students a desire for health, they are also there to sell health educators the book. Therefore, health educators should take some time examining the representations in these texts, while questioning their own definitions of who is healthy and who can become healthy. Do they actually wish to imply that access to health is limited to young, white, slim, middle-class, physically abled, and physically active people? If health educators are committed to increasing the potential for health for *all* people, then the focus should not be directed primarily at those for whom health is most easily attained and maintained. Rethinking the images that represent health may help restructure health educators' goals.

It is an interesting exercise to try to envision alternative healthy-image photographs. Here is one of my choices for a cover photograph: An old woman of color, sitting on a chair with a book in her lap, is looking out at a small garden that has been reclaimed from an urban backlot.

Acknowledgments. I would like to thank Nancy Worcester, Julie D'Acci, Sally Lesher, and Elizabeth Ellsworth for their critical readings of this chapter and their valuable suggestions.

Notes

1. Cars appear in health textbook photographs primarily in the context of either environmental concerns or the stresses of modern life.

2. Occasionally, photographs used were actually taken for advertising purposes. For example, in a chapter on exercise there is a full-page color photograph of a runner with the credit "Photo by Jerry LaRocca for Nike" (Insel & Roth, 1988, p. 316).

3. Examining the wages of disabled women can give a sense of the potential economic problems: "The 1981 Census revealed that disabled women earn less than 24 cents for each dollar earned by nondisabled men; black disabled women earn 12 cents for each dollar. Disabled women earn approximately 52 percent of what nondisabled women earn" (Saxton & Howe, 1987, p xii).

4. "Supercrip" is a term sometimes used among people with disabilities to describe people with disabilities who go beyond what would be expected of those with no disabilities. It should not be necessary to be a one-legged ski champion or a blind physician to prove that people with disabilities deserve the opportunities available to the able-bodied. By emphasizing the individual "heroes," the focus shifts away from societal barriers and obstacles to individual responsibility to excel.

5. I am using "old" rather than "older" for two reasons that have been identified by many writing about ageism. "Older" seems a euphemism that attempts to lessen the impact of discussing someone's age, along with such terms as senior citizen or golden ager. The second point is the simple question: "Older than whom?"

References

Barsky, A.J. (1988). The paradox of health. *The New England Journal of Medicine, 318* (7), 414–418.

Barthes, R. (1977). *Image-music-text.* (S. Heath, Trans.). New York: Hill and Wang.

Berger, J. (1972). *Ways of seeing.* London: British Broadcasting Corporation and Penguin Books.

Coser, L.A., Kadushin, C., & Powell, W. (1982). *Books: The culture and commerce of publishing*. New York: Basic Books.

Israel, P., & McPherson, C. (1982). Introduction. In G.F. Matthews, *Voices from the shadows: women with disabilities speak out* (pp. 13–21). Toronto: Women's Educational Press.

Leiss, W., Kline, S., & Jhally, S. (1986). *Social communication in advertising: Persons, products and images of well-being*. Toronto: Methuen.

Matthews, G.F. (1983). *Voices from the shadows: Women with disabilities speak out*. Toronto: Women's Educational Press.

Norsigian, J. (1986, May/June). dieting is dangerous to your health. *The Network News*. National Women's Health Network, 4, 6.

Overman, S.J., Mimms, S.E., & Harris, J.B. (1987). Readability of selected college personal health textbooks. *Health Education, 18* (4), 28–30.

Saxton, M., & Howe, F. (EDs) (1987). *With wings: An anthology of literature by and about women with disabilities*. New York: Feminist Press at the City University of New York.

Sidel, R. (1986). *Women and children last*. New York: Viking Penguin.

Sternhell, C. (1985, May). We'll always be fat but fat can be fit. *Ms.*, pp. 66–68, 141, 154.

Whatley, M.H. (1988). Photographic images of blacks in sexualiaty texts. *Curriculum Inquiry, 18* (2), 137–155.

Worcester, N. (1988). Fatophobia. In N. Worcester & M.H. Whatley (Eds.), *Women's health: Readings on social, economic, and political issues*. Dubuque, IA: Kendall/Hunt.

Worcester, N., & Whatley, M.H. (1988). The response of the health care system to the women's health movement. In S. Rosser (Ed.), *Feminism within the science and health care professions: Overcoming resistance* (pp. 117–130). New York: Pergamon.

Appendix:
Textbooks examined for this chapter

Carroll, C., & Miller, D. (1986). *Health: The science of human adaptation* (4th ed.). Dubuque, IA: Wm. C. Brown

Dintiman, G.B., & Greenberg, J. (1986). *Health through discovery* (3rd ed.). New York: Random House.

Hales, D.R., & Williams, B.K. (1986). *An invitation to health: Your personal responsibility* (3rd ed.). Menlo Park, CA: Benjamin/Cummings Publishing Company.

Insel, P.M., & Roth, W.T. (1988). *Core concepts in health* (5th ed.). Mountain View, CA: Mayfield Publishing.

Levy, M.R., Dignan, M., & Shirreffs, J.H. (1987). *Life and health*. (5th ed.). New York: Random House.

Mullen, K.D., Gold, R.S., Belcastro, P.A., & McDermott, R.J. (1986). *Connections for health*. Dubuque, IA: Wm. C. Brown.

Payne, W.A., & Hahn, D.B. (1986). *Understanding your health*, St. Louis: Times Mirror/Mosby.

Ω

Super Women
by Edward Dolnick

Look at a school photo of a fifth-grade class, the boys in their coolest T-shirts, the girls just starting to grow gangly. Look at the nursery in a big-city hospital, at row upon row of swaddled babies. Look at the teenagers working at McDonald's or at the 60-year-olds trundling off the bus behind their tour guide at the Washington Monument.

Then look again in a few years. In every case, if you tried to put together a reunion, you'd find that more males than females had died. If you could take an immense group snapshot of everyone in the United States today, females would outnumber males by 6 million.

In this country, women outlive men by about seven years, and the figure is close to that in all industrialized nations. Throughout the modern world, cultures are different, diets are different, ways of life and causes of death are different, but one thing is the same—women outlive men.

It starts even before birth. At conception, male fetuses actually outnumber females by about 115 to 100; at birth, the ratio has already fallen to about 105 boys to every 100 girls. By about age 30, there are only enough men left to match the number of women. And from there on, women start building a lead that just grows and grows. Beyond age 80, there are twice as many women as men.

"What's dramatic," says Deborah Wingard, an epidemiologist at the University of California at San Diego, "is that if you look at the top ten or twelve causes of death, *every single one* kills more men." She runs a finger down this melancholy Top Ten and rattles off one affliction after another—heart disease and lung cancer and homicide and cirrhosis of the liver and pneumonia. Each kills men at roughly twice the rate it does women.

"Diabetes," Wingard resumes after catching her breath, "is the only one that even comes close to being"—she

By Edward Dolnick. Reprinted from *In Health*, July/August © 1991.

pauses, in search of a nonjudgemental word—"to being equitable."

Women's superiority extends far beyond merely living longer. Women are better than men at distinguishing colors. They have a sharper sense of taste and a better sense of smell. Would any child, confronted with a dubious-looking glass of milk, be so foolish as to give it to his father, rather than his mother, to sample?

The differences between men's and women's sexual capacities are much too familiar to need repeating here. Mark Twain once devoted a bitter essay to satirizing the workmanship of a Creator who had come up with two such mismatched creatures. "After fifty, [a man's] performance is of poor quality, the intervals between are wide, and its satisfactions of no great value to either party," Twain lamented in his old age. "Whereas his great-grand-mother is as good as new."

In outdoor athletics, women aren't much match for men. But one trend is worth noting: The more a competition requires stamina, the better women fare. The first woman to win a mixed-sex national championship did so in a 24-hour endurance race. Ann Trason ran 143 miles' worth of circles around a track, four miles more than the (male) runner-up. Helen Klein, a 68-year-old who considers a 50-mile race routine, holds all the "ultramarathon" records in her age group. Women win so many long-distance dogsled races that one musher has designed a "Save the Males" T-shirt.

In real-life ordeals, too, women seem at least as durable as men. One man trapped in the Warsaw Ghetto by the Nazis kept a journal in which he recorded the growing misery of his fellow Jews. "At 14 Ostrowska Street is a house where there are only women and children," he wrote in the cold and hungry winter of 1942. "All the menfolk have died. In general, men have a markedly higher mortality—the reason being that men have less endurance, work harder, and so forth." Six miserable months later, the diarist continued to marvel at "the courage and endurance of our women" who were now "coming forward to replace the men, who fall out exhausted."

In bad times, women may also be psychologically more resilient than men. A study of areas of London heavily bombed during World War II, for example, found that 70 percent more men than women became psychiatric casualties. The study's (male) author summarized its findings: "It may be true that women are more emotional than men in romance, but they are less so in air raids."

Women have more acute hearing than men, and keep their hearing longer. Women have colder hands and feet than men, but complain and suffer less when exposed to bitter cold.

Are you beginning to detect a pattern?

Men out-stutter women four to one. Men go bald, and sprout hair from their ears to make up for it. They're more likely to be color-blind, 16 to one, and are especially prey to ulcers and hernias and back problems. Faced with such a list of defects, any conscientious manufacturer would have issued a product recall.

WHY ARE MEN SO PUNY? A century ago, the question would have made no sense. In 19th century America, men outnumbered and outlived women. This situation presented no challenge to conventional wisdom. Women were, authorities from the Bible to Shakespeare agreed, "the weaker vessel."

God was in *His* heaven, all was right with the world. But in the 20th century, the trend reversed itself. Women began living longer than men, primarily because pregnancy and childbirth had become less dangerous. The gap grew steadily through the decades. In 1950, for the first time ever in the United States, females outnumbered males.

That made for some wrinkled brows. If men were so strong, why were they all dying? Part of the damage turned out to self-inflicted. Overall, statisticians figure that one-third of the longevity gap can be attributed to the ways men act. Men smoke more than women, drink more, and take more life threatening chances.

Men are murdered (usually by other men) three times as often as women are. Overall, they commit suicide at a rate two to three times higher than that of women. This fact holds for every age group, without exception, whether you compare teenagers or the middle-aged or the elderly.

If men don't have guns or knives, they make do with cars. Men have twice as many fatal accidents per mile driven as women do. Men are more likely to drive through an intersection when the light is yellow or red, less likely to signal a turn, more likely to drive after drinking. Men drivers!

But behavior doesn't explain away the longevity gap. Women seem to have an innate health advantage. Even among people who have never smoked regularly, for example, the death rates from heart disease, lung cancer, and emphysema are between two and four times higher for men than women.

As the fifties drew to an end, conventional wisdom finally came up with an explanation. Men's problem wasn't biology so much as a newly discovered killer called stress. Heart disease was claiming more and more male victims, and the reason, according to the new way of thinking, was that stress lurked in office buildings and corporate boardrooms, the very places *men* spent their days.

Breadwinning in earlier eras may have had more panache—slaying a lion with a spear called for a certain flair—but earning a living in the modern workplace was portrayed as just as dangerous. A popular book called *Stress and Your Heart*, published in 1961, summed it all up: "It seems that being the breadwinner—whether man or woman—is a difficult job. Tension is inevitable. The job of homemaker, on the other hand, gives the woman some time—if she desires it—to relax and let some things go."

Let women be so foolish as to venture out of the home and into the line of fire, the good doctors thundered, and they would begin dying at the same rate as men. But a funny thing happened on the way to the funeral.

Between 1950 and 1985, the percentage of employed women in the United States nearly doubled. Those working women, study after study has found, are as healthy as women at home. And where differences between the two groups have been reported, the advantage have gone to the working women.

The doomsayers had predicted that employed women would collapse under the stress of "role overload," as they tried to juggle work, children, and homemaking. The extra stress is there, surveys confirm, but it hasn't brought ill health along with it. The reason, it seems, is that paid work provides women with feelings of self-esteem, responsibility, and camaraderie that outweigh its drawbacks. Work is no picnic—that's why they call it work—but it appears to beat staying home.

Scientists who have studied the female-male health gap find that all the data point to one conclusion: Mother Nature is a bigot. "In comparison with the female," according the one zealous researcher, "there can be little doubt that the male has a higher mortality rate in almost all forms of animal life studied thus far, in nematodes, mollusks, crustacea, insects, arachnids, birds, reptiles, fish, and mammals." Whether you're a man or a mouse, a fruit fly or an alligator or a pheasant, females live longer. Not that studying mortality tables for spiders will shed much light on the human gender gap.

Every living thing *is* assembled according to instructions on its chromosomes, though, and considerable work has been done on the ways male and female chromosomes differ. Humans have 23 pairs of chromosomes. Males have one nonmatching pair, denoted XY, while the corresponding pair in females is XX. This XX pairing is often cited as the secret of women's superiority.

The reasoning is straightforward: The two chromosomes of a matching pair are nearly but not quite identical, like two neighbors' recipes for the same dish. Even if there is a mistake in one chromosome's recipe—if egg whites aren't listed among the ingredients for chocolate suffle—dessert may still turn out fine, because the other chromosome has its own recipe.

But males have only a single X chromosome—one recipe—and so they are more vulnerable than females to any errors on it. If their one recipe omits egg whites, the souffle is going to be a flop. If their single X chromosome is defective, it's possible for a serious genetic disorder to appear.

That makes for a whole list of genetically determined and predominantly male foul-ups. These can be innocuous, like color-blindness or the inability to ask for directions even when hopelessly lost. But they can also be devastating. Hemophilia and muscular dystrophy, for instance, are diseases caused by a defect in a single gene on the X chromosome. They are far more common in males than females.

The chromosome theory has problems, though. For one thing, in birds, butterflies, and moths, it is males who have the double chromosome and they still die before females. More importantly, there just aren't enough cases of the most feared genetic diseases to account for more than a tiny bit of longevity gap between men and women. Ingrid Waldron, a biologist at the University of Pennsylvania and an authority on the gender gap, puts it succinctly: "Most of the common X-linked diseases aren't fatal, and most of the fatal X-linked diseases aren't common."

Even so, there still are researchers who believe chromosomes are the culprits. Some pin the blame directly on the Y chromosome, the male chromosome. At a 1987 conference on aging, for example, John Hopkins's Kirby Smith reported on four generations of an Amish family he has been studying. The men appear absolutely normal, but they are missing part of their Y chromosome. For unknown reasons, these men not only outlive their male neighbors but also live several years longer than Amish women. With a flair for tabloid prose too rarely seen in science, Smith summarized his finding as "Too much Y and you die."

Most scientists think the answer lies elsewhere. They focus on hormones, and though the hormone theory doesn't account for all of women's advantages over men, it goes a long way toward explaining a crucial one. For both sexes, heart disease is the leading cause of death. The difference is that women have an extra decade of immunity before they start to succumb.

Estrogen (from the Greek for "producing frenzy"!) seems to be the key. Before age 40, when virtually all women are still producing estrogen, heart disease kills three men for every woman. But from that point onward, the odds in favor of women drop steadily.

To buttress the argument, instead of comparing men and women of the same age, compare premenopausal and postmenopausal women of the same age. Again, the women whose ovaries are producing estrogen are the ones with the healthy hearts. Moreover, postmenopausal women who take estrogen supplements seem to have less heart disease than matching groups.

And just as estrogen seems to be the heroine of the story, testosterone, the male sex hormone, seems to be the villain. Until puberty, boys and girls have the same cholesterol levels. But when boys hit adolescence and testosterone kicks in, their level of HDL cholesterol, "good cholesterol," plunges. In girls, HDL levels hold steady. Women maintain that advantage throughout their lives.

The story of LDL cholesterol, "bad cholesterol," is similar. In both sexes, LDL levels start a steady rise at puberty. But the increase is steeper, and therefore more dangerous, in men. When menopause begins (and estrogen production plummets), women's LDL levels climb higher than men's. This raises the risks for women, but their high HDL levels still leave them better protected than men are.

One moral seems to be that testosterone has hung on past its glory days. The hormone, which seems to cause aggressiveness and which certainly produces big muscles, may have been a nifty innovation when man's major duty was hurling rocks at the next tribe. Back then, a 30-year-old ranked as a tribal elder.

Today we live decades past our reproductive prime. We hunt only if someone has misplaced the remote control clicker. We tend to go light on the nuts and berries and heavy on the cheeseburgers and chili dogs. Testosterone doesn't seem like such a bargain anymore.

Testing the testosterone-as-the-bad-guy theory is tricky, because recruiting volunteers is so tough. Veterinarians have provided one clue. Neutered tomcats, it turns out, live about two years longer than their intact brothers. Part of the reason is that they are less likely to die in fights, but even if you look only at cats that died of natural causes, the neutered cats lived longer. Spaying females doesn't affect their lifespans.

The obvious place to look for more evidence is at accounts of the thousands of eunuchs who served through the centuries as palace guards in Europe and Asia. As late as 1896, the Emperor of China employed 3,000 eunuchs, and the Ottoman Empire, which lasted until 1923, never abandoned the practice. At the centers of European culture, *castrati* were operatic superstars, whose unearthly singing inspired cries of *"Viva il coltello!"* ("Long live the knife!") But no one ever studied the longevity of these men.

For that, we have to turn not to ancient Rome or imperial China, but to Kansas only a few decades ago. There and elsewhere, mental hospitals and homes for the retarded sometimes castrated their inmates, usually with the intent of rendering them more docile. One research team studied 297 men who had been castrated at an institution for the mentally retarded in Kansas. The last operations were performed in 1950.

Except for having had the bad luck to fall into the surgeons' hands, the researchers claimed, the eunuchs were strictly comparable to the other men in the study. But on the average, the castrated men outlived a matching group of male inmates by nearly 14 years. Even more surprising, they also outlived a peer group of female inmates. "It is probably impossible to devise any [other] way to select a group of males that would outlive females," the authors observed.

Not every difference between the sexes favors women. On average, men are taller than women and have heavier bones and bigger muscles. Men will die sooner, but we'll have hit more home runs by the time we go.

Men have sharper eyes and quicker reaction times. And psychologists who spend their days tormenting volunteers claim that men have a higher threshold of pain. This will come as a surprise to any father who has fainted in a delivery room.

Men are leaner, with about 10 percent less body fat than women. The reason presumably lies in our evolutionary history—women's bodies are designed so that, even in hard times, there will be an easy-to-tap fuel reserve for pregnancy and nursing. Estrogen lends a hand by helping the body convert food to fat. (When unscrupulous chicken growers wanted plump, tender birds in a hurry, they added estrogen to the feed. Testosterone would have made for tough, stringy birds, with a tendency to get in bar brawls.)

It's a good system if there's a risk of famine. In ordinary circumstances, though, the effect is that men have an easier time than women losing weight. Holding to a steady weight is easier, too, because men are bigger and our metabolism is about 6 percent faster. We gulp in more oxygen and throw off more heat.

As a result, men have the luxury of burning twice as many calories as women do. Men stay thin because we're gas guzzlers; we're puffed with pride because we hardly get any miles to the gallon.

The headstart in fighting paunch favors men, but it has more to do with vanity than health. Men do have one undisputed advantage over women that is far more than cosmetic. Autoimmune diseases, illnesses in which the immune system attacks the body rather than protects it, strike women disproportionately. Multiple sclerosis, for example, affects twice as many women as men. For lupus, a sometimes fatal disease in which the immune system can disable any of the body's organs, the ratio is nine women to one man. For rheumatoid arthritis, three to one.

Even here, there is speculation that the problem is too much of a good thing. Some scientists believe that females have more robust immune systems than males do. That would make for a better defense against illness, usually, but it might also increase the odds that the immune system would turn traitor, by shifting into overdrive or going haywire.

The case is hardly airtight. It's true that prenatally and in infancy, boys are more vulnerable to fatal infections than girls are. But, later on, there's no evidence that women are better than men at fighting off disease. Overall, cancer's death toll, for example, is roughly equal in both sexes.

Day in and day out, in fact, women feel sicker than men do. Women make more visits to the doctor, take more prescriptions and nonprescription drugs, and spend more days stuck in bed. This is not a new phenomenon. In 1676 one diarist noted in passing, "I have heard physicians say that they have two women patients to one man."

Since women nonetheless manage to outlive men, this has made for a nasty but entertaining debate among medical scholars. One faction contends, essentially, that women feel sick so often because they are "in touch with their bodies." Men, on the other hand, are too brutish or too proud to notice they're not feeling well. This is reminiscent of a story I was told when I was little, about how dinosaurs were so dumb that they walked around for a week after they had died, because it took that long for the message to make its way to their brains.

The contrary view is just as unflattering, though *it* slanders women. This position can be summed up as follows: Do women complain more, or what?

But the resolution of the great "Who's sicker?" debate seems easy enough. Women turn out to be less vulnerable than men to life-threatening diseases, but more vulnerable to everyday sickness and pains. Women are plagued by arthritis and bunions and bladder infections and corns and calluses and constipation and hemorrhoids and menstrual woes and migraine headaches and sleepless nights and varicose veins.

In the meantime, men get heart attacks and strokes. Women are sick, but men are dead.

When it comes to mental health, more or less the same picture holds. Women are more likely than men to be miserable day to day, but men are more likely to have devastating illnesses. Women bend and men break.

Depression, for example, is about twice as common in women as in men. But schizophrenia, the most debilitating mental illness, is twice as common in men. And (in part because of schizophrenia) men in mental hospitals outnumber women three to two.

After a spouse dies, men fare far worse than women. They are more depressed, more likely to seek psychiatric help and to need tranquilizers, and more likely to fall ill. In the first months that they are alone, according to several studies a few years back, men are more likely than women to follow their partners into the grave.

Some social scientists skeptical of this work refused to believe that the men were dying of grief. They proposed, instead, that the widowers' problem was malnutrition, because they didn't know how to cook. More recent studies have settled the question—the men died so soon after their wives that grief had to be the cause; they hadn't had time to starve.

Men fare poorly, it seems, because in many cases their wives were their sole confidantes. Without spouses to share problems and fears, newly widowed men are left alone to founder and sink. Women who lose their husbands, in contrast, often have a circle of close friends to confide in and count on.

The conventional explanation for differences in male and female psychology is by way of analogy. Women respond to every dip and bump in the road, like cars with springy suspensions. Men, who are trained to keep stiff upper lips, roar over minor divots like cars with rigid shock absorbers. On good roads men do well, but when they come to speed bumps or potholes, watch out.

But behavior changes. As a result, the health gap between men and women isn't a fixed feature of the landscape, like the Grand Canyon. In recent decades, the gap between men and women's lifespans has narrowed. It reached its maximum of 7.8 years in 1970 and is now seven years. The explanation is not that women's health is deteriorating. Women's health is improving, but men's is improving faster.

Men, or some of them, are smoking less than they used to, drinking less, and eating better. Gloomy forecasts about how women would start dropping like flies as they moved into the workplace got things exactly backward. "The gap isn't shrinking because women are acting like men," says Wingard, the University of California epidemiologist. "It's shrinking," she goes on, with barely concealed mirth, "because men are behaving more like women."

But for all their advantages, women reap a cruel reward. Eleven women in 12 outlive their husbands. Men die too young, and women end up sick and alone in their old age.

It is a hard game, and there is no winning. William Randolph Hearst once suggested to Dorothy Parker that her short stories were too sad. "Mister Hearst," she told him, "there are two billion people on the face of the earth, and the story of not one of them will have a happy ending."

Ω

119

Images and Gender Roles

1. Make a list of characteristics which get identified as "masculine" and "feminine." By each characteristic write "yes" or "no" as to whether this is a characteristic which is valued and rewarded by our society.

female characteristics	valued?	male characteristics	valued?

2. In what ways is it just as dangerous or more dangerous for women to say, "Women are more nurturing than men" as it is for people to say that "Men are better at certain things."

3. A longtime peace activist has said, "A prerequisite for being president of the USA should be that a person has to be a mother before they can be president." Describe your reaction to this statement and problems with such statements.

4. Check below which strategies you think are likely to help improve the role of women in society?

_____Trying to eliminate differences between sexes/genders

_____Trying to make men more like women

_____Trying to make women more like men

_____Making it possible for both men and women to explore both masculine and feminine sides of themselves

_____Trying to make society value a much wider range of characteristics and behaviors

Briefly comment on why you made the choices you did:

5. Compare the messages girls and boys in your family got about "appropriate" vs. "inappropriate" behavior for their sex. When were girls praised for feminine behavior? for masculine behavior? Were boys ever praised for feminine behavior?

6. As you read through the "Super Woman" article, make a list of the characteristics which Edward Dolnick identifies as having a large female:male difference. For each of these characteristics, think of societal influences which you think contribute to the large sex/gender gap and note this in column a. In column b, identify societal changes which you think could help narrow the sex/gender gap.

characteristics	a contribute to gap	b narrow the gap

7. If average untrained college-age men and women are tested for physical fitness, the men are likely to appear to be more fit, particularly in the area of strength. These results fit with the assumption that many make that women naturally have less physical potential than men. However, exercise physiologists find very different results. For example, men tend to have greater strength in both upper (back, arms, shoulders) and lower body, but when the measurement is adjusted relative to body weight, the differences in lower body strength disappear. When untrained men and women begin to do weight-training, the women often progress much faster because they are farther below their potential. Androgens are needed for muscle proliferation, so the fact that the average women has lower levels of androgens than the average man means there is some limit on her muscle bulk. However, this does not mean much in terms of strength limitation since women can increase greatly in strength without "bulking" (muscles increasing in size). Right now we have no idea what the strength capability of women is since women are so undertrained in terms of strength.

    Women have a great capacity for developing endurance. Leading women marathoners can beat all but the best male runners and would, in fact, have won many past Olympic men's marathons with their current times. Women do even better in relation to men in ultra marathons (50 or 100 miles). Women hold many long-distance swimming records and compete directly with men.

    When boys and girls are tested for physical performance, they are matched up to ages 10 to 12. In fact, girls are often faster than their male classmates in elementary school. After age 12, boys tend to increase in strength and cardiovascular fitness more than girls. Exercise physiologists believe these differences may be more social than biological in origin. It is not hormones that make women weaker but social and cultural processes.

Discussion Questions

a. Untrained males and females show little difference in lower body strength but larger differences in upper body strength. Show how this situation might arise by examining the activities from early childhood through adulthood that males and females might engage in that are likely to develop upper or lower body strength.

b. Differences in physical performance between males and females generally first appear around puberty. What are the changes in physical activity around puberty that might affect this? What are the social and cultural messages that may limit girls' activities at puberty? Compare your own forms of exercise before and after puberty.

c. How does the definition of women as "weaker" limit women's lives? Examine such issues as work, recreation, safety. Who benefits from the definition of women as weaker?

4

Mental Health

Many formerly battered women who have been close to death with life threatening physical injuries have said the physical violence had less impact on them than the day to day psychological/emotional abuse they survived. Many women with chronic fatigue syndrome so severe that taking a shower became a major goal have said that the worst part of their condition was that people (including doctors) would not believe they were ill and had said the condition was "all in their head." Mental and physical health issues have so much impact on each other that in many cases it may be misleading to try to make a distinction and in other cases it can be very dangerous to confuse mental and physical health ramifications of a situation. Readers will notice that mental health components are central to every topic in this book.

"Women and Mental Health" provides an overview of definitions of mental health, gender differences in patterns of mental ill health, women and depression, women and mental health services, and positive suggestions for change. In "Gender Issues in the Diagnosis of Mental Disorder," Paula Caplan describes specific examples of how sexism among mental health professionals results in "serious oversights, inadequate treatment, and even mistreatment and harm—primarily to females but also sometimes to males." While portraying the dangers of the Diagnostic and Statistical Manuals of Mental Disorders' (DSM) "dangerously misogynist" psychiatric labels used against women, Caplan questions why there are no equivalents where male socialization becomes defined as a mental health issue. For educational and consciousness-raising purposes, Margrit Eichler and Paula Caplan have proposed

a new DSM category of Delusional Dominating Personality Disorder!

"Co-dependency: A Feminist Critique" looks at how the co-dependency label gets put on many of the same behaviors which our society encourages as positive for women and then, "because co-dependency so accurately describes what many of us experience in our lives; we blame ourselves for the behaviors."

In "Sexual Abuse by Psychotherapists," Estelle Disch, a therapist who is also a survivor of sexual abuse by a therapist, outlines both the ramifications of this serious issue and steps a woman can take if she questions whether she has been treated so inappropriately by a therapist. The article provides useful guidelines for finding a new therapist.

Now that many women who choose to be in therapy have identified that they want counseling which relates to their socialization in a sexist society, consumers need to be alerted to the trend for some therapists to market themselves as "feminist therapists" even if their therapy techniques are fairly traditional. Guiding philosophies a woman seeking feminist therapy should be able to expect are outlined in the next article, "Basic Concepts of Feminist Therapy."

The last article in this chapter, "Mental Patients' Liberation Front: Seeking Control" provides an introduction to mental health activism by people who have been mental patients, their critiques of the present mental health system, and alternatives for more patient controlled or patient-useful services.

Women and Mental Health

by Marian Murphy

What We Mean by Mental Health

Mental health, as opposed to mere absence of mental illness is a complex and often controversial subject. What defines mental health? Who defines it? In terms of women, notions of mental health carry an added burden of value judgments and traditional beliefs. It is my view that mental health is a concept that needs constant redefinition in the light of new knowledge and, within the framework of this discussion, mental health refers not simply to the absence of symptoms or problems but to the presence in a woman of *well-being* and *growth* and the ability of a woman to solve problems in a reality-based way.

A healthy and growing person can be described as moving towards increased acceptance of and openness to herself and others; increased self-support and self-esteem; growing capacity to give and receive love; increased intellectual competence and creativity; greater freshness of perception and richness of feelings (both joy and pain); a more aware, autonomous, and caring value system; a growing sense of closeness to the natural world; a greater frequency of moments of transcendence; a growing enjoyment of living in her present experience. Using this kind of standard, most people live in a state of permanent mental ill health.[1] At the very least, it is estimated that on average we each fulfil less than 10 per cent of our potential for this kind of growth. The extreme forms of this general ill health are reflected in the increasing numbers of people using psychiatric and counselling services and increasing rates of suicide, alcohol/drug abuse and crime.

In the case of women, this situation is compounded by the very standards used to define mental health/illness. There are differing standards of mental health for women than for men among mental health professionals. An often-cited study carried out by Broverman and colleagues (1970)[2] showed that a double standard is employed when assessing the mental health of women and men. Behaviour that was regarded as healthy for an adult, sex unspecified, and thus viewed from an ideal absolute standpoint, was identical to behaviour considered healthy for men, but not for women. This finding that psychiatrists, psychologists and social workers ascribe male-valued stereotypic traits more often to healthy men than to healthy women conceals a powerful, negative assessment of women in general. For instance, these professionals were more likely to suggest that healthy women differ from healthy men by being more submissive; less independent; more easily influenced;

more excitable in minor crises; less competitive. Such a combination of traits is a most unusual way of describing any mature, healthy individual.

Another important factor here is the notion of health itself that is used by many professionals working in health services, i.e., an adjustment notion of health. This would suggest that one of the most important factors involved in mental health is adjustment to one's environment. This, together with the existence of different norms of female and male behaviour, also leads to different standards of mental health for women and men. Thus for women to be healthy from an adjustment viewpoint, we must adjust to and accept the behavioural norms for our sex, even though these behaviours are generally less valued socially and are considered less healthy for the generalised competent, mature adult. Acceptance of this adjustment notion of health places women in the difficult position of having to decide whether to exhibit those positive characteristics considered desirable for men and adults such as assertiveness and ambition, thus calling our 'femininity' into question; or to behave in the prescribed 'feminine' manner, accept second-class adult status and possibly live a lie to boot. This strongly suggests that mental health professionals should be concerned that the influence of sex-role stereotypes on their professional activities actually reinforces social and psychological conflict.

Thus, before we even get to the point of looking at the different mental health statistics of women and men, we can begin to consider the possible effects of this double standard of health. A possible implication is that (a) behaviours and feelings exhibited by women and considered 'normal' for us, (e.g., low self-esteem, feelings of depression) and thus not requiring treatment, would be seen as 'symptoms' in men and would be treated; (b) women exhibiting behaviour which did not conform to these female stereotypes (non-nurturing, lack of interest in childbearing) would be considered 'abnormal' and in need of psychiatric treatment. There is much evidence that this is in fact the case. There are, therefore, numerous implications for both sexes, in the way in which they view themselves and how they should deal with life problems and also in the kinds of treatment they receive from the mental health and medical professions.

Differences in Patterns of Mental Ill Health

The worldwide picture is that the majority of clients for mental health services are women. In North America, for example, women comprise 60-75 percent of clients. In Canada, it has consistently been demonstrated that women receive more prescriptions for all drugs than men and this

Reprinted with permission from PERSONALLY SPEAKING ed. Liz Steiner Scott, Attic Press Dublin, 1985.

difference is even more noticeable in the case of psycho-tropic (mood-changing) drugs, with between 67–72 per cent of these drugs going to women. In Britain, 12 per cent of women take tranquillisers daily for a month or more each year. Although there are no statistics for Ireland, doctors' reports would suggest an equally high level of usage of tranquillisers by women. Women have consistently higher levels of medical consultations than men, both with general practitioners and specialist consultants. What is even more striking than these overall rates of usage of mental health services, which, after all can sometimes be dismissed as differences in help-seeking patterns and willingness to talk about distress etc., is the different patterns of illness displayed by women and men.

In community studies in Britain and the USA where people who have not sought help at all are studied, women consistently report more distress, anxiety and depression. In diagnostic terms, doctors are treating large numbers of women with such clinical conditions as hysteria, eating disorders such as anorexia nervosa(under eating) and bulimia (binge eating) and, most particularly, depression. The incidence of depression in women (matched only by rates of alcoholism in men in Ireland) illustrates the internalised way in which women deal with problems, whereas it appears that men cope by externalising their frustrations. As depression is the most prevalent mental illness among women and has been extensively studied, it may be useful to spend some time on it here.

Women and Depression

Is there something inherent in being a woman that predisposes us to developing an emotional illness? There are a number of possible answers to this question. Firstly, it is suggested that the incidence of depression is actually more equally divided between women and men but that each sex expresses it differently. It is suggested that men often develop mechanisms such as excessive drinking, or have outbursts of violence. Many treated alcoholics do have symptoms of depression so it would not be unreasonable to infer that men may use alcohol to hide their symptoms of depression. For others, chronic alcohol abuse and the cause and effect factors have not yet been sorted out and, although it is possible to speculate that there are large numbers of depressed men in the community who are simply not visible because of the masking effects of alcoholism, there is no evidence that this is the case.

The differing ratios of depressive ill health in women and men is often accounted for by the fact that women perceive, acknowledge, report and seek help for stress and its related symptoms more readily than men. However, recent studies have shown that women do not experience or report more stressful events than do men nor do we evaluate the standard lists of life events (death of a spouse, separation, change in jobs, etc.) as having greater impact than do men. We must, therefore, conclude that women do actually experience more frequent and more severe symptoms of depression than men.

Could women's depression be accounted for by biological factors? While there is now some evidence to suggest that there is a genetic factor operating in depression, the samples that have been studied are few and there is insufficient evidence to draw conclusions about the way depression is transmitted or to explain the sex differences. Similarly, while there is good evidence that premenstrual tension (PMT) increases rates of depression, it is not a major cause. Also, the amount of female depression that is attributable to the possible effects of oral contraceptives is extremely small indeed.[3] There is excellent evidence that the period following childbirth does induce an increase in depression. However, contrary to widely held views, there is now evidence to show that the menopause has virtually no effect in increasing depression rates.[4] While, therefore, some portion of the sex differences in depression, probably during the child-bearing years, may be explained by reference to biological and hormonal factors, it is not sufficient to account for the consistently large differences.

Sociologists, psychologists, feminists and others concerned with women have become increasingly occupied with explaining why more of us become depressed. The conventional belief is that our long-standing disadvantaged social status causes women to become depressed. The persistence of social status discrimination for women therefore is proposed to explain the greater numbers of us suffering from depression. One extensive study on depression in women[5] suggests that there are two main reasons why we become depressed. This study holds that many women find their situations depressing because of the real social discrimination we experience in our everyday lives; this makes it difficult for us to achieve control by direct action and self-assertion, further contributing to our psychological distress. Such discrimination leads to legal and economic helplessness, dependency on others, chronically low self-esteem, low aspirations and ultimately clinical depression. The second reason why women become depressed is that our socialisation discourages assertiveness. Young women learn to be helpless while we are growing up and thus develop a limited ability to respond when under stress. Instead of learning to act out in frustration or anger as young men do, young women internalise these feelings and become depressed.

Attempts to test these hypotheses have focused on the different rates of mental illness among married and unmarried women.

If these hypotheses are correct, marriage should be of greater disadvantage to women than to men, and since married women are more likely to embody or find themselves in the traditional stereotyped role, they should, therefore, have higher rates of depression. In one study it was found that the higher overall rates of many mental illnesses for women are largely accounted for by higher rates for married women.[6] In every other marital status category, single, divorced and widowed women have lower rates of mental illness. It concludes that being married has a protective effect for males but a detrimental effect for women. Similar conclusions have been reached by researchers in several different countries.

This study and others attribute the disadvantage of the married women to several factors: role restrictions (most men occupy two roles and therefore have two sources of gratification whereas many women have only one); the low prestige of housekeeping and its frustrating effect for many women; the unstructured role of 'housewife', allowing time for brooding and the fact that even if a married woman works, her position is usually less favourable than a working man's.

There are, of course, other important intervening factors such as family size and financial resources. Other researchers have examined the relationship between psychological stress and subsequent affective disorders.[7] They found that working-class married women with young children living at home had the highest rates of depression. Subject to equivalent levels of stress, working-class women were five times more likely than middle-class women to become depressed. Four factors were found to contribute to this class difference: loss of a mother in childhood; three or more children under the age of fourteen living at home; absence of an intimate and confiding relationship with partner; lack of full- or part-time employment outside the home. The first three factors were more frequent among working-class women. Employment outside the home, it was suggested, provided some protection by alleviating boredom, increasing self- esteem, improving economic circumstances and increasing social contact.

From these studies, it can be concluded that the excess of depressive symptoms in women is not entirely due to biological factors inherent in being female, but is contributed to by the conflicts generated by the traditional female role, and the isolation that this role may bring.

The Mental Health Services: How Women Use Them and How Women Are Treated by Them

Given that more women than men experience symptoms of depression and other mental ill health, how is this manifested when we look at the mental health services? To begin with, as already noted, rates of consultation are higher. The usual avenue to the health services is through contact with general practitioners. In this country general practitioners say that at least 25 per cent of consultations are due to psychological factors and that they have neither the training, the time nor the resources to provide appropriate treatment. Moreover, many problems which result from a way of life or a particular difficulty or habit has come to be regarded as diseases rather than problems. Some women's problems which may actually be social, economic, ethical or legal, may be misidentified or wrongly regarded as psychiatric disturbances.

However, there have been few attempts by any western governments to introduce professionals with other than medical training into the first line of contact with people suffering from these kinds of problems and similarly, no attempts have been made to implement programmes of primary prevention and mental health education. The most likely form of treatment, therefore, that a woman will receive for a variety of these problems, is medical, in the form of mood-changing drugs. In fact doctors are more likely to offer tranquillisers to us than to men who present the same complaints, specifically complaints which involve the client being: unhappy, crying, depressed, nervous, worried, restless and tense. For these kinds of complaints men are more likely to receive a more physical therapies, laboratory tests and referrals to specialists. Here again the double standard is apparent.

A major contributing factor to this scenario is women ourselves who, in fact, frequently request our doctors to prescribe drug treatment for such symptoms. It has been suggested that this comes about as a result of women's view of our situation, a view which society teaches us. Women have learned to see our resentment and despair about our place in the social structure, as an individual problem, an emotional disorder. Women are trained to invalidate our own experiences, understanding and feelings and to look to men to tell us how to view ourselves. Ideas, concepts, images and vocabularies available to women to think about our experiences have been formulated from the male viewpoint by universities, professionals, industries and other organisations. These are reinforced by images of women in the media: women's magazines, women's novels, women as depicted in advertisements, children's stories and much more. These views are supported by the findings of a Vancouver study that questioned groups of women about their understanding of the uses of minor tranquillisers. Women felt that tranquillisers were sometimes needed to help them cope; coping, for them, meant the management of their roles as housewife and mother. In retrospect, some women expressed doubts about the role of illness that they had accepted and wondered about other options. One woman said: 'I feel that, essentially, when a doctor prescribes a pill for me, it's to put him out of my misery'. Another commented that a prescription for babysitters would have been more useful than a prescription for tranquillisers.[8]

When we look at the training attitudes and practices of doctors and psychiatrists, we see even more blatant examples of sex-bias in treatment. In 1974 a study highlighted the process by which medical schools teach demeaning and derogatory attitudes to women, both as patients and as students.[9] Physicians are taught that women's illnesses are not worth understanding, are unimportant and are of emotional origin. The woman 'patient' is objectified and made fun of. These assumptions about women are part of the very fabric of our society—this appears to be borne out by several studies in the USA on the amount of sex-bias and sex-role stereotyping involved in psychotherapeutic practice. In July 1974, responding to requests by the American Psychological Association Committee on Women in Psychology, a task force was established to look at this whole area. The task force identified four general areas affecting women as clients. The first of these was in the area of support for traditional sex roles. Here the therapists assumed that resolving of problems and self-fulfillment for women come from marriage or perfecting the role of wife without any recognition of women's other potential roles in society. The second general area was the above-mentioned bias in the medical profession's expectations and devaluation of women. This was exemplified in practice by the use of theoretical terms and concepts (e.g., masochism), to ignore or condone violence towards and victimisation of women; and by the use of demeaning labels such as manipulative, hysterical etc. when describing female patients. The third general area was the sexist use of psychoanalytic concepts, e.g. labelling assertiveness and ambition with the Freudian concept of penis envy. The fourth area of discrimination identified was the therapist's response to women as sex objects, e.g., heavily weighing physical appearance in the selection of patients or having a double standard for male and female sexual activities and even going as far as seducing female clients.

In view of these findings the American Psychological Association subsequently advocated a whole range of educational efforts to overcome these appalling practices and injustices. There is little evidence to show that these findings have had any effect on the practice of many psychiatrists. In fact, the realisation that 'feminine' characteristics can, in fact, be seen as those of any oppressed group of people tends to be astounding to the psychiatrist.

It is obvious then that the three interacting sets of factors briefly discussed here (a) the medical and mental health systems and the process of medicalisation; (b) the mental health professionals and their attitudes and theoretical backgrounds and (c) the woman and her socialisation; perpetuate a situation which predisposes women to mental, and particularly depressive, illness. Women's problems are treated only as psychological problems, without any prospect of addressing and dealing with the root causes.

Where Do Women Go from Here?

Internationally, the future for our mental health is bleak. In Ireland, as everywhere, additional stress factors such as high unemployment rates and the consequent lack of access to work outside the home for many women, interact with a traditionally male medical and psychiatric culture emanating from a society that clings stubbornly to a view of woman as homemaker and mother. Realisation of the need for a new medical model is appearing, however, and the supposed scientific basis of psychiatry has been greatly criticised. Psychiatrists are beginning to see sexism as a barrier to our understanding of the family and to acknowledge that 'much patriarchal rhetoric has masqueraded as theory.'[10]

Theoretical and practical alternatives are emerging that approach women's problems in ways that are more closely connected with our life experiences. Worldwide, feminist therapy is developing to such a degree that it has been suggested that it has some of the characteristics of a school of psychotherapy. The increased equality of client and

therapist, the main focus on environmental interpretations, the movement away from sex-role prescriptions and the role of the features of this new therapy. In Ireland some alternatives to traditional psychotherapy are available but only in urban centres. Women's self-help groups and consciousness-raising groups can be particularly useful here. Women in groups can come to realise that cultural values we have accepted unquestioningly such as maternal success, complete devotion of self to motherhood, and consumerism, as a major source of our tensions and dissatisfactions. Researchers have found that consciousness-raising groups provide a forum in which mildly depressed women with low self-esteem can explore our feelings about ourselves and our life situations. Obviously, participation in such groups is not a substitute for psychotherapy for those women whose problems are long-standing and severe. However, they can provide a useful starting point for women who are beginning to take more personal responsibility for the quality of our lives.

A range of other resources has also begun to emerge which provide support and reduce the isolation of women in extended families. These include family and community resource centres which often provide mother and child clubs, pre-school and day-care facilities, discussion and personal development groups, employment counselling, assertiveness training and legal clinics. 'Return to work' courses, creches in a variety of educational facilities and opportunities for women to come together to work at co-operative ventures are playing a vital role in preventing the development of further mental illness among women. In Ireland, there are few counselling centres which provide education and treatment that is not sex biased, but beginnings are being made.

For women undergoing particular crises, facilities such as rape crisis centres supply practical help, enabling us to confront our anger and avoid chronic and disabling shame and embarrassment. Advice is also available on possible legal action and its implications. Transition houses provide shelter for battered women and their children and have served to alert the community to the enormity of this problem.

Notwithstanding these developments, a great deal still needs to be done. Generally, we need to be more aware of the factors leading to stress and mental ill health. Preventive programmes should be established to help people discover and use their own coping mechanisms and recognise the value of yoga, relaxation techniques, akido, a balanced lifestyle, and other alternatives to the traditional medical response to mental illness.

Caution must be exercised by women anxious to develop alternatives outside the traditional framework of 'the home'. They should not swing to the opposite extreme and create new kinds of 'career' and other pressures that can equally cause an imbalance—to behave like men under stress is not a solution. The ideal would be to redistribute nurturing and work roles between women and men allowing for more balanced lifestyles for all. It is also vital that the new kinds of services already discussed at some length be encouraged and recognised as viable sources of help for women who have hitherto all too often been seen as in need of psychiatric treatment.

Finally, it is imperative that those working in the mental health professions be encouraged, both at pre- and post-qualifying levels, to employ the following guidelines in their dealings with women and that we in turn begin to seek and insist upon a service that embodies the following principles: (1) an equal relationship with shared responsibility between counsellor and client; (2) provision of help in differentiating between the politics of the sexist social structure and those problems over which, realistically, we have personal control; (3) provision of help in exploring our personal strength and how we can use it constructively in personal, work and political relationships; (4) provision of help in confronting unexpressed anger in order to combat depression and to make choices about how to use our anger constructively; (5) provision for helping women to redefine ourselves apart from our relationships to men, children and home including exploration of fears about parental role changes; (6) encouragement to women to nurture ourselves as well as caring for others, thereby raising self-confidence and self-esteem; (7) encouragement of the development of a range of skills to increase women's competence and productivity. This may include assertiveness training, economic and career skills and advice on how to reeducate family and friends who resist change. Although not every counselling situation with women will necessarily incorporate all of these principles they provide a basis for mental health professionals as well as a standard which can be used by women to evaluate the treatment we receive. Women clients, no less than men, have a right to mental health services that are sex-fair, competent and ethical.

Conclusion

Moving from an 'ideal-type' definition of mental health, through some of the examples of ill health in women, and how these are currently treated, I have arrived at suggestions which I believe would help to promote better levels of mental health in women. These suggestions are underlined by a view of people and their psychological needs which I, together with others, working in the mental health services, hold. This view presupposes that mental health involves a balance between three basic areas of life (see diagram): love, based on self-acceptance and self-esteem; work, providing opportunities for a sense of achievement, recognition and status; play, allowing for relaxation and forgetting of self and other preoccupations.

Traditionally, women have loved and worked, men have worked and played. This imbalance has impoverished the lives of both sexes. Ironically, now that some men are beginning to learn to feel and show emotions, affection in relationships is being awarded a status it did not enjoy when found predominantly among women. Women, however, must not only achieve recognition status for the work we do, we must also learn to look after

our own needs for relaxation, play and satisfying work and above all for a sense of self that is not defined for us either by society or by our relationships with others. For each individual woman this means maximising existing opportunities for looking at and, if necessary, reordering her lifestyle. For members of the health profession, it means reorganising and eliminating sex-biased practices.

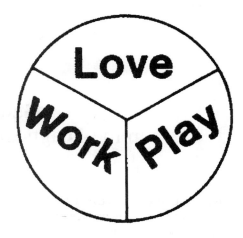

For the community as a whole, it not only means making a commitment to programmes of prevention in the mental health field, but also rejecting the rigid adherence to the stereotypical division of roles, responsibilities and acceptable behaviours between women and men.

It has been because of the growth of feminist thinking and 'psychotherapy' that changes and reanalysis of women and mental health have begun to take place. This development must be guided and supported. It is important for women to recognise our own strengths and contributions in this field and to look to each other for the shared experience and discussion which will allow greater control and responsibilities in our lives.

Questions for Discussion

1. Do you think that the family as we know it is to blame for a considerable amount of mental ill health in women? Discuss.
2. Some women become depressed after childbirth. Why? What other events in women's lives might be the cause of their depression?
3. From your own experience, how does the medical profession treat women as clients? How might you change that attitude?
4. Is it in women's 'nature' to be more prone to mental ill health, especially depression, than men? Discuss.
5. If you have ever taken tranquillisers for any length of time, can you assess how they affected you? Did they help? How? Was it difficult to stop taking them?
6. In what ways can women's groups be a positive force for mental health?
7. If you were in need of professional help, where would you go? Can you think of any alternatives to professional help that might be of use?

131

Suggested Reading

Ann Dicksons *A Woman in Your Own Right: Assertiveness and You* (London: Quartet 1982).

Phyllis Chesler, *Women and Madness* (London: Avon 1974).

Luise Eichenbaum and Susie Orbach, *What Do Women Want?* (London: Fontana 1983).

Elizabeth Howell and Majorie Bayes (eds), *Women and Mental Health* (New York: Basic 1981).

Ann Kent-Rush, *Getting Clear: Body Work for Women* (London: Wildwood 1974).

Ann Kent-Rush and Anica Vessel Mander, *Feminism as Therapy* (New York: Moon Publications 1974).

Ω

Gender Issues
in the Diagnosis of Mental Disorder

by Paula J. Caplan

Historically, it has been considered acceptable—indeed, womanly—for two or more women or girls to band together to help the poor, the sick, the helpless, the oppressed, children, or men. The only time it has not been considered acceptable for women to do this has been when the help was for themselves or for other women. Women who have done the latter have been branded as selfish, unwomanly, belligerent, strident, and so on; they have been accused of complaining too much or of ignoring the needs of other people. They have been threatened with ostracism by the host culture.

In spite of such threats, some women have continued to insist that women's concerns be given high priority. It was high time for a feminist conference on gender, science, and medicine—like this one—which Dr. Elaine Borins so beautifully put together.

I shall present a very brief sampling of some of the ways in which sexism among mental health professionals has resulted in serious oversights, inadequate treatment, and even mistreatment and harm—primarily to females but also sometimes to males. It is important to keep in mind that sexism is not the only bias that profoundly skews and twists the process of diagnosis. Racism, ageism, classism and homophobia are some of the other deep-seated prejudices that are reflected in the creation and assignment of diagnostic labels by mental health professionals.

Although there is space here to mention only a few examples, I've chosen these carefully to provide a sense of the enormous range of diagnostic problems and harm that result from sexism.

Learning Disabilities

In my earliest years as a clinical psychologist, I specialized in children's learning problems (Kinsbourne & Caplan, 1979). One of most widely accepted bits of "wisdom" in that field was, and still is, that far more boys than girls have learning disabilities. Recent research (Shaywitz, Shaywitz, Fletcher, & Escobar, 1990) suggests that, in fact, learning disabilities are equally common in both sexes. Nevertheless, in virtually all clinical settings, more boys than girls are brought in with complaints about learning problems; and I wondered whether that pattern of *noticing* and referral for learning disabilities reflected the pattern of *real* learning disabilities. My own research (Caplan, 1973, 1977; Caplan & Kinsbourne, 1974) a number of years ago suggested that girls' learning disabilities and other academic problems are more likely than boys' to be overlooked and underdiagnosed, and there seemed to be several reasons for this:

First, since it is considered less important for girls than for boys be academically successful, low academic performance by girls appears less likely to be labeled a problem than low academic performance in boys; therefore, girls' learning difficulties are unnoticed or, when noticed, not considered to warrant referral, remediation, or any other kind of treatment (this is the "As long as she's pretty and nice she'll get a husband. She doesn't need to be smart" attitude).

Second, girls are socialized to deal with frustration and failure in less disruptive, antisocial ways than are boys. As a consequence, a learning disabled girl is more likely than an equally learning disabled boy to deal with that frustration in ways that lead her teachers or parents to take her to professionals in the hope that they can "do something" to keep her under control.

Paula L Caplan, PhD, is author of *Between Women: Lowering the Barriers*, *The Myth of Women's Masochism*, and *Don't Blame Mother: Mending the Mother-Daughter Relationship*.

This pattern is harmful to girls and to boys in different ways. Many girls' learning problems are simply never noticed, and boys who already have one problem (e.g., learning disability) develop a second problem (disruptive behavior) as part of their attempt to cope in a sex-appropriate, traditionally masculine way. Canadian psychologist Meredith Kimball (1981) has identified the deep-seated sexism in North American educational systems' allocation of funds for remediation of learning disabled children. Kimball points out that it is commonly believed (although by no means based on solid evidence) that boys have more reading disabilities than girls and that girls have more trouble (although, interestingly, these are not usually dignified with the term "learning disability") with so-called "visual-spatial tasks," which are assumed to be important for doing math and sciences.

Where do public monies for remediation go? Overwhelmingly, they are poured into remedial *reading* programs, and little or no remediation is provided for children with visual-spatial problems. A similar disproportion characterizes the research that is done on learning disabilities: Overwhelmingly, it is focussed on reading problems, the problems thought to plague boys far more than girls. Although some might argue that reading is the most important school-related skill and therefore deserves more attention and funding, even North America's post-Sputnik stress on the importance of education in mathematics and sciences did not result in any substantial increase in a focus on visual-spatial problems.

Psychiatric Diagnoses

When the American Psychiatric Association last revised its massive handbook, *Diagnostic and Statistical Manual of Mental Disorders* (DSM)—which is probably the most widely used listing of psychiatric labels—they included two new, dangerously misogynist diagnostic categories. A great deal has been written elsewhere (see Caplan, 1987, for details and additional references) about the numerous problems and dangers involved in these categories, which are "self-defeating personality disorder" (SDPD) and "late luteal phase dysphoric disorder" (LLPDD), but I shall briefly mention some of the major ones here.

Self-defeating personality disorder was initially to be called, "masochistic personality disorder," and even though the title was changed, the criteria and the implications are the same. The criteria applied to these people include putting other people's needs ahead of their own, not feeling appreciated even though they really are, and settling for less when they could have more.

This diagnostic label is dangerous because:

1. It applies to what I call the "good wife syndrome": Women in North America are traditionally raised to put other people's needs ahead of their own and to settle for less when they could have more (it's called being unselfish, not being a demanding shrew, and/or having poor self-esteem so that one doesn't *realize* that one could do better), and it has been well-documented that women's traditional work (housework and childcare) in fact is *not* appreciated. Thus, after a woman has conscientiously learned the role her culture prescribes for her, the psychiatric establishment calls her mentally disordered. It does *not* do anything similar for men. It does not classify as a psychiatric disorder the inability to identify and express a wide range of emotions, a "disorder" which has been proven to characterize enormous numbers of North American males.

2. It is a description of the typical battered or severely emotionally abused woman. Such women characteristically experience dangerous plummeting in their self-esteem because of the abuse, and, trying to be good women and good wives, they try to become even more self-denying, giving, and undemanding than other women in an attempt to persuade the abuser to stop the abuse. Applying the label of "self-defeating personality disorder" to these women is a pernicious form of victim-blaming. Although users of the DSM are cautioned not to apply this label when abuse was the major cause of the woman's apparently "self-defeating" behavior, it has been well-documented (see Firsten, 1991, for a review) that therapists almost never ask their clients about abuse, and when they do, clients are reluctant (ashamed, scared) to talk about it. As Poston and Lison (1989) report, "Many would sooner ask a client if she is hearing voices than ask her if she has sexual abuse in her background, even though figures would indicate that the chances of an abusive background far outweigh the occurrence of hearing voices" (p. 21).

3. The label is dangerous because it leads both therapists and the women so diagnosed to believe that the problems come from within, that the women have a sick need to be hurt, humiliated, unappreciated, etc. Since my book, *The Myth of Women's Masochism*, was published (1987), hundreds of women have told me that in years of traditional psychotherapy, their therapists told them regularly that they brought all their problems on themselves. When the women say, for instance, "But Fred was wonderful to me when we were dating. It wasn't until our wedding night that he started to beat me," the therapist all too often replies, "Ah, yes! So *consciously* you didn't choose an abusive man. But your self-defeating motives are *unconscious!*" Such "treatment" is, I believe, a major cause of depression in women: They are unjustifiably given the message that there is no point in their trying to get out of an abusive or otherwise distressing relationship or situation, because their sick, unconscious motives will inevitably lead them straight into more trouble.

4. Prime movers of the DSM revisions have themselves pointed out that people diagnosed in this way typically have what is called a "negative therapeutic reaction," that psychotherapy makes them worse (Kass, MacKinnon,

& Spitzer, 1986). No surprise, I say, because if I have a broken leg, and the doctor puts a cast on my arm instead, my leg will certainly get worse. If a woman is being abused or severely emotionally neglected and unappreciated by her intimate partner, then a therapist who takes the approach that she enjoys her misery and has an unconscious need to suffer not only does not help but actively makes her worse.

The other misogynist diagnosis, LLPDD, is a fancy term for premenstrual syndrome as a psychiatric disorder. What's wrong with that? Several things.

1. While we all know women who have genuine physical or mood problems that seem to be regularly associated with their menstrual cycle, the danger is in calling these troubles psychiatric problems. Robert Spitzer, chief author of the most recent DSM revisions, told a press conference that psychiatrists don't know any psychiatric treatment that will help women with PMS but that PMS as a psychiatric diagnosis is essential to enable psychiatrists to figure out what they can do for these women. Although Spitzer may have good intentions, since psychiatric labelling tends to have negative and even dangerous consequences, until there is reason to believe that PMS is a psychologically caused problem *and/or* is helped by psychiatric treatment, there is no justification for using this label. Women who have PMS have enough trouble without having to worry that they are crazy. Furthermore, our society typically seizes on any suggestion of women's emotional weakness to justify keeping women out of well-paying, responsible jobs. (By contrast, although it is known that men's job performance varies according to predictable cycles, since there is no easy-to-pinpoint marker like monthly bleeding with which to associate those changes, men are regularly allowed to work at such dangerous jobs as piloting airplanes without being checked for where they are in their cycles.)

2. Nutritional, vitamin, and exercise treatments of various kinds have been shown to be helpful to many women who have PMS. These forms of treatment are not widely recommended (perhaps not even known) by the psychiatric and medical community, and calling PMS a psychiatric problem makes it less likely that women will be told about such useful courses of action.

Perhaps the most striking feature of SDPD and LLPDD is that the DSM includes no equivalent diagnostic categories for males, that is, there is no male SDPD parallel in the sense of having a category that describes an extreme form of males' socialization, such as "Macho Personality Disorder," and there is no male equivalent of LLPDD such as "Testosterone-Based Aggressive Disorder."[1]

Why Isn't the Health Insurance Industry Scared?

The health insurance industry ought to be up in arms about both of these diagnoses. Why? Because most nice women and virtually all battered women could be erroneously given the label of "self-defeating personality disorder," and once they are in psychiatric treatment, since they are not psychiatrically disordered they will be unlikely to "get well"; thus, the therapy is likely to be interminable. Women who enter psychiatric treatment for their PMS will, of course, experience little or no improvement for this physiologically-based disorder, and since they don't "get well," they may regularly lie on a psychiatrist's couch—until they reach menopause, at which time they will no doubt be considered in need of psychotherapy for their menopausal disorder. I have repeatedly contacted the health insurance lobby in the United States and the Canadian department of Health and Welfare, but they have chosen not to express any opposition to these categories, even though one would think that they would be worried that their coffers will be rapidly drained.

The Abuse of Mothers of Sexually Abused Children

After a few, brief years during which many brave adults revealed that they had been sexually abused as children and were believed, there has been a dangerous, unbelieving backlash. The media are filled with allegations that children claim they are sexually abused by their fathers only because the children's nasty, scheming mothers forced them to say it, in an effort to hurt their ex-husbands. Some mental health professionals, egged on by an enthusiastic legal profession, have legitimized this backlash through the use of the psychiatric label "Munchausen's syndrome by proxy." The label "Munchausen's syndrome" is a psychiatric diagnosis applied to people (usually women) who are described as going from one physician to another in the mistaken belief that they have something physically wrong with them, that they have a pathological need to believe they are physically ill. Typically, I have heard psychiatrists describe such a person as "never being satisfied until she gets someone to operate on her." Now, "Munchausen's by proxy" is being applied to a woman whose child reports being sexually abused. The diagnosis is supposed to indicate that the woman has a need to believe that something terrible is happening not to her but rather to her child.

This is a particularly terrifying, nauseating development. For so long, mothers have been damned by therapists for *not* reporting sexual abuse in their children—mothers' explanations that they *did not know* it was happening are ignored, and therapists say they *must have known unconsciously*—and now, they are being damned and pathologized if they *do* make the report. When their children are being seriously harmed, the harm to the children is too often ignored and disbelieved, while the spotlight is turned on the allegedly sick mother. This is one of the more vicious and irresponsible forms of mother-blaming, a phenomenon whose pervasiveness among mental health professionals has been well-documented.

Conclusion

The sheer variety of gender biases in diagnoses represented in this brief paper reflects the power and the pervasiveness of sexism in the realm of diagnosis. This means that both conclusions drawn from research mired in these biases and the clinical and human applications of biased categories need rapid and radical transformation.

NOTE

1. After this paper was presented at the 1988 Gender, Science, and Medicine Conference, Margrit Eichler and I proposed, for educational and consciousness-raising purposes, the diagnostic category described in the Appendix as a way to redress the sexist imbalance in the DSM. Curious to see what would happen, we submitted the category to the DSM-IV Revisions Task Force, and excerpts from the disturbing, sometimes hilarious, but always revealing correspondence from some of the Task Force members about this category have now been published in a paper called "How *Do* They Decide Who Is Normal? The Bizarre, But True, Tale of the *DSM* Process" (Caplan, 1991). A comprehensive review of the research relevant to the category has also been published (Pantony & Caplan, 1991). We note that, in our hurry to get the proposal circulated, we inadvertently omitted a great many possible criteria that we feel ought to have been included, such as some related to homophobia, racism, classism, materialism, ableism, weightism, and so on.

References

Caplan, Paula J. (1973) The role of classroom conduct in the promotion and retention of elementary school children. *Journal of Experimental Education, Spring. 41(3).*

Caplan, Paula J. (1977) Sex, age, behavior, and subject as determinants of report of learning problems. *Journal of Learning Disabilities, 10,* 314–316.

Caplan, Paula J. (1987). *The myth of women's masochism.* NY: Signet.

Caplan, Paula J. (1991) How *do* they decide who is normal? The bizarre, but true, tale of the *DSM* process. *Canadian Psychology 32(2),* 162–170.

Caplan, Paula J., & Kinsbourne, Marcel. (1974) Sex differences in response to school failure. *Journal of Learning Disabilities, 7,* 232–235.

Firsten, Temi (1991). Violence in the lives of women on psych wards. *Canadian Woman's Studies, 11(4),* 45–48.

Kass, Frederic, Mackinnon, Roger A., & Spitzer, Robert L. (1986). Masochistic personality: An empirical study. *American Journal of Psychiatry, 143,* 216–218.

Kinsbourne, Marcel, & Caplan, Paul J. (1979). *Children's learning and attention problems,* Boston: Little, Brown.

Kimball, Meredith (1981). Women and science: A critique of biological theories. *International Journal of Women's Studies, 4,* 318–335.

Pantony, Kaye Lee, & Caplan, Paula J. (1991) Delusional dominating personality disorder: A modest proposal for identifying some consequences of rigid masculine socialization. *Canadian Psychology, 32(2),* 120–133.

Poston, Carol, & Lison, Karen. (1989) *Reclaiming our lives: Hope for adult survivors of incest.* Boston: Little, Brown.

Shaywitz, Sally E., Shaywitz, Bennett A., Fletcher, Jack M., & Escobar, Michael. (1990) Prevalence of reading disability in boys and girls: Results of the Connecticut longitudinal study. *Journal of American Medical Association, 264(8),* 998–1002.

Appendix

*Delusional Dominating Personality Disorder (DDPD)**

Individuals having this disorder are characterized by at least 6 (?) of the following 14 criteria (note that such individuals nearly always suffer from at least one of the delusions listed):

1. Inability to establish and maintain meaningful interpersonal relationships

2. Inability to identify and express a range of feelings in oneself (typically accompanied by an inability to identify accurately the feelings of other people)

3. Inability to respond appropriately and empathically to the feelings and needs of close associates and intimates (often leading to the misinterpretation of signals from others)

4. Tendency to use power, silence, withdrawal, and/or avoidance rather than negotiation in the face of interpersonal conflict or difficulty.

5. Gender-specific locus of control (belief that woman are responsible for the bad things that happen to oneself, and the good things are due to one's own abilities, achievements, or efforts)

6. An excessive need to inflate the importance and achievements of oneself, males in general, or both. This is often associated with a need to deflate the importance of one's intimate female partner, females in general, or both

7. The presence of any one of the following delusions:

    A. the delusion of personal entitlement to the services of
        1. Any woman with whom one is personally associated
        2. Females in general for males in general
        3. Both of the above

    B. the delusion that women like to suffer and to be ordered around

    C. the delusion that physical force is the best method of solving interpersonal problems

    D. the delusion that sexual and aggressive impulses are uncontrollable in
        1. Oneself
        2. Males in general
        3. Both of the above.

---

*The Criteria for Delusional Dominating Personality Disorder was first printed by *Canadian Psychology* 32(2), pp. 120–133.

E. the delusion that pornography and erotica are identical

F. the delusion that women control most of the world's wealth and/or power but do little of the world's work

G. the delusion that existing inequalities in the distribution of power and wealth are a product of the survival of the fittest and that, therefore, allocation of greater social and economic rewards to the already privileged are merited (Note: the simultaneous presence of several of these delusions in one individual is very common and frequently constitutes a profoundly distorted belief system)

8. A pronounced tendency to categorize spheres of functioning and sets of behavior rigidly according to sex, e.g., belief that housework is women's work

9. A pronounced tendency to use a gender-based double standard in interpreting or evaluating situations or behavior (e.g., a man who makes breakfast sometimes is considered to be extraordinarily good, but a woman who sometimes neglects to make breakfast is considered deficient)

10. A pathological need to affirm one's social importance by displaying oneself in the company of females who meet any three of the following criteria:

A. are conventionally physically attractive

B. are younger than oneself

C. are shorter in stature than oneself

D. weight less than oneself

E. appear to be lower on socioeconomic criteria than oneself

F. are more submissive than oneself

11. A distorted approach to sexuality, displaying itself in one or both of these ways:

A. A pathological need for flattery about one's sexual performance and/or the size of one's genitals

B. An infantile tendency to equate large breasts on women with their sexual attractiveness

12. A tendency to feel inordinately threatened by women who fail to disguise their intelligence.

13. Inability to derive pleasure from doing things for others

14. Emotionally uncontrolled resistance to reform efforts that are oriented toward gender equity

Note: In keeping with the stated aims of the DSM, the proposed category is atheoretical, but there is little or no evidence that it is biologically based. In fact, there is a great deal of evidence that it is an extremely common disorder that involves a great deal of psychological upset both to the patient and to those with whom the patient deals. There is also evidence that the disorder is socially-induced and ... that the younger the patient when ... treatment is begun, the better the prognosis.

Ω

Co-dependency: A Feminist Critique

by Bette S. Tallen

Graduate Studies in Education and Human Development
Rollins College

Thanks to Elliott, Donna Langston, Mara, Rosemary Curb for comments and suggestions although only I am responsible for the opinions expressed here.

I live in a community where co-dependency is big business, where women have had in-hospital treatment for it, where many belong to Co-dependents Anonymous, where therapists advertise in the women's community as specialists in co-dependent treatment. Many women have described themselves to me as co-dependent. This behav-

ior is neither new nor unique. In 1989 when I worked in a Women's Studies Department in a state university in southern Minnesota, we offered a one-credit workshop on co-dependency, we were so flooded by student demand for the course that we had to schedule a second section. This was in a community of less than 40,000 people. Moreover, the more I talk to other women around the country the more I realize none of this behavior is all that unusual. Books on co-dependency are best sellers, not only in feminist bookstores but on national best-seller lists. Women-only and lesbian-only co-dependent groups abound. Treatment centers for women advertise in newspapers as well as on TV.

In short, co-dependency is an idea whose time has come. Sharon Wegscheider-Cruise defines co-dependents as "all persons who (1) are in a love or marriage relationship with an alcoholic, (2) have one or more alcoholic parents or grandparents, or (3) grew up in an emotionally repressive family." (Wegscheider-Cruise, as quoted in Anne Wilson Schaef, *Co-Dependence: Misunderstood—Mistreated*, p.14.) Feminists and non-feminists alike embrace the concept of co-dependency to describe a phenomena that, according to Wegscheider-Cruise affects 96% of the population. (*Ibid.*)

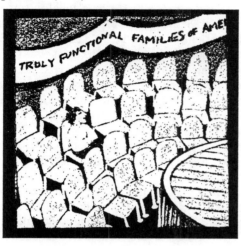

From *Sojourner: The Women's Forum*, (January, 1990). Illustation © 1990 by Linda Bourke.

Startlingly few critiques of the concept of co-dependency have emerged from our lesbian and feminist communities. We have no sustained analysis of the history of the term and have had little or no discussion of the political implications of using it as a method of understanding women's lives. Recently, I heard a woman describe another woman who is dying of cancer as only sick because she was co-dependent (cancer being one of several fatal diseases that co-dependency "causes," at least according to Anne Wilson Schaef. (*Co-Dependence*, p.8.) I was enraged, both as a cancer survivor and as a teacher of courses on women and health, I know only too well about the environmental and political issues that are critical to any discussion of cancer. African-American women and men suffer from and die from cancer in far greater numbers than do white people. Women continue to die from such drugs as DES. Are we all co-dependent? Or are we all suffering from a system that systematically targets certain groups as expendable? In short, what do we as women gain from explaining aspects of our lives as stemming from co-dependency?

Who is a co-dependent person? Who gets to say? Who has the appropriate credentials and skill to label someone as co-dependent? The list of symptoms of co-dependency sounds like a catalogue of our lives. Anne Wilson Schaef,

for example, lists the following as characteristics of co-dependency: dishonesty, not dealing with feelings in a healthy way, control, confusion, thinking disorders, perfectionism, external referenting, dependency issues, fear, rigidity, judgmentalism, depression, inferiority/grandiosity, self-centeredness, loss of personal morality, stasis and negativism. (*Co-Dependence*, pp. 42–43.) Who hasn't experienced these feelings? John and Linda Friel argue,

Is it not true that almost everyone had some form of dysfunction in their childhood that could lead to co-dependent symptoms? And if everyone has "it," does it not lose its conceptual and diagnostic meaning. . . . The [DSM–III–R] always describes symptoms, but asks us to look at length and severity of symptoms . . . before we make a definite diagnosis. (*Adult Children: The Secrets of Dysfunctional Families*, p.161)

Since apparently only the "experts" can label co-dependents and since all of us potentially suffer from "it," we are all forced to seek their "expert" advice, treatment, and workshops in order to "get well," or opinion to determine if we are sick in the first place.

Co-dependency as a concept emerged during the late 70's from the therapy community. Melody Beattie suggests that the term emerged simultaneously from several treatment centers in Minnesota. (*Co-dependent No More*, p. 29.) With the concept of co-dependency the therapeutic community attempts to co-opt both the feminist movement and the Twelve Step movement represented by Alcoholics Anonymous.

Alcoholics Anonymous, one of the most successful grassroots movements of our time, was founded in 1935 by two upper-middle-class white males, Bill Wilson and Dr. Robert Smith. It has literally saved the lives of thousands of men and women who would have otherwise died because of their drinking. Much is quite admirable about Alcoholics Anonymous, its offshoot organizations, and the Twelve Steps themselves. However, feminists and lesbians need to examine the roots of AA, et. al. We must also make distinctions between those groups that are under the AA umbrella (such as Al-Anon and Alateen) and are therefore governed by AA's Traditions and those that are not (such as Co-dependents Anonymous). Alcoholics Anonymous attempts to combine the medical knowledge of alcoholism with the pragmatism of William James ("Keep on coming back! It works!") and a form of Christian fundamentalism which is peculiarly American ("Let Go. Let God.")* The founders of AA believed in scaring the alcoholic by hitting "him" (in its early days AA did not admit women) with the medical facts about *his* "disease." Only when the alcoholic had sunk as low as possible, would *he* be amenable to treatment. Underlying the Twelve Step approach to the treatment of alcoholism is a conversion experience, being "born again," after one hit rock bottom. This can involve either a religious experience, as traditionally understood (belief in a patriarchal

*For a more detailed discussion of the history and roots of AA see my paper, "Twelve-Step Programs: A Lesbian-Feminist Analysis," in *NWSA Journal*, Summer 1990.

God) or can also mean an immersion in a community (the community of those recovering) or any number of possibilities in-between. AA historian, Ernest Kurtz, describes it as a, "*salvation* attained through a *conversion*, the precondition of which was the act of *surrender*." (Ernest Kurtz, *Not-God: A History of Alcoholics Anonymous*, p.182.) Critical to this conversion is not only an understanding of the Twelve Steps but also its grounding in the Twelve Traditions of Alcoholics Anonymous.

The Twelve Traditions are the governing principles of AA, they express many of the principles of first century Christian anarchism on which AA was based. They were designed to keep AA a grassroots, member-focused organization. Not only do the Traditions distance the organization from experts and from treatment approaches, but they also address the forms of self-aggrandizement and endorsement that are seen at the core of alcoholic behavior. They fully explain the Anonymous part of the AA name. Twelve Step groups not under the AA umbrella are not bound by the Traditions. And it is precisely these traditions, to my mind the most positive features of AA, that are getting lost in the Recovery Industry.

It does not take a particularly astute observer of American life to realize how big the Recovery Industry is, judging from its numerous publications, workshops, treatment centers, best-selling books, etc. Its big names are major media stars: their words and ideas come at us from all directions. We are literally bombarded with their messages. And what they have done to the Twelve Step movement is most interesting indeed.

Recently a friend and I visited one of the largest treatment centers for women in southern Minnesota, we were both suitably impressed by the presentation. It was slick, the brochures impeccable, the grounds immaculate, and of course, the facility spacious and inviting (providing the patient was not on medicaid or public assistance, they treat only those with adequate insurance or cash). Critical to the center's treatment program is its in-patient Twelve Step groups. In fact, one of the therapists mentioned that because the center was not given enough time and money from insurance companies to provide truly adequate de-tox (e.g., for some addicted to prescription medications it could take months to bring them safely off the drug but most insurance plans pay only for no more than thirty days in-hospital treatment), groups (along with individual counseling) were the primary treatment. When I questioned the head psychiatrist about requiring patients to attend Twelve Step meetings, since required attendance is antithetical to AA practice, she replied, "Yes, that is a problem," and changed the subject. Questions about how the therapists (many of whom were neither recovering substance abusers nor self-identified co-dependents) could participate in recovery groups were met with the same gracious stonewall of polite avoidance. The presence of therapists as experts, qualified only by training and not by experience, in such meetings, and the compulsory attendance contradict the Traditions and practices of AA (e.g., therapists cannot remain anonymous in group meetings when they see the same clients in individual counseling). Further, this takes place, not in a grassroots setting accessible to all who need help, but in an expensive facility which is enormously profitable. One of the therapists frankly admitted that she had never even heard of the Twelve Traditions. She stated that the only reason the hospital had started the women's unit was because they knew it would make money. And lots of money it makes.

Co-dependency and its treatment lie at the heart of how the Recovery Industry seeks to manipulate and control women. Ostensibly the concept arises out of the Al-Anon movement, the group started by Lois Wilson and Anne Smith that was initially composed of wives of men in AA. Al-Anon was founded on the concept that those who lived with alcoholics were affected by alcohol in some of the same ways as the alcoholic. However, at no time during its founding or since, was it held that alcohol affected the spouse physically, as it affected the alcoholic. The behaviors of the alcoholic were the primary issues. Enabling behaviors of the significant other were not seen as a disease or an addiction, but as a stumbling block to the alcoholic's recovery. The current concept of co-dependency varies from this quite significantly.

First, and perhaps most important, co-dependency is seen as a disease, a progressive, definable disease, with an inevitable outcome, and which, if not treated will result in death. Schaef even argues that, left untreated, the co-dependent will likely die before the addict. (*Co-Dependence*, p. 6.) There is the implication that co-dependency may actually be a more serious condition than addiction to a substance. Co-dependency is characterized as an addiction that produces significant physical symptoms, which some experts believe occur before the co-dependent becomes involved with the substance abuser. As the Friels argue, "[W]e are stating clearly that we do not believe that people become co-dependent because they have been living with an addict. Rather we are stating that they are in a relationship with an addict *because* they are co-dependent." (*Adult Children*, p.157.) The difference between the stance taken by the Recovery Industry and that of Al-Anon is huge. People in Al-Anon, are encouraged to create a healthy distance between themselves and the behaviors of the alcoholic, but they are not viewed as being ill prior to the relationship. Feminists and others who have critiqued Al-Anon say it too often focuses only on the alcoholic and not enough on the significant other.

Second, almost all the behaviors ascribed to co-dependents are traditionally seen as feminine behaviors in this society. How the experts on co-dependency handle this, I believe, underlies much of how the co-dependent movement itself seeks to de-politicize feminism. Melody Beattie, for example, describes the characteristics of co-dependent behavior as low self-worth, repression, obsession, controlling, denial, dependency, poor communication, weak boundaries, lack of trust, anger, and sex problems. (*Co-dependent No More*, pp. 35-47.) These behaviors form feminine identity in American culture. Growing up female means identifying ourselves as weaker, less-worthy, dependent on men, etc., in order to survive. If we resist these messages, we are penalized for our anger and lack of trust.

Because co-dependency so accurately describes what many of us experience in our lives, we blame ourselves for the behavior. In an introductory women's studies class I taught, a student talked about how much she learned from the book *Women Who Love Too Much* and how it helped her understand her feelings about her ex-husband, who battered her. I made an off-handed comment that perhaps the best book would not be on women who love too much but one on men who hit too much. In her journal, she wrote about how my comment "blew her away;" she never thought she could hold him responsible for his own behavior. Co-dependency, thus teaches us that femininity is a pathology, and we blame ourselves for self-destructive feminine behavior, letting men evade any real responsibility for their violent and abusive behavior. The Friels state, "If some one tried to make love to me when I said I didn't want to, this would be an individual boundary invasion." *(Adult Children,* p. 58.) I would call that rape. (They consider incest the result of "weak intergenerational boundaries," p. 60.) Redefining rape as weak boundaries on the part of both victim and perpetrator blames the victim.

Critical to co-dependency analysis is the view that you cannot control the behavior of the addicted person. Although obviously it is true that no one can control anyone else's behavior, the extension of the argument is that a co-dependent cannot even criticize the behavior of the addicted person rather they are taught to focus exclusively on their own health. Anne Wilson Schaef states that responsibility should no longer imply any kind of obligation, but rather should only be seen as the ability to respond, to explain one's own behavior. She writes, "responsibility is the *ability to respond.* In the Addictive System responsibility involves *accountability and blame.*" *(When Society Becomes an Addict,* p. 42.) In this view, women's responsibility is to look at their own behavior: they can neither blame nor hold men accountable for violent and abusive behavior. Sexism, and by extension, any system of oppression, becomes only the problem of the victim; the perpetrator can no longer be held responsible.

Third, the therapy community de-politicizes feminism by insisting that the root cause of co-dependent behavior is being raised in a dysfunctional family. The concept of dysfunctional family is based on the idea that it is possible to have a warm, loving, close nuclear family within the context of racist, capitalist, heteropatriarchy. It betrays the fundamental feminist insight that the patriarchal family itself is the primary institution in the oppression of women. As Simone de Beauvoir states, "Since the oppression of women has its cause in the will to perpetuate the family and to keep the patrimony intact, woman escapes complete dependency to the degree in which she escapes from the family." *(The Second Sex,* p. 82.) Not only does the concept of dysfunctional family ignore the sexism and heterosexism involved in the reality of family life, but it also renders invisible the racism and classism inevitably underlying the "warm, loving, family" conceived of by family therapists and psychologists. It creates, in Audre Lorde's term, a "mythical norm:" a standard by which we all judge ourselves to be wanting. ("Age, Race, Class and Sex: Women Redefining Difference," in *Sister Outsider,* p. 116.) The fantasy of the "functional" family imagines a well-employed father, and perhaps now, an equally well-employed mother, and children, able-bodied and well-adapted to society's definition of their race, class and gender. Families, such as the single-parent African-American family or gay and lesbian families, are seen as dysfunctional by definition and are therefore dismissed without any understanding of how those families may function far better for their members than the white, middle-class, "ideal" family. As Donna Langston has pointed out to me, many of the characteristics of co-dependent behavior, when seen in a working-class context, are actually critical aspects of survival skills. To learn to depend on others is what enables poor and working-class people to survive. To work only on healing the pain from having been raised in an "dysfunctional" family, holds out the hope that it is possible to achieve a fundamentally healthy family in this society without challenging the basic institutions of capitalism, heterosexism, sexism, racism, and classism that produced the patriarchal family in the first place. When we, as feminists, work on our issues of childhood abuse and neglect, part of the purpose is healing our own pain, but we also must seek to understand the political context that makes such abuse widespread, accepted, and an everyday occurrence, and fight collectively to stop it. The lack of any racial or class analysis in any of the literature on co-dependency underlines the white, middle-class nature of its roots in the therapy community and reinforces my belief that it represents an attempt to de-politicize feminism. Co-dependency adherents argue that we can get "well" without fundamentally altering the very institutions that created the situation in the first place. Beattie goes so far as to argue, that a preoccupation with injustice is a further proof of addiction. *(Co-dependent No More,* p.33.)

Why then is the concept of co-dependency so attractive to so many feminists and lesbians? A primary reason, in my view, is that co-dependency theory so accurately describes the reality of many of our lives. We feel powerless and unhappy. We live in a woman-hating culture where we pay a high price for resisting internalizing messages of feminine weakness and unworthiness. We are taught to depend on men for our survival. Co-dependency treatment offers hope that we can achieve our own private health. It allows those privileged by race, class, or sexual identity, among others to avoid looking at our privileged statuses. Co-dependency theory feeds on our complacency: we are no more responsible for behavior oppressive to others than any man is for his behavior to women. It teaches us that only we are responsible for our fate, that social activism and discontent are merely further symptoms of our "disease." When white women are confronted by women of color about their racism, they can now claim that racism is another symptom of their addiction, and their major task is to "get well." White people are not racist because they are sick, they are racist because they benefit from a system of racial superiority, they are privileged.

Co-dependency offers a relatively safe haven for those who can afford treatment. Its theory addresses many of the same concerns that we as feminists address, but without asking us to pay the high personal price of challenge and criticism. How many times have we felt judged wrongly or trashed in feminist groups without being given adequate space to explain? Co-dependency treatment offers a context of personal support that is all too often missing in our communities.

Co-dependency provides another way to resist the messages of femininity without fundamentally questioning the values of the racist, capitalist, heteropatriarchy we live with. We can get well, are encouraged to resist on a personal level, without ever really having to examine what made us "ill" in the first place. Therefore as we get "better," millions of other women will continue to be born into a culture that is misogynist to the core. Co-dependency theory offers a way to achieve a personal peace without examining the cost of that peace to others.

Bibliography

Melody Beattie, *Co-dependent No More*. New York: Harper/Hazelden, 1987.

Simone de Beauvoir, *The Second Sex*. New York: Bantam, 1961.

John Friel and Linda Friel, *Adult Children: The Secrets of Dysfunctional Families*. Pompano Beach, Florida: Heath Communications, 1988.

Ernest Kurtz, *Not-God: A History of Alcoholics Anonymous*. Center City, Minn.: Hazelden, 1979.

Audre Lorde, *Sister Outsider*. Trumansburg, N.Y.: Crossing, 1984.

Anne Wilson Schaef, *Co-Dependence: Misunderstood—Mistreated*. Minneapolis: Winston, 1986.

Anne Wilson Schaef, *When Society Becomes an Addict*. San Francisco: Harper & Row, 1987.

Ω

Sexual Abuse by Psychotherapists

by Estelle Disch

Anna* finds a male therapist to work on issues in her marriage and a deep depression which has settled in on her since her father's death a year earlier. She is just realizing that her depression is related to the fact that she never addressed the sexually seductive behavior and other emotional abuse she suffered with him in childhood. The therapy seems to progress well until she begins to work on the childhood abuse. In the midst of the work she begins to have sexual feelings toward the therapist. He reciprocates her sexual response, and they begin having sex during the therapy sessions.

Lillian encounters her therapist at a social event a month after terminating therapy. They chat a while and the therapist asks Lillian for a date. On the date, they end up in bed. Lillian feels both attracted and awkward. She has always liked her therapist and now she can't understand the confusing feelings she's having.

Ruth attends a therapy group with other women. The therapist encourages the group to socialize outside of the therapy sessions and often invites group members to social events at her home. In individual sessions with Ruth, the therapist initiates sexual activity but asks Ruth to keep their behavior a secret, emphasizing that Ruth is special and that the others would be jealous if they were to find out. When Ruth finally musters the courage to break this secret, she discovers the same thing has happened to other group members.

Therapist X approaches most women clients with the same line: "Your basic problem is sexual repression. If you work on that, your other problems will disappear. I can help you if you let me make love to you. I realize that this is unorthodox treatment, but I have studied it in depth and I am convinced it will help you. But you have to agree not to tell anyone about this or the treatment won't be possible." Sometimes Therapist X expresses deep love and commitment to his clients. Some have left their husbands for him, expecting him to leave his wife and marry them.

From *Sojourner: The Women's Forum*, (April 1989,). Copyright © 1984 by Sojourner, Inc. Reprinted by permission.

Estelle Disch does feminist therapy as a clinical associate at Tapestry, Inc., in Cambridge, Massachusetts, and teaches sociology at U.Mass./Boston. She is a survivor of sexual abuse by a psychotherapist. The author gratefully acknowledges the helpful feedback of Kathleen Kelley and Rita Arditti in the preparation of this article.*

*All names are fictitious and the stories presented here are composites of the most typical situations I have heard in five years of work with survivors of sexual abuse by therapists. Any similarity to real individuals is purely coincidental.

Sexual involvement with clients is a violation of the ethics codes of all professional psychotherapy associations in the United States. It is even part of the criminal code in several states. Sexual involvement may include anything from a sexualized atmosphere (such as seductiveness or a voyeuristic interest in the client's sex life) to overt sexual acts such as prolonged sexual hugging or kissing, genital contact, intercourse, etc.

The regulations against sexual involvement in therapy exist for three reasons: 1) A therapist who is sexually involved loses his or her ability to think clearly about the client's needs; 2) Sexual feelings are often a normal part of the therapy process. The client cannot begin to make sense of her feelings if the therapist provides an opportunity for her to act them out; 3) Clients are "vulnerable" adults. Because of a phenomenon called transference, feelings experienced in childhood, often toward parents, are reexperienced in response to the therapist. Thus, the client takes on some of the characteristics of a child in the therapy process and, therefore, cannot make fully adult decisions in relation to the therapist. The concept of sex between mutually consenting adults is highly questionable when one of them is the other's therapist.

Transference usually persists long after the therapy ends, making post-therapy sexual involvement equally risky for the client. In some cases, the therapist maneuvers a premature termination in order to develop a sexual relationship with the client when the therapy ends. In others, what appears to be a serious mutual relationship starts during the therapy and the therapy is either continued in the form of a lover relationship, or the therapy is ended so that therapist and client can pursue their romantic involvement. When these post-therapy social relationships end, the client is often struggling to figure out what went wrong years later.

According to the substantial clinical literature on sexual involvement between therapists and clients, as many as 12 percent of professionals (depending on the group studied) admit to having had sexual contact with at least one client. In a study of psychiatrists conducted by Nanette Gartrell, Judy Herman, and Silvia Olarte, 65 percent of respondents knew of cases of sexual abuse, the vast majority of which had not been reported. The Walk-In Counseling Center in Minneapolis, Minnesota, which has responded to more than 800 cases of sexual abuse since 1974, finds that most reported cases are of male therapists abusing female clients (over 80 percent), followed by cases of females abusing females (over 10 percent), males abusing males (under 5 percent), and females abusing males (about two percent).

Clients who have experienced sexual abuse in therapy suffer from a range of feelings much like those experienced by incest survivors. Guilt, shame, and a profound sense of betrayal are common, along with confusion about whether to "protect" the therapist or to confront him/her about the abuse. Often clients have themselves betrayed spouses or lovers via the sexual involvement with the therapist. The secretive nature of most sexual involvement makes it feel like a form of incest and, in fact, incest survivors appear to be especially vulnerable to this abuse: more than half of the women who have attended workshops I run for survivors of sexual abuse by therapists know themselves to be incest survivors. The boundary violations which occurred in childhood seem so much a part of many women's lives that continued boundary violation somehow feels normal. Many women lack the clarity and power to stop the abuse by the therapist, even though many have felt that something was "wrong" when the sexual activity began.

Boundaries are limits on behavior—rules for how people in various roles ought to behave, and statements from each individual as to what kinds of behaviors she can accept or tolerate without feeling violated. Boundary violations are often thought of as physical (e.g. crowding, unwanted touch, real or threatened physical and sexual violence), but can be emotional or intellectual as well (role reversals between parents and children or therapists and clients, emotional enmeshment, telling others what they think or feel, etc.). A helpful booklet on boundaries by Rokelle Lerner is listed in the resources below.

Clear boundaries in therapy include: sessions which occur at prearranged times and which start and end on schedule, ordinarily without interruptions; a clear fee arrangement; clear (but re-negotiable) treatment goals; a therapy hour focused on the client (i.e., the therapist does not use the time to get attention concerning his or her own problems); clarity on the part of the therapist as to how his or her values impact the therapy; a clear contract about confidentiality, so that the client will know who else knows about her (i.e., supervisors); no sexual involvement between therapist and client; no social contact outside the therapy hour except in those cases where overlapping political or social circles demand it, in which case the rules for interaction should be defined as clearly as possible, and the effects of any outside contact carefully monitored in the therapy.

If the therapist's boundaries are clear (i.e., the therapist knows who she or he is and respects the guidelines of ethical therapy), the client can be free to feel and express whatever she experiences without fear of being invaded or fear that her own behavior might violate the boundaries of appropriate therapy. Unclear boundaries on the part of the therapist can lead either to boundary violations of various sorts (not always sexual) or to inhibitions/censorship on the part of the client because at some level she knows that the therapist isn't trustworthy on certain topics. Either of these experiences leads, at best, to a limited therapy experience or, at worst, to a disaster.

If reading this article leads you to question a current or former therapy experience, you might want to think about some of these questions: Does the therapist seem overly interested in your sex life? Have you and the therapist kissed in a sexual way? Has there been breast or genital contact with the therapist? Does the therapist give or send you love letters or frequent presents? Does the atmosphere seem sexually charged from the therapist's side? Does the therapy feel like some sort of sexual affair, even if it isn't overtly sexual? Does the therapist talk about his or her sex life? Does the therapist talk about being lonely or does he or she appear needy and vulnerable?

If there has been no overt sexual activity, I suggest that you try discussing your feelings and see how your therapist responds. The therapist should help you sort out whether your sense of the sexualized nature of the relationship is coming entirely from you or whether he/she is somehow participating in what seems seductive or sexual to you. If you remain confused about whether or not the therapy is good for you, you might consider consulting with another therapist to help you sort out what you need to do. If there is or has been overt sexual contact in the relationship, I recommend that you get out of the "therapy" as soon as you can.

The primary goal of the therapy is to help women empower themselves as much as possible within the limits of the social order in which we find ourselves. The saying "give a person a fish and she eats for a day; teach her to fish and she eats for a lifetime" is applicable here. Sex on the couch, even if the client thinks that is what she really wants is the equivalent of giving the client food and undermining her opportunity to learn how to feed herself in her own way, in her own environment. It is a form of "quick fix," often an expression of addictive sexuality on the part of the therapist. The "fix" may appear to meet an immediate need, but it will not heal the issues that the client needs to address; it robs her of the opportunity to encounter her pain and loneliness and to figure out how she's going to solve those problems in her life. And, usually, the sexual relationship with the therapist turns out to be a disappointment, leaving the client with an unfinished therapy experience and the additional burden of having to figure out what went wrong.

Survivors of sexually abusive therapy are usually as much in need of therapy as they were when the sexual involvement began, but are now in the difficult position of having to risk trusting another therapist. Common feelings at this point include anger or rage, depression, distrust of therapists, and grief over lost time, money, and opportunity for help.

If you have been sexually involved with a therapist and feel ready to discuss it with others, there are several things you can do: 1) Talk to people you trust about what happened. Choose confidants carefully because many people don't understand this issue and will either blame you for what happened or minimize its importance. 2) Find a support group or therapy group focused on this issue. 3) Arrange to confront the therapist, ideally in the presence of a neutral third party who understands the issue. 4) Get politically involved in client or therapist education or in lobbying for more effective education/discipline of offending therapists. 5) File a complaint with a licensing board, a professional association, an agency where the therapist works, or in court.

Complaints filed with licensing boards, professional associations, and agencies usually will not cost much money unless you elect to hire your own lawyer to help you through the complaint process. Finding a lawyer to work with you in a court case is more complicated, since someone has to pay the lawyer and many survivors do not have the money to do that. Malpractice insurance policies often have sexual abuse exclusions (too many cases were filed) so you can't count on the therapist's insurance to pay damages and legal fees. Most malpractice lawyers are willing to work on a contingency fee basis if the therapist has some assets and if your case is one that the lawyer thinks can be won.

If you are seriously considering filing a complaint, I urge you to try to find out what the process is like from someone who has gone through it. Nearly everyone I know who has filed a complaint has felt more empowered after doing so, but the experience of going through the process is often humiliating, frustrating, and time-consuming, and the outcome is sometimes disappointing. There is a "rape trial" aspect to the experience in that you have to discuss very personal, deeply painful parts of your life with total strangers.

If the therapist belongs to no professional organizations, is not licensed, is not employed by an agency, and has no assets, you will not be able to file a complaint unless you can pay a lawyer to handle your case in court.

If you have been sexually abused in therapy and are considering finding a new therapist, try to protect yourself by asking some questions about the therapist's ethics and way of working (e.g., a touch-oriented therapy may be risky after sexual abuse). Find out what kind of training the therapist has, to which professional associations the therapist belongs, what kind of supervisory back-up the therapist has, what experience the therapist has working with survivors of sexually abusive therapy, whether or not the therapist has ever been sexually involved with a client and where she or he stands on this issue. A competent therapist should answer these kinds of questions without getting defensive. Any therapist who does not seem appropriately upset when you describe what you've been through should be avoided. And if you are a survivor of sexual abuse in childhood, I would look for a therapist with intact personal and therapeutic boundaries who also has clinical expertise in that area.

Consumers of therapy are at risk of abuse by incompetent therapists, since many times they don't know what to expect of therapy. There are books available to help you understand what to expect of the process (see resources). Women who go to therapy to grow and empower themselves are often derailed from their goals by therapists who are caught in their own illness or ignorance. We deserve the support and knowledge to choose our therapists carefully, to get out of abusive situations, and to get the help we need in order to survive as well as possible in a social order that already abuses women in too many ways.

Resources

Clinical Literature

Brown, L. "Power, Responsibility, Boundaries: Ethical Concerns for the Lesbian Feminist Therapist," *Lesbian Ethics*, Vol. 1, No. 3, 1985, pp. 30–45.

Bruckner-Gordon, F. et al. *Making Therapy Work: Your Guide to Choosing, Using, and Ending Therapy.* Harper and Row, 1988.

Gartrell, N. et al. "Reporting Practices of Psychiatrists Who Knew of Sexual Misconduct by Colleagues," *Am. J. Orthopsychiatry,* Vol. 57, No. 2, April 1987, pp. 287–295.

Hall, M. *The Lavender Couch: A Consumer's Guide to Psychotherapy for Lesbians and Gay Men.* Boston: Alyson Press, 1985.

Lerner, R., *Boundaries for CoDependents.* Center City, MN: Hazelden Foundation, 1988.

Vasquez, M. and Kitchener, K, Eds. "Special Feature: Ethics in Counseling: Sexual Intimacy Between Counselor and Client" (6 articles), *Journal of Counseling and Development,* Vol. 67, No. 4, Dec. 1988, pp. 214–241.

Schoener, G., et al. *Psychotherapists' Sexual Involvement with Clients: Intervention and Prevention.* Minneapolis, MN: Walk-In Counseling Center, 1989 (forthcoming).

Accounts by Survivors

Bates, C. and Brodsky, A. *Sex in the Therapy Hour.* NY: Guilford, 1989.

Freeman, L. and Roy, J. *Betrayal.* NY: Stein & Day, 1976.

Plasil, E. *Therapist.* NY: St. Martin's, 1985.

Walker, E. and Young, P. *A Killing Cure.* NY: Henry Holt & Co. 1986.

———————————————————————————————— Ω

♀

Basic Concepts of Feminist Therapy

by Joan Berman

Feminist therapy is a philosophical approach to the conduct of therapy, counseling, and consultation. It presents a new set of ground rules which is in the process of being developed from the ideas of political feminism and the women's liberation movement. Some of the basic ideas include:

- The personal is political. All behavior and experience is viewed in a sociopolitical context as part of a pattern of socialization. This idea helps clients to look outward as well as inward in order to differentiate what belongs to society and is being imposed, and what is internal.
- Sexism and sex-role stereotyping limit options available to both women and men.
- The therapist is aware of and explicit about her personal value systems, recognizing that there is no such thing as value-free therapy.
- Feminist therapists have a commitment to developing an egalitarian relationship with clients.

Issues in Feminist Therapy

- The importance of identifying external sex-role-related causes of difficulties, and separating these from internally related problems.
- The necessity of taking personal responsibility for change without blaming oneself.

- The importance of expanded sex-role definitions and options.
- The rejection of traditional diagnostic labels, along with the personality tests used to assist the process of putting women into categories. Many diagnostic terms applied to women have sexist implications and assumptions.
- The adoption of an androgynous model of mental health in which the individual integrates the positive aspects of "feminine" and "masculine" roles. For example, a person could be both compassionate and assertive, intelligent and nurturant.

Themes in Feminist Therapy

Anger

Generally, women are taught to suppress their anger. Sometimes it is turned inward as depression, or as somatic symptoms. In feminist therapy, a client may learn new ways of expressing and channeling these feelings, perhaps as a source of motivation for collective action and social change.

Self-nurturance

Women are taught to care for others, their family, friends, and often they work in service professions. They tend to ignore their own needs, viewing them as unimportant. Feminist therapy emphasizes the importance of caring for oneself, which is not selfish, but self-loving. The client learns to become aware of her own needs and desires, and how to express them to others.

From *Network Newsletter,* (newsletter of The New Mexico Affiliate of the National Women's Health Network) Winter 1986. Copyright © by National Women's Health Network. Reprinted by permission.

Autonomy

A therapist confirms the client's own experience and trusts the client's judgment, helping her to trust her own perceptions. She learns how to choose from expanded options. Career counseling may be used to expand a woman's freedom of vocational movement.

Applications

Power

Women are taught that they lack power, both economically and interpersonally (as seen in language, gesture, and invasion of personal space). Feminist therapy can provide a place for a woman to challenge her beliefs about her own lack of personal power and to experiment with powerful behavior that falls outside the generally acceptable patterns for women. This might include assertion training, martial arts, or other physical training activity.

Sexuality

Feminist therapy explicitly validates all sexual choices for women and views awareness and expression of sexu-

ality as a right. It offers opportunity to explore bases of current sexual attitudes, values, and behaviors, and to think about options for future sexual choices without being sexually exploited (e.g., by the therapist).

Victims of Violence

Feminist therapy rejects explanations of violent incidents (such as rape, molestation, incest and battering) which blame the victim, suggesting the seductive child or the woman who provokes her own beating. Rather, feminist therapy views these acts as the results of living in a sexist society where abuse of women is tolerated.

Depression

The high rates of depression among women indicate that sex-role constraints may socialize women into depressive symptoms. (These symptoms may be seen as an exaggeration of expected female behavior.) It is also related to issues of power and self-nurturance. Therapy rarely includes drugs, and never includes electro-shock therapy.

Ω

Mental Patients' Liberation Front: Seeking control
by Susan Shapiro

Judy Chamberlin is the author of *On Our Own,* an enlightening and empowering book which outlines not only problems in the existing mental health system, but also clear suggestions for patient-controlled alternatives. Chamberlin, who spent about five months as a patient in six different mental hospitals, says, "It was years before I allowed myself to feel anger at a system that had locked me up, denied me warm and meaningful contact with other human beings, drugged me, and so thoroughly confused me that I thought of this treatment as helpful." But out of her anger—and with the support of others in the mental patients' liberation movement—has come strength and action.

SHAPIRO: What is Mental Patients' Liberation Front?

CHAMBERLIN: MPLF is an organization of people who have been mental patients. It's been around Boston since 1971, and is now part of a network of 50 or more

groups in North America that are unified by the idea that people who've been patients should control their own lives and shouldn't have their rights taken away from them. We're in contact with groups all over the world who are doing similar kinds of work

What kind of activities is MPLF involved in?

We do a lot of different things—advocacy, giving advice, information, and referrals. We also do a lot of just talking and listening to people. With this new Massachusetts Commissioner of Mental Health, there's a good possibility that we'll get funding within the next year to start a drop-in center or residence of some sort.

In *On Our Own,* it was interesting how you broke down the psychiatric system into mental institutions, halfway houses, and private therapy—and rejected all three.

A lot of people think that the only problems are in the public mental health system, and that if you can get people out of institutions, the problems disappear. But they don't, because once people get labelled "psychiatric patients"— whether they're in private therapy, halfway houses, community treatment centers, or hospitals—they get very much discredited as people. Usually it's done with benevolent intentions—you are "confused," you don't know what's best for you—and somebody else has to take on a paternalistic role. But it ends up that the patient has no power, and the treater has all the power. And that's very dangerous, because when you lose control of your own life, anything can happen to you. When you start objecting, you can be told that the only reason you're objecting is that you're sick and can't see clearly.

Can you talk about some of the ways in which patients are disempowered?

Basically by not being taken seriously. There are stories about people who find out that their date of birth or some bit of information on their records is wrong. If they say, "I wasn't born on May 13, I was born on June 13," they're believed to be having a delusion. Somebody is always scrutinizing you, figuring out what you really mean. You're not taken as an equal, as another human being who has some troubles, but as somebody who is totally untrustworthy. It's very scary—you begin to lose your sense of who you are. They say that feelings of depersonalization are one of the prime symptoms of schizophrenia, yet everything they do to you, including the drugging, makes you feel depersonalized.

One of the things that seems to happen to a lot of people in the system is that they don't trust themselves anymore. They think you have to be a staff member to be a competent person. There are thousands of decisions that you have to make just to live in the world—you know, am I going to buy Wheaties or Cornflakes—but at an institution, you're considered a good patient if you don't do any of that stuff, if you let yourself be steered through the day always doing what other people want you to do.

Do you feel that the current mental health system is harmful for everybody?

It has that potential. It reinforces the sense that what's wrong with you is wrong with *you*. There are a lot of things that are wrong out there which make us unhappy, and I really think that most people are going to feel much better about themselves when they get involved in action rather than in "fixing themselves."

I know many women who have had positive experience in private therapy, and I wonder if it's because they are feminists (who have rejected traditional values) often with similar backgrounds to their therapists' (educational, political, etc.). Do you think these areas of commonality make a difference in terms of a significant power imbalance?

Sure. If your vision of a good life and your therapist's vision are the same, therapy can be very comforting. That situation is the least likely to have a big power imbalance. Everybody has problems that are personal in combination with problems that are really political and social. If you can isolate a specific thing that you're doing to yourself and can learn to do it differently, that can certainly be helpful. The problem is that you get into all these other situations, the power trips and the confusing of what's your own personal problem with what isn't.

Can you describe a viable alternative to the current mental health system?

I always talk about alternatives, because there's no one thing that's going to be good for all people. If people would just talk more about their problems, their feelings, maybe we'd short-circuit some of the crises. But in order to do that right now, you have to define yourself as having something wrong with you. There have to be ways to talk about feelings, problems, and anxieties without being labelled or having a record established. When you do get to the point of crisis, there should be hotlines and places you can walk into with a minimum of formalities and get somebody to talk to and, most important, listen to you.

Do you think it's best to have that "somebody" be a professional or somebody who has been through a similar experience?

Certainly the whole self-help aspect is really important. Being a mental health professional doesn't necessarily mean you're a good listener. The kind of centers I'm talking about would have no power to do anything to anybody. They'd have to let somebody walk out even if he or she said, "I'm going to kill myself." They could say, "We have a nice place here where you could stay and relax for a while, and maybe after a while you wouldn't want to kill yourself. Would you like that? Yes? Fine. No? Okay." That's very hard to do. But if there were places available that were non-punitive and non-restrictive of people's liberties—which you could walk out of at any time—I think more people would go to them.

Are portrayals of mental institutions in movies like *Cuckoo's Nest* and *Frances* accurate?

Both of those movies told part of the truth. There were a couple of major fallacies in *Cuckoo's Nest*. The absolute, total power of the nurse was just not true. There are certainly nurses with absolute power over patients, but she was shown as having total power over the doctors, too, and that has to do with Ken Kesey's hatred of women. The patients, with the exception of McMurphy and the chief, were all stereotyped mental patients whom we're supposed to recognize as types and not see as whole human beings. But the institution as it was portrayed—yeah, that's what institutions are like. They're not the snakepits that they show in *Frances,* which apparently was true of institutions in the '30s and '40s. They're a different kind of horrible place now, in a sterile, numbing way. *Frances* was the most accurate description I have ever seen in movies or literature of how they take somebody who doesn't fit in and transform her not fitting in into an illness. She became less and less what she had been, and more and more a mental patient. In the end, they defeated and destroyed her.

"Hill Street Blues" showed an episode about a mental patient who, upset because a butcher wouldn't give him a bone for his dog, crashed a stool into something. Soon after the judge let him go, the man committed a murder.

Statistically that's so wrong. Most mental patients are not violent, but the media link of mental patients and violence is very strong. In most cases, if mental patients are accused of a violent act, it's violence against themselves. But most people are not even accused of a violent act; they are accused of being incapable of taking care of themselves by reason of mental illness.

What are the problems in using a medical model for non-medical problems?

It fits in very well with most people's conception of things in this age of science, and solving problems through scientific means. Labels like "schizophrenic" or "manic depressive" put things in a category for people: "Well, now I know what it is. So-and-so is sick, so we'll turn her over to the doctors." And the doctors take charge and put her in the hospital.

Also, the person who's suffering doesn't know what she's going through, either. For some people, being told that they're sick is okay, because it explains what they're going through. A lot of people embrace the medical model at one point or another in their episode because for a while it seems to answer those questions better than any other model.

But if this is an illness, what part is diseased? Now they're trying to pin that down; there's all this research on brain chemistry. But I think ultimately we're going to look back on this later in the same way we look back at debates over how many angels can dance on the head of a pin.

Has the theory of chemical imbalance ever been proved?

There are hundreds of theories, and they all point to different chemicals. Because they need brain chemicals to fit their model, researchers are out there madly looking for brain chemicals. And they're finding them, but nobody can duplicate anybody else's research. The fact that there are hundreds of theories shows how invalid this is as science. It's not that they're on the track of something and getting closer and closer.

People are accustomed to thinking that this is the way we're going to solve these problems. But if you go back 400 or 500 years in western history, you find that people were accustomed then to seeing problems as religious, able to be solved by theological means. Just as we can now say that it's ridiculous to look for the devils that possess crazy people, I think that later we will be able to say, "It's silly to be looking in people's brains instead of looking at people's lives."

Do you know what percentage of institutionalized people are women?

You hear in the women's movement that there are many more women than men. That may be true for all therapy contacts, because women are vastly overrepresented in private practice. But in hospitals, you get different statistics on that.

Are female patients treated differently in hospitals?

Yes. It's a very sexist system. Of course, it depends on whom you run into and what their theoretical schooling has been, but you still get a lot of people who think of women in traditional roles, with a different emotional makeup. There's also a tremendous amount of sexual abuse, and if women in general can't get themselves to be taken seriously when they complain about sexual abuse, how can women mental patients?

You pointed out in the book how, in institutions, sweeping the floor becomes "industrial therapy" and going to the movies becomes "recreation therapy." Is there any real therapy going on?

If there is such a thing as "therapy," I think it by definition has to be something that's contracted to between two parties who have a somewhat equal relationship. What's really therapeutic is regaining control of your life. You can call anything "therapy." Most of the things that are called therapy in institutions are very infantilizing; you do all this kindergarten stuff, like cutting out colored paper. It's a relief from boredom, but it shows how little respect people have for you as an individual and as an adult. There's "milieu therapy"—you're *there,* and they call that milieu therapy. It's "chemotherapy" to be taking drugs, even if it's against your will. It's very strange.

Whatever you were when you went into the hospital—housewife, student—is supposed to be your goal when you get out, what you're supposed to want to go on doing. But a lot of people come into mental hospitals when their whole lives are changing. That can be very painful and difficult and frightening, but to make them *not* change, to have the idea of changing be seen as part of their sickness—just pushes people back to whatever it was that drove them crazy in the first place.

Is there any particular experience that you had in a mental hospital that you want to share with *Sojourner* readers?

I'm debating whether to pull out my juiciest horror story. You know, I think it really goes beyond horror stories, because even people who've had fairly decent experiences in mental hospitals have experienced the same thing—the routinized disrespect for personhood, the sense that you really don't count, the sense that just about everybody you come into contact with doesn't take you seriously as a whole adult human being, the sense of always being patronized. You can go through that whole experience without meeting even one single person who takes you as a unique human being, instead of just somebody who can be summed up by, you know, "24-year-old schizophrenic." How the hell is anybody supposed to feel better in a place where they get you up at 7:00 in the morning and put you to bed at 9:00 at night, where you line up and eat this not-very-good or sometimes extremely awful food, and where you don't have a moment's privacy?

If a woman came to you and said she was in a terrible crisis and felt like she couldn't cope, what would your advice be?

To provide her with other people she could talk to, who could confirm her feelings. It's an awful world, and people are in really desperate situations. To feel desperate when you don't have enough money to feed your kids or the landlord's throwing you out on the streets doesn't mean there's anything wrong with you. It doesn't mean that you're a weak person and that some stronger person could get through it. Janet Gotkin, a movement activist and good friend of mine, was asked in a group how she got through her parents' dying, and she said, "Badly." And I think that's how we get through crises—badly. We suffer and cry and stay up all night, and we eat too much and pace the floor, and we talk crazy and do all kinds of things, because somehow we're getting through the crisis. Nobody sails through it well, healthy, strong—that's a myth that cripples all of us. It's okay to cry and scream and curse fate and do any one of five trillion crazy things that people do to get through a crisis. Confirm people's feelings. Let them know that when you feel weird, it's okay to act weird. And don't trivialize or romanticize it. There was a lot of that in the late '60s; going crazy was the ultimate trip. It's very, very painful. Let somebody know how much it hurts, and let them cry.

What if there is someone who feels like she just can't be alone and really does need a place to go?

That's where the big lack is. There's a tremendous need for respite. You don't need a hospital or a medical staff to give somebody shelter and good food and human contact. It can be done. One of the things I talked about in the book was the crisis center that did it right and did it cheaper than any hospital. Talking to you is the last thing the staff in a hospital is doing. There aren't very many of them, and they're all busy running around, doing paperwork, making sure that everybody gets her lunch, and all the stuff that has to do with running an institution.

Is there anything else you want to say to *Sojourner* readers?

I'd like people to think about their attitudes toward therapy and craziness and mental patients. There are a lot of people who are pretty sensitive and aware who just never have thought about this issue. People have to start thinking about their own prejudices, their own feeling that crazy people are to be dealt with by somebody else. Most people have had feelings at one time or another that could have ended up with them getting labelled. We need to see that unity, instead of the "us/them" separateness. People need to see that we're all connected.

Author's Note: *For more information about MPLF, call 617-628-8438 or write: P.O. Box 514, Cambridge, MA 02238. On Our Own is published by McGraw-Hill and can be ordered by sending $5.60 to MPLF. Make checks payable to Judi Chamberlin.*

Ω

Mental Health

1. Stress is defined as the non-specific response of the body to demands made on it. These demands can be physical or emotional. The response is non-specific in the sense that, no matter whether the stressor (cause of stress) is seemingly negative or positive, the body responds the same way physiologically. On scales that measure stress of life-events, marriage, graduation, and promotion get high stress ratings, along with break-up of a relationship, death in the family, and a jail sentence. If we cannot find ways to manage stress, there can be many possible long term health consequences, such as high blood pressure, high cholesterol (both of which increase the risk of heart disease), lowered resistance to infectious diseases, more migraines if prone to them, various disturbances of the digestive system (including ulcers and colitis), and sleep problems.

    a. List five stressors in your life.

        1.
        2.
        3.
        4.
        5.

    b. List five ways you cope with or manage stress.

        1.

        2.

        3.

        4.

        5.

    c. If any of the answers in b. have potential negative consequences, identify an alternative positive approach. For example, some people deal with stress by shopping, but a shopping spree can create more stress when the bills have to be paid. Others may turn to alcohol or binge eating. What are "healthy" alternatives to these strategies?

    d. Are there differences in the stressors women and men in this society may experience? Are there differences in the way women and men may choose to or be able to deal with stress?

2. Mental health is said to be related to maintaining a balance of work, play and love in our lives.

    a. How do these elements balance out in your life?

    b. Thinking through the roles that women and men play in this society, and by reading Lesley Doyal's "Hazards of Hearth and Home" article in chapter 3, think of whether there may be differences for women and men in trying to maintain a balance in their lives. If so, describe some specific differences:

3. What does it mean that mental health professionals give similar definitions for healthy adults and healthy men but describe healthy women as more submissive, less independent, more easily influenced, less competitive?

    a. Does this mean "the only mentally healthy women are the ones who adjust to a world where women are considered inferior?"

    b. Does questioning sexism mean that someone is mentally unhealthy?!

Chapter

5

Alcohol, Tobacco, and Other Drugs

The "war on drugs" in the United States has targeted illegal drugs, especially cocaine. However, if we examine which drugs are responsible for the majority of drug-related health problems, the focus changes to legal drugs. Use and abuse of alcohol, tobacco, and psychoactive prescription drugs are responsible for more deaths and disease than the well-publicized "crack epidemic." The first article in this section, "Addictive Behaviors" from *The Women's Health Data Book,* presents an excellent overview of the use of these common drugs by women and what is known about the ways in which women's physiology (hormones, menstrual cycle, total water content) must be considered to understand the effects of these drugs. Unfortunately, women are often under pressure to use legal drugs (medical prescriptions for psychoactive drugs; alcohol and tobacco advertising targeted at women) and then receive information on the dangers only when pregnant. The protection of the fetus is often presented as more important than the health of the woman herself. "Alcoholics Invisible: The Ordeal of the Female Alcoholic," a classic article by Marian Sandmeier, demonstrates the ways in which the health care system has failed to deal appropriately with women's problems with alcohol. The next article, "Women and Children Last," expands and updates issues raised by Sandmeier, discussing the barriers women face in attempting to obtain alcohol and other drug treatment. In the article "The Twelve-Step Controversy," Charlotte Davis Kasl, a psychologist and former member of 12-step programs, continues this discussion by examining programs modeled after Alcoholics Anonymous, which was originally designed for and by men. She provides a 12-step model built on the reality of women's lives, which may be more useful to women trying to heal and move from "*r*ecovery to *dis*covery." Susan Janicki's essay adds a very personal perspective on the process of recovery, and also examines some specific issues for lesbians around alcohol abuse, dependency, and recovery. The

devastation of fetal alcohol syndrome (FAS) in Native American communities is analyzed by Charon Asetoyer, a Native American health activist and educator. She emphasizes the need to end victim-blaming approaches and repressive measures (such as forced sterilization) and calls for leadership to examine and correct the underlying societal and economic factors that lead to alcohol abuse among Native Americans. A follow-up letter to Asetoyer's article by Ruth Hubbard adds research data to support the importance of the role of economic and social factors in FAS.

"How Women are Targeted by the Tobacco Industry" examines the drug that has helped women reach parity with men in the areas of lung cancer and other respiratory diseases. The article examines the ways women, especially younger women, have been targeted by the tobacco industry as an important market, both in the United States and internationally. Advertising approaches and themes are described, and the article concludes with some specific ground rules for women's magazines around tobacco advertising. This chapter ends with a positive note as an article from the *Journal of the American Medical Association* describes anti-smoking activism, particularly against the targeting of specific groups (women, people of color, teens) by the tobacco industry.

It is important to emphasize that the women's movement has been slow to recognize that the battle against the tobacco industry must be seen as a feminist issue and also needs to be placed in an international context, as the tobacco industry has targeted many Third World nations in response to dwindling U.S. markets. As the women's health movement confronts this problem, it must be recognized that we are fighting against the exploitation of women and *not* attacking women who smoke. As with the issues around FAS, a feminist approach to drug education and policies should never be victim-blaming.

Addictive Behaviors

from The Women's Health Data Book

Alcohol Use

The use of alcohol by women is prevalent in American society. The limited data that are available indicate that alcohol affects women differently than men. Regarding alcohol use by women, the Report of the Public Health Task Force on Women's Health Issues notes that "there are few areas in which conclusions can be stated categorically, and fewer still in which our knowledge . . . is more than fragmentary."

Survey results cited in this section are often based on small numbers of subjects, which may produce unstable estimates. Self-reports of alcohol consumption are often used in surveys. These estimates are more often underestimates than overestimates of consumption.

Discussion of the complex issues surrounding alcohol use by women is hampered by the fact that scientific research has often ignored differences in alcohol use by women and men. In studies that have examined these differences, the research findings have often been inconclusive because of small sample size. Furthermore, the interrelationships between physiology, social factors, and alcohol use are not well understood. Although it is convenient to discuss prevalence, causal factors, and correlates of alcohol use separately from issues related to mental and emotional problems, these problems are often interrelated and frequently occur together.

Two national surveys have filled some of the gaps in our knowledge. One is a periodic survey called the National Household Survey on Drug Abuse and is conducted by the National Institute of Drug Abuse. It measures the prevalence of drug use among the household population aged 12 years and over, using a random sample of the population to provide the latest data. This survey includes persons living in some group quarters, such as college dormitories and homeless shelters. The 1991 survey also included Alaska and Hawaii for the first time. Another survey is the National Survey of Drinking, which is conducted by the National Institute of Alcohol Abuse and Alcoholism. This survey, based on self-reported information, was designed to represent adults over 18 years of age.

Use of Alcohol by Women

Women who consume alcohol have been stigmatized since ancient times, particularly if their drinking was excessive according to the prevailing standards of their society. This stigmatization has led to an unwillingness on the part of women, as well as clinicians and researchers, to acknowledge the problem of alcoholism in women, making it difficult to estimate the magnitude of the problem.

It is agreed that women drink less than men. At all ages, women are less likely than men to have consumed alcohol in their lifetime, in the past year, or in the past month. On the other hand, women are more likely than men to be lifetime abstainers. In one study, 45% of women reported that they had never used alcohol, compared with 18% of men. While there is agreement that women on average drink less alcohol than men, there is mounting evidence that when they drink comparable amounts they are likely to be more impaired than men, both immediately and over longer periods of time.

It has been reported that one reason alcohol has a greater intoxicating effect on women than on men is that total body water content differs between the sexes. In general, women have smaller body water quantities than men of similar size because they have a higher proportion of fatty tissue. The result is higher blood alcohol concentrations in women. It has also been reported that women respond differently to alcohol throughout their menstrual cycle, but the mechanisms involved are not fully understood. Further study is needed on the basic processes involved in alcohol metabolism during the menstrual cycle and the role that estrogen levels play, since lower peak blood alcohol levels and alcohol clearance rates have been found in women taking oral contraceptives.

Alcohol-Related Morbidity and Mortality

Alcohol abuse is the principal cause of cirrhosis of the liver, which is the ninth leading cause of death in the United States. There is some evidence that women are more likely than men to develop advanced liver disease, even with similar drinking histories. One of the few longitudinal studies of alcoholic women estimated that their average life span is reduced by 15 years because of both alcohol-related disorders such as liver disease and a higher incidence of alcohol-related accidents and suicides. In that study, more than 30% of the alcoholic women had died after 12 years of follow-up, a rate 4.5 times higher than the controls selected from other hospital patients.

Although the liver is the organ most seriously affected by alcohol consumption, women experience many other alcohol-related disorders, including hypertension, obesity, anemia, malnutrition, and gastrointestinal hemorrhage. Rates of obstetric and gynecologic conditions, including amenorrhea, miscarriage, early menopause, gynecologic surgery, and infertility, are higher than expected in alcoholic women than in other women. The reasons for these increased rates are unclear, although both biologic and psychosocial factors are thought to be involved.

Alcohol Use During Pregnancy

Alcohol use during pregnancy has been identified as the leading preventable cause of birth defects. Although alcohol crosses the placental barrier, its effects on the developing fetus are variable because of differences in the degree and timing of exposure, genetic differences in maternal metabolism of alcohol, maternal nutritional status, and possible interaction with other drugs.

Fetal alcohol syndrome is a set of birth defects characterized by abnormal features of the face and head, growth retardation, and central nervous system abnormalities often reflected in mental retardation. It has been noted in some of the babies born to mothers who drank heavily during their pregnancy. Babies with milder symptoms are said to have fetal alcohol effects, which may not be apparent until the child is older. The most common fetal alcohol effects are learning disabilities, retarded growth, and mental retardation.

It is disturbing to find in one study that, although the prevalence of alcohol consumption reported by pregnant women in the United States showed a relative decline of 38% from 1985 to 1988, women who drank during pregnancy did not decrease the number of drinks consumed. This study also found that the prevalence of alcohol use remained highest among women who may be at higher risk for poor pregnancy outcome: pregnant smokers, single mothers, and the youngest and the least-educated women in the study showed no reduction in their use of alcohol.

Minority Women

Seventy-five percent of black women, 70% of Hispanic women, and 83% of white women have reported that they have used alcohol at some point in their lives. In general, regardless of age, white women are more likely than black women to report alcohol use. Black and white women are equally likely, however, to drink heavily. In one study, binge drinking reported by mothers was higher among whites (11%) than among blacks (9%). At the same time, the rate of fetal alcohol syndrome among blacks in another study was seven times that among whites. The reason for this apparent contradiction is not understood, and further research is needed. Despite the overall lower reports of use, black alcoholic women who were followed for 12 years after treatment were found to have higher mortality than the white alcoholic women in the same study (6.7% versus 3.9%). Black women also report more alcohol-related health problems than white women.

High rates of fetal alcohol syndrome have also been found in some American Indian tribes in the Southwest. Several factors, including cultural influences, patterns of alcohol consumption, and nutrition, are thought to be associated with the prevalence of fetal alcohol syndrome in this population.

Adolescents and Young Adults

Self-reports of alcohol use by young females aged 12–25 years indicate that drinking is widespread in this age group. In 1990, 53% of women aged 18–25 years and 24% of girls aged 12–17 years reported that they had used alcohol in the past month. Although the proportion of young females reporting that they currently use alcohol has declined from a peak (76%) in 1979, these levels of alcohol use remain high. Furthermore, about 35% of female college students report patterns of recent heavy drinking, defined as five or more drinks in a row in the past 2 weeks. Among high school seniors, 29% of females and 46% of males report similar heavy drinking patterns.

The leading cause of death among young people in the United States is accidents and injuries. Alcohol has been implicated in nearly half of all deaths caused by motor vehicle accidents, suicides, and homicides and in one-third of all drownings and boating accident deaths.

The complex interaction of biologic differences and psychosocial factors seem to influence women's patterns of alcohol use. It is readily apparent, however, that additional research efforts are required to increase the limited knowledge that is currently available.

Drug Use

Females use virtually all types of illicit drugs, but they use them less frequently than males. Data from the 1991 National Household Survey of Drug Abuse indicate that among persons 12 years of age and older, females are less likely than males to have ever used, or to have used in the past year or the past month, any illicit drug. Illicit drug use by women in all three of these categories (lifetime use, use in the past year, and current use) is highest among women during their peak childbearing years. Perhaps the most striking statistic is that 53–57% of women aged 18–34 years reported using an illicit drug at least once in their lifetime.

Medical and Nonmedical Use of Psychotherapeutic Drugs

Incidence of Use

The major exception to the generalization that drug use by men exceeds that by women is in regard to the use of medically prescribed psychotherapeutic drugs (sedatives, tranquilizers, stimulants, and analgesics). Prescribed medications may be used medically to serve a legitimate therapeutic function, or they may be used nonmedically, that is, in a manner inconsistent with prescribed instructions. It is not possible from the data available to determine how much of the reported use of prescribed drugs in men and women is appropriate and medically justified.

Almost without exception, regardless of age, women who reported that they had used psychotherapeutic drugs at some time in their lives were more likely than men to have had the drug prescribed for them. Seventy-one percent of adolescent females who reported that they had used a tranquilizer during their lifetime indicated that they had received it as a prescribed medication. Women over 18 years of age reported higher use of stimulants than men. Among youths aged 12–17 years, females had higher rates than males of nonmedical use of sedatives (54% versus 48%), stimulants (79% versus 55%), and analgesics (13% versus 8%).

Consequences of Use

Women are more likely than men to become addicted to prescription drugs and to use them, often with alcohol, to medicate themselves to cope with anxiety, depression, and painful reactions to life stresses. Adverse consequences associated with the medical use of psychotherapeutic drugs are infrequently reported. However, persons who misuse psychotherapeutic drugs are more likely to report problems such as depression and argumentativeness.

Drug-Related Morbidity

Drug-related morbidity is difficult to estimate. The Drug Abuse Warning Network (DAWN) is a surveillance system designed to monitor drug-related visits to hospital emergency rooms in 21 metropolitan areas of the United States. In 1990, there were more than 370,000 emergency-room episodes related to drug abuse. Provisional data indicate that the total number of drug-related visits to emergency rooms increased from more than 89,000 in the fourth quarter of 1990 to more than 100,000 in the second quarter of 1991. During the same period, cocaine-related visits increased by 31%, from nearly 20,000 to more than 25,000. In addition, there was a 26% increase in the number of emergency-room visits related to heroin use.

It is not clear whether these changes represent an increase in cocaine and heroin abuse or whether they reflect the severe medical complications that may result from prolonged drug use. Changes in the rate of drug overdoses could also contribute to greater use of emergency-room services. In contrast, data available for 1988–1989 show that there was a decrease in visits to emergency rooms for cocaine-related problems among young women of all races and ethnic groups. In the same year, however, there was an increase among older women, particularly among older white women. More recent data on these trends are not available at this time.

Drug Abuse During Pregnancy

Thirty percent of women of childbearing age report that they have used marijuana at least once in their lifetime, and at least 3% have reported that they are current users. No studies have demonstrated abnormal pregnancy outcome attributable to the effects of marijuana use during pregnancy.

Opiate (heroin) addiction is less common than marijuana use among women, but the health risks to the mother and baby are serious. Women who are addicted to opiates are often in poor general health. They have a higher incidence of chronic infections, gynecologic problems, anemia, and sexually transmitted diseases, including human immunodeficiency virus (HIV) infection.

Because these women often use other drugs, have poor nutrition, and lack adequate prenatal care, serious obstetric complications can occur. Women using opiates during pregnancy are at higher risk for preterm labor, intrauterine growth retardation, and preeclampsia. Use of opiates close to the end of pregnancy can result in babies who suffer from drug withdrawal after birth. Unfortunately, opiate-dependent women are less likely to seek treatment than opiate-dependent men, and those who do seek treatment often find that services to meet their needs are almost nonexistent.

In 1991, 9% of women reported that they had used cocaine (including crack cocaine) at some point in their lives. Cocaine is highly addictive and produces an immediate but brief period of intense euphoria followed by a period of severe depression and agitation. Cocaine users frequently use various combinations of drugs and alcohol to prolong the period of euphoria. Cocaine has severe behavioral and biologic effects, including impulsivity, hypertension, seizures, cardiac arrhythmia, tachycardia, myocardial infarction, and sometimes death. Decreased interest in food over a long period can lead to malnutrition.

During pregnancy, cocaine can affect the fetus, resulting in an increased incidence of spontaneous abortion and fetal death. A higher risk of preterm labor, precipitous delivery, placental abruption, and fetal distress with meconium staining has been observed among women using cocaine. Higher rates of congenital malformations have also been noted in babies born to mothers who used cocaine. An increased rate of sudden infant death syndrome among infants born to mothers who used cocaine during pregnancy has also been observed.

Special Populations

Minority Women

The National Household Survey on Drug Abuse found that white women were more likely (35%) than black (33%) or Hispanic (25%) women to have used an illicit drug at some point in their lives. Current use of any illicit drug was also found to be slightly higher among black females (7%) than among white or Hispanic females (5%).

Elderly Women

Although the elderly are generally not users of illicit drugs, they are recognized as having high levels of legal drug use. Elderly women constitute 11% of the population, yet 25% of all prescriptions are written for this group. It has been reported that older patients may have as many as 30 drugs prescribed for them each year. Prescriptions for elderly women often include estrogen replacement therapy, sedatives, hypnotics, antianxiety drugs, antihypertensive drugs, vitamins, analagesics, diuretics, laxatives, and tranquilizers, which are prescribed for elderly women at a rate 2.5 times that of elderly men.

It is clear that the potential for harmful drug interactions is a serious threat to older women. Research has shown that women experience more adverse drug reactions than men, possibly due to the large number of drugs they take. Other health consequences associated with drug use in the elderly are suicide, insomnia, affective disturbance, and impairment of cognitive and motor function, which can be severe enough to lead to institutionalization.

Currently, it appears that drug misuse, rather than abuse, is more common in the elderly. However, some experts believe that as more people who were drug abusers in their early years reach older ages, they may be more likely to abuse psychoactive drugs that may be prescribed for them.

Although the available evidence suggests that women's experience with drug use and abuse is different from men's, the data are limited. More research is essential to provide an understanding of the physiologic, psychosocial, and behavioral dimensions of drug use throughout women's lives.

Smoking

The fact that the year Eleanor Roosevelt smoked a cigarette in public is recorded (1934) is an indication that such an event was rare. At that time there were little national data available on the prevalence of smoking, but it was estimated that 17% of adult women in the United States were smokers. By 1965, 34% of American women smoked, an all-time high.

Although the rate of cigarette smoking has never been as high among women as among men, the rate for both men and women has declined. The decline has been less dramatic for women, and the latest data show that 27% of women in the United States currently smoke. About one in every four women under 25 years of age is a current smoker. After age 25, approximately one in every three women smokes. Of great health significance is the fact that between 1965 and 1985, the percentage of women who are heavy smokers, defined as those who smoke 25 or more cigarettes a day, increased from 13% to 23%.

The good news is that there has been a 21% decline in the prevalence of smoking among women since 1965. Current female smokers are more likely to be separated or divorced women, women who have less than 12 years of education, and women with annual family incomes of less than $20,000. The highest proportion of former smokers are found among college-educated women, women who are married, and those with high incomes.

Smoking Initiation

Fifty-six percent of all adult women have never smoked. Fewer females than males start smoking before age 20, but regardless of the age at which they begin to smoke, women are more likely to continue to smoke.

Furthermore, the younger a woman is when she starts to smoke, the more likely she is to be a current smoker.

Between 1965 and 1985, the percentage of former smokers has increased among adult women. The percentage of lifetime smokers (both current and former smokers), however, has remained constant since 1970, suggesting that the proportion of women who start to smoke has not declined.

Smoking Cessation

Seventeen percent of all adult females are former smokers. Smoking cessation may be accompanied by a wide range of withdrawal symptoms that vary considerably among individuals. Data about withdrawal and smoking cessation strategies in women versus men, however, are scarce. National data indicate that both former and current smokers cite present and future health concerns as reasons for quitting. Women smokers report more concern than men about gaining weight as a result of quitting.

Smoking-Related Morbidity and Mortality

Because cigarette smoking by women did not become widespread until during World War II, women are just now facing the increased morbidity and mortality associated with cigarette smoking. Cigarette smoking contributes to one of every five newly diagnosed cases of cancer and up to one-fourth of all cancer deaths among women.

As a result of the increase in cigarette smoking among women, the rate of deaths from lung cancer has increased dramatically in women. In 1988, lung cancer exceeded breast cancer as the leading cause of cancer death in white women. It has been estimated that it takes about 15 years after a smoker quits for her risk of lung cancer to return to that of a nonsmoker. A marked increase in deaths from chronic obstructive pulmonary disease (COPD) among women is expected in the next few decades, because an estimated 82% of all COPD deaths are attributable to cigarette smoking.

Heart disease is the leading cause of death for both men and women in the United States. Women with smoking patterns similar to those of men experience similar rates of cardiovascular morbidity and mortality, although studies have shown that women have a protective factor for heart disease prior to the age of menopause. Other cardiovascular conditions associated with smoking in women include lower levels of high-density lipoproteins, peripheral vascular disease, subarachnoid hemorrhage, and severe or malignant hypertension. Like their male counterparts, current female smokers have an increased incidence of sudden death. Women smokers over the age of 35 years are advised not to use oral contraceptives because their risk of heart attack and stroke is increased.

Smoking and Pregnancy

Cigarette smoking has been implicated as a risk factor in about one-quarter of all births of babies weighing less than 2,500 g at birth. Babies born to women who smoke are, on average, 200 g lighter than babies born to comparable non-smoking mothers. Increasing levels of maternal smoking result in an increased risk of obstetric complications such as abruptio placentae, placenta previa, premature or prolonged rupture of membranes, and preterm delivery. The risk of miscarriage, stillbirth, and neonatal death increases directly with increasing levels of smoking during pregnancy. Further study of the role of smoking and other factors that may confound the relationship with perinatal outcome is warranted.

A recent study used cross-sectional data obtained by telephone interview from the Behavioral Risk Factor Surveillance System (BRFSS), a system of participating state health departments collaborating with the Centers for Disease Control. It was found that 21% of pregnant women and 30% of nonpregnant women were current smokers at the time of the study. Because the prevalence of having ever smoked was similar in the two groups, the difference in the current smoking rates was due to the fact that the pregnant women had quit smoking rather than to differences in when smoking had commenced.

These findings were supported by another study in which it was found that one-third of white women aged 20–44 years smoked prior to pregnancy and 39% of the smokers indicated that they quit while pregnant. Among current smokers in the BRFSS study, 38% of pregnant women and 53% of nonpregnant women reported that they were heavy smokers (smoking 20 or more cigarettes per day). Pregnant women over 30 years of age were less likely to smoke than women in their 20s. Unmarried pregnant women were more likely than married women to be smokers both before and during pregnancy. The prevalence of smoking decreased sharply with increasing education. Seventy percent of the women who quit smoking while pregnant resumed within 1 year, with the majority relapsing in the first 3 months after delivery.

Special Populations

Minority Women

Although the prevalence of smoking is high among all women, black and Hispanic women have lower overall current and lifetime rates of cigarette use than white women. The 1988 National Household Survey on Drug Abuse found lifetime use of cigarettes to be higher among white females (73%) than either Hispanic females (52%) or black females (63%). In this survey, similar patterns of current smoking were found. Only 20% of Hispanic and 24% of black women reported that they were smokers at the present time, compared with 26% of white women. This represents a decline among white and black women from the 1987 National Health Interview Survey findings. In that survey, an equally high percentage of current smokers was found among black and white females (27%). It is not clear whether this difference between the two surveys is due to methodologic factors or whether it represents a real decline.

Black women have consistently been shown to have a lower prevalence of smoking during pregnancy than whites. It has also been found that black women are less likely to quit after they become pregnant. This suggests that the difference in the prevalence of smoking among black pregnant women is due to the lower prevalence of ever having smoked in that population. Because other data suggest that there is no racial difference in prevalence of ever having smoked, however, these findings await further clarification.

Adolescent women

Despite all of the publicity given to the health risks associated with cigarette smoking, adolescent females are more likely to smoke than their male counterparts in high school and in young adulthood, whether or not they are in college. Studies have shown that students who smoke are also more likely to use alcohol and illicit drugs, particularly marijuana.

A 1987 follow-up study of adolescents in the southeastern United States showed that among teenagers who did not smoke in 1985, more whites than blacks started smoking. White females in the study were more likely than blacks to start smoking at 12 years. Peer pressure was correlated with the likelihood that a white teenager would smoke, but this factor was not important for black teenagers in this study.

Tobacco use has been identified as the single most preventable cause of death and disease. Although progress has been made in social interventions to decrease smoking, the adverse health effects of smoking become apparent over a long interval, and the effects of the increased use of tobacco by women are just beginning to be felt. There is an immediate need for vigorous action to decrease smoking among women in order to improve health outcomes in the years ahead.

Ω

Alcoholics Invisible:
The Ordeal of the Female Alcoholic

by Marian Sandmaier

Even under the best of circumstances, the ability to turn away from a drug to which one is physically and psychologically addicted requires uncommon courage and determination. But most of the women whom I interviewed recovered from alcoholism in the face of an appalling lack of support from the doctors, therapists, alcoholism personnel, and others charged with diagnosing and treating their illness. With a few notable exceptions, these women were discouraged by the health system from embarking on alcoholism treatment to begin with, and once involved in treatment, were denied supports and services important to their recovery. They discovered what most alcoholic women who seek help are forced to recognize: that contemptuous attitudes and sheer ignorance about women with alcohol problems pervade the health system as thoroughly and destructively as any other segment of society. There, as anywhere, the real needs and the very humanity of alcoholic women remain invisible.

Within the health system, the first person an alcoholic woman is likely to encounter is her own doctor. And at first glance, he* would seem to be in an excellent position to identify her alcohol problem and steer her toward appropriate treatment.

Diagnosis

Yet physicians appear highly unlikely to diagnose alcoholism in their female patients. In a 1975 survey of 89 women in Alcoholics Anonymous, fully half of the women surveyed said they had tried to discuss their drinking problem with someone who told them they couldn't possibly be alcoholic; twelve received such advice from physicians, five of these psychiatrists.[1] Of the 50 women I interviewed, 45 had been seen by doctors while they were drinking alcoholically, but only seven were ever confronted by their physicians about their alcohol abuse. A 54 year-old Boston woman recalled: "In all of the times I landed in the hospital during my drinking years, no doctor ever said anything to me about alcoholism. I always either had colitis or a kidney problem or pneumonia, and when they couldn't think of anything else, I would have nerves. Twice I attempted suicide and once wound up in a hospital afterward for three months. And in those three months, I

saw a psychiatrist every day and not once did he say a word to me about being alcoholic. And at that point I had been drinking almost around the clock."

Some physicians fail to respond to even clear-cut evidence of alcohol problems in their women patients. "I used to carry a big purse full of beer into my psychiatrist's office and drink right through the sessions," recalled a young social scientist from Virginia. "He never said a word to me about it. As I look back, I think I was probably challenging him to say something, to do something, to help me. But he never dealt with it." A Detroit homemaker who had a drinking problem while still in college encountered the same kind of reaction from her therapist at a university health service. "There were times when my husband called my psychiatrist in the middle of the night because I'd be so out of control and drunk and hysterical. . . . But when I would come in for my next session . . . the drinking would never get mentioned as a problem in itself."

Probably the primary reason for many doctors' failure to confront alcohol problems in their patients is, perhaps surprisingly, sheer ignorance of alcoholism itself. Although alcohol abuse affects at least 10 million persons in the United States and is considered the third largest health problem in the country, it is one of the most neglected areas of study in medical schools. Although this situation is slowly being corrected, few medical schools even today offer more than one course on the subject, and many limit their coverage to a single lecture. This gap in education is largely due to alcoholism's heritage as a moral problem rather than a medical one, despite its obvious physical and emotional consequences. In a 1972 nationwide survey of 13,000 physicians who treat alcoholism, 70 percent declared alcoholics to be difficult and uncooperative patients, while a sizable minority believed alcoholism indicated a "lack of will or morality."[2]

Further, as the research of Phyllis Chester and others has demonstrated, doctors as a group hold notably stereotypical attitudes about appropriate behavior for women.[3] Consequently, many physicians who believe that alcoholism is a sign of moral laxity may well also subscribe to the double standard rendering alcoholism—i.e., immorality— more shameful in a woman than a man, and thus more discomfiting to discuss with a female patient. Indeed, a study of the attitudes of 161 physicians toward their alcoholic clients revealed that a substantial number of doctors believed that, compared to the alcoholic man, the alcoholic woman "had loose sexual morals, had more psychosexual conflict such as homosexuality, and was more likely to get into social difficulties."[4]

From *Social Policy*. Jan/Feb 1980, pp. 25–30. Reprinted with permission from THE INVISIBLE ALCOHOLICS, McGraw Hill, New York.

*I use the pronoun "he" deliberately because the medical profession is still overwhelmingly masculine; at present only 12 percent of physicians are women.

But if a doctor is unable or unwilling to diagnose a woman as alcoholic, he may give her condition another label instead. All too often, a physician notes the distraught state of his alcoholic female client, makes a primary diagnosis of "depression" or "anxiety," and proceeds to prescribe a pill to alter her mood, most commonly a tranquilizer, sedative, or antidepressant. Consequently, many alcoholic women walk out of their doctors' offices not only with their alcoholism undiagnosed but with a second powerful potentially addictive psychoactive drug in hand. A 50-year-old Maryland woman who abused both alcohol and a variety of pills described her introduction to mood-altering drugs: "I was incredibly jumpy from all the booze I was drinking, so my doctor put me on both Librium and Nembutal—one to calm me during the day and the other to get me to sleep at night. Then about a year later, he put me on Dexedrine to get me going in the morning, to counteract the effects of the pills—and the alcohol. He actually knew I was drinking, but he never seemed to see it as a major problem." A young Black woman from Washington, D.C. recalled her first visit with a psychiatrist during one of her worst periods of drinking. "I told this man I was depressed and exhausted all the time, but I also told him I thought my drinking might be getting a little out of hand. He told me to be cool about it and handed me a prescription for an antidepressant. In three months, I was going through a month's worth of that prescription every ten days."

Both their professional training and prevailing societal attitudes influence doctors and therapists to view women as inherently less stable emotionally than men by virtue of their female biology, and therefore more prone to psychological disturbances. Consequently, many doctors may be likely to misread a number of serious medical problems in women—including alcoholism—as merely "nerves," depression, or another emotional ailment. This image of women as "naturally" given to mental disorders is the content of much of the advertising by which the powerful American drug industry, at a cost of 1 billion dollars per year—approximately $5,000 per physician—tries to persuade doctors to prescribe mood-altering drugs to their patients.

Psychoactive drug use is not risk free for anyone, but it is especially dangerous for problem drinkers for several reasons. Perhaps the most obvious danger is that of mixing a mood-altering drug with alcohol. The combination of alcohol and certain psychoactive drugs produces a supra-addictive effect substantially more powerful than the effects of any of the drugs taken alone, and consequently increases the possibility of accidental death by an overdose. Access to both alcohol and psychoactive drugs also makes suicide attempts a relatively easy matter, a serious concern in view of the high rate of such attempts—many of them successful—among alcoholic women.

The other major danger of prescribing mood-altering drugs to an alcoholic is the possibility of cross-addiction, that is, dependence on both alcohol and one or more other drugs. Anyone who habitually uses psychoactive drugs

may become addicted to them, but the alcoholic is a particularly high risk as she has already established an addictive drug use pattern with alcohol. Cross addiction sometimes keeps a woman drinking for a longer period of time, because she may be able to switch to Valium or another pill temporarily when the effects of alcohol become too staggering for her body to bear. And a woman addicted to both alcohol and pills is likely to face more difficulties in treatment, because she must withdraw and recover from the effects of two or more powerful drugs instead of alcohol alone.

Yet despite these multiple dangers, many physicians distribute these drugs to alcoholic women with an alarmingly free hand. According to Dr. LeClair Bissell, chief of the Smithers Alcoholism Center of New York City's Roosevelt Hospital, it is so easy for alcoholic women to get prescriptions for these drugs that, once addicted, many obtain their maintenance supply from several physicians simultaneously. "If a doctor is giving an alcoholic woman pills, don't imagine he is her only source. He is probably part of a long succession of people who are prescribing for her. For instance, the gynecologist is quite capable of writing prescriptions for Librium and Valium. The general practitioner, if there is one, will hear some of her problems and prescribe pills too. If there's been an emergency room afterward, that may result in yet another prescription for tranquilizers. Even the ophthalmologist taking care of the glasses can prescribe pills. The possibilities are endless."

Since physicians prescribe psychoactive drugs for women in the general population at almost twice the rate they prescribe them for men,[5] it is perhaps not surprising that alcoholic women are far more likely to be cross-addicted than alcoholic men. A 1977 nationwide survey of more than 15,000 Alcoholics Anonymous members showed that 29 percent of the women but only 15 percent of the men were addicted to other drugs besides alcohol. Of new AA members 30 years old or younger, a startling 55 percent of women were cross-addicted, compared to 36 percent of men.[6] Smaller surveys report similar findings: a study of residents in 36 alcoholism halfway houses in Minnesota, for example, found that nearly twice as many women as men were addicted to both alcohol and drugs.[7] Studies of individual treatment programs report similar female-male ratios for cross-addiction.[8]

Treatment

Not every physician, of course, acts as an obstacle to treatment. Some doctors are not only impressively knowledgeable about alcoholism, but will forthrightly confront any patient, regardless of sex, who shows symptoms of the illness. But even if an alcoholic woman is fortunate enough to come into contact with such a physician—and the odds are not good—he can provide no guarantee that she will ultimately receive caring and effective treatment. For once a woman acknowledges her alcohol problem and is ready to seek help, she is then faced with an alcoholism treatment system that, by and large, neither welcomes nor understands her.

The first challenge a woman may confront is simply finding an alcoholism program that has room for her. A 1976 study conducted by the Association of Halfway House Alcoholism Programs of North America reported that of a representative nationwide sample of 161 alcoholism halfway houses, 56 percent served men only, 35 percent were coed, and only nine percent were open only to women. Further, and perhaps more important, women occupied only 19 percent of all available beds in the 161 houses, because the "coed" units reserved only ten to 30 percent of their beds for women.[9] Another survey, conducted by the New York State Commission on Women and Alcoholism, found that in 45 inpatient alcoholism facilities in the state, only 17 percent of all beds were allocated for women. Some surveyed centers refused to treat women at all, citing inadequate budgets and, in one case, the lack of space for a second bathroom.[10]

The scarcity of treatment space for women stems largely from the long-standing assumption by the health system that alcoholism is essentially a male illness. Prior to 1970, the year Congress passed legislation requiring alcoholism programs to offer services to women as a criterion for receiving federal funding, relatively few alcoholism programs admitted women on any basis. And even after the legislation was enacted, many programs added only a few token beds for women rather than providing space on a par with the actual numbers of alcoholic women in the population. It is not uncommon, even today, for a 30-bed treatment center to reserve only four or five beds for women clients.

Consequently, some women seeking help for alcoholism become names on waiting lists, or are forced to travel far out of their communities to find programs with room for them. Others, like the many women in our society who are considered troublesome and who lack other options, end up in mental institutions. Although they are resorted to less often now than in the past, psychiatric hospitals are still used as dumping grounds for some women with drinking problems. Dr. LeClair Bissell described the typical experience of an alcoholic woman consigned to a psychiatric ward: "First of all, it's usually not hard to get her in there because women have always been willing to self-define as mentally ill more readily than men, especially if the alternative is to be called an alcoholic. And as for her drinking, it plays right into the psychiatric approach that says, 'Find the underlying cause, get a lot of insight, pull up your socks, honey, and guess what? You won't be drinking like that anymore and you'll be having two drinks before dinner just like everybody else.' Never mind that she is physically addicted to alcohol."

The "treatment" of alcoholic women in mental wards is sometimes marked not only by ignorance but outright brutality. A Washington, D.C. businesswoman remembered: "My husband told me he was taking me to a hospital and I went willingly, no questions asked. I was diagnosed as alcoholic. My husband left and I was told to follow the man who was carrying my bags. And as we walked along I noticed that he was locking doors behind him and I said: 'What are you doing that for?' And he said, 'Don't you know where you are?' And I said, 'No' and he said, 'You're at a federal facility for the insane.'

"It turned out that the hospital had an alcoholism program for men but none for women, so if you were unfortunate enough to be taken there as an alcoholic woman, you got thrown in with the violently insane. I will never forget it. I was put in a ward where people were defecating in the corner and ladies were walking around nude. And the people working there were just brutal. Really brutal. Full of contempt. I was treated like an animal just like everyone else there. There were no doors on the johns. You had to take a shower with somebody watching you. The blanket on my bed smelled like urine. For the first three days I just shook—I was having junior grade DTs. I was withdrawing from alcohol for the first time in my life and they didn't give me any drugs or any other kind of help. I just lay on my cot and shook."

But even if a woman is able to avoid the route of the psychiatric ward and finds an alcoholism program that has room for her, adequate treatment is by no means guaranteed. For by and large, the alcoholism treatment system is still very much a man's world, with most recovery programs primarily used, staffed, and directed by men and designed to meet male needs. As Rita Zimmer, director of a New York Bowery area alcoholism program, summarized the situation: "Just because most facilities now admit some women doesn't mean that most of them make any attempt to develop programs that relate to women. It doesn't mean they really try to reach out to find alcoholic women in the community. It doesn't even mean they hire staff who have an interest in working with women or who have any knowledge of how to work with women." Consequently, many women find themselves in treatment programs which are neither prepared nor committed to meeting many of their fundamental psychological and practical needs.

Perhaps more than anything else, a woman beginning treatment for alcoholism needs to feel cared about and believed in. In most cases, she has weathered years—sometimes decades—of a brutalizing addiction that has left her overwhelmed with feelings of failure and hopelessness about the possibility of acceptance by others. Dr. Edith Gomberg, professor of psychology at the University of Michigan and a pioneering researcher on women and alcoholism, noted from her experience: "... in a deviance disorder like alcoholism, the attitude (conscious and unconscious) of the therapist toward women and toward alcoholism and the enthusiasm and interest of the therapist seem far more related to outcome than the technique used."[11] Given the importance of these factors, the attitudes of many treatment professionals toward alcoholic women are deeply disturbing. A survey of 161 physicians involved in alcoholism treatment revealed that they generally believed that "women have more basic personality disorders: they are more hostile, angry, unhappy, self-centered, withdrawn, depressed and more subject to mood swings; they are more emotional, lonely, nervous; they have less insight, and are not as likable as men alcoholics."[12] Other surveys note similar negative views of women among treatment personnel, in particular the notions that alcoholic women are more emotionally unbalanced than alcoholic men, and by implication, more difficult to treat. Such attitudes are deeply destructive to recovering women because they are likely to become self-fulfilling prophecies.

As the theory that women are more psychologically maladjusted than men appears to be widespread among alcoholism-treatment personnel and can seriously undermine a woman's successful recovery, its origins need to be examined more closely. It is possible that on the average, an alcoholic woman may actually enter rehabilitation more emotionally impaired than an alcoholic man, due to the psychic strain of the particularly harsh stigma attached to female alcoholism. But it is also likely that the "sicker" label springs from deeply sexist notions about the psychology of women held by mental health professionals. In the study most clearly illustrating these attitudes, conducted in 1970 by Dr. Inge Broverman and Dr. Donald Broverman, a group of psychotherapists was asked to define, respectively, a mature healthy man, a mature healthy woman, and a mature healthy adult. The clinicians, who displayed a high level of consensus in their conclusions, described a healthy male and a healthy female in very different terms. Specifically, they characterized a healthy, mature woman as more submissive, less independent, less adventurous, less competitive, more excitable in minor crises, more easily hurt and more emotional than a mature, healthy man. Equally significant, their description of a healthy adult closely paralleled their characterization of a healthy man, and thereby differed radically from their assessment of a healthy woman.[13] This landmark study, along with others which have replicated its findings, indicates that the standard of mental health in our culture is a clearly masculine one, and conversely, that feminine behavior is basically inconsistent with society's concept of adult mental health.

Stereotypical views of women among alcoholism professionals not only earn many women the damaging labels of "sick" and "hard to treat" but almost inevitably shape the criteria used for women's recovery. If a "healthy" woman is considered relatively submissive, dependent, and noncompetitive, such behaviors are likely to be urged on alcoholic women as evidence of emotional maturity, while behaviors that fail to conform to conventional feminine norms are apt to be punished. When Ardelle Schultz first joined the staff of a drug-alcohol program near Philadelphia in the early 1970s, she found that the staff—until her arrival entirely male—was bent on such a "reeducation" program for women clients:

Women were being taught a new set of behaviors to please males. They were told to give up their sleazy bitch ways.... If a woman happened to be naturally sexy and sensuous, she was accused of seducing the men and chastised. If she was unfemininely aggressive and angry, she was told she was treacherous and that she was losing her sensitivity and humanity. If she was lesbian, she was accused of being a man-hater and "sick." In other words, she was learning, again, to repress a part of herself that belonged to her and to become an "honest paper doll" cut out in man's image.[14]

Pressure to conform to such narrowly sexist standards of behavior is seriously damaging to any woman, but it is apt to be particularly destructive to a woman who is alcoholic. The heavy load of guilt, self-hatred, and worthlessness that an alcoholic woman drags with her into treatment is inextricably linked to her failure to live up to a self-denying and impossible ideal of womanhood—the sexual innocent, the nurturing mother, the dutiful wife, the consummate "lady." To be assaulted in treatment with further accusations of her sins against femininity—whether blatantly or subtly conveyed—can only reinforce her already profound conviction of failure as a woman.

Indeed, therapy that imposes a stereotyped vision of femininity on recovering women may also intensify the very kinds of conflicts that triggered their abusive drinking in the first place. Recent research by Dr. Sharon Wilsnack and others indicates that many women who become alcoholic suffer painful sex-role conflicts, usually between a consciously desired "feminine" self-image and unconscious "masculine" strivings which they experience as unacceptable and acutely threatening to their identities. This research shows that drinking may stifle this conflict, allowing a woman to temporarily integrate the masculine and feminine sides of her personality, and that uncontrolled drinking may be activated by a crisis that forces her forbidden "unfeminine" feelings to the fore.

The Social Context

Insensitivity to the psychological needs of alcoholic women is often coupled with apparent indifference to some of their most urgent practical concerns. For example, the typical woman entering an alcoholism treatment program is in serious financial difficulty and badly needs job training. More often than not, she is divorced, has custody of her children, and is receiving little or no support money from her ex-husband. Her job skills are likely to be minimal and she probably has been unable to work steadily for some time. A 1977 survey by the National Institute on Alcohol Abuse and Alcoholism revealed that of the some 60,000 women in federally funded treatment programs, approximately 30 percent were unemployed at the time of entering treatment, and only about seven percent held professional-level jobs. The mean household income of all the women surveyed was about $7,000.[15]

Yet, regardless of these stark financial realities, few alcoholism programs offer serious job training to recovering alcoholic women, either within the facilities themselves or through arrangements with outside agencies. The myth appears to linger among program staff that women don't really need jobs, that their own and their children's survival are never wholly or even primarily dependent on their own wage-earning abilities. This obliviousness to the economic realities of women's lives was underscored in a recent study of staff attitudes toward clients at a Newark, New Jersey, drug-alcohol program, in which researchers asked the 25 male and nine female staff members their perceptions of the major problems faced by their clients. Less than a quarter of the staff believed that lack of job training was a significant problem for women, although it was seen as a major need for male clients. But when the clients themselves were asked what they perceived as their most serious problems, an overwhelming 96 percent of the women named lack of job training. No other single problem was named by as many women.[16]

When job training is offered to women at all, it is usually for low-paying "women's work" such as typing and other clerical functions, while men in the same program are often trained for more lucrative, highly skilled occupations. Many alcoholism programs provide no job training opportunities whatever for women, instead assigning them the "occupational therapy" of household chores within the program residence, or brush-up courses on cooking, sewing, and home management. Although these skills may be useful and even necessary to some women, to offer them in lieu of hard-nosed job training almost ensures continuing financial hardship for many women once they leave a treatment program. Unable to find a job that pays enough to support themselves and possibly children as well, many find themselves on welfare shortly after completing treatment, or are forced to work two jobs simply in order to pay the bills. Clearly, it is not a way of life conducive to staying sober.

Child care is another service crucially needed by recovering women and almost never provided by alcoholism programs. As most recovery facilities are designed for and by men, this gap is not altogether surprising, since men who enter rehabilitation programs ordinarily leave their children in the care of their wives. But women who begin alcoholism treatment have no such convenient caretakers. Even if a woman's husband is still living with her, which is unlikely, he is rarely able or willing to undertake primary care of the children while she gets help for her alcoholism. Foster care is generally a risky choice, since poor women in particular may be declared "unfit mothers" on the basis of their alcoholism and lose custody of their children, sometimes permanently. As for private day care and other kinds of child care services, New York City family alcoholism counselor Sheila Salcedo observed: "Day care centers are prohibitively expensive and have incredible waiting lists, and the homemaker services charge so much money that your average woman could never afford it. So if you have a lady in need of immediate detoxification and other treatment and she happens to have children, you're really in trouble."

Despite this clear and pressing need for child care services, to date only two alcoholism programs in the entire country offer in-house child care, and few others offer even minimal outside arrangements. Consequently, many women are literally prevented from getting any kind of alcoholism treatment because they can't find anyone to take care of their children. And if a woman tries to begin treatment without having made workable child care arrangements, her recovery is undermined from the start. Salcedo noted: "It is very difficult for most women to get the rest they need in treatment if the kids aren't in good hands. It's easy enough to say, 'OK, let's send the woman into rehab', but if she's got five kids at home, one of whom is on drugs and another who is failing school, and a husband who never really wanted her to go into treatment in the first place, nothing that happens in that treatment program is going to make any kind of impression on her. She gets phone calls from home, she worries, she feels guilty. What kind of treatment does that amount to?"

The realities of women's lives are such that they also may need more intensive follow-up than men after completing a formal program of treatment. In general, women are likely to both face greater pressures than men and receive less support from others once they return from a rehabilitation program to the "real world." Dr. LeClair Bissell observed: "There is much less support from the family of the alcoholic woman than the man. As soon as she returns from treatment she is expected to begin taking care of the children and cooking dinner for the husband and whatnot. And AA (Alcoholics Anonymous) sometimes rather blandly advocates '90 meetings in 90 days' at the beginning, which is fine in theory, but what about the woman who has a job and whose babysitter leaves every day at five o'clock? Or whose husband refuses to take care of the kids every night? How is she going to work the mechanics of that?"

The acute stress and isolation faced by many women following treatment can seriously threaten their sobriety. "You can't just treat a woman, show her how to stop drinking and then tell her to go out and do her own thing," said Clara Synical, founder and director of Interim House, a halfway house for alcoholic women in Philadelphia. "You have to go step by step, follow through, and keep in touch with her so she knows she has a home where she can get support at all times." Yet few alcoholism facilities provide any sustained follow-up services to clients once they complete treatment, in terms of either counseling or practical help in rebuilding their lives. Without such support, many women become quickly overwhelmed by the multiple pressures of their new situations and, sometimes within a few months or even weeks of completing treatment, turn back to the bottle for relief.

The disregard for women's concerns which marks many rehabilitation programs has sparked a small but vigorous movement within the alcoholism field to develop treatment programs specifically designed for women. These programs, which are often staffed and used entirely by women, are committed to providing alcoholic women with a strongly supportive, caring environment and to approaching their recovery needs in the context of women's total experience in society.

Yet, within the alcoholism field, support for women's programs has been grudging at best. Organizers of such programs have found funding hard to come by in a field that has yet to fully recognize the extent of female alcoholism, much less the inability of many traditional programs to meet women's needs. The National Institute on Alcohol Abuse and Alcoholism has funded only 29 women's programs in a total of some 500 treatment facilities, and although some of these federally supported programs are excellent, they clearly do not begin to meet the extent of women's needs. At present, many major metropolitan areas and even entire states are without a single women's program or even a coed program that has instituted special services for female clients.

Since alcoholism programs sensitive to women's concerns still comprise only a tiny percentage of existing programs, the vast majority of women continue to be treated in facilities that fail to meet many of their most pressing needs. Many women drop out of these programs before completing treatment. The reasons they cite are varied: lack of emotional support from staff, an inability to make suitable child care arrangements, diffuse feelings of alienation and isolation, sometimes simply an overwhelming sense that "it's not helping." Occasionally, women leave because of sexual harassment or abuse from male staff or residents. Of those who complete treatment, most studies show a significantly lower rate of recovery by alcoholic women than men, in some cases less than half the rate for men.[17] A good number of women who resume abusive drinking after leaving treatment become part of the "revolving door" syndrome, making their way in and out of treatment programs over and over again for years, endlessly searching for a way out of their addiction, and endlessly failing to find it.

Notes

1. Jane E. James, "Symptoms of Alcoholism in Women: A Preliminary Survey of A. A. Members," *Journal of Studies on Alcohol*, 36 (1975), p. 1567.
2. Robert W. Jones and Alice R Heinch, "Treatment of Alcoholism by Physicians in Private Practice: A National Survey," *Quarterly Journal of Studies on Alcoholism*, 33 (1972), pp. 117–131.
3. Phyllis Chester, *Women and Madness* (New York: Avon Books, 1972).
4. Marilyn W. Johnson, "Physicians' Views on Alcoholism with Special Reference to Alcoholism in Women." *Nebraska State Medical Journal*, 50 (1965), p. 380.
5. Herbert I. Abelson et al., *National Survey on Drug Abuse: 1977*, vol. 1 (Rockville, Md.: National Institute on Drug Abuse. U.S. Department of Health, Education and Welfare, 1977). p. 102.
6. John L. Norris, "Analysis of the 1977 Survey of the Membership of Alcoholics Anonymous" (Paper presented at the Thirty-second International Congress on Alcoholism and Drug Dependence. Warsaw, Poland Sept. 3-8, 1978), p. 20.
7. Luise K Forseth, "A Survey of Minnesota's Halfway Houses for the Chemically Dependent" (Unpublished paper, 1976), p. 9.
8. Ingrid Waldron, "Increased Prescribing of Valium, Librium and Other Drugs: An Example of the Influence of Economic and Social Factors on the Practice of Medicine," *International Journal of Health Sciences*, 7 (1977), p. 55.
9. Association of Halfway House Alcoholism Programs of North America, "Statistical Survey of Full Member Halfway House Alcoholism Programs" (St. Paul, Minn.: 1976), pp 6-7.
10. Cheryl Gillen *et al.*, "Report on Survey of Eighty-Eight New York State Outpatient Detoxification Halfway House and Rehabilitation Facilities" (New York: Committee on Women and Alcoholism in New York State, 1977), p. 1.
11. Edith S. Gomberg, "Women and Alcoholism," in V. Franks and V. Burtle (ed.), *Women in Therapy* (New York: Brunner/Mazel, 1974), p. 183.
12. Johnson, "Physicians' Views on Alcoholism," p. 380.
13. Inge Broverman *et al.*, "Sex Role Stereotypes and Clinical Judgments of Mental Health," *Journal of Consulting and Clinical Psychology*, 34 (1970), pp. 1–7.
14. Ardelle M. Schulz, "Women and Addiction" (Paper presented to Ohio Bureau of Drug Abuse, Cleveland, Oh., June 17, 1974), pp. 23–24.
15. National Institute on Alcohol Abuse and Alcoholism, U.S. Dept. of Health, Education and Welfare, *Women in Treatment for Alcoholism in NIAAA Funded Facilities*, 1977 (Rockville, Md.: 1978), p. 8.
16. Stephen J. Levy and Kathleen M. Doyle, "Attitudes Toward Women in a Drug Treatment Program," p. 431.
17. David A. Pemberton, "A Comparison of the Outcome of Treatment in Female and Male Alcoholics," *British Journal of Psychiatry* , 133 (1967), pp. 367–373.

Ω

Women and Children Last
Barriers to Drug Treatment for Women

by LaRay Brown

Drug abuse often compounds the immense difficulties that the poor face in finding jobs, housing, child care, education, and health care. For many, drug abuse effectively precludes the constructive resolution of all other problems. Drug abuse has strained many already overburdened community institutions to the breaking point and destroyed the economic and social strengths of many neighborhoods. The effects of increasing drug and alcohol abuse among women is particularly devastating because of their pivotal position in both family and community structure in poor neighborhoods. Between 1970 and 1984, the number of Black and Hispanic families headed by women more than doubled. Among the poorest third of Black families, over 70 percent were headed by women in 1990.

Clearly, women's drug and alcohol use devastates the women themselves, many already rendered physically and mentally vulnerable by the circumstances of poverty and lack of access to health care. The effects on their children are also tragic, both because they affect the health of the child-to-be at the prenatal level and because women, as the traditional caregivers, affect their children. Yet, at the same time that women's needs for mental health and drug treatment services are growing (see side-bar), existing public health systems are are suffering cutbacks and dismantling. Moreover, the services that exist, particularly drug and alcohol treatment, are not designed to serve women and their children effectively.

Although much attention has been focused on the rise of crack cocaine use, alcoholism and alcohol use continue to be significant problems for women and their children. The combination of both alcohol and drug use or the use of many types of drugs at once poses particular problems for treatment providers. Moreover, chemical dependency is often accompanied by other significant mental health problems, further exacerbating women's difficulties in obtaining the services they need to achieve relief and recovery.

In New York City, as elsewhere, the need for drug treatment far exceeds the resources available. The full extent of the unmet need is unknown, since there is no central clearinghouse that maintains information about vacancies and waiting lists for drug treatment programs. However, it is known that methadone programs currently reach, at most, 15 percent of the heroin-using population. Other treatment modalities are available for only about 2 to 4 percent of those addicted to other drugs.

The present system of drug treatment for women is not only costly, but it strains and disrupts families because there are so few services that allow women to receive appropriate treatment while continuing to raise their children. Although some drug users would not accept treatment even if it were available, some experts believe that the existence of comprehensive drug treatment centers that provided outreach, immediate evaluation and referral, and on-site assistance would encourage greater numbers of drug users to seek treatment. This article highlights the obstacles that women in New York City face in getting treatment for drug and alcohol abuse and concludes with a model of the type of comprehensive services they and their families need to help them attain recovery and sobriety.

From *Health/PAC Bulletin,* Summer 1992, pp. 15–19. Copyright © 1992 by Health/PAC Bulletin. Reprinted by permission.

LaRay Brown is Assistant Vice-President of Mental Health and Chemical Dependency Services at the New York City Health and Hospitals Corporation and a member of the Health/PAC Board. Her positions in this article are based on work she has done with women working toward recovery and economic self-sufficiency. This is a revised version of a presentation given at the Health/PAC forum on Women antd Health at the American Public Health Association annual meeting, Atlanta, GA, November 11, 1991.

Women, Children, and Drug Use

- An estimated 500,000 children in New York State have parents who are drug users. Half the clients of residential drug treatment programs and two-thirds of methadone program clients have children.

- There were an estimated 10,000 drug-addicted mothers in New York City in 1991, a more than threefold increase since 1988.

- More than 90 percent of women who use drugs fail to get drug treatment before giving birth.

- There was an increase of 3,746 percent in substance abuse by pregnant women in New York City between 1980 and 1988, with increased use of cocaine a contributing factor.

- An estimated 1 in 60 newborns are infected with HIV in some areas of New York City, primarily as a result of maternal drug use.

- The number of women in prison New York State increased 59 percent from 1988 to 1989, largely as a result of drug abuse.

- The major cause of deaths among women ages 15 to 44 in New York City are drug abuse, AIDS, and homicide.

- Fetal alcohol syndrome occurs in approximately 1 in 400 live births in New York State. Another 2,000 children are born with alcohol-related birth defects each year. Fetal alcohol syndrome now leads Down's syndrome and spina bifida as the country's major cause of birth defects with associated mental retardation. Of the three, only fetal alcohol syndrome is totally preventable.

Obstacles to Treatment

Chemically dependent women who are trying to get help from public mental health programs, such as those provided by New York City's Health and Hospitals Corporation, face basic and specific barriers to recovery due to the fragmentation and lack of coordination of services among provider agencies. In New York City, women must negotiate at least four different bureaucracies, since agencies for addictions treatment are separate from departments of child and family welfare, housing, and other entitlement services. Women face additional obstacles in dealing with the Department of Employment.

When a woman in New York City enters a residential treatment program, she often has no alternative but to place her children in foster care through the Child Welfare Administration (CWA) if she has no family to keep them. If she is in a day treatment program, she needs homemaker services, which are provided through CWA, but she often has no one to coordinate the provision of these services with her treatment or medical needs.

The Department of Welfare tries to coordinate housing and services for homeless women and their families through entitlement programs such as Aid to Families with Dependent Children (AFDC) and the Women, Infants and Children nutrition program (WIC). But here, as at every point in the bureaucratic maze, there is no coordination and no assistance provided in obtaining drug treatment services.

Even without the confusion and institutional barriers that women using public programs face, the treatment services offered by the City of New York suffer from a grave lack of readily available slots of every kind. Although there have been increases in funding within the last two years for the development of programs for women, particularly pregnant addicts, access to treatment remains difficult. There are virtually no treatment programs able to accommodate them as women with families, on either an inpatient or outpatient basis, and no comprehensive residential services for women that can include their partners, and their children. In New York City there are less than a handful of residential rehabilitation services for women and children—The United Bronx Parents' La Casita and Odyssey House's MABON may be the only existing examples. Thus, a major conflict for most women in obtaining inpatient detoxification or residential treatment services is that, because of this programmatic disregard for their family life and the often mandated placement of their children in foster care, their attempts to obtain treatment can involve a choice between their own well being and that of their children.

Once women participate in drug treatment and their children are placed in foster care, the women find little institutional support for their attempts at recovery. The child welfare system has no comprehensive plan or organizational structure for the stages of mental health recovery or recovery from drug dependency. For example, there are no protocols to deal with relapses into substance abuse, which are common. Because the rules are inflexible, a relapse causes the continued disruption of families as the family members and welfare and foster care agencies try to contend with the changing circumstances.

In addition, families are assigned to different workers within the Child Welfare Administration at different stages of intervention, further contributing to fragmented casework planning. The system also fails to provide intensive therapeutic services to women who are trying to regain custody of their children. Foster care workers generally do not have time to do the intensive therapy work that is needed, and social workers, working with preventive services and boarder babies, focus primarily on providing treatment for women who have not yet lost their children. Women struggling to regain their children after losing them during drug treatment are mostly viewed as "incompetent" by the system and written off.

Mothers seeking treatment avoid the foster care system as much as possible. They rely on family and friends to take care of their children, if they are not mandated by law to use foster care. But placement of children with relatives can promote intergenerational, financial, and emotional conflicts that can undermine the mother's authority and exacerbate the stress of her recovery, and thus serve as a disincentive to continue treatment. While extended family placements are often helpful and sometimes essential, they are also made difficult because support benefits are greater for children in foster care than on welfare.

Women who are homeless have an additional layer of bureaucratic difficulty. Residential treatment programs are not coordinated with permanent housing options for those who are homeless, and after treatment these women are thrown back into situations that invite relapse or may prevent treatment in the first place. Women with their children in the shelter system must confront pervasive drug use there. Yet, if they choose to enter treatment, placing their children in foster care, they face a Catch-22 situation. Once they leave the shelter system for any reason, even to enter drug or mental health treatment, they forfeit their place on the long waiting lists for housing and must start all over again, which may mean months or a year more wait to obtain an apartment. And, once they leave residential treatment, having placed their children in foster care, they cannot get them back again, because they have no permanent housing. Moreover, because the women do not have current custody of their children, the housing agency gives them lower priority for permanent housing. This is true for women who are mandated to place their children, as well as for those who do so voluntarily. This Catch-22 situation would frustrate and demoralize the strongest of people. Those who are poor, without community or family support, and in need of treatment can easily lose the ability to persevere.

Much of this difficulty could be avoided if there were adequate numbers of publicly subsidized child care arrangements and slots in most drug treatment or preventive service agencies. Specialized care for medically fragile newborns is especially needed. Ideally, these child care services would be designed as a comprehensive parenting program within each drug treatment setting.

Besides the insuperable obstacles to treatment, to continued custody of their children, and to permanent housing, women who have drug and mental health treatment needs also face considerable difficulties in getting benefits from entitlement programs, such as welfare and WIC. These programs are often unavailable to women and their newborns during the medically critical first months after birth due to perpetual delays in the opening of new cases, often caused by the slow acquisition of vital documents.

For women in day treatment, homemaker services, like child care, are essential. Such services are not easy to obtain and are often withdrawn after six months, at a time when most women are in very early and fragile stages of sobriety. (Drug users often need a full 18 months of rehabilitation in order to avoid relapse.)

As a final obstacle and indignity, federal welfare policy discourages—if not prohibits outright—women in recovering from applying to long-term educational and vocational programs following treatment by threatening to close a recipient's case, reduce their benefits allocation, or withdraw support services altogether if they apply for additional help from such programs. This avenue closed, women are forced to accept coercive work incentive programs that offer few long-term opportunities for economic independence and low wages that maintain the women in poverty.

Comprehensive Services

Women who depend on the public mental health system for help with substance abuse need a complete range of treatment, health, and social support services. A woman must not be forced to choose between separation from her children and treatment. Services must be developed that focus on women, their children, and their partners, treating all these individuals simultaneously.

Program models must be assessed by their impact on two key areas: family cohesion and the long-term economic stability of program participants. Recovery is a process of empowerment, based on long-term development and self-awareness, with the goal of individual autonomy. Self-sufficiency is critical to long-term sobriety.

Community-based centers of consortia of providers designed to provide a complete package of necessary support services for women in a central location must be funded and implemented. These centers or consortia should combine drug and alcohol treatment for women, as well as other mental health services, with support services ranging from housing, to job training and skills, primary health care, and child care services. At the same time, the program must work with the women's children, providing necessary educational, developmental, health, and preventive services. Such a comprehensive treatment program would offer a continuum of treatment, with the following specific components:

Intensive Residential Treatment

Many women in the early stages of withdrawal from addiction need to begin treatment in intensive treatment programs especially designed to meet their needs. The program should consist of highly structured drug and alcohol abuse treatment services that concentrate on overcoming the addiction. Daily activities should center on group and individual therapy. Support and direction from peers is a key component of successful residential treatment programs, with women assuming greater responsibility as they progress through the program. Thus, a specific focus on women who are pregnant or have children is essential in encouraging their recovery.

Children who have a parent who abuses drugs and alcohol often have not had the attention and care that is necessary for healthy development. Because women in treatment need to focus on overcoming their own addiction, much of the initial care of the children will need to be provided by care givers in the residential program. Services that should be available for children include individual assessment, child care, specialized nurseries, recreation, and age-appropriate prevention and treatment (when appropriate) to deter substance abuse later in life.

Poor health usually accompanies substance abuse. Pregnant women who are drug and alcohol users present particularly difficult medical problems at a time when even healthy women can have trouble getting adequate obstetrical care. Medical services are a necessary component of the program for both women and children. Needed services range from well child care to emergency services. Health services should be provided on site where possible, and the program must establish connections to services provided in the community when more intensive medical services are required.

Supportive Living Facilities

A supervised residence for women and their children should be available as an alternative level of care for women who graduate from intensive residential treatment so that they may continue their progress toward independence or for women who do not need intensive treatment services but are not ready to leave a supported community. This component in the continuum of treatment should begin to focus on the family's life after treatment to promote adjustment to a drug-free life-style.

In this stage of treatment, women would choose to receive drug counseling and begin to develop skills that will enable them to maintain a self-sufficient family. For example, women might participate in appropriate educational and vocational programs so that they could apply for and maintain steady employment. As they progress, women would assume increasing responsibility for the care of their children.

With the continued support and guidance of program staff, women would then develop a discharge plan for themselves and their family to provide for a smooth and successful transition to the next stage of treatment and beyond to independent living within the community. The discharge plan should integrate the concept of case management to ensure that the women and their families are connected with support services outside the treatment program.

Services available to residents of the supportive living facilities would include:

- In-house drug treatment services, including individual and group counseling and HIV prevention and education services.
- Day care, recreation, family counseling, and support services for the children.
- Case management, to being to link women to services in the community.
- Health care for both women and children, similar to that provided in the intensive residential treatment component.
- Vocational and employment services and education.
- Life skills training, including stress management, household management, money management, and the development of parenting skills.
- Discharge planning.
- Mutual self-help and peer support.

Although most of these services should be provided on site, some could be made available near the residential facility. They must be guaranteed, however, and coordinated through individual case management on behalf of each woman and her children.

Independent Apartments

Another level of care may be needed in some communities to continue the process of helping the reunited family unit make the transition to total independence.

At the independent apartment stage of the treatment continuum, services would be designed to make independent living possible and successful. Women would live in an apartment and assume primary responsibility for caring for their children and maintaining the household. Apartments should be clustered to allow peer support. Treatment staff would no longer be on site 24 hours a day, but many support services would remain available.

Program staff should make frequent visits, and case management staff would ensure continued connection to social, vocational, and educational services and outpatient drug and alcohol abuse treatment. Homemaker services and child care are provided so that women could go to school, work, or community programs. Children would continue to receive counseling and participate in age-appropriate educational and recreational programs.

Before the women graduate to truly independent living, staff would work with each woman and her children to develop a comprehensive discharge plan to ensure that arrangements were made for permanent housing and community services, including enhanced outpatient services.

Permanent Housing

As part of the discharge-planning process, the program's case managers, working with state and local housing and social service agencies, would assist families in obtaining permanent housing. Once in permanent housing, the families would continue to receive enhanced outpatient and case management services determined by the family's needs.

Enhanced Outpatient Slots

As part of the effort to provide continued care and treatment in the community, the program must provide outpatient services that meet the particular needs of women who are pregnant or have children. Enhanced outpatient services should include child care, specialized nurseries for children, and case management to ensure women's access to health, social support, educational, and vocational services.

These enhanced outpatient services should also be available to women in the community who need support and treatment but do not require residential intervention. Reaching women before they require residential treatment is cost-effective and allows the family to maintain ties to the community and support networks.

Outreach Services

Community outreach services should be available to identify and reach women and children in need of the services because of emergencies or relapse.

The development of a comprehensive treatment continuum for chemically dependent women in family support communities will eliminate existing barriers to treatment, reduce the number of children placed in foster care, and provide a cost-effective means of keeping families together. By adding new components to treatment and coordinating other support services needed by these families, the public mental health and drug treatment systems will be more effective in assisting this high-risk population.

The goal of the public system should be to make treatment available to all those who need it and, through active outreach efforts, to increase the number of substance abusers who seek help. Limited resources necessitate hard choices about who is to receive treatment and how that treatment is to be provided, but women deserve priority and comprehensive attention.

Pregnant substance abusers desperately need prenatal care and are often motivated to accept treatment to improve the health of their babies. Mothers at risk of losing custody of their children are similarly motivated. Women should have the opportunity to be treated, to reach their full potential, to keep their families intact, and to protect their children from addiction, HIV infection, and developmental impairments. The destruction of the health and lives of babies and children by their mothers' drug use represents an unacceptable cost in terms of medical care, foster care, special education, and long-term social problems.

Ω

♀

The Twelve-Step Controversy

by Charlotte Davis Kasl

Drug addiction, codependency, incest, compulsive eating, sex, gambling, and shopping—multitudes of people are using 12-step programs modeled after Alcoholics Anonymous (AA) to recover from these problems. But beneath the surface of this massive movement, women are asking, is this really good for women? While female dissatisfaction with AA is not new (Jean Kirkpatrick founded Women for Sobriety in 1976), widespread questioning of these programs has only begun recently.

In workshops and group interviews, women repeatedly expressed fear about opening up the sacrosanct 12-step institution to scrutiny: "I'm afraid if we talk about this I'll lose something that helped me," or "I questioned the steps in my training program and they said I'd have to leave if I kept that up."

Women who question "the program," as it's often called, have been shamed, called resistant, and threatened with abandonment. They have been trained to believe that male models of nearly anything are better than whatever they might create for themselves.

Some women are grateful for what 12-step programs have given them: a generally available peer model providing support and understanding at no cost. Yet no one way works for everyone. The steps were formulated by a white, middle-class male in the 1930s; not surprisingly, they work to break down an overinflated ego, and put reliance on an all-powerful male God. But most women suffer from the *lack* of a healthy, aware ego, and need to strengthen their sense of self by affirming their own inner wisdom.

Research strongly indicates that alcohol addiction has links to genetic predisposition. A vital point that seems overlooked in AA is that in the case of nearly all substance abuse, the brain chemistry and the body ecology need extensive healing in order to prevent the protracted withdrawal syndrome of depression, anxiety, volatile emotions, and obsessive thinking that can last for years. Too often women endlessly attend groups, have psychotherapy, or take antidepressants when their emotions are actually being influenced by a chemical imbalance that could be helped by proper nutrition and exercise.

Other addictions, and codependency (as well as the will to recover), are influenced by cultural *oppression,* which includes poverty, battering, racism, sexism, and

Charlotte Davis Kasl is the author of "Women, Sex, and Addiction: A Search for Love and Power" (Harper & Row 1990) and is currently writing "Many Roads, One Journey; Moving Beyond the Twelve Steps" (Harper & Row, to be published in 1992). Her monograph, "Paths of Recovery," is $7.00, from Box 7073, Minneapolis, Minn. 55407.

homophobia. Treatment programs need to incorporate understanding—and advocacy—regarding these concerns.

As a psychologist and a former member of 12-step programs, I have encouraged women to write steps that resonate with their own inner selves, putting the focus on self-empowerment.

Here are the 12 steps (as published by AA World Services) followed by a critique and by some possible empowerment steps:

1. "We admitted we were powerless over [our addiction]—that our lives had become unmanageable." The purpose of this step is to crack through denial or an inflated ego and acknowledge a destructive problem. It can be helpful to say "I am powerless to change my partner," but many women abuse chemicals or stay in harmful relationships *because* they feel powerless in their lives. Thus, many women prefer to affirm that they have the power to *choose* not to use chemicals or have dependent relationships. So, alternatively: *We acknowledge we were out of control with _____ but have the power to take charge of our lives and stop being dependent on others for our self esteem and security.*

2. "Came to believe that a Power greater than ourselves could restore us to sanity." I believe that spiritual power is neither higher nor lower but all pervasive. I would replace the passivity implied in this step—that something external will magically restore us to sanity—with "affirmative action": *I came to believe that the Universe/Goddess/Great Spirit would awaken the healing wisdom within me if I opened myself to that power.*

3. "Made a decision to turn our will and our lives over to the care of God *as we understood Him.*" This conjures up images of women passively submitting their lives to male doctors, teachers, ministers, often with devastating consequences. Instead: *I declared myself willing to tune into my inner wisdom, to listen and act based upon these truths.*

The following steps are grouped together here because they all ask women to focus on negative aspects themselves:

4. "Made a searching and fearless *moral inventory* of ourselves."

5. "Admitted to God, to ourselves, and to another human being the exact nature of our *wrongs.*"

6. "Were entirely ready to have God remove all these *defects of character.*"

7. "*Humbly* asked Him to remove our *shortcomings.*"

8. "Made a list of all *persons we had harmed,* and became willing to *make amends* to them all."

9. "*Made direct amends* to such people wherever possible, except when to do so would injure them or others." (All emphases mine.)

We women need to make a searching and fearless inventory of how the culture has mired *us* down with guilt and shame, recognizing how hierarchy has harmed *us* and how *we* have been complicit in harming ourselves and only then look at how we have harmed others. So, instead:

We examined our behavior and beliefs in the context of living in a hierarchal, male-dominated culture.

We shared with others the ways we have been harmed, harmed ourselves and others, striving to forgive ourselves and to change our behavior.

We admitted to our talents, strengths, and accomplishments, agreeing not to hide these qualities to protect others' egos.

We became willing to let go of our shame, guilt, and other behavior that prevents us from taking control of our lives and loving ourselves.

We took steps to clear out all negative feelings between us and other people by sharing grievances in a respectful way and making amends when appropriate.

10. "Continued to take personal inventory and when we were wrong promptly admitted it." As one woman said in a group, "Admit that I'm wrong? I say I'm wrong for breathing air. I need to say I'm *right* for a change." *Continued to trust my reality, and when I was right promptly*

admitted it and refused to back down. We do not take responsibility for, analyze, or cover up the shortcomings of others.

11. "Sought through prayer and meditation to improve our conscious contact with God *as we understood Him*, praying only for knowledge of His will for us and the power to carry that out." Instead of looking to an external power, women need to reach inside and ask, What do I believe, what feels right to me? For example: *Sought through meditation and inner awareness the ability to listen to our inward calling and gain the will and wisdom to follow it.*

12. "Having had a spiritual awakening as the result of these steps, we tried to carry this message to [others], and to practice these principles in all our affairs." The desire to reach out to others is a natural step that comes with healing, but women need to remember to first care for and love themselves and then to give from choice, not from guilt, emptiness, or to prevent abandonment.

Most important is that we not identify ourselves with such labels as codependent or addict, or get stuck in chronic recovery as if we were constantly in need of fixing.

The goal is to heal and move on, embrace life's ups and downs, and move from *re*covery to *dis*covery. Then we can break through the limitations imposed by hierarchy, work together for a just society, and free our capacity for courage, joy, power, and love.

— Ω

Alcoholism: A Recovering Perspective
by Susan Janicki

I am a recovering alcoholic. I use the word recovering in lieu of recovered so that I don't forget that alcoholism is a disease that never goes away no matter how much I have it under control. People forget this all of the time; that it is a disease and that I am controlling it for the moment.

In my quest for support and information concerning my drinking problem I discovered many things. First, that I could say the words, "I have a disease" but that it took five years for this to finally sink in and to understand just what the implications were. My initial belief was that the label of disease was finally levied by the medical status quo as a last-straw measure: maybe if we relieve the alcoholic of their guilt by making them think it's not their fault, they will make an attempt to "get well".

I told myself over and over again all the right things that were supposed to help: It's *not* my fault. I was born with this. It's hereditary (after all, how could I hope to be the first of three generations to get sober?). After many years of this internal bantering mixed with self-hatred I still wasn't convinced. Below it all were my true feelings. I just "knew" that I was a weak-willed, slobbering drunk with a hopeless lack of self-discipline. It was this self-pity and the beginnings of mental and physical breakdown that literally forced me to stop drinking. I had one choice, disease or not. I felt it death to continue. I had no spirit left, no strength but I did have the freedom of choice. I *chose* to stop drinking. This was when I realized that alcoholism was truly a disease affecting my physical body and manipulating my ability to think clearly about alcohol and about all aspects of my life including attitudes about my work, my art, relationships and people.

Much is written and available for people who want to stop drinking, people generally being defined as the heterosexual population. My first visit to an AA meeting exemplified this. One of the first drunk-a-logs (an alcoholic sharing thoughts and details of their bouts under the influence) I listened to was from a man, aged between 35 and 45, who realized, finally, that he had "hit bottom" after fifteen years of abusing and humiliating his wife and two young daughters. While I can empathize with the lack of control manifesting itself in a violent manner, (I had, on occasion, battered my fists through many a pane of glass) I could only hear the screams of fear and pain from the woman in his life and their two daughters. I left that meeting, went to a bar and had a drink for each of them and, of course, a couple for myself. While I am aware that each AA meeting is made up of different community members, all diverse people, and that AA is responsible for helping millions get sober, it didn't seem the way for me to go. It became apparent to me that while I could identify with the disease; its symptoms and signs, I could never identify with the "straight" community and the matter-of-fact ways that mysogyny crept into their daily existence and was accepted. These were not my people. I realized then that I either had to do this alone or find other lesbians with the same problem.

Four years passed. Obviously, alone was not my answer. But how could I share this terrible secret with anyone? The community of lesbians was small enough. Part of the reason I drank was loneliness—how could I alienate them by confessing to being an alcoholic? My anguish and isolation were topped only by the progression of the disease as I began to enter the second stages. I tried out the line on a few close friends, "I think I may have a drinking problem." Some heard this, some didn't. I tried again over the course of several months, testing new phrases and getting bolder and more desperate. The responses ran the gamut from, "Don't be silly of course you're not an alcoholic," to "Nah, stop being so hard on yourself. You're making it a bigger problem than it is." Actually, I did have friends that recognized and labelled my disease correctly. I screamed inside, aching to be validated for my illness, yet it wasn't from them that I sought validation. Finally, I confessed, "I'm sick!" They hugged me. Some consoled me and some wondered, but I don't think they knew what to believe. Neither did I. After all, alcoholism didn't strike creative, intelligent, productive individuals like myself. Alcoholics were helpless, weak, miserable people who lacked self-respect and discipline. *I* couldn't be an alcoholic.

Meanwhile, I kept drinking, alone, in my apartment, tormented with confusion, pain, self-pity and emotional helplessness. My ex-lover, who had courageously but none too gently identified our past relationship as a co-dependent one (One where the partner of the alcoholic is just as sick as the alcoholic) sent me the book, "Out From Under; for Sober Dykes and Their Friends," an anthology of writings edited by Jean Swallow and written by lesbians struggling with alcohol and drug issues. At the same time,

one of my long-time friends, now living out of state and dealing with some of the same issues around alcohol, sent me the book, "Selfwatching," by Ray Hodgson and Peter Miller. It was these two books, combined with the sources of love that sent them, timing and a gentle nudge from the goddess that encouraged me to try again.

The most empowering of thoughts I learned at this time was that alcoholism is indeed a predictable, progressive and, most importantly, *treatable* disease and that I was not alone. Alcoholism plays a devious role in the lesbian population and is slowly being identified and dealt with. Until recently, the only places where lesbians could meet other lesbians were gay bars. Alcohol plays an enormous role in these social scenes where drinking helps diffuse the feelings and insecurities that accompany the stresses involved in coming out as a lesbian. AA now has meetings (mostly in large cities, however) for lesbians. Amethyst Women, located in Boston, started organizing "Chem-free" social events to support sobriety and yet provide that lesbian-only social space that we need so desperately to help combat isolation. Even Meg Christian got sober and shared it with us in "Turning It Over" (at last, a good lesbian/alcoholic role model!). I was beginning to feel less alone.

Despite my new-found support and resources, I still drank. Why?, you say. It was simple. I could not stop. Or should I say, I could and did stop. Every day I quit and vowed I would come home at night without stopping off for a beer or a bottle of wine to enhance my solitary meals. But each and every afternoon, as twilight drew nearer, the disease which pervaded my thinking helped me rationalize my way into a grocery store liquor display with thoughts of ambiance in the form of one small glass of wine to accompany the linguine with clam sauce menu planned and, of course, candle light. This is taking care of myself, I thought. Bullshit! That was the disease. I went on for months like this, embellishing my rationalizations with more and more excuses until I was drinking as heavily as before (which. by the way, was not all that much for a *non*-alcoholic person). Oh, I was clever; getting the house clean, work and errands done all before five or six o'clock because I knew (not consciously, of course) that I would be incapable of anything except emotional outbursts and sleep after nightfall.

Depression hit harder than ever. Thoughts of suicide slithered in like heat into a cool room on a hot day. I wasn't fooling myself. I knew now more than ever how this disease operated. I had no control; knowledge, yes, but I just couldn't stop. The harder I tried the more I whipped myself, the harder it got. You see, I believed that with my new found understanding of alcoholism and my persevering personality that I would never "hit bottom," at least not what I perceived bottom to be. I also thought that I could moderate or control my drinking, a definite clue that the disease "theory" had not yet fully sunk in.

Emotional tragedy times two and a new job that mattered greatly to me . . . all within the same week was more than I could deal with. I hit my bottom, literally, overnight.

The next day, sick and drained, I surrendered to the knowledge that either I get professional help or death was my only acceptable option. I called a crisis line and a woman answered the phone. That was over eight months ago. I have not had a drink since.

Now, the hardest part begins. As I said before, much is written for the alcoholic; the active alcoholic. In sobriety I have found little support beyond the perfunctory "congratulations" when I bring up the fact that I have persevered for yet another month. Of course, other recovering alcoholics truly understand the magnitude of what I have done and how it affects and will continue to affect my life. However, most of my friends are *not* alcoholics. In general, the people I meet who may or may not become important to me in my life are not alcoholics. The woman I've chosen to befriend and may even allow myself the vulnerability of involvement and intimacy is not an alcoholic. How can I convey to them what recovery is like for me?

My past involvement with alcohol was, perhaps, the most intimate of all my relationships. When I was in pain and needed a friend, when friends weren't around . . . the bottle was there. I trusted that soothing blurring of the edges. I thought I preferred it. Now, I have a new-found self and the rediscovery of what it is like to feel pain without the use of alcohol as an anesthetic. At times, my feelings are jumbled and I've even lost some ability to articulate, with words becoming cumbersome, sometimes elusive. When I push too hard to understand, thoughts racing, feelings on overload, depression settles in like a warm blanket. I can't move my arms. Words come out in sighs. I become inert, unfocused. This is a part of my recuperation.

Many women drink to escape pain; the emotional pain of abandonment and abuse, feelings of helplessness, fear of loss of control .... You name it. Pain is familiar to all of us. It weaves in and out of our lives like a spider web in a dark corner. During recovery, previously covered over pain oozes out as from an abcess. It cannot be controlled, no matter how hard you may try. The smallest of incidents can trigger memories blocked by years of drinking. An expression on someone's face can unlock an excruciating recall of a moment or feeling previously stored away for your own survival. The recovering alcoholic savors these moments of memory recall. It is by re-feeling those feelings never understood, that the recovering alcoholic can fit together the broken pieces of their life and accept the realities they cannot change. This is an important part of the recovery process.

These incidents have no patterns or respect for timing. Friends and lovers of recovering alcoholics can give support only with acknowledgements that help validate the importance of struggle for self-awareness being rediscovered through sobriety. Hugs help too.

Sometimes I am impatient with the "new" me. My wit is slower, less caustic. Perhaps it's just better timed. My interpretations of situations and occurrences are more serious. Sometimes, I lack patience or clarity and burst with frustration. I am more intense, sometimes too intense. Meanwhile, I plug on; proud of myself for "treating" my own disease on an every day basis. May 1st, 1986 I celebrate one year of sobriety.

Ω

Fetal Alcohol Syndrome:
A Nation in Distress

by Charon Asetoyer

And indeed, if it be the design of Providence to extirpate these Savages in order to make room for cultivators of the earth, it seems not improbable that Rum may be the appointed means. It has already annihilated all the tribes who formerly inhabited the sea coast.

—from the diary of Ben Franklin (1700s)

Let us put our minds together and see what kind of life we can make for our children.

—Sitting Bull (1800s)

It becomes clear who was the savage and who was the civilized man.

Historical Overview

In 1973, two doctors from Seattle, Washington, David Smith and Kenneth Jones, identified an irreversible birth defect that occurs when alcohol is consumed during pregnancy. They called it fetal alcohol syndrome (FAS) and noted its effects: mental retardation, deformed facial features, and stiff joints in the hands, arms, hips, and legs.

From *Sojourner: The Women's Forum,* March, 1993, Copyright © 1993 by Sojourner, Inc. Reprinted by permission.

Charon Asetoyer is the founder and director of the Native American Women's Health Education Resource Center in Lake Andes, South Dakota. She is on the boards of the National Women's Health Network and Women Organized for National Health Care Campaign.

This naming of FAS by "modern man," however, was not our first knowledge of the connection between alcohol and the birth of unhealthy children. As early as 428–347 B.C., in the Laws of Plato, we find warnings about alcohol consumption during pregnancy: "Any man or woman who is intending to create children should be barred from drinking alcohol." Plato believed that all citizens of the state should be prohibited from drinking alcohol during the daytime and that children should not be made in bodies saturated with drunkenness. He went on to say: "What is growing in the mother should be compact, well attached, and calm."

In 322 B.C., Aristotle was quoted as saying: "Foolish, drunken, hair-brained women most often bring forth children like themselves, morose and languid." In ancient Sparta and Carthage, the laws prohibited bridal couples from drinking on their wedding night for fear of producing defective children. Even in the Bible (Book of Judges 13:7), an angel warns the wife of Manoah: "Behold, thou shalt conceive and bear a son, and now drink no wine or strong drink."

If the great philosophers were aware of the relationship between alcohol and birth defects, why has it taken so long for modern medicine to reach the same conclusion?

Ben Franklin's diary serves as a reminder that the colonial governments of what are now referred to as the United States, Africa, and Australia all used alcohol, in one form or another, to manipulate and control the local inhabitants of the continents they invaded. Alcohol was often used as a form of money with which to barter with local inhabitants for land, food, and animal hides. Colonial governments knew that indigenous people had no experience with alcohol and, therefore, were vulnerable to its effects. As Franklin makes clear, annihilation of indigenous people through alcohol became the unofficial policy of the colonial (U.S.) government.

Throughout U.S. history, the government has continued to use alcohol to control, manipulate, and murder Native Americans. Alcohol has been legal, illegal, and legal again at the whim of various presidents. The most recent change in the law pertaining to alcohol use among Native Americans was in 1953, when the Eisenhower administration once again legalized the sale of alcohol to Native Americans. Knowing this history, we should not be surprised that alcoholism remains a major health problem among Native Americans, nor that alcoholism results in the birth of significant numbers of children with FAS.

The Women and Children in Alcohol Program

Of all women who drink alcohol during pregnancy, 40 percent will give birth to children suffering from either FAS or a lesser condition known as fetal alcohol effects (FAE). FAE occurs four to six times more often than FAS, and though a less serious birth defect, we must not underestimate it. The effects are: below average intelligence; learning disabilities; visual, speech, and hearing problems; hyperactive behavior; and a short attention span. FAE may also be accompanied by some of the same physical disabilities as FAS. FAE children usually are not detected until they enter school, where they are often seen as children with discipline problems. On Native American reservations, it is estimated that anywhere from one in nine to one in four children are born with FAS or FAE.

To address the problems of alcohol consumption among Native American women and its impact on their children, the Native American Community Board (NACB), a nonprofit project based on the Yankton Sioux Reservation in Lake Andes, South Dakota, developed the Women and Children in Alcohol program. NACB was founded in 1985 to improve the quality of life for indigenous people and to ensure the survival of our culture through increasing awareness of health issues pertinent to our communities and encouraging community involvement in economic development efforts.

Women and Children in Alcohol was the first program of the NACB, and this focus resulted in NACB opening the first Native American Women's Health Education Resource Center in 1988. Located on the Yankton Sioux Reservation, the center addresses many of the unmet needs of women and children identified during the initial program, including child development; nutrition; adult learning; women's health issues, especially reproduction, AIDS and other sexually transmitted diseases, and cancer prevention; and environmental issues. It is not enough to go out into the community and spread the word about FAS/FAE. Information is important; however, there is more to it than that.

Blaming the Women

Early on, we discovered that when people learned of FAS/FAE, they were quick to blame mothers and their children. No one wanted to examine the larger picture, to ask questions about why women drink when pregnant. What about men's involvement in this, the peer pressure to drink in a community where alcohol use has become the accepted norm? What about the idle time in communities where the unemployment rate is often as high as 85 percent and the high school drop-out rate is over 60 percent? What about the high rates of domestic violence and sexual assault in our communities and the lack of community agencies to address these issues? It is easy to say that a mother's drinking causes an FAS/FAE child to be born, but it is far from the whole truth.

Women who are chemically dependent don't plan to get pregnant and give birth to unhealthy children. They are often the products of abusive childhoods or of homes where their parents drank. They were introduced to alcohol at an early age—I've known children on reservations addicted by the time they were ten or eleven years old. As adults, these women have many health problems of their own—liver damage, diabetes, and other conditions related to alcohol abuse. But these are not uncaring mothers. Chemically dependent mothers love their children as much as other mothers—no matter how unlikely this may seem to outsiders. They must also live with the guilt that society imposes upon them for having given birth to imperfect children. Every day they are reminded that had they not consumed alcohol during pregnancy, their children would probably have been normal and healthy. Chemically dependent women who seek treatment find one barrier after another blocking their paths. Only a small number of alcohol and drug treatment centers take pregnant women. In our four-state area, there is only one such center designed for Native American women. The Kateri program, in St. Paul, Minnesota, will take women through their sixth month of pregnancy (due to complications with Title 19, women cannot receive medical coverage if they stay beyond this point). This program, however, is in the process of being closed down because of problems with state and county funding.

Even if a woman is able to find a treatment center, in most cases, she will be unable to have her children there with her. If she is lucky enough to have supportive and available family members, she can leave her children with them; otherwise, she must turn them over to foster care, where she may fear that they will be abused and neglected. Most Native American women will not turn their children over to foster care unless ordered to do so by the courts.

Of course, someone must pay for women to enter treatment centers. Often, for poor women, the only means of gaining access to treatment is through a court order. But more often than not, when a woman is prosecuted for crimes related to chemical dependency, the courts find it easier and cheaper to terminate parental rights or to sentence a woman to jail than to provide treatment.

In recent years, it has become more and more common for prosecutors to charge women with child abuse or with giving a controlled substance to a minor in cases where a woman has continued to drink or take drugs during pregnancy. Judges want to punish women for engaging in what they consider self-indulgent behavior. They see these mothers as abusive rather than ill. The court may not even consider the fact that the woman being prosecuted may have tried to gain access to unavailable services.

Women of color are reported to authorities eight times more often than white women for giving birth to babies who are drunk or who have controlled substances in their blood. These women are often brought to the attention of authorities by social workers or doctors who deliver their children. But what have these service providers done to help these women deal with their addictions? In our communities, it is a sad fact that social-service and child-protection workers are often aware of alcohol problems among children and adults but are unwilling to intervene because those in need of assistance are part of their own extended family or the family of a tribal council member. Because of the politics involved, a social worker may lose his or her job for trying to assist a child in need of services.

Several years ago, a doctor at the Indian Health Services Hospital on our reservation diagnosed a child with FAS. It turned out to be the tribal chairman's child. The doctor was transferred out of our hospital. It is easier for the problems of families and children to be ignored, for the entire system to become dysfunctional, and for all of the blame to fall on alcoholic mothers, who are given little or no support in the first place.

Sterilization Abuse

Since the courts are rarely interested in helping women to overcome their additions, they have instead focused on how to prevent alcoholic and drug-addicted women from having children. Although judges have shied away from permanent surgical sterilization of women because of fear of violating women's civil rights, new contraceptive technologies have allowed judges to order women to be temporarily sterilized. This, too, is a violation of civil rights.

Norplant, a surgically implanted contraceptive that prevents pregnancy for up to five years, has become the sterilization method of choice among judges. Norplant must be implanted, and removed, by a physician; thus, the woman who is subjected to Norplant has no control over her fertility. She is sterilized. The same is true with the contraceptive Depo-Provera (an injected contraceptive that lasts for approximately three months), which was used to sterilize mentally ill Native American women in the 1980s. Not only were these Indian women injected with Depo-Provera without their approval, but they were given the contraceptive before the FDA had even approved it for use in this country.

The first case in which a judge, as part of a plea bargain, ordered a woman to use Norplant, was in California in 1991. The woman, Darlene Johnson, was African American. The judge had little, if any, understanding of the potential harm that Norplant might do to this woman. He did not know that Johnson had health conditions that could become life-threatening if she were to be given Norplant. Should court officials who have no medical background be prescribing powerful medications? Will the courts assume legal responsibility if they endanger a woman's life in prescribing a potentially harmful drug?

Poor women, many of them women of color, have been targeted for sterilization not only through the courts but through bills in a number of states that require the use of Norplant as a condition for receiving welfare. Clearly, society takes the attitude that you reduce the risk of FAS/FAE babies by sterilizing women at high risk for giving birth to these babies. Reducing the risk of alcoholism and drug addiction among women of color and providing treatment for those in need is not a priority. This means that FAS/FAE and chemically dependent children often end up as orphans, dependent on the state for medical treatment as well as other social services.

Addicted mothers end up absent from home because they are still "using" and are out in the streets, in jail, or are dead after many years of substance abuse. Others must care for the children who may end up in foster homes or state facilities for the remainder of their lives. I have a close family member who has FAE. He lost his mother when he was seven years old due to an alcohol-related car accident.

By the time he was fourteen, he had been in ten foster homes. Some were so bad that he experienced sexual abuse, drug abuse, and neglect. He is now 25 and has many problems with chemical dependency as well as with the law.

Society must take some responsibility for allowing a system to continue to function in this manner. It seems that it is easier to allow a system to be ill than to assist it in trying to get healthy. Both tribal and state courts have overstepped their authority in recommending or sentencing women to use Norplant or Depo-Provera. The bottom line is that this is sterilization, whether short-term or permanent, and such a policy carries with it strong connotations of racism and genocide when women of color are the intended targets. We cannot forget that in the mid '70s, the surgical sterilization of Native American women was common practice, with estimates running as high as 25 percent of all child-bearing age women having been permanently sterilized against their will.

Conclusion

It is easier to blame women for being alcohol- or drug-addicted than to admit that society has failed to provide services that will help these women to work toward a healthy lifestyle. Though not entirely surprised by the response of the courts, I have been shocked by hearing health care professionals support sterilization policies. In a recent interview with an Indian Health Service doctor concerning Norplant and Native American women, he said that he "would support court ordering of Norplant for the prevention of FAS/FAE." Never during the entire interview did he mention or suggest that the system had failed in trying to assist women who are alcohol or drug addicted.

Fetal alcohol births are an indicator of a Nation in distress. What does this mean for the future of a Nation? For the existence of a culture? The quality of a Nation's leadership is derived from its people and the vulnerability of a Nation lies in its leadership. Health care professionals, social service workers, tribal leaders, lawyers, and judges—people in a position to create a positive response to this issue—have chosen not to do so. Thus, they must share the burden of guilt each time an FAS/FAE or chemically dependent baby is born.

Ω

Fetal Alcohol Syndrome Class Related
by Ruth Hubbard

Readers of Charon Asetoyer's article about fetal alcohol syndrome in the March health supplement might like to know about a paper published in the journal *Advances in Alcohol and Substance Abuse* in summer 1987. The article, written by Nesrin Bingol and six others and entitled "The Influence of Socioeconomic Factors on the Occurrence of Fetal Alcohol Syndrome," reports the results from a study comparing the children of 36 upper-middle or upper-class chronic alcoholic women and the children of 48 chronic alcoholic women receiving public assistance in New York City. The authors found that whereas 4.6 percent of the children of the affluent mothers exhibited Fetal Alcohol Syndrome and other alcohol-related effects, 71 percent (or 15 times as many) of the children of the poor mothers did. Both groups of women were heavy drinkers, but their lives differed in many ways. For example, the poor women were more likely to have had alcoholic parents and grandparents and less likely to eat regular and balanced meals than the affluent women. The results of this study show clearly that Fetal Alcohol Syndrome is not just the result of pregnant women drinking too much alcohol, but of the economic, social, and physical neglect entire segments of our population experience all their lives.

Ω

From *Sojourner: The Women's Forum*, April 1993, Vol. 18, No. 8, page 5. Copyright © 1993 by Sojourner: The Women's Forum. Reprinted by permission.

♀

How Women Are Targeted by the Tobacco Industry

by Amanda Amos

If women in many parts of the world are smoking in greater numbers than ever before, it is probably no coincidence. Women represent a fresh and lucrative target group for the tobacco industry, which has learned to tailor its products and promotion to women's presumed tastes. The promotion images, themes and devices used are analysed in the following article, which also suggests some healthy ground rules for women's magazines to consider adopting.

In the last few years the tobacco industry has aimed both its products and its advertising increasingly at women. Tobacco companies have always been keen to develop the female market. Given the decline in smoking in many developed countries (especially among men) and the fact that tobacco kills off a quarter of its consumers, however, these companies are resorting more than ever before to the creation and expansion of new markets. Women are key target groups in both developed and Third World countries.

Items in the tobacco and advertising press are explicit about the importance attached to targeting women. Articles entitled "Suggesting that retailers should 'look to the ladies',"[1] "Women—a separate market,"[2] and "Creating a female taste,"[3] have appeared in the British journal *Tobacco*, as have similar articles in the United States press.[4,5] The international journal *Tobacco Reporter*, which has featured such articles as "Targeting the female smoker,"[6] concludes that "women are a prime target as far as any alert European marketing man is concerned."[7]

How Are Women Targeted?

The overall objective of any campaign is to make smoking cigarettes in general, and one brand in particular, more appealing. This is achieved by tailoring the marketing mix to specific groups, which may involve altering the product, its price, its availability and its image through packaging and promotion. The particular marketing strategy used to target women will vary with factors such as: the tobacco company; the country—its culture, smoking patterns and trends, and its restrictions on advertising and promotion; and whether the campaign is aimed at a particular subgroup of women, defined by characteristics such as age, ethnicity and affluence.

In the USA and Europe several complementary strategies have been adopted, the most important being:

— promoting images designed to appeal specifically to women;
— producing new brands for women only;
— using women's magazines to direct advertising at women.

From *World Health Forum*, Vol. 11, 1990, pp. 416–422. Copyright © 1990 by World Health Organization. Reprinted by permission.

Dr. Amos is Lecturer in Health Education, Department of Community Medicine, Usher Institute, University of Edinburgh Medical School, Teviot Place, Edinburgh EH8 9AG, Scotland.

Creating the Right Image

"The image is luxury and sophistication, confidence and style, as manufacturers pursue half of America's smokers: the women." *Tobacco Reporter*[6]

Since the 1920s, when women first began to be targeted, various attractive images and themes have been used to encourage smoking, promote its social acceptability, and highlight the supposed desirable attributes of particular brands of cigarettes. A number of times smoking has been advertised as being glamorous, sophisticated, fun, romantic, sexually attractive, healthy, sporty, sociable, relaxing, calming, emancipated or liberated, rebellious and—last but definitely not least—an aid to slimming.[8–10] These images and themes have been conveyed by a variety of means ranging from straightforward verbal and visual messages, for example, advertisements featuring young attractive women and slogans such as "You've come a long way, baby", to the more subtle visual imagery of luxury represented by silk or satin and by symbols of success or high style such as expensive and exotic locations.

The message that smoking helps you stay slim appeared very early in the USA with the infamous ad of the 1930s encouraging women to reach for a cigarette "instead of a sweet". This message continues to be promoted today, although more subtly, through the association of slender female models with slender cigarettes. For example, in a recent German advertisement that depicted three people smoking different versions of the same brand of cigarette, it was the woman who was smoking the "slim line" cigarette.

Even in the United Kingdom and other countries that have more stringent restrictions on the content of tobacco advertisements, words such as long, slim and slender frequently appear in advertising copy. While they supposedly describe the merits of the cigarettes, clearly they also serve to associate the product with the aspirations of a large section of the target audience: women.

Cigarette manufacturers and advertisers argue that these messages and imagery merely encourage brand-switching or sustain brand loyalty among those who already smoke. However, there is increasing research evidence that such advertisements serve to encourage and reinforce smoking among the young.[11–13] A recent report by the New Zealand Toxic Substances Board[13] has concluded that brand-switching accounts for only 7% of the economic return from maintaining tobacco advertising and sponsorship. In the developing world, enormous amounts of money are spent on tobacco ads directed at women—even in places such as Hong Kong, where only some 3% of women are smokers.

> Given the decline in smoking (especially among men) and the fact that tobacco kills off a quarter of its consumers, tobacco companies are resorting more than ever before to the creation and expansion of new markets. Women are a key target group.

Women are targeted through a variety of other promotional activities as well. These have included special offers such as free silk stockings, contests, free cosmetics, and clothing carrying the brand logo. Another popular method is the sponsorship of women's sports (e.g., tennis) which receive widespread media coverage, and of women's events such as fashion shows. Again, the aim is to enhance the brand's image by associating it with socially valued activities.

> At various times smoking has been advertised as being glamorous, sophisticated, fun, romantic, sexually attractive, healthy, sporty, sociable, relaxing, calming, emancipated or liberated, rebellious and—last but definitely not least—an aid to slimming.

For Women Only—Women's Brands

"Question—what have Kim, Benson and Hedges Longer Length, and More got in common? ... All three brands are calculated to appeal to the growing women's sector of the cigarette market.
Tobacco [1]

The targeting of women entered a new phase in the late 1960s with the launch in the USA of Kim, the first of a new wave of brands aimed solely at women. These "women only" brands use advertising and packaging which emphasize feminine characteristics and positive female images. For example, Eve—with its archetypal female name—has a filter tip decorated with a flower motif; Satin has a special luxury satin-like paper tip. Then there are the "designer" brands such as Ritz, which carries the logo of Yves St. Laurent, and Cartier. As mentioned above, there has also been an explosion in the number of extra-long (over 100 mm) cigarettes, which are particularly popular among women. A recent arrival in Europe is Vogue, a new brand described by *Tobacco* as a "stylish type of cigarette with obvious feminine appeal, being slim and therefore highly distinctive."[14] This has been followed by Capri, the world's first "ultra-slim" cigarette, and Dakota, launched in the USA for "virile females."[15]

Women's Magazines—Readers' Health or Magazines' Wealth?

"For a number of years women's magazines have been a favourite advertising medium for all the best selling uni-sex brands."
Tobacco [16]

In many countries, particularly where tobacco advertising is banned from television, the most popular medium for targeting women is women's magazines. Cigarette advertising in these magazines has grown substantially. In the USA eight of the twenty magazines receiving the most cigarette advertising are women's magazines.[9] In the United Kingdom revenue from tobacco ads in women's magazines increased by 50% in real terms between 1977 and 1982[17] and by 10% between 1984 and 1988.[18] In 1988 nearly £9.7 million was spent on cigarette advertisements compared with some £7.2 million in 1984. A recent survey of the top women's magazines in 14 European countries found that 72% of them accepted cigarette advertisements.[19]

There are several reasons why women's magazines are so popular with tobacco advertisers.

Magazines in the European survey which did not accept cigarette advertisements, 1988.

		Reason for non-acceptance		
		Total media ban	Partial media ban	Magazine's policy
Finland	Gloria	x		
	Me Naiset	x		
France	Vogue			x
Greece	Domino			x
	Seventeen			x
Ireland/	Company	x		
United	Cosmopolitan	x		
Kingdom	Elle	x		
	Just Seventeen	x		
	Marie Claire	x		
	Smash Hits	x		
	Vogue	x		
Italy	Vogue	x		
Netherlands	Yes			x
Portugal	Elle	x		
	Guia	x		
	Maria	x		
	Marie Claire	x		
	Maxima	x		
	Muhler Moderna	x		
Spain	Greca			x
Sweden	Frida	x		

Source: reference 19 and unpublished data.

- They have an enormous number of readers. In the United Kingdom around half of all women are regular readers of women's magazines.[17, 18]
- They are read by women of all ages and backgrounds. Hence, through the careful selection of magazines, specific groups such as young women or black women can be reached. A recent survey in the USA found more tobacco ads in women's and youth magazines than in magazines targeted at other population segments.[20]
- Magazines can lend a spurious social acceptability or stylish image to smoking. In a British study the health editor of high-fashion magazine said that publication of an ad in that magazine was "as good as a stamp of acceptability."[17]
- The presence of tobacco ads in a magazine may dilute the impact of articles on tobacco and health. Alternatively, they may induce magazine editors to downplay this issue or avoid covering it altogether. There are numerous examples of magazines in the USA which have allegedly lost tobacco advertising because they reported on the adverse health effects of smoking, or which have reportedly refused to cover this health issue or altered articles to de-emphasize its importance because they were worried about losing lucrative sources of advertising revenue.[21] New evidence from the USA shows that women's magazines as a group are more sensitive to the presence of cigarette advertising than are other magazines.[22]

Thus women's magazines represent a battleground between the competing interests of, on the one hand, the tobacco companies and advertisers wishing to target their massive female audience and the magazines wishing to maximize their own revenues, and, on the other, editors and journalists wishing to report the facts without bias and to protect the health of their readers. At present, the tobacco interests seem to be winning the battle.

> In the developing world, enormous amounts of money are spent on tobacco ads directed at women—even in places such as Hong Kong, where only some 3% of women are smokers.

Recent studies of women's magazines in the USA[23], the United Kingdom[18], and in Europe[19] have found that smoking, a major cause of ill-health and premature death among their readers, is receiving scant coverage in the medium most trusted by women—women's magazines. Only 29% of British women's magazines had published a major article on smoking and health in the year preceding the survey.[18] The preliminary findings of a survey of the top women's magazines in 14 countries in Europe showed that only half had recently covered this issue.[19] Indeed, some of the editors said that they would never cover it or had stopped covering it. The coverage that was given was often brief and considerably less than that given to tobacco

advertisements. In the top French magazines, for example, only 24 articles appeared in 1988, as compared with 123 pages of tobacco advertisements.

> The targeting of women entered a new phase in the late 1960s with the launch of the first of a new wave of brands aimed solely at women.

Magazines' attitudes to coverage of the health hazards of smoking varied considerably, both in the United Kingdom and in other European countries. One key factor was the personal interest and commitment of the editor with regard to smoking and health. Another factor, though many editors denied its importance, was the desire not to offend tobacco advertisers. The following candid comments came from the advertising department of one of the top-selling British women's magazines. "The difficulty is that we take money from these people. It does not matter how much we take from them, it's difficult for us to endorse anything that goes against the companies. Even editorially, they have to go carefully. The tobacco companies are very sensitive about their image."[17]

In the British and United States studies, the magazines that were most dependent on tobacco advertising gave least coverage to the health hazards of smoking. As remarked by a well-known editor who has come herself from the advertising world, "I think 'who needs somebody you're paying millions of dollars a year to come back and bite you on the ankle'?"[23]

Not only do many magazines avoid reporting on smoking and health while giving considerable space to tobacco ads. They also feature pictures of glamorous models smoking in their fashion pages. The European survey found that a third of the magazines had no policy on the editorial portrayal of positive images of smoking.[19] Fewer than half said that they would not publish such pictures. Magazines in Denmark, France and Spain had the worst records. For example, in 1988 one major French fashion magazine published 20 fashion photos depicting models smoking, and another published 25. The double standards of many magazines was illustrated in one issue of a Spanish magazine, where an article on the health of Spanish women—which included a section on smoking—was sandwiched between cigarette advertisements and photos of fashion models smoking.

The Way Forward

Numerous expert national and international bodies that have looked at the issue of tobacco and health, including the WHO Expert Committee on Smoking Control[24] and the Royal College of Physicians in London[25], have all reached the same conclusion. Smoking and smoking-related disease will decline only if a comprehensive approach is taken to tackling the problem. This includes a ban on all tobacco advertising and promotion.

Many countries have already adopted such a ban and many more are considering it. In the meantime, action should be taken to reduce the tobacco industry's ability to target key groups such as young people and women. Just as many women's magazines now play a negative role by allowing companies to promote their lethal product, they can also play an important positive role by encouraging their younger readers not to start smoking and helping their older readers to kick the habit. Women's magazines throughout the world could take the lead in protecting and improving the health of their readers by adopting these ground rules.

- Follow the example of several magazines in Europe and refuse to accept cigarette advertisements (see table). Although most of the magazines listed in the table were not allowed to accept advertisements because of national laws or regulations, five had voluntarily decided to refuse tobacco advertisements. These were French *Vogue*, Greek *Domino* and *Seventeen*, Spanish *Greca*, and Netherlands *Yes*.
- Give regular coverage to aspects of smoking including health hazards, how to give up smoking, and non-smokers' rights.
- In the case of a teenage or youth magazine, make a special effort to increase awareness of the special risks that smoking poses to young women, such as smoking while being on the pill, and smoking and pregnancy.
- Avoid the use of glamorous pictures of people, including fashion models, smoking.

References

1. Reisman, E. Suggesting that retailers should "look to the ladies". *Tobacco* March 1983, pp. 17–19.
2. Cole, J. Women—a separate market. *Tobacco*, March 1988, pp. 7–9.
3. Gill, B. & Garrett, S. Creating a female taste. *Tobacco*, March 1989, pp. 6–7.
4. Sobczynski, A. Marketers clamor to offer lady a cigaret. *Advertising age*, 31 January 1983. pp. 14–16.
5. O'Connor, J.J. Women top cig target. *Advertising age*, 28 September 1981, pp. 9, 93.
6. Anon. Targeting the female smoker. *Tobacco reporter*, April 1983, pp. 44–45.
7. Rogers, D. Editorial. *Tobacco reporter*, February 1987, p. 8
8. Ernster, V.L. Mixed messages for women: a social history of cigarette smoking and advertising. *New York State journal of medicine*, 85: 335–340 (1985).
9. Davis, R.M. Current trends in cigarette advertising and marketing. *New England journal of medicine*, 316: 725–732 (1987).
10. Jacobson, B. *Beating the ladykillers*. London, Gollancz, 1988.
11 Aitken, P.P. et al. Cigarette brand preferences of teenagers and adults. *Health promotion*, 2: 219–226 (1988).
12. Chapman, S. & Fitzgerald, B. Brand preferences and advertising recall in adolescent smokers: some implications for health promotion. *American journal of public health*, 72: 491–494 (1982).
13. Toxic Substances Board. *Health or tobacco*. Wellington, New Zealand Department of Health, 1989.
14. Cole, J. For a special occasion. *Tobacco*. December 1988, pp. 15–16.
15. Specter, M. Uneducated white women are target of new cigarette. *Washington Post*, 17 March 1990, pp. D1, D10.
16. Anon. Are there now more women smokers than men? *Tobacco*, November 1985, pp. 29–32.
17. Jacobson, B. & Amos, A. *When smoke gets in your eyes: cigarette advertising policy and coverage of smoking and health in women's magazines*. London, British Medical Association/Health Education Council, 1985.
18. ASH Women and Smoking Working Group. *Smoke still gets in her eyes—a report on cigarette advertising in British women's magazines*. London, British Medical Association/ASH, 1990.
19. Amos, A. Women's magazines and tobacco—preliminary findings of a survey of the tobacco policies of the top women's magazines in Europe. In: *Proceedings of the 7th World Conference on Tobacco and Health*, Perth, Health Department of Western Australia (in press).
20. Allright, C.C. et al. Cigarette advertisements in magazines: evidence for a differential focus on women's and youth magazines. *Health education quarterly*, 15: 225–233 (1988).
21. Warner, K.E. Cigarette advertising and media coverage of smoking and health. *New England journal of medicine*, 312: 384–388 (1985).
22. Warner, K. et al. The economics of cigarette advertising: impacts on magazines' revenues and editorial practice regarding coverage of smoking and health. In: *Proceedings of the 7th World Conference on Tobacco and Health*. Perth, Health Department of Western Australia (in press).
23. White, L. & Whelan, E.M. How well do American magazines cover the health hazards of smoking? *ACSH news and views*, 7(3): 1, 8–11 (1986).
24. *Controlling the smoking epidemic. Report of the WHO Expert Committee on Smoking Control*. Geneva, World Health Organization, 1979 (Technical Report Series, No. 636).
25. Royal College of Physicians. *Health or smoking?* London, Pitman 1983.

Ω

If you know of any women's magazines that carry tobacco advertising you might like to bring this article to the attention of their Editors.

Tobacco Foes Attack Ads That Target
Women, Minorities, Teens, and the Poor

by Paul Cotton

From ghettos to ski slopes, tobacco advertisements are coming down.

Advocates for minors, minorities, women, and the poor are on the offensive, scoffing at tobacco company claims that cigarette promotions are not aimed at the groups most at risk for acquiring nicotine addiction.

Antismoking activists are adopting what they see as the industry's own tactics, moving away from wide-angle warnings about the long-term health threats and focusing instead on specific brands, the smoker's self-image, and the short-term social consequences, in messages tailored to specific groups.

"We've done a good job of reaching middle-class white America, but not the groups most at risk," says American Cancer Society (ACS) spokesman Steve Dickinson. So new ACS ads twist the tobacco industry's images of success and sophistication. As a beautiful, dark-skinned woman smoking a cigarette becomes covered with a gloppy substance, the ad asks, "If what happened on your insides happened on your outsides, would you continue to smoke?"

Initiative in the black community has been ignited by a virtual wallpapering of inner-city areas with tobacco and alcohol billboards and by now-aborted plans to market a brand of cigarettes, called *Uptown*, to urban blacks.

"When our people desperately need the message of health promotion, Uptown's message is more disease, suffering, and death for a group already bearing more than its share of smoking- related illness and mortality," complains Department of Health and Human Services Secretary Louis W. Sullivan, MD, who helped keep the brand off the market—though a similar campaign is being used for a brand called *Salem Box*.

Nicotine addiction afflicts 34% of black adults vs 28% of whites and 27% of Hispanics, according to a 1989 survey by the Simmons Market Research Bureau. That is why lung cancer and heart disease rates are higher among blacks, says Sullivan, who hopes the victory against Uptown is "just the beginning of an all-out effort."

Women's groups are similarly outraged over a campaign for *Dakota* cigarettes that said they would be marketed to "virile females."

Native Americans, who suffer very high addiction rates to many substances, are also incensed at the misuse of the word *Dakota*, which means *friend*, says Shirley Butts, RN,

of Fort Totten, ND, a Turtle Mountain Chippewa and member of Dakotans Against Dakota Cigarettes.

Uptown and Dakota "made it very clear tobacco companies are targeting, and gave us something we can rally around as women and minorities," says Virginia Ernster, PhD, an epidemiologist at the University of California, San Francisco, who has testified before Congress on the tobacco industry's efforts at recruiting women.

"The industry does target women, minorities, and youth. They know the statistics on who's going to replace the 2.5 million smokers the industry loses each year," 400,000 of them to tobacco-related deaths, says Michele Bloch, MD, PhD, director of the Women vs Smoking Network in Washington, DC.

"Those replacement smokers are always children," with the average age for starting now 12.5 years, she says.

"If present trends continue, by 1995 women will outnumber men because more girls start smoking than boys and women quit less often," says Bloch. Among high school seniors, 20% of females smoke vs 16% of males, with higher rates for high school dropouts. By 2000 only 5% of college graduates will smoke vs 30% of high school dropouts, all largely due, says Bloch, to targeting.

Opposition to Uptown and Dakota, though, created "a one-two punch that has made the climate in Congress acceptable for legislation limiting tobacco ads in a way no one would have anticipated a year ago," she says, particularly a bill that would ban pictures of people.

"Adults respond to claims of low tar and nicotine, whereas kids respond to the Marlboro man," says John Madigan, a spokesman for the cancer society's Washington office.

Those associations can last a lifetime, as organizers of a boycott against Marlboro cigarettes and Miller beer are finding out, AIDS (acquired immunodeficiency syndrome) activists want gay and lesbian bars to stop stocking both products because of parent company Philip Morris' support for Sen. Jesse Helms (R, NC). But while patrons "don't bat an eye" when a bartender says there is no Miller, they go next door to buy Marlboro when it is removed from vending machines, says Frank Smithson, boycott coordinator in New York. "People are very fond of their cigarette brands. The graphics are part of who and what they are."

A total ad ban is not likely soon because there is little grassroots support, says Mark Pertschuk, executive director of Americans for Nonsmokers Rights in Berkeley, Calif.

Canada and other countries do have such bans, but Sheila Banks, media affairs director for Philip Morris

From JOURNAL OF THE AMERICAN MEDICAL ASSOCIATION, Sept. 26, 1990, Vol. 264, No. 12, pp. 1505–1506. Copoyright © 1990 by the American Medical Association. Reprinted by permission.

USA, says the bans do not cut youth smoking rates. Finland, for example, has the world's highest rate of smoking among teenage boys despite a dozen years without tobacco advertising, she says.

And in the United States there is "a very basic First Amendment issue," says David Fishel, senior vice president for public relations for the R.J. Reynolds Tobacco Company.

Pertschuk says banning ads for products that are deadly or harmful "in no way violates the First Amendment."

But Fishel warns that such an effort would engender a "backlash from smokers. It's getting to the point where you have to say, 'Hey, this is still America.'"

Fishel and Banks both insist they scrupulously avoid any pitch to the underaged. Banks says the fact that teens and preteens account for nearly 90% of new smokers is "probably true because kids try that which they associate with being an adult. The harder you tell them not to do something the more they want to do it."

Pertschuk's group uses that fact to turn tobacco ads inside out. "Children hate to be manipulated. We harness that and use the industry's own ads to ridicule" the ideas in them.

Only ridicule can counteract the seductive adult mystique surrounding cigarettes, says Alan Blum, MD, founder of Doctors Ought to Care (DOC), which attacks specific brands on a *Mad Magazine* level, for example, "Barfboro" and "Wimpston."

"People say it's so sophomoric, but how else are we supposed to appeal to kids other than to be juvenile?" asks Blum, a family practitioner and assistant professor at Baylor College of Medicine in Houston.

"I've never seen a kid go into a store and say 'A pack of cigarettes, please.' Kids are 'branded' for Marlboro and Camel," says Blum. "You're not going to get to kids by talking about the danger or the smell. But no one wants to be associated with a brand name that's ridiculed."

In the adult world, no one wants to be associated with a brand promoting itself to children. That fact is helping DOC get tobacco ads off popular Rocky Mountain ski slopes.

The Jackson Hole Ski Resort at Teton Village in Wyoming is removing Marlboro flags from a coin-operated race-course there after DOC surveyed all the fourth and fifth graders in town, says DOC member Brent Blue, MD, a family practitioner in Jackson Hole. "We got a much higher correlation of kids who raced at Teton Village knowing Marlboro than those who did not."

The Aspen Skiing Company in Colorado is also dropping Marlboro sponsorship. And Jackson Hole Ski Corp president Paul McCollister plans to propose a nationwide ban on tobacco sponsorship to the United Ski Industries Association. "When you stop and think about it, it's ridiculous not to," he says.

That sentiment is not shared by many other sports businessmen, though. Houston Astrodome officials had security guards remove Blum and other protesters at a Camel-sponsored Cinco de Mayo celebration there, which Blum says was aimed at Hispanic children.

DOC is campaigning against tobacco billboards in sports arenas as well, on the grounds that they constitute illegal television advertising.

A protest in August against such ads in San Francisco's Candlestick Park got support from many smokers, says Susan Smith, administrator of Tobacco-Free California. "They don't want their kids exposed even if they themselves smoke."

A letter-writing campaign to US Attorney General Richard Thornburgh is under way, asking him to assess the $10,000-per-violation fines. Blum says the word *Marlboro* was televised during virtually half the 93-minute Marlboro Grand Prix.

"If they'd keep track of all sporting events over the next 6 months we could erase the national deficit," says DOC president Rick Richards, MD, of Augusta, Ga. "The Federal Trade Commission ignores the ads, even though the amount companies pay is based on the number of exposures they are likely to get during the telecast," says Richards. Enforcement would "require no new legislation, just sitting down with a videotape player."

Existing legislation is one tool black leaders in Baltimore, Md, are using against the ubiquitous billboards pushing legal drugs in low-income areas there. Many billboards came down when neighborhood organizations found a 20-year-old residential area zoning restriction, says Robert Blackwell, an inspector in the city's zoning office.

Whitewashing of billboards by black leaders in New York helped get the attention of Philip Morris, which plans to turn over some billboards it rents to community groups, says Banks.

Advertising to minorities is a "catch-22" issue, says RJ Reynolds' Fishel. "In the past we've been criticized for not including blacks, now they're saying we funnel too much."

Tobacco support for minority organizations is also under fire. The National Association of Black Journalists turned down a $40,000 Philip Morris donation.

"It was a tough decision because tobacco companies have long been supporters of black media when very few others have. But we couldn't take money from an organization deliberately targeting minority populations with a substance that clearly causes cancer," says the group's president, Thomas Morgan. "We simply became more aggressive in our fund-raising so we could do without it."

That option does not exist for many minority publications, which would fold without tobacco dollars.

Tobacco revenues cause self-censorship of antismoking stories, says Kenneth Warner, PhD, professor of public health policy at the University of Michigan School of Public Health, Ann Arbor. Last April, at the Seventh World Conference on Tobacco and Health in Perth, Australia, he presented an analysis of 99 magazines over 25 years that found a statistically significant negative correlation between cigarette ad revenue and coverage of smoking, especially in women's magazines.

A "favorite tactic" of the American Medical Women's Association is "cleaning these magazines out of our waiting rooms," says president Susan Stewart, MD. (See *JAMA*. 1989;262:1290–1295.)

Women's organizations also often take tobacco money because "so little other money is available. Many corporations that earn money from women do not support women's groups," says Bloch. Both she and Banks agree that Virginia Slims put women's tennis on the map when no one else would.

"It is ironic that a product which causes major damage to the heart and lungs is associated with a sport requiring top physical fitness and aerobic capacity,"says Stewart, accusing Virginia Slims of "taking advantage" of the inadequate funding of women's sports.

DOC's answer is its own tennis tournament, the Emphysema Slims, held September 15 and 16 in Santa Fe, NM. It is billed as the world's largest throw-tobacco-out-of-sports protest.

Morgan feels other organizations will drop tobacco sponsorship " as time goes on, simply for the sake of principle." But tobacco company attempts at targeting will also intensify, he says. "Where are they going to turn but to the people least equipped to fend off the attractions of advertising, the poor and uneducated?"

Ω

Drugs, Alcohol, and Smoking

1. The last two articles in this chapter examined the marketing of cigarettes to specific groups. Collect cigarette advertisements from magazines or other sources.

    a. Compare the strategies in the ads that seem to be directed at women with those aimed at men. Are there recurring themes you can identify (such as smoking associated with being thin)?

    b. Do any of these ads seem to be directed at specific ethnic or racial groups?

    c. Most adult smokers begin smoking before they are 20. Are there any educational strategies you can think of to counter the ads aimed at young women?

2. A friend's use of alcohol can sometimes cause a dilemma in a social situation. Think of a situation (real or hypothetical) in which you are concerned about a friend's drinking. For example, your friend has had too much to drink and she's planning to drive her car home from the party, or she's drinking late into the night and you know she has to be at work early the next morning. How can you, as a supportive friend, interrupt this behavior?

    How would the situation be different if this was a frequent occurrence with her as compared to an event that happened only once?

    Would there be any different issues if your friend were a man instead of a woman?

3. You have been asked to consult on a new alcohol and drug treatment center for your community. All the other "experts" on the committee have years of experience in setting up treatment centers for men. Drawing on "Alcoholics Invisible" and "Women and Children Last," and other information or experience, identify a number of issues which you may need to address to insure that this new facility will be appropriate for women.

6

Menstruation

The normal physiological process of menstruation has been defined and redefined by male "experts." It has been labeled a disability or illness, as a barrier to higher education for women, as a weakness that justified keeping middle-class women from working outside the home (working class women were expected to continue their work). Later, menstrual cramps were identified as psychogenic in origin, brought on by the fear of femininity or sexuality. Now hormonal fluctuations are blamed for a wide range of symptoms premenstrually, from acne and water retention to homicidal behavior and self-mutilation. The first article in this section, "Women, Menstruation, and Nineteenth Century Medicine," puts the changing definitions and meanings of menstruation within their historical contexts, while at the same time addressing a recurring theme in medical history—"the reluctance of physicians to accept new scientific findings." In "The Meaning of Menstruation," Louise Lander examines what the social sciences say about the meaning of menstruation, concluding that the meanings will always change because menstruation will always be one aspect of what it means to be a woman in a given cultural and historical context.

With all the changes in labels and definitions, one view of menstruation has remained relatively constant in recent years: menstruation is a big money-maker, with a huge market of healthy women for various industries to target. For example, when it was discovered that cramps were not in our heads, but in our uteruses and the causal agent, prostaglandins, was found, pharmaceutical firms began putting a lot of advertising dollars into selling over-the-counter anti-prostaglandin drugs. While this has largely been a benefit for women who experience dysmenorrhea, we should be alert to potential problems whenever any new groups of drugs are mass-marketed to healthy people. PMS provides an even more dramatic example relating to

menstruation, as "The Selling of Premenstrual Syndrome" clearly explains. We selected this article for several reasons: it is a classic, the basic issues it addresses go well beyond PMS to include much of women's health, and it is an excellent way to remember Andrea Boroff Eagan, a women's health activist and writer, who recently died. PMS clinics sprang up all over the country and progesterone is prescribed without any solid data on effectiveness or risks. While a small percentage of women may suffer from severe PMS and benefit from this treatment, there is a clear attempt to convince a lot more women that they have this "disease" and need treatment.

Since women went "off the rag" and began using disposable menstrual products, there has been a large profitable business in tampons, napkins and pads (see worksheet on menstrual products for a clearer view of the amount of money a woman may spend on these products). While these are products most women want to keep on the market, the competition and profit motive have sometimes meant that consumer health and safety receive minimal attention.

In spite of all these negative views, women have been redefining menstruation for ourselves—as a normal, healthy physiological process. Some women have even developed celebratory menstrual rituals. (It is important to note, however, that many women cannot menstruate and for women who are trying to become pregnant, menstruation can be viewed with great disappointment and sadness).

This chapter concludes with a view of menstruation that clarifies the role of social and cultural factors in defining the process. The classic "If Men Could Menstruate" by Gloria Steinem also is an answer to the old question, "Do feminists have a sense of humor?"

♀

Women, Menstruation,
and Nineteenth-Century Medicine

by Vern Bullough and Martha Voght

One of the recurrent themes in medical history is the reluctance of physicians to accept new scientific findings. This may well be due to the innate conservatism of medical practitioners and their unwillingness to use patients as guinea pigs for treatment about which they are unsure. Sometimes, too, the reluctance comes because new findings demonstrate that previous practices might have been harmful to the patient; this turn of events is difficult to accept. Often, however, the reluctance is not attributable to any medical reason but results when new findings upset the emotional attachments, some would say political prejudices, that most physicians hold and which have little to do with medicine itself. This paper is concerned with this kind of of position.

When the belief structure of the physician is threatened, even in fields outside of medicine, he often uses his medical expertise to justify his prejudices and in the process strikes back with value-laden responses which have nothing to do with scientific medicine. Unfortunately, since he is assumed to speak with authority, his response, perhaps as he intended, has influence far beyond that of ordinary men. One of the best examples of this is the controversy over the physical disabilities of women which took place in the last part of the nineteenth century as women began to demand more education and greater political equality and to challenge many of the male stereotypes about woman's place. Since medical practitioners were almost all men, and many of them were hostile to any change in the status quo in male-female relationships, they inevitably entered the struggle with arguments which not only appear today as ludicrous, but even in the period they were writing were not based upon any scientific findings and in fact went contrary to those findings. This is particularly true in their understanding of the consequences of menstruation.

During the last part of the nineteenth century American physicians toyed with several theories of menstruation. In general they were aware of the theories of John Power of London who postulated that ovulation and menstruation

were connected. American medical journals also made an attempt to keep their readers current on the English research which tended to support his theories.[1] At the same time, however, many physicians seriously discussed various folk theories about menstruation, retaining with little change in content ideas which appear in the Hippocratic corpus or in Aristotle. Many still held that it was the effect of the moon upon women that caused them to menstruate; others held that the fetus was formed from the menstrual flow. The popular underground pseudonymous marriage manual *Aristotle's Masterpiece* held that menstruation was due to the casting out of the excess blood which would have nourished the embryo if pregnancy had occurred.[2] Even as late as the 1890s when the first experimental work leading to the understanding of human hormones was taking place, American physicians were still discussing the question of whether the ovaries triggered menstruation, whether the uterus was an independent organ and performed the menstrual function without external aid, or whether the fallopian tubes were responsible for the monthly flow.[3] A few, however, perhaps influenced by the Victorian disgust at the sexual and reproductive processes, considered menstruation a pathological condition. These physicians believed that in Paradise humans had reproduced asexually and it was only when man had fallen that perfection had been replaced by the evil of sex. An article in the *American Journal of Obstetrics* in 1875, for example, argued that menstruation was pathological, proof of the inactivity and threatened atrophy of the uterus. As evidence of its unnaturalness the author claimed that conception was most likely when intercourse occurred during the monthly flow, but intercourse at such times was dangerous and forbidden because the menstrual blood was the source of male gonorrhea. Since menstruation therefore stood in the way of fruitful coitus it obviously had not been ordained by nature.[4]

In 1861 E.F. Pflüger demonstrated that menstruation did not take place in women whose ovaries had been removed, a finding which reinforced the ovarian theory but did not end the debate since Pflüger himself in 1863 hypothesized that there was a mechanical stimulus of nerves by the growing follicle which was responsible for congestion and menstrual bleeding. This led him to believe that menstruation and ovulation occurred simultaneously.[5] It was not until the twentieth century and a better understanding of the hormonal process that the timing of ovulation was fully understood. In the meantime, many American physicians accepted Pflüger's theory that nervous stimulation triggered menstruation, and it was this

From BULLETIN OF THE HISTORY OF MEDICINE 47 (1973): 66–82. Copyright ©1973 by Johns Hopkins University Press. Reprinted by permission.

This article is also reprinted in the excellent collection *Women's Health in America*, edited by Judy Walzer Leavitt, University of Wisconsin Press, 1984.
VERN L. BULLOUGH is Dean of the Faculty of Natural and Social Sciences, State University of New York College, Buffalo, New York. MARTHA L. VOGHT is a free-lance writer of educational materials in Bishop, California. Reprinted with permission from Bulletin of the History of Medicine 47 (1973): 66-82.

belief which led large numbers of physicians to express opposition to any emancipation of women.

This paper is not the place to discuss the movement for female emancipation, but even a brief synopsis must point out that women were much more assertive of their rights in the last part of the nineteenth century than earlier. Though traditionally women in the United States had received some sort of primary education, if only to learn to read the Bible, they had been denied entrance to any of the grammar schools or colleges. In 1783, for example, twelve-year-old Lucinda Foote was examined for admission to Yale and found capable of giving the "true meaning of passages in the *Aeneid* of Virgil, the *Select Orations* of Cicero and the Greek *Testament*." She was, however, declared unqualified to enter the college because of her sex.[6] Physicians of the time were generally more inclined to favor female education than oppose it. Perhaps the best example is Benjamin Rush. He urged female education on the grounds that it would allow women to better fulfill their familial responsibilities, be less prone to superstition, have talent in managing their family's affairs, and be better teachers for their sons. Rush also pointed out to his fellow males who might be somewhat hesitant to accept his ideas that the ignorant were the most difficult to govern and an educated wife could, by virtue of her education, be more easily shown the wisdom of her husband's orders and decisions.[7] It was only later that a significant portion of the medical community appear in opposition to female education.

During the first part of the nineteenth century the female academies and seminaries began to multiply, and in the 1830s full-fledged colleges were proposed for women and Oberlin College opened its doors to both sexes.[8] Soon medical schools also found themselves under attack for failure to admit women, and a few women such as Elizabeth Blackwell managed to receive medical training. Most women, however, turned to nursing as an alternative to challenging the male bastion of medicine,[9] but it is perhaps no accident that medical opposition to feminine emancipation began to increase as the physician himself felt threatened by the few women attempting to enter medical school. About 1870 several medical writers began proclaiming that education for women was a disastrous error since girls between twelve and twenty could not stand the strain of higher education, in large part because of the physiological strains which puberty and ovulation put upon them.

Among the first theorists of menstrual disability, by far the most influential was Edward H. Clarke, a professor of materia medica at Harvard and a fellow of the American Academy of Arts and Sciences. In 1873 he wrote that though women undoubtedly have the right to do anything of which they are physically capable, one of the things they could not do and still retain their good health was to be educated on the pattern and model of men. He held that while the male developed steadily and gradually from birth to manhood, the female, at puberty, had a sudden and unique period of growth when the development of the

reproductive system took place.[10] If this did not take place at puberty, it would never occur, and since the system can never do "two things well at the same time," the female between twelve and twenty must concentrate on developing her reproductive system. To digest one's dinner, he held it was necessary to temper exercise and brain work; likewise, during the growth of the female reproductive system, brain work must be avoided. The overuse of the central nervous system would overload the switchboard, so to speak, and signals from the developing organs of reproduction would be ignored in favor of those coming from the overactive brain. Even after puberty females were not to exercise their minds without restriction because of their monthly cycle. The menstrual period was vital, Clarke held, and any mental activity during the "catamenial week" would interfere with ovulation and menstruation,[11] the necessary physiological processes of being female.

He then proceeded to demonstrate, at least to his own satisfaction, that higher education left a great number of its female adherents in poor health for life. He was alarmed that the increase in the number of young women being educated would so deplete the population that within fifty years "the wives who are to be mothers in our republic must be drawn from trans-Atlantic homes."[12] For proof of his assertion he offered as evidence the cases of young women he had as patients whose ill health he ascribed to hard study. One had entered a female seminary at fifteen in good health but after a year of application to her studies and following the routine of the school, which included standing to recite, she was pale and tired "every fourth week." A summer's rest restored her but by the end of the second year she was not only pale but suffering from an "uncontrollable twitching of a rhythmical sort" in the muscles of her face. On the advice of the family physician she was taken for a year of travel in Europe and returned cured. Unfortunately she then returned to school where she studied without regard to her menstrual periods and, though she graduated at nineteen as valedictorian, she was an invalid and it took two years in Europe for her to recover. Her illness, according to Dr. Clarke's diagnosis, resulted from making her body do two things at once. He reported the case of another young woman, a student at Vassar, who began to have fainting spells and suffer painful and sparse menses. Inevitably she graduated at nineteen as an invalid, suffering from constant headaches. Dr. Clarke believed this was because she suffered from the arrested development of her reproductive system due to her education. As evidence he claimed she not only had menstrual troubles but was rather flat chested. Another young college woman came to him with a history of diminishing menstrual flow, constant headaches, mental depression, acne, and rough skin. Eventually Dr. Clarke committed her to an asylum.[13] It was also of some concern to Dr. Clarke that young women of the lower classes were expected, during puberty, to take jobs in domestic service or in factories. In his practice he had seen evidences of ill health among such women which he blamed upon their work. Yet, he concluded that labor in factory at a loom was far less damaging than study to a woman, because it worked the body, not the brain. It was primarily brain work which destroyed feminine capabilities.[14]

Women who concentrated upon education rather than the development of their reproductive system also underwent mental changes, according to Clarke. Not possessing the physical attributes of a man, they also tended to lose the "maternal instincts" of a woman to become coarse and forceful. By educating women, said Dr. Clarke, we were creating a class of sexless humans analogous to eunuchs. To solve this alarming problem, he recommended strict separation of the sexes during education, particularly after elementary school. He urged that female schools provide periodic rest periods for students during their menstrual periods. The young women would also have shorter study periods since they were by nature weak and less able to cope with long hours.

A girl cannot spend more than four, or, in occasional instances, five hours of force daily upon her studies, and leave sufficient margin for the general physical growth that she must make. . . . If she puts as much force into her brain education as a boy, the brain or the special apparatus (i.e., the reproductive system) will suffer.[15]

He held up as models some reports on German education, showing that menstrual rest for female students was practiced.[16]

Though there was immediate unfavorable reaction to Clarke's thesis, it still became widely accepted. His critics pointed out, for example, that Clarke had done no scientific study on the matter, that he generalized from a few clinical cases in his own practice, and that his description of periodic rests in European education were totally untrue. One critic commented that "Dr. Clarke has thrown out to a popular audience a hypothesis of his own, which has no place in physiological or medical science. . . . His whole reasoning is singularly unsound."[17] There was some suspicion that Clarke's argument was designed to end speculation at Harvard about admitting female students.[18] Nevertheless, the popularity of his message is indicated by the fact that within thirteen years, *Sex in Education* went through seventeen editions.

Those physicians who followed Clarke tended to exaggerate his position and to ascribe far more harm to the education of women than even he had dared. T.S. Clouston, a physician of Edinburgh, Scotland, wrote a lengthy series for the *Popular Science Monthly* to demonstrate to the public the dangers of the education of females. He pointed out that it was medically accepted that the "female organism is far more delicate than that of men; . . . it is not fitted for the regular grind that the man can keep up." Overstimulation of the female brain causes stunted growth, nervousness, headaches and neuralgias, difficult childbirth, hysteria, inflammation of the brain, and insanity. The female character is likewise altered by education; the educated woman becomes cultured, but "is unsympathetic; learned, but not self denying." Clouston admitted the weak point of his argument, "that it is not founded on any basis of collated statistical facts," based only upon observations of physicians of their own patients. Nonetheless, he expressed the hope that research to gather the facts would be carried on in the future.[19]

This, in fact, began to happen but the results were not what Clouston anticipated. The Massachusetts Labor Bureau made the first report on the health of American college women based upon statistical evidence and not the "haphazard estimate of physicians and college instructors."[20] The results indicated that of 705 college women, 78 percent were in good or excellent health, 5 percent were classed as in fair health, and 17 percent were in poor health. When these women had started college, 20 percent were in poor health. The report concluded that there were no marked differences in health between college women and the national average.[21] John Dewey, in his analysis of the report, decided that worry over personal matters was more harmful to health than overstudy.[22]

In spite of the publicity given the study, there was little change in attitudes among those who believed women and education made a dangerous mixture. In the same year that it appeared, Henry Maudsley wrote in *Sex in Mind and in Education* that the concurrence of puberty and higher education meant that mental development was accomplished at the expense of physical. While acknowledging that there were no facts to provide an answer to the question—what are the effects of coeducation?—he nonetheless answered the question by citing Clarke and declaring that girls educated in the traditional ways were losing "their strength and health." The imperfect development of the reproductive system interfered with the development of the feminine character leaving the educated woman without a sufficiently feminine frame of mind. The education of women must be designed to prepare them for their proper sphere.

It will have to be considered whether women can scorn delights and live laborious days of intellectual exercise and production, without injury to their functions as the conceivers, mothers, and nurses of children. For, it would be an ill thing, if it should so happen that we got the advantage of a quantity of female intellectual work at the price of a puny, enfeebled, and sickly race.[23]

Clarke and most of his imitators subscribed to the Pflüger theory of menstruation, but it was not a necessary preliminary to the belief in the physical disability of women. John Goodman, a Louisville physician, believed that the ovular theory of menstruation was untenable. Instead menstruation was "presided over by a law of monthly periodicity," a "menstrual wave" which affected the entire female being and from whose dictates women could not escape.[24] This theory, although in conflict with that of Pflüger, was appropriated to the cause of those who opposed female education. A good example is George J. Englemann who, in his presidential address before the American Gynecological Society in 1900, expressed the opinion that female schools should heed the "instability and susceptibility of the girl during the functional waves which permeate her entire being," and provide rest during the menstrual periods. At the same time he said that menstruation was controlled by "physical conditions and nerve influences," and that the first menses were accelerated by mental stimulation. His observations contradicted those of Clarke, since while Clarke found educated women ceasing menstruation, Englemann found that mental work increased the frequency of menstrual flow.[25] Nevertheless he would agree with Clarke that women could not endure the rigors of higher education.

J.H. Kellogg, whose *Plain Facts for Old and Young* was responsible for inculcating vast numbers of Americans with the idea that masturbation led to insanity, added also to the public misinformation about menstruation. Part of Kellogg's success was due to the fact that he appeared to be so scientific:

There has been a great amount of speculation concerning the cause and nature of the menstrual process. No entirely satisfactory conclusions have been reached, however, except that it is usually accompanied by the maturation and expulsion from the ovary of an ovum, which is termed ovulation. But menstruation may occur without ovulation, and vice versa.[26]

He then stated that the first occurrence of menstruation is a very critical period in the life of a female, that each recurrence renders her specially susceptible to morbid influences and liable to serious derangements, and that she must carefully watch out during these periods.

There is no doubt that many young women have permanently injured their constitutions while at school by excessive mental taxation during the catamenial period, to which they were prompted by ambition to excel, or were compelled by the "cramming" system too generally pursued in our schools, and particularly in young ladies' seminaries.

He added, however, that a moderate amount of study would not be injurious, and he had no doubt that a large share of the injury which has been attributed to overstudy during the catamenia was caused by improper dress, exposure to cold, keeping late hours, and improper diet. Kellogg also wondered about women workers and felt that female workers should be protected during their periods. He felt it was wrong that women in order to keep their situations were required to be on hand daily and allowed no opportunity for rest at the menstrual period.

In many cases, too, they are compelled to remain upon their feet all day behind a counter, or at a work table, even at periods when a recumbent position is actually demanded by nature. There should be less delicacy in relation to this subject on the part of young women, and more consideration on the part of employers.[27]

As the movement for female emancipation grew, the physicians who discussed the frailties of the female did so with increasing emotional fervor. The president of the Oregon State Medical Society, F.W. Van Dyke, in 1905, claimed that hard study killed sexual desire in women, took away their beauty, and brought on hysteria, neurasthenia, dyspepsia, astigmatism, and dysmenorrhea. Educated women, he added, could not bear children with ease because study arrested the development of the pelvis at the same time it increased the size of the child's brain, and therefore its head. The result was extensive suffering in childbirth by educated women. Van Dyke concluded by declaring that the women who were remembered in history were faithful wives and good mothers such as Penelope, Cornelia, St. Elizabeth; and these would still be remembered when "the name of the last graduate of the woman's college shall have faded from the recollection of men forever."[28]

Dr. Ralph W. Parsons in the *New York Medical Journal* in 1907 cited many of the above authorities to show that the results of higher education for women could lead only to ill health. He claimed college women suffered from digestive disorders as well as nervous and mental diseases.

The nervous system has been developed at the expense of other bodily organs and structures. The delicate organism and sensitive and highly developed nervous system of our girls was never intended by the Creator to undergo the stress and strain of the modern system of higher education, and the baneful results are becoming more and more apparent as the years go by.[29]

He offered as proof the fact that in 1902, 42 percent of the women admitted to New York insane asylums were well educated, while only 16 percent of the men admitted had gone beyond grade school He concluded that women "who have undergone the strain of the modern system of education, are much more liable to become victims of insanity than men of the same class."

One of the mental diseases to which college women were prone was the modification of feminine traits of mind. These women developed distaste for the duties of home life, were egotistical, assumed independence of speech and manner, and were not attentive to the advice of their parents. Educated women neglected to cultivate refined speech, had loud voices, laughed with gusto, and sometimes even used slang and profanity. "They do not exhibit," said Dr. Parsons, "the modesty of demeanor which we have been taught to believe is one of the most admirable traits of the feminine character." Colleges encouraged unwomanly behavior. At one school girls publicly appeared on stage in knee breeches, and in the performance used such words as "devilish" and "damned." Such women as these would never be able to fulfill their female functions, for not only was their reproductive apparatus stunted by education, but no man would ever love them. This was because men had deep sentiment for women with "feminine traits of character with which God intended they should be endowed."

Parson's solution went far beyond anything proposed in the nineteenth century by medical men. Girls, he decided, should not learn Latin, Greek, civics, political economy, or higher math, for these subjects could be of no use to them in their proper sphere. They should have shorter school hours than boys, and spend most of their time in home economics classes.[30]

All of these twentieth-century physicians had available to them a careful study on the health of college and noncollege women, printed in the *Publications* of the American Statistical Association, 1900–1901. This study, carried out during the 1890's, compared college women, not to the "average" woman of the census, as past projects had done, but to a control group of noncollege women composed of their own relatives and friends of their own social class. The study found that though college women married two years later than noncollege women there was a growing tendency to marry later among both groups. Noncollege women had "a slightly larger number of children," but college women had more children per years of married life. There were no differences in problems of pregnancy and mortality of children. The health of the children was roughly equal; although among college-educated mothers the researchers felt they detected slightly fewer delicate children and slightly more robust children. The study found no significant difference between the health of the two groups of women before or after college age. Seventy-five percent of the college women had been employed before marriage, while only 34 percent of the noncollege women had had outside employment. The college women chose different kinds of husbands than the control group. Seventy-five percent of them married college men, while their noneducated cousins married a college-educated husband in only half the cases. Sixty-five percent of college women married professional men, while only 37 percent of the noncollege women had husbands in the professions.[31]

The physicians who persisted in accepting the theories of Clarke et al. simply ignored such studies. G. Stanley Hall who, though one of the outstanding psychologists of the early twentieth century, strongly believed that woman's place was in the home, simply dismissed the statistical studies as inaccurate. Instead, he felt, physicians who treated overeducated women were more likely to see the true circumstances. Inevitably Hall's classic *Adolescence* repeated all the fears and superstitions concerning female education. For example, he connected menstruation to mental exercise. As proof he offered the fact that American girls had their first menses at an average of 14 years of age, while European girls were, on the average, 15.5 years of age before menstruation started. This precocity of American girls was "due chiefly to mentality and nerve stimulation," in other words, education. "Education," theorized Hall, "in a temperate or subartic zone is more productive of precocity than in the south, and if general nervous stimulus is the cause, the same schooling is more dangerous in the city than in the country."[32] Hall was heavily influenced by Clarke's concept of rest during the menstrual periods, and suggested that the female, rather than observing the weekly Sabbath, should have rest periods of four successive days per month. These days would be devoted to leisure and religion, since during menstruation the female was inclined "to a natural piety and sense of dependence" which accounted for the fact that women were more religious than men.[33] Women were by nature intuitive, Hall claimed, not mental. By being "bookish" woman lapsed into male manners and fashions, declined from "her orbit," and obscured her "original divinity."[34]

He believed with Goodman that the ruling factor of female life was periodicity. For most of her life a woman had no alternative but to give way to its dictates, and for this reason special schools should be established for girls. Under no circumstances should coeducation exist, for putting adolescents in the intimacy of the classroom destroyed "the bloom and delicacy" of the girls. Female schools should be in the country, with plenty of places for exercise and privacy. All students should observe the "monthly Sabbath" during their menstrual periods, during which time

the paradise of stated rest should be revisited, idleness be actively cultivated; reverie, in which the soul, which needs these seasons of withdrawal for its own development, expatiates over the whole life of the race, should be provided for and encouraged in every legitimate way, for in rest the whole momentum of heredity is felt in ways most favorable to full and complete development. Then woman should realize that *to be* is greater than *to do*; should step reverently aside from her daily routine and let Lord Nature work.[35]

Such opinions as this were unlikely, in 1905, to go unchallenged by the feminists. Martha Carey Thomas, president of Bryn Mawr College, attacked this lyrical report on periodicity as "sickening sentimentality" and "pseudo-scientific." She held that the seventh and seventeenth chapters of Hall's work were more degrading to womanhood than anything written since Michelet's *La Femme*. She recalled her student days, when she was "terror-struck lest I, and every other woman with me, were doomed to live as pathological invalids in a universe merciless to woman as a sex." Now "we know" that it is not "we," but the "man who believes such things about us, who is himself pathological, blinded by neurotic mists of sex, unable to see that women form one-half of the kindly race of normal, healthy human creatures in the world."[36]

Serious research also questioned the point of view Hall represented. One such study hypothesized that if the menstrual cycle had such influence on women, it ought to show up on tests comparing motor and mental abilities of both men and women. When the results were analyzed it was found that none of the efficiency curves correlated with the menstrual cycles and that the males in the tests had varying efficiencies similar to the females rather than being stable and unvarying as had been thought. In fact, the curves produced by the two sexes were indistinguishable when the notations of the menstrual periods were removed. How, asked the researcher Leta Stetter Hollingworth, was such a striking disparity from what had been the accepted scientific position to be accounted for. Two possible explanations were offered. First the scientific and medically accepted facts were not facts at all but traditions carried on by mystic and romantic writers that "woman is a mysterious being, half hysteric, half angel," and this attitude had somehow found its way into the scientific writing. Scientists seeking to justify this had "seized" upon the menstrual cycle as the probable source of the alleged "mystery" and "caprice of womankind." Once formulated, then, the dogma became cited as authority from author to author until the present day. A second possible explanation of the error was that physicians had not based their conclusions upon accurate evidence. She postulated that normal women did not come under the care and observations of physicians but rather only those with mental and physical diseases. Physicians generalized from these patients, and determined that women were chronically ill. Moreover, once these observations were accepted, experiments to disprove them were difficult since, until the end of the nineteenth century, all investigators were men and the taboo upon mention of the menstrual function made such research next to impossible.[37]

In actuality the explanation is probably far more complex than this. It is quite possible that physicians were simply blind to what was gong on and were so prejudiced than they refused to see reality. There is also the possibility that during the nineteenth century young women did have more than their share of menstrual difficulties. One source of such problems was undoubtedly diet. It was generally believed a century ago that certain foods, especially highly flavored dishes and meats, aroused the sexual appetites. It was, accordingly, desirable to regulate the diets of young girls so as to protect them from unhealthy desires, and physicians found that protein deprivation was a successful cure for female masturbation.[38] Female boarding schools, to minimize sexual interest among their charges, were likely to follow such a prescribed vegetable diet. A study of female higher education in the 1890s deplored the low state of boarding school health, due, it was believed, to diet and lack of exercise, as well as the pressures of the curriculum.[39]

Clelia Mosher, whose research into menstruation among college women spanned several generations between 1890 and 1920, found that girls in the earlier period probably did have greater menstrual difficulties than those in the 1920s. She at first concluded that the reason for this was that during the nineteenth century girls were taught that they were going to be sick during menstruation and the result was a self-fulfilling prophecy. She also found, however, that there was a correlation between dress and menstrual difficulties. During the 1890s and the early years of the twentieth century most young women were put into tight corsets, banded clothing, and unsupported heavy skirts. This clothing interfered with the respiration, made the abdominal muscles flabby, restricted physical activity, and deformed the body on the same principle that the binding of feet in China did. The result was, Mosher held, chronic disturbances of the organs and prolonged menstrual flow.[40] She prepared tables correlating menstrual pain among college women with the width and weight of their skirts and the measurements of their waists. Her figures showed that as the skirt grew shorter and skimpier, and the waist larger, the functional health of women improved. In 1894, 19 percent of the college women were free form menstrual difficulties; in 1915–16, 68 percent considered their periods no problem. In the earlier period the average skirt was 13.5 feet around the hem, the average waist measurement was twenty inches, and the woman also wore several petticoats, some fifteen pounds of clothing hanging from a constricted waist. By the beginning of

World War I women wore their skirts above the ankle, skirts were narrowed, petticoats fewer, and waist measurements had increased by 40 percent.[41]

Such studies did much to ease the traumas inflicted by some of the male medical writers of the last part of the nineteenth century. Increasing reassurance came from the growing numbers of college-educated and career women who seemed none the worse for their years of hard study or work. While the generation of Martha Thomas had been haunted by the "clanging chains of that gloomy little specter," Dr. Edward H. Clarke's *Sex in Education,* several generations of educated women tended to prove that "college women were not only not invalids, but that they [were] better physically than other women in their own class of life."[42] In part too, the development of the sanitary pad in the aftermath of World War I also freed women from some of the more confining aspects of menstruation. Not all physicians, however, adjusted their thinking to correspond with the latest scientific findings. At the beginning of the twentieth century most sex manuals warned against exciting lives and mental stimulation for pubertal girls.[43] Perhaps this was to be expected but, when the same sort of material was still being published thirty years later, it is possible to wonder what motivated the physicians who wrote it. William J. Robinson's book, for example, in 1931 in its twenty-second edition, still warned that only a minority of women were free from illness during their menstrual periods, and that most should rest at least two days, avoid dancing, cycling, riding, rowing, or any other athletic exercises, and probably postpone travel by auto, train, or carriage.[44]

That some of the medical hesitation to change seems political, a hesitation to accept women as equals, is evident even in the 1970s. After all it was in 1970 that Edgar Berman, previously best known as the friend and physician of Hubert Humphrey, remarked that women could not fill leadership roles because of the influences of their periodicity, that is their menstrual cycles and menopause.[45] This statement cost him his position in the Democratic Party and made not only him but Humphrey an object of attack by the militant members of women's lib. That the belief still has currency is also indicated by the fact that the first issue of the new woman's magazine *Ms.* found it relevant enough to counter with an article on male cycles and gave hints to women on how to discover whether the men in their lives were ebbing or flowing.[46]

This is not the place to argue the existence of male cycles, however, but only to indicate that it is very possible for medical concepts to get mixed up with political and social beliefs. Perhaps this is inevitable since we are human, but it ought to make the physician a little more cautious in distinguishing his biases from his objective findings. In retrospect it does seem that the nineteenth-century physician grew somewhat more shrill in his emphasis on the instability of the female at the very time that women and their male allies were challenging the old stereotypes. A few physicians jumped into the controversy citing their own clinical observations as evidence in ways that today we can regard only as ludicrous. This in fact happened with a whole series of physiological functions and human activities but was particularly harmful when such sexual topics as menstruation, masturbation, or birth control were dealt with. Obviously women are anatomically different from men, and they do have monthly periods, but to generalize from this and a few isolated patients to a whole theory of female inferiority seems to be an example of poor medical theorizing. The difficulty with past medical theory, whether good or bad, however, is that it often remains a part of the popular ideology of a later generation. One of the things that women of today have to overcome is some of the mistaken concepts about menstruation and its effect.[47]

Notes

This paper was presented at the 45th annual meeting of the American Association for the History of Medicine, Montreal, Canada, May 4, 1972. Research sponsored by the Erickson Educational Foundation, Baton Rouge, La.

1   John Power, *Essays on the Female Economy* (London: Burgess and Hill, 1831); G.F. Girdwood, "Theory of menstruation," *Lancet*, 1842–43, i: 825–30; J.Bennet, "On healthy and morbid menstruation," *Lancet*, 1852, i: 35, 65, 215, 328, 353.

2   Aristotle [pseud.], *The Works of Aristotle in Four Parts, containing I. His complete Master-piece; . . . II. His Experienced Midwife; . . . III. His Book of Problems; . . . IV. His Last Legacy . . .* (London: published for the bookseller, 1808), 126.

3   See M.M. Smith, "Menstruation and some of its effects upon the normal mentalization of woman," *Memphis Medical Monthly*, 1896, *16:* 393–99; C. Frederick Fluhmann, *Menstrual Disorders, Diagnosis and Treatment* (Philadelphia: W.B. Saunders, 1939), 17–26.

4   A.F.A. King, "A new basis for uterine pathology," *American Journal of Obstetrics*, 1875–76, *8:* 242–43.

5   E.F.W.Pflüger, *Ueber die Eierstöke der Sügethiere und des Menschen* (Leipzig: Englemann, 1863).

6   Thomas Woody, *A History of Women's Education in the United States,* 2 vols. (New York: The Science Press, 1929), 2: 137.

7   Benjamin Rush, *Essays, Literary, Moral and Philosophical* (Philadelphia: Thomas & Samuel Bradford, 1798), 75–92.

8   Woody, *History of Women's Education,* 2: 231.

9   See Vern Bullough and Bonnie Bullough, *Emergence of Modern Nursing* (New York: Macmillan, 1969), passim.

10   Edward H. Clarke, *Sex in Education; or, A Fair Chance for Girls* (Boston: James R. Osgood & Co., 1873), 37–38.

11.   Ibid., 40–41.

12   Ibid., 63.

13   Ibid., 65–72.

14   Ibid., 133.

15   Ibid., 156–57.

16   Ibid., 162–81.

17   George F. Comfort and Anna Manning Comfort, *Woman's Education and Woman's Health* (Syracuse: Thomas W. Durston & Co., 1874), 154.

18   G. Stanley Hall, *Adolescence, Its Psychology and Its Relations to Physiology, Anthropology, Sociology, Sex, Crime, Religions and Education,* 2 vols. (New York: D. Appleton and Co., 1904), 2: 569.

19   T.S. Clouston, "Female education from a medical point of view," *Popular Science Monthly* 24 (Dec. 1883–Jan. 1884): 322–33.

20   John Dewey, "Health and sex in higher education," *Popular Science Monthly* 28 (March 1886): 606.

21   Annie G. Howes et al. *Health Studies of Women College Graduates: Report of a Special Committee of the Association of Collegiate Alumnae* (Boston: Wright & Potter, 1885),9.

22   Dewey, "Health and sex in higher education," 611.

23   Henry Maudsley, *Sex in Mind and in Education* (Syracuse: C.W.Bardeen, 1884), 14.

24   John Goodman, "The menstrual cycle," *Transactions,* American Gynecological Society, 1877, *2:* 650–62; "The cyclical theory of menstruation," *American Journal of Obstetrics, 1878. 11:* 673–94.

25   George J. Englemann, "The American girl of today: the influence of modern education on functional development," *Transactions,* American Gynecological Society, 1900, *25:* 8–45.

26   J.H. Kellogg, *Plain Facts for Old and Young* (Burlington, Iowa: I.F. Segner, 1882), 83.

27   Ibid., 86.

28   F.W. Van Dyke, "Higher education a cause of physical decay in women," *Medical Records,* 1905, *67:* 296–98.

29   Ralph Wait Parsons, "The American girl *versus* higher education, considered from a medical point of view," *New York Medical Journal,* 1907, *85:* 116.

30   Ibid., 119.

31   Mary Roberts Smith, "Statistics of college and noncollege women," *Publications,* American Statistical Association, 1900–1901, *7, nos. 49–56:* 1–26.

32   Hall, *Adolescence,* 1: 478.

33   Ibid., 1: 511.

34   Ibid., 2: 646.

35   Ibid., 2: 639.

36   M. Carey Thomas, "Present tendencies in women's college and university education," Feb., 1908, in *The Woman Movement: Feminism in the United States and England,* ed., William O'Neill (Chicago: Quadrangle Books, 1969), 168.

37   Leta Stetter Hollingworth, *Functional Periodicity: An Experimental Study of the Mental and Motor Abilities of Women during Menstruation,* Teachers College, Columbia University Contributions to Education, No. 69 (New York: Columbia University Press, 1914), 44, 66, 93, 95.

38   John Tompkins Walton, "Case of nymphomania successfully treated," *American Journal of the Medical Sciences,* 1857, *33:* 47–50.

39   Anna C. Brackett, ed., *Women and the Higher Education* (New York: Harper, 1893), 90.

40   Clelia Duel Mosher, "Normal menstruation and some of the factors modifying it," *Johns Hopkins Hospital Bulletin,* 1901, *12:* 178–79.

41   Clelia Duel Mosher, *Women's Physical Freedom* (New York: The Woman's Press, 1923), 1, 29.

42   Thomas, "Present tendencies in women's college and university education," 169.

43   See, for example, William H. Walling, *Sexology* (Philadelphia: Puritan Publishing co., 1904), 207.

44   William J. Robinson, *Woman: Her Sex and Love Life,* 22d ed. (New York: Eugenics Publishing Col., 1931), 80–81.

45   *New York Times,* July 26, 1970; *Los Angeles Times,* Feb. 21, 1972.

46   Estelle Ramey, "Men's cycles," *Ms.* Spring 1972, 8–15.

47   For a survey of some recent research on the topic see Mary E. Luschen and David M. Pierce, "Menstrual cycle, mood and arousability," *Sex Research* 8 (February 1972): 41–47.

Ω

The Meaning of Menstruation

by Louise Lander

In our search for the hidden treasure that is the meaning of menstruation for modern women, we have so far found some clues in the realm of biology: that cyclicity is a function of life, not of femaleness; that hormonal influences affect both sexes and operate in extremely complex ways, with the causal arrows between hormones and behavior pointing in both directions; and that from an evolutionary perspective the way modern human females experience menstruation is anomalous. If biological science has this to offer, what help can social science provide?

Social Science as Spinning Wheels

The short answer is, not a lot. Social scientists concerning themselves with menstruation have had to expend large amounts of energy discrediting a body of masculinist research that was on its way to entrenching menstrual stereotypes as scientific fact. Having accomplished that task, they have been expending their energies trying to design methodologically sound research that fits the human experience of the menstrual cycle into neat social scientific categories—dependent and independent variables, correlations and tests of statistical significance. Contradictory findings abound, perhaps because the subjects and their lives are more complex than the methodology by which they are being examined. A mass of material yields only a little of interest, that concerning the different ways human beings explain how they feel, depending on the social context of their being asked. But in fairness to the social scientists, we should note that the interesting material from biology has come less from studies of the menstrual cycle itself than from work that incidentally casts light on that phenomenon; when it has looked at menstruation directly, biomedical science has given us the morass we examined in Chapter 5.

Social scientists used to be fascinated with the subject of mood changes as a function of the menstrual cycle, using elaborate questionnaires to ask batteries of women how they felt during the various stages of past menstrual cycles and coming up with findings that served to buttress the concept of a premenstrual syndrome. By now that body of research has been pretty thoroughly discredited: It has been well established that a study that asks women to record their moods day by day produces different results from one asking them to record their moods from memory of the past; that women taking part in a study they know concerns the menstrual cycle will give different answers

from those in a study whose purpose is disguised; that looking at data in terms of group averages frequently presents a different picture from that produced by individual responses; and that negative moods found in the premenstrual stage of the cycle may reflect stresses that are themselves changing the length of the cycle and determining when the premenstrual stage occurs.[1]

Attempts to construct new bodies of social scientific research concerning menstruation have been less successful than attempts to discredit the research of the past. Studies looking for correlations between personality types or socialization categories and the experience of menstruation have given us a wealth of contradictions: High femininity scores on a personality test, for example, have been found to correlate positively, negatively, or not at all with severity of menstrual symptoms, depending on the study. Some studies, in other words, suggest that women identifying with those characteristics traditionally defined as feminine (being nurturant, supportive, and deferential) experience greater menstrual distress than less conventional women, other studies suggest the reverse, and still others find no association between such personality measures and the degree of menstrual discomfort.[2]

Research attempting to correlate cultural attitudes surrounding menstruation with the extent of menstrual distress has been similarly inconclusive.[3] One study, which hoped to correlate stress and traditional socialization with menstrual symptoms and attitudes, found that its strongest correlation reflected what might be called the reality effect: Women with the most severe menstrual symptoms had the most negative attitude toward menstruation. "Thus," concludes the researcher, "it appears that menstrual attitudes are not merely a product of socialization but also a function of women's experiences with symptoms that disrupt their lives."[4] Apparently it surprises social scientists to find that women are in touch with reality, that menstrual experience is more than a web of outdated taboo.

Menstruation as Label

But just as menstrual pain is real, so other—perhaps more subtle but no less real—feelings may or may not be labelled menstrual by the women experiencing them. A study comparing women taking oral contraceptives with women not taking them, for example, inquired about conditions such as headache, backache, irritability, abdominal and breast swelling, cramps, depression, and happiness, and asked the subjects to what they attributed these various conditions—tension, illness, the menstrual cycle, a good or bad day, something else, or unknown. It turned out that during the premenstrual phase of the cycle, women on the pill were more likely to connect their state of being to their menstrual cycle than women not on the pill. This finding logically reflects the fact that the contraceptive pill creates an artificial menstrual cycle in which menstruation is totally predictable, unlike the usual situation for women whose cyclicity is not under artificial control; thus the explanation of being premenstrual is more readily available to women on the pill as a way to make sense of how they feel.[5]

This analysis, called attribution or cognitive labelling theory, harks back to the research described in the chapter on hormones in which subjects were injected with adrenalin thinking it was a vitamin supplement, sometimes told and sometimes not told that they might experience certain physical effects, and then put in a room with a stooge who acted either euphoric or angry. The subjects who had access to a physiological explanation for the way they felt experienced less anger or euphoria than those who were uninformed.[6] Other research has found that negative behavior described as occurring during a woman's premenstrual period is likely to be attributed to the menstrual cycle but that positive behavior is more likely to be attributed to factors in the woman's personality or situation.[7]

There are a number of states and actions, in other words, that are sufficiently ambiguous that they might or might not be a function of menstrual cyclicity; whether or not they are put in that category has something to do with the availability of cyclicity as an explanation and something to do with the positive or negative nature of what needs to be explained— biology, especially menstrual biology, being seen as a negative element in a woman's life, and the concept of premenstrual syndrome being a conveniently available label to attach to any negativity that occurs during the premenstrual phase.[8]

To say that attribution theory is about all the social sciences have to offer us is to say as much about the complexity of human beings as about the deficiencies of researchers. Human beings stubbornly refuse to keep their variables well separated—the premenstrual phase, for example, which social scientists would like to assume "causes" certain states, may itself be determined by certain states, as when the stress of, say, final exams accelerates the start of one's period. In that case, a state is causing the premenstrual phase, rather than the reverse.[9] Or negative premenstrual feelings may be a realistic reflection of painful experiences of menstruation in the past rather than a psychological expression of a hormonal state in the present.[10]

Menstruation as Synchrony

One of the most fascinating findings of menstrual cycle research—some of it conducted by psychologists, some by biologists—is located precisely on the border between biology and culture. This is the phenomenon known as menstrual synchrony, an old wives' tale become scientifically established fact. Three studies of college women have found that close association between women over a number of months leads to a significant coming closer together of the dates their periods start. Two studies found this convergence operating among roommates and among pairs of women who identified each other as closest friends; the third study used a population of women living in single rooms and thus dealt only with closest friends.

The first menstrual synchrony study, conducted in the early seventies at a women's college, also looked at the correlation between contact with men and the length of the menstrual cycle. Comparing women who spent time with men at least three times a week with those whose association with men was less frequent, the women who interacted infrequently with the opposite sex had significantly longer menstrual cycles. The other two studies were unable to duplicate this finding, but they were carried out at coeducational institutions and thus could not replicate the extent of the separation of the sexes; they distinguished their subjects in terms of frequency of social contact with men, but all of the subjects were seeing men as fellow students every day.[11]

The phenomenon of menstrual synchrony is a perfect example of the convergence of the biological and the social, a social situation shaping a biological process. As we saw was often the case with hormones, this phenomenon is the opposite of the conventional assumption that female biology affects conduct; here conduct—being in close association with another woman—is affecting biology—the endocrine events that determine the timing of the menstrual cycle.

What causes menstrual synchrony? No one knows, but some speculate about the possibility of substances known as pheromones. These are a class of chemicals used by many species to effect communication between members of the species, one individual releasing the substance into the environment and another receiving it and reacting to it. It is not clear whether human pheromones exist, but one intriguing study took underarm perspiration from one woman and applied it to the upper lip of several other women; a control group received plain alcohol instead of sweat. After four months, the women in the experimental group but not in the control group showed a significant shift in the timing of their menstrual cycle toward that of the donor of the perspiration.[12]

Menstrual synchrony is not the only example of social situations affecting menstruation, although it is the most elegantly established. Wartime has provided an unwanted laboratory for studying the effects of extreme situations, and wartime catastrophes including air raids, internment, and the threat of extermination have been seen to bring about the cessation of menstruation in women with previously normal cycles. Among women in concentration camps, the frequency of amenorrhea has seemed to vary with the harshness of conditions and the danger of death, although there is some evidence that malnutrition also played a part. Peacetime studies have found a connection between food intake and menstruation, with the menses stopping among women who are malnourished and among obese women who lose substantial amounts of weight.[13]

Less drastic life changes, such as going away to a new environment—a convent, the armed forces, or a residential school—have also been found to trigger amenorrhea in a substantial percentage of women.[14] Anxiety about exams can have the same effect.[15] In social-scientific terms, menstruation turns out not to be an independent variable; in real-life terms, menstruation is an integral part of what it means to live as a human being, a creature of culture as much as biology, the two merging and mutually interacting so that the distinction becomes meaningless.

Menstruation as Pain

But then there is the problem of pain—and it exists across cultures, an apparently irreducible biological core of menstrual negativity. A study conducted by the World Health Organization in the early eighties surveyed women in ten countries in various stages of development (Egypt, England, India, Indonesia, Jamaica, Korea, Mexico, Pakistan, the Philippines, and Yugoslavia) and found that women all over the world, rural and urban, of low and high social status, experienced physical discomfort in connection with menstruation, with frequencies ranging from 50 to 70 percent. Younger women tended to experience discomfort during their periods; older women, before bleeding began. Women using an IUD were more likely to complain of discomfort that women using no contraception or using some other method—suggesting that a total escape from the cultural into the biological is impossible after all. The most commonly reported symptoms were back pain and abdominal pain.

The reported experience of mood changes in connection with menstruation was much more varied than was the case with physical discomfort—ranging from 23 percent among the Sudanese in Indonesia (surveyed separately from the Javanese) to 71 percent in England (home of the doyenne of PMS, Katharina Dalton) and 73 percent among the Moslems in Yugoslavia (surveyed separately from non-Moslems). The Indonesian Sudanese reported both the lowest incidence of mood changes (23 percent) and the highest incidence of physical discomfort (71 percent); this intriguing pattern provides another suggestion that total escape from the cultural is impossible, for it might mean that this is a culture in which somatic symptoms are more socially acceptable than changes in mood.[16]

The general response to menstrual discomfort, it might be noted, is apparently stoicism—most women reported doing nothing by way of treatment (the minority who took analgesic drugs tended to be urban, better-educated women), and, outside of India, menstruating women made little change in their daily routine, inside or outside the home. (In India the concept of menstrual pollution leads most women to avoid many household tasks during menstruation.)[17]

Pain as Culture

But even to the extent that there is an irreducible, crosscultural core of menstrual pain, looking like a purely biological phenomenon—ignoring for the moment the cultural elements that crept into the WHO data—pain itself turns out to be a cultural phenomenon, its extent and meaning shaped by the surrounding circumstances. Perhaps the most clear-cut demonstration of pain as culture is a classic study, conducted in the forties and fifties, comparing the experience of pain of soldiers wounded in battle and male patients coming out of surgery. Both groups were asked whether they were in pain and, if so, were asked to rate their pain as slight, moderate, or severe; those experiencing pain were also asked if they would like something to relieve it. Both groups had suffered wounds, battle wounds or surgical wounds, in the areas of the chest and abdomen or in the bones.

Although the damage to tissue inflicted on the soldiers by high explosive shell fragments was far greater than the damage inflicted on the surgical patients by their surgery, the experience of pain was far greater for the patients than for the soldiers: 83 percent of the patients, but only 32 percent of the soldiers asked for something to relieve their pain; 14 percent of the soldiers, but only 4 percent of the patients claimed not to be in pain at all.[18]

What was clearly more important than traumatized nerve endings to the experience of pain was the meaning of what was happening at the source of the pain. For the soldiers, being wounded was a blessing; having been in constant danger of imminent death, to be wounded and still alive was an immense relief, heightened by the awareness that their wounds had taken them away from the battlefield for good. For the surgical patients, having surgery was a disaster, upsetting the order of their lives, instilling a fear of death or disability— in general, a source of enormous anxiety. Thus the positivity or negativity of what was underlying the tissue trauma shaped the extent to which that physiological condition was experienced as pain.

For menstruating women, the experience of menstruation is negative or at best ambivalent—just as the experience of being female has reason to be negative or at best ambivalent. An irregularly contracting uterus—or whatever physiological process may be generating a pain stimulus—has no favorable context, no positive meaning to alleviate its effect. Far from being a route off the battlefield, menstruation is another sector of the battlefield—a symbol, in a masculinist culture, of a woman's inferior position.

The Negativity of Female Physicality

Menstruation also reminds a woman of her body, and women generally live in their bodies in a state of uneasy alliance at best. There is some evidence that athletes suffer less menstrual discomfort than sedentary women,[19] which may have something to do with lower levels of prostaglandins or higher tolerances for pain, but may also have something to do with athletes being on better terms with their physicality. To a person who is physically fit, her body is both more important and less important than to the sedentary— more important in the sense that its being in peak condition is something she values, less important in that her attitude toward her body is more detached, more that of an outside observer. She simultaneously lives in her body more comfortably and can step outside her body and analyze its condition, good or bad, more matter-of-factly.

The estrangement that most women feel from their bodies was nicely demonstrated by a study in which women and men were shown nine line drawings of women and men ranging from extremely thin to extremely heavy and asked to note which represented themselves, which the body they would like to have, which the body they thought was most attractive to the opposite sex, and which drawing of the opposite sex was most attractive to them. Women consistently rated their own bodies as heavier than what they would like to be and what they thought was attractive to men, whereas for men the three ratings were almost identical. (What women rated as the ideal male body was lighter than the male ratings, but what men rated as the most attractive female body was heavier than what women rated as ideal and what they thought was attractive to men.) Another statistical tidbit suggesting women's estrangement from their bodies is the fact that about 90 percent of cases of anorexia and bulimia are women.[20]

Studies comparing high school and college women athletes with nonathletes, on the other hand, have found that the athletes have a much more positive image of their bodies than the nonathletes; one such study also found the athletes expressing much more satisfaction with life in general than the nonathletes.[21]

None of this is to promote jogging or yoga as a sure-fire cure for menstrual cramps or premenstrual bloating, only to suggest that the experience of menstrual discomfort may frequently be part of a package that includes estrangement from our physicality and that learning to inhabit our bodies more comfortably, a lesson that athletics can teach, might make the experience of menstruation less problematic. Attaining a state of physical fitness can demonstrate that there is more to the female body than the capacity to grow babies, can impart a sense of strength and self-assurance that, among other benefits, can make coping with physical inconveniences a more matter-of-fact proposition.

Biomedicine versus Holism

Still, we are faced with the lesson—and the problem— of the previous chapter that regular menstrual cyclicity, month in and month out for years at a time, is a condition that the human female body has not had time to adapt to on an evolutionary time scale, and that menstrual discomforts of various kinds may be the price we pay for that disjunction between human evolution and human culture. Just as high blood pressure, for example, is a disease of civilization, reflecting the damage wrought by the fight-or-flight response as evolutionary anomaly, so menstrual distress might be called a discomfort of civilization. But just as one can take a high-tech route or a holistic route to coping with one's hypertension, taking medication or doing meditation, so one can make similar choices about coping with menstrual distress.

A few studies by psychologists, for example, starting from the premise that menstrual cramps have something to do with painful contractions of the uterine muscle, have explored the possibility that learning to relax one's musculature can alleviate menstrual pain. In one study, subjects were trained to achieve a state of deep muscle relaxation and at the same time to imagine scenes relating to menstruation, in all of which they remained calm and comfortable while thinking of all that they had to do during their period, just as it was beginning. The participants were instructed to carry out this procedure on their own at least twice a day. Two months after the training, symptoms that subjects had reported feeling often on a before-and-after questionnaire were being experienced only rarely.[22]

Another study used a different relaxation technique combined with biofeedback measuring the temperature of the vagina; this because muscle relaxation is accompanied by dilation of blood vessels and a rise in temperature (and there is a common artery supplying the uterus and the vaginal wall) and the researcher hypothesized that temperature biofeedback would reinforce the relaxation training. After eight weekly training sessions, with instructions to do the relaxation exercises daily on their own, subjects' scores on an index designed to measure dysmenorrhea went down by more than two-thirds.[23]

As we saw in Chapter 5, one can also take antiprostaglandin pills for cramps. The difference, of course, is that pills merely reinforce our typical alienation from our physicality—our body becomes something to chemically zap when it misbehaves—whereas an approach like visualization or deep muscle relaxation promotes the integration of psyche and soma, the mind coaxing the muscles to relax, the pleasurable feeling of relaxed muscles then alleviating the anxiety in the mind that was caused by the pain and was also intensifying the pain, the lessened anxiety then making it easier for the muscles to relax further, which further alleviates the anxiety, and so on. All of which is not to provide a primer on the holistic treatment of menstrual distress, only to note that anomalous human states, whether hypertension or dysmenorrhea, can be coped with in ways that reflect humankind's technological alienation from itself or in ways that reflect humankind's complex integration of soma and psyche, biology and culture.

Menstruation as Culture

The problem of culture outpacing evolution and the physiological quirks that accompany that phenomenon is a problem of the human species, not a problem unique to women. What is uniquely a problem of women is being put down for our biology—or, more precisely, being put down for other reasons and our biology then being called upon as a convenient justification of the putdown. Men's problems with their prostate glands or their greater susceptibility to heart attacks have never been thought reason to disbar them from full participation in social and political life. President Jefferson suffered from migraines; President Kennedy had Addison's disease, which is a serious hormonal disorder, and a bad back.[24] When people are valued, their physiological problems are taken in stride. If women were valued, their menstrual aches and pains would be inconsequential—-and the fact of being valued would itself have the effect of reducing those aches and pains.

Modern women's constant menstrual cyclicity is a result of, is symbolic of, our escape from compulsory motherhood. When that escape becomes threatening—when the alternative to compulsory motherhood is female encroachment on formerly male domains—it becomes useful to call menstrual cyclicity a disability. Then women are disabled from full participation in social and political life either because they are having babies or because they are not having babies.

But if regular menstruation is a concomitant of our escape from compulsory motherhood, it does not define modern women any more than a high rate of heart disease defines modern men. It does illustrate that modern human societies, like earlier ones, are places where biology and culture are inseparable—where menstruation is both a biological event whose nature is profoundly shaped by cultural forces and a biological event that is frequently used as a political weapon by cultural forces.

Thus menstruation per se has no meaning, for menstruation per se does not exist. The physical flow that comes monthly—the evolutionary anomaly—only exists as one aspect of what it means to be a woman at the turn of the twenty-first century. As that meaning changes, the meaning of menstruation will change—will become more negative, more positive, more ambivalent, or perhaps free of emotional baggage altogether. Ultimately, the question of menstruation is not a problem to be solved, it is an issue that needs to become a nonissue, like the question of how many angels can dance on the head of a pin; for it would and will become a nonissue if and when women are fully accepted as full-fledged human beings.

Ω

♀

The Selling of Premenstrual Syndrome
Who Profits from Making PMS "The Disease of the 80s"?
by Andrea Eagan

In the summer of 1961, I was working as a laboratory assistant at a major pharmaceutical firm. Seminars were regularly given on recent scientific developments, and that summer, one of them, on the oral contraceptive, was given by an associate of Dr. Gregory Pincus, who was instrumental in the development of the Pill. As a rule, only the scientists went to the seminars. But for this one, every woman in the place—receptionists and bottle washers, technicians and cleaners—showed up. Oral contraception sounded like a miracle, a dream come true.

During the discussion, someone asked whether the drug was safe. Yes, we were assured, it was perfectly safe. It had been thoroughly tested in Puerto Rico, and besides, you were only adjusting the proportions of naturally occurring substances in the body, putting in a little estrogen and progesterone to fool the body into thinking that it was "just a little bit pregnant." The Food and Drug Administration had approved the sale of the birth-control pill in

the United States the year before. News of it was everywhere. Women flocked to their doctors to get it. The dream, we now know, was much too good to be true. But we learned that only after years of using the Pill, after we had already become a generation of guinea pigs.

Since then, and because of similar experiences with DES and with estrogen replacement therapy (ERT), because of the work of the women's health movement and of health activists like Barbara Seaman, we have presumably learned something: we have become cautious about medical miracles and scientific breakthroughs. To suddenly discover, then, that thousands of women are rushing to get an untested drug to cure a suspected but entirely unproved hormone deficiency which manifests itself as a condition with a startling variety of symptoms—known by the catch-all name premenstrual syndrome (PMS)—is a little shocking.

Often when a drug suddenly makes the news, or when a new "disease" for which there is a patented cure is discovered, it is fairly easy to find the public relations work of the drug manufacturers behind the story. As just one example, estrogen replacement therapy for the symptoms of menopause had been around since the 1940s. But in 1966, a Brooklyn physician by the name of Robert Wilson wrote a book called *Feminine Forever,* which extolled the benefits of ERT in preventing what the author called "living decay." Wilson went on TV and radio, was interviewed for scores of articles. He claimed that *lifelong* ERT, starting well before menopause, would prevent or cure more than 20 different conditions, ranging from backaches to insomnia and irritability. Wilson ran an operation called the Wilson Research Foundation that put out information to the media and received grants from drug companies. Among those contributing to the Wilson Foundation was Ayerst Laboratories, the largest manufacturer of the estrogen used in the treatment of menopause symptoms. Ayerst also funded a group called the Information Center on the Mature Woman, from which regular information bulletins were sent to the media.

Many doctors had misgivings about ERT (the link between estrogen and cancer had been reported since the 1930s), but the information that the public received about ERT was almost entirely positive. One of the few warnings against ERT appeared in *Ms.* in December, 1972. Three years later, in 1975, a study was published in the *New England Journal of Medicine* reporting that estrogen users had a five to 14 times greater incidence of uterine cancer than did nonusers. This *was* news, and it made the papers. (The *New England Journal,* like several other prestigious medical journals, sends out advance issues to some news services, which is why the networks all have the same story on the same day.)

Women, needless to say, were concerned about ERT. Many simply stopped taking the drug, and sales of Premarin (the brand name of Ayerst's ERT preparation, which accounted for 80 percent of the market) dropped.

Soon after this, Ayerst received a memo on media strategy from Hill & Knowlton, its public relations firm. This memo, the sort that is supposed to be absolutely confidential, became public when someone sent a copy to the New York women's newspaper, *Majority Report. MR* published the entire memo under the headline, "New Discovery: Public Relations Cures Cancer." The first part of the plan was to take the spotlight off estrogen and refocus it on menopause. The "estrogen message," said the memo, "can be effectively conveyed by discreet references to 'products that your doctor may prescribe.'" Articles on menopause were to be placed in major women's magazines. Information was also to be fed to syndicated women's page columnists, general magazines and prominent science writers and editors.

The second part of Hill & Knowlton's plan was to counter anticipated negative publicity. A list of potentially damaging events—research reports (one was expected from the Mayo Clinic), FDA announcements, lawsuits—was given. News releases were to be prepared *in advance* of the "damaging commentary . . . in as much detail as possible." When this memo became public (Jack Anderson picked it up after *MR*'s publication), Ayerst denied any

intention of following its recommendations, but the memo actually outlines the kinds of steps some drug manufacturers take to bring their products to the attention of the public and to counteract criticism.

The same story, with only minor changes, can be told for a number of other drugs, so when I began seeing articles about PMS and progesterone treatment, I immediately had some questions. Why was PMS suddenly "news"? What do we really know about progesterone? And who are the advocates of this treatment?

PMS stories began appearing rather suddenly about two years ago, after two Englishwomen claimed PMS as a mitigating factor in their defense against murder charges. When the stories about these cases appeared, many American women who suffer from cyclical problems naturally became interested in finding out all they could about the condition.

PMS itself is not news. It was first mentioned in the medical literature in the 1930s, and women presumably had it before then. Estimates on the numbers of women affected by PMS vary wildly. Some claim that as many as 80 percent are affected while others place estimates at only 20 percent. Similarly, doctors' opinions vary on the number and type of symptoms that may indicate PMS. They cite from 20 up to 150 physical and psychological symptoms, ranging from bloating to rage. The key to recognizing PMS and differentiating it from anything else that might cause some or all of a woman's symptoms is timing. The symptoms appear at some point after ovulation (around mid-cycle) and disappear at the beginning of the menstrual period. (It should not be confused with dysmenorrhea or menstrual discomfort, about which much is known, and for which several effective, safe treatments have been developed.)

While PMS is now generally acknowledged to be a physical, as well as a psychological disorder, there is little agreement on what causes it or how it should be treated. There are at least half a dozen theories as to its cause—ranging from an alteration in the way that the body uses glucose to excessive estrogen levels—none of which have been convincingly demonstrated.

One of the most vocal proponents of PMS treatment is Katharina Dalton, a British physician who has been treating the condition for more than 30 years. Dalton believes that PMS results from a deficiency of progesterone, a hormone that is normally present at high levels during the second half of the menstrual cycle and during pregnancy. Her treatment, and that of her followers, relies on the administration of progesterone during the premenstrual phase of the cycle.

Progesterone is not absorbed effectively when taken by mouth. Powdered progesterone, derived from yams or soybeans, can be dissolved in oil and given in a deep, painful muscular injection. Or the powder can be absorbed from vaginal or rectal suppositories, a more popular form. (In this country the Upjohn Company is the major manufacturer of progesterone, which they sell only in bulk to pharmacies where pharmacists then package it for sale.

Upjohn makes no recommendation for the use of progesterone and is conducting no tests on the product.)

Although she promotes the progesterone treatment, Dalton has no direct evidence of a hormone deficiency in PMS sufferers. Because progesterone is secreted cyclically in irregular bursts, and testing of blood levels of progesterone is complicated and expensive, studies have been unable to show conclusively that women with PMS symptoms have lower levels of progesterone than other women. Dalton's evidence is indirect: the symptoms of PMS are relieved by the administration of progesterone.

Upon learning about Dalton's diagnosis-and-cure, many women concluded that they had the symptoms she was talking about. But when they asked their doctors for progesterone treatment, they generally got nowhere. Progesterone is not approved by the FDA for treatment of PMS (the only approved uses are for treating cessation of menstrual flow and abnormal uterine bleeding due to hormone imbalance); there is *nothing* in the medical literature showing clearly what causes PMS; and there has never been a well-designed, controlled study here or in England of the effect of progesterone on PMS.

Despite some doctors' reluctance to prescribe progesterone, self-help groups began springing up, and special clinics were established to treat PMS. Women who had any of the reported symptoms (cyclical or not) headed en masse for the clinics or flew thousands of miles to doctors whose willingness to prescribe progesterone had become known through the PMS network. And a few pharmacists began putting up progesterone powder in suppository form and doing a thriving business.

How did PMS suddenly become the rage, or what one New York gynecologist called "the hypoglycemia of the 1980s"? At least part of the publicity can be traced to an enterprising young man named James Hovey. He is reported to have claimed he had a B.A. in public health from UCLA despite the fact that, aside from extension courses, he had been there less than a year. (UCLA does not even have a B.A. program in public health.) He met Katharina Dalton in Holland several years ago at a conference on the biological basis of violent behavior. Returning to the United States, he worked with a Boston physician who opened the first PMS clinic in Lynnfield. A few months later, Hovey left the clinic. He then started The National Center for Premenstrual Syndrome and Menstrual Distress in New York City, Boston, Memphis, and Los Angeles—each with a local doctor as medical director.

For $265 (paid in advance), you got three visits. The initial visit consisted of a physical exam and interview, and a lengthy questionnaire on symptoms. During the second visit, the clinic dispensed advice on diet and vitamins, and reviewed a monthly record the patient was asked to keep. On the third visit, if symptoms still persisted, most patients received a prescription for progesterone.

Last year, James Hovey's wife Donna, a nurse who was working in his New York clinic, told me that they were participating in an FDA-approved study of progesterone, in conjunction with a doctor from the University of Tennessee. In fact, to date the FDA has approved only one study on progesterone treatment of PMS, which is conducted at the National Institute of Child Health and Human Development, an organization unrelated to James Hovey.

Similar contradictions and misrepresentations, as well as Hovey's lack of qualifications to be conducting research or running a medical facility, were exposed by two journalists last year. Marilyn Webb in the *Village Voice* and Jennifer Allen in *New York* magazine both dug into the operation of the clinic and Hovey's past to reveal him as a former Army medical corpsman turned entrepreneur. Hovey left New York and gave up his interest in the New York and Boston clinics. He is currently running a nationwide PMS referral service out of New Hampshire.

In a recent interview, Hovey said that the clinic business is too time-consuming, and that he is getting out. His "only interest is research" he says. He was associated with two scientists who applied to the FDA for permission to do progesterone studies but who were rejected because the FDA considered the doses of progesterone to be too high. At last report, Hovey still headed H and K Pharmaceuticals, a company founded in 1981 for the manufacture of progesterone suppositories, and it is as a supplier that his name has appeared on FDA applications.

Hovey's involvement in PMS treatment seems to have centered on the commercial opportunities. Others, such as Virginia Cassara, became interested in PMS for more personal reasons.

Cassara, a social worker from Wisconsin, went to England in 1979 to be treated by Dalton for severe PMS. The treatment was successful and Cassara returned to spread the good news. She invited Katharina Dalton to Wisconsin to speak and notified the press. Though only one article appeared, it brought women "out of the closet," Cassara says. Cassara began counseling and speaking, selling Dalton's books and other literature. Her national group, PMS Action, now has an annual budget of $650,000, 17 paid staff members, and 40 volunteers. Cassara spends most of her time traveling and speaking.

Cassara's argument is compelling, at least initially. She describes the misery of PMS sufferers, and the variety of ineffective medical treatments they have been subjected to in their search for relief. For anyone who is sensitive to women's health issues, it is a familiar tale: a condition that afflicts perhaps millions of women has never been studied; a treatment that gives relief is ignored. Women, says Cassara, are pushed into diet and exercise regimens that are difficult to maintain and don't always work. One valid solution, she feels, lies in progesterone.

According to FDA spokesperson Roger Eastep, Phase I studies—those that determine how much a particular substance is absorbed by the body and how it works—have yet to be done for progesterone. But in the meantime, more and more doctors are prescribing the hormone for PMS.

Dr. Michelle Harrison, a gynecologist practicing in Cambridge, Massachusetts, and a spokesperson for the National Women's Health Network, is one physician who does prescribe progesterone to some women, with mixed feelings. "I've seen it dramatically temper women's reactions," she says. "For those women whose lives are shattered by PMS, who've made repeated suicide attempts or who are unable to keep a job, you have to do something. But I have a very frightening consent form that they have to sign before I'll give progesterone to them." Harrison also stresses that a lot of PMS is iatrogenic; that is, it is caused by medical treatment. It often appears for the first time after a woman has stopped taking birth-control pills, after tubal ligation or even after a hysterectomy, in which the ovaries have been removed.

When doctors do prescribe progesterone, their ideas of the appropriate dosage can vary from 50 to 2,400 mg. per day. For some women, dosages at the lower end of the scale do not bring relief from their symptoms. It has also been reported by women taking progesterone and in medical literature that the effect of a particular dose diminishes after a few months. Some women are symptom-free as long as they are taking the drug, but the symptoms reappear as soon as they stop, regardless of where they are in the menstrual cycle.

For all these reasons, some women are taking much higher doses than their doctors prescribe. Michelle Harrison had heard of women taking 2,400 mg. per day; Dalton had heard about 3,000; Cassara knows women who take 4,000. Because PMS symptoms tend to occur when progesterone is not being taken, some women take it every day, instead of only during the premenstrual phase. Some bleed all the time; others don't menstruate at all. Vaginal and rectal swelling are common. Animal studies have shown increased rates of breast tumors and cervical cancer. Marilyn Webb, a reporter who began taking progesterone while working on a story about PMS, developed chest pains after several months. She asked all the doctors she interviewed whether any of their patients had experienced chest pains. Every one said that she or he had at least one patient who had.

Reminding her of the history of the Pill, of DES, and of ERT, I asked Virginia Cassara whether she was concerned about the long-term effects of progesterone on women. "I guess I don't think there could be anything worse than serious PMS," she responded. "Even cancer?" I asked. "Absolutely. Even cancer." Later, she said, "I think it's paternalistic of the FDA to make those choices for us, to tell us what we can and cannot put in our bodies. Women with PMS are competent beings, capable of making their own choices."

I don't have severe PMS, and I don't think I fully understand the desperation of women who do and who see help at last within reach. But given our limited understanding of how progesterone works, I do not understand why women like Cassara are echoing drug company complaints of overregulation by the FDA. I'm alarmed to see women flocking to use an untested substance about which there is substantial suspicion, whose mode of action is not known, to treat a condition whose very cause is a mystery. And I fear that, somewhere down the line, we will finally learn all about progesterone treatment and it won't be what we wanted to know.

One doctor, who refused to be quoted by name, cheerfully assured me that progesterone was safe. "Even if a woman is taking 1,600 milligrams per day, the amount of circulating progesterone is still only a quarter of what is normally circulating during pregnancy." And I couldn't help but think of the doctor at the seminar more than 20 years ago: "Of course it's safe. It's just like being a little bit pregnant."

The Vitamin Cure

Diet and vitamin therapies are, according to many doctors, effective in the large majority of PMS cases. Michelle Harrison has found that most of her patients will respond to a hypoglycemia diet: whole grains, no caffeine, lots of water, no sugar, frequent small meals. To this, she adds up to 800 mg. per day of vitamin B6 during the premenstrual phase. Harrison has written a clear and useful 50-page booklet, *Self-Help for Premenstrual Syndrome* ($4.50, plus $1.50 postage and handling, from Matrix Press, Box 740M, Cambridge, Massachusetts 02238), which includes charts for keeping track of symptoms and lots of good advice about diagnosis and treatment, as well as a look at the social and political questions raised by PMS.

Dr. Marcia Storch (author of *How To Relieve Cramps and Other Menstrual Problems*, Workman Publishing, $3.95) and her associate, Dr. Shelley Kolton, believe that reducing salt intake helps to curb water retention and headaches that result from it. They also prescribe 300 to 500 mg. daily of vitamin B6. Kolton says that this therapy is effective in about 80 percent of all cases, though it may take several months for the treatment to work. (Storch and Kolton do not recommend progesterone because of safety concerns.) —*A.E.*

Ω

♀

If Men Could Menstruate— A Political Fantasy

by Gloria Steinem

A white minority of the world has spent centuries conning us into thinking that a white skin makes people superior—even though the only thing it really does is make them more subject to ultraviolet rays and to wrinkles. Male human beings have built whole cultures around the idea that penis-envy is "natural" to women—though having such an unprotected organ might be said to make men vulnerable, and the power to give birth makes womb-envy at least as logical.

In short, the characteristics of the powerful, whatever they may be, are thought to be better than the characteristics of the powerless—and logic has nothing to do with it.

What would happen, for instance, if suddenly, magically, men could menstruate and women could not?

The answer is clear—menstruation would become an enviable, boast-worthy, masculine event:

Men would brag about how long and how much.

Boys would mark the onset of menses, that longed for proof of manhood, with religious ritual and stag parties.

Congress would fund a National Institute of Dysmenorrhea to help stamp out monthly discomforts.

Sanitary supplies would be federally funded and free. (Of course, some men would still pay for the prestige of commercial brands such as John Wayne Tampons, Muhammad Ali's Rope-a-dope Pads, Joe Namath Jock Shields—"For Those Light Bachelor Days," and Robert "Baretta" Blake Maxi-Pads.)

Military men, right-wing politicians, and religious fundamentalists would cite menstruation ("*men*struation") as proof that only men could serve in the Army ("you have to give blood to take blood"), occupy political office ("can women be aggressive without that steadfast cycle governed by the planet Mars?"), be priests and ministers ("how could a woman give her blood for our sins?"), or rabbis ("without the monthly loss of impurities, women remain unclean").

Male radicals, left wing politicians, mystics, however, would insist that women are equal, just different, and that any woman could enter their ranks if only she were willing to self-inflict a major wound every month ("you *must* give blood for the revolution"), recognize the pre-eminence of menstrual issues, or subordinate her selfness to all men in their Cycle of Enlightenment.

Street guys would brag ("I'm a three-pad man") or answer praise from a buddy ("Man, you lookin good!") by giving fives and saying, "Yeah, man, I'm on the rag!"

TV shows would treat the subject at length. ("Happy Days": Richie and Potsie try to convince Fonzie that he is still "The Fonz," though he has missed two periods in a row.) So would newspapers. (SHARK SCARE THREATENS MENSTRUATING MEN. JUDGE CITES MONTHLY STRESS IN PARDONING RAPIST.) And movies. (Newman and Redford in "Blood Brothers"!)

Men would convince women that intercourse was *more* pleasurable at "that time of the month." Lesbians would be said to fear blood and therefore life itself—though probably only because they needed a good menstruating man.

Of course, male intellectuals would offer the most moral and logical arguments. How could a woman master any discipline that demanded a sense of time, space, mathematics, or measurement, for instance, without that in-built gift for measuring the cycles of the moon and planets—and thus for measuring anything at all? In the rarefied fields of philosophy and religion, could women compensate for missing the rhythm of the universe? Or for their lack of symbolic death-and-resurrection every month?

Liberal males in every field would try to be kind: the fact that "these people" have no gift for measuring life or connecting to the universe, the liberals would explain, should be punishment enough.

And how would women be trained to react? One can imagine traditional women agreeing to all these arguments with a staunch and smiling masochism. ("The ERA would force housewives to wound themselves every month": Phyllis Schlafly. "Your husband's blood is as sacred as that of Jesus—and so sexy, too!": Marabel Morgan.) Reformers and Queen Bees would try to imitate men, and *pretend* to have a monthly cycle. All feminists would explain endlessly that men, too, needed to be liberated from the false idea of Martian aggressiveness, just as women needed to escape the bonds of menses-envy. Radical feminists would add that the oppression of the nonmenstrual was the pattern for all other oppressions ("Vampires were our first freedom fighters!") Cultural feminists would develop a bloodless imagery in art and literature. Socialist feminists would insist that only under capitalism would men be able to monopolize menstrual blood....

In fact, if men could menstruate, the power justifications could probably go on forever.

If we let them.

Ω

Menstruation

This worksheet must be optional. Some parts of this worksheet are designed for women who go through reproductive cycles. Women who do not have reproductive cycles and men may or may not want to interview women about the personal questions asked in I and III.

1. Your menstrual cycle

Observe changes your body goes through during a monthly cycle. Here are a few things you may want to note. You may think of others you would find interesting to record (cravings, water retention, etc.). See if you can identify when you are ovulating/have ovulated. If you are on oral contraceptives, how will your observations differ from those of women not on synthetic hormones?

Temperature Record body temperature (by mouth is fine) first thing in the morning before you get up, have anything to drink or smoke. You are more likely to note changes if you have a fairly regular schedule and if you use a very accurate thermometer.

Mucus (secreted by the cervical glands) Observe changes in mucus. Choose your own words to describe what you feel. Words like much, some, scant, clear and watery like egg-whites, and sticky are sometimes useful. Remember that contraceptive gels, creams, and foams and semen in the vagina will mask much of what you might notice about mucus.

Breasts—Fuller, less full, lumpier, tender, "What I think of as 'normal'", and sore may be words useful to describe breast changes.

Date	Temperature	Mucus	Breasts	Other Observations
1				
2				
3				
4				
5				
6				
7				
8				
9				
10				
11				
12				
13				
14				
15				
16				
17				
18				
19				
20				
21				
22				
23				
24				
25				
26				
27				
28				
29				
30				
31				
32				
33				
34				
35				

II. Menstruation Products

Calculate how much you or an "average" woman spends on menstruation products in a lifetime. (These calculations can be based on today's prices.) Check current prices for one or two brands of tampons, napkins, or other "menstrual hygiene product". Estimate how much of this product is used each menstrual period. (A woman with a heavy flow will use many more than a woman with a light flow.) For your calculations you will need to figure how many years a woman will menstruate (age of menopause—age of menarche), and how many times a year a woman menstruates. Show your work. (For a very accurate estimation, you would want to think about how pregnancies, lactation, choice of contraception, and menstrual changes at different ages would influence your calculations, but you do not need to do this for this question.)

III. Premenstrual syndrome

The publicity about premenstrual syndrome (PMS) and advertising for drugs promising a medical-fix for PMS have worked to make women and men regard the days pre-menstrually as "the bad time of the month" for women.

    A. If a few days are regarded as the relatively "bad" days, then other parts of the month must be viewed as relatively "good". Identify "good" things you associate with different parts of your cycle. (These might include such things as times of high energy, times when you require less sleep, times when you most enjoy how your body feels, times when you especially enjoy exercising, times when you find it easy to resist sweet foods.)

    B. Some women identify very positive things about their premenstrual days. For many women this is a time when they are most creative, their dreaming is most vivid, they are the most sexually aroused, they find it easiest to "justify" taking time for themselves, they feel most in touch with things in their life which need changing. Identify positive things you, your friends, or your mother notice about premenstrual days.

7

Aging, Ageism, Mid-life and Older Women's Health Issues

When younger students suggest that the issues of aging are not relevant to their lives, it is very appropriate to point out that we are all, constantly, in the process of aging! Patsy Murphy's "Ageing" article bring this point home by looking at the issues of aging from the vantage point of a 43-year old. The excerpt from "An Open Letter to the Women's Movement" by Barbara Macdonald is necessary since the women's movement must include work on ageism, as well as unlearning racism and other oppressions, if it is to be a movement truly representing all women.

Ageism can have a damaging effect on health in a number of ways and the next two articles specifically look at the intersection of ageism and sexism. Ruth Sidel's "The

Special Plight of Older Women" shows how economic policies in this country are particularly harmful to older women. In "The Need for Intimacy", Jane Porcino emphasizes the emotional deprivation of many older women.

"The Colours of Menopause" looks at the diversity of experience which women have related to this time of transition in their lives, and encourages discussion and research on the cultural vs. physiological influences on menopausal changes.

"The Selling of HRT: Playing on the Fear Factor" summarizes many of the debates which *should* be taking place on the use of hormonal products for mid-life and older women.

Ageing

by Patsy J. Murphy

I cried bitterly when I reached my twenty-third birthday because everyone else in my year in college was nineteen or thereabouts and I felt life passing me by. I dreaded thirty with a passion which in retrospect was idiotic—I had the happiest time of my life between thirty and thirty-five. I walked the beach at Dunquin on my fortieth birthday on a lovely June day and felt terrific, and when asked at forty-three to write on ageing I felt resentful—it's hip to be over forty in New York and ageing is something I wasn't thinking about anyway. Now I've been thinking about it for the last month and what I feel about ageing is GUILT. Lots of Guilt and mostly about the things that I haven't done that I thought I would have—I haven't written a book, made a movie, seen Vienna—I haven't, in short sorted out my life and it's time I did. . . . On the other hand, I've enjoyed myself, reared a daughter (almost), supported us both and today I am starting to sort out my life.

I believe that most of the time ageing isn't so dreadful. A friend of mine told me crisply that ageing is what other people notice about you—you don't monitor its progress. My daughter used to carefully count the lines on my forehead when I was thirty-three and I know they've increased and multiplied, but I remain unaware of it until I pass a shop window and see this Winnie-the-Pooh-shaped middle-aged woman and then I reel in horror at the vision that is me.

But the vision isn't as dreadful as the guilt, which has to do with things I've left undone. At my back I always hear time's winged chariot. I've run a questionnaire amongst some of my contemporaries, who are, as a French woman I know puts it, 'happy in their skin'—that is doing what they want to do and liking themselves. They don't mind ageing. I asked the cleverest woman I know how she felt about it and she said that 99 percent of the time she was totally unconscious of ageing—ageing was no bother But the one per cent was the awful, awful nostalgia about the past. I'll come back to the past later, but 99 per cent is OK. The message for me is to do things that make me like myself and avoid the many, many things that make me hate myself—drinking too much, not making dental appointments. The message is the same for us all, sisters.

I asked a psychologist about guilt—it's normal he says, but it's useless: 'Take it out into the back garden and get rid of it,' he says. So, guilt apart, what does ageing mean? It means the body ain't what it used to be, but what the hell—the mind has more information and the body more experience. Ageing means that situations don't scare you

Reprinted with permission from PERSONALLY SPEAKING, ed. Liz Steiner-Scott, Attic Press, Dublin, Ireland 1985.

as much as they did when you were young. I no longer feel terror when I walk into a room full of people. I no longer dread having to speak in public. I no longer think that someone else is going to sort out my life for me though I often wish that someone would.

For many women ageing brings freedom—a time to do things for themselves, by themselves, things that family responsibilities excluded for years. You don't have to be twenty to be knocked out by Venice, and the southern sun beams as benignly on your back at forty as at eighteen. A good book is still a good book. A glass of wine is still a glass of wine.

I've convinced myself that ageing has its compensations, but I'm still frightened of old age. I'm frightened of all the things that I presume everyone fears, being on my own, having no one to love, no one loving me, not being able to manage, the fear that the whole structure that one calls one's life, which I often feel I have small control over, will collapse around me and that I won't have the health or the energy to put it together again. Old age is not a subject one hears discussed. People on the radio and in books talk to the old, not about being old, but about their past, their part in the revolution, their girlhood, their village long ago. My fear of old age is the fear of death, which I have only experienced as the loss of other people, particularly the dreadful loss of my father. I couldn't bear his death—I hated to think of him in the cold ground. I still cannot face the idea of my own death.

I can face the more immediate horrors, though. I don't believe that the menopause is such a big deal or that it's going to make me feel useless. I imagine it must be quite a relief—no more periods—and it can hardly make me more evil-tempered than I can be now. So what is it that worries me? I'm back where I started. I'm back with my friend talking about the awful nostalgia. I'm there in my past looking at a photograph of us all sitting on a wall in Paris in 1958, skinny, happy, hopeful. . . . Or I'm back in a place of which I can say, like Edna O'Brien's green-eyed girl, 'I was happy here' and I feel my ghost, I see my former self, before motherhood, before mortgages, before security mattered. This is agony, the skewer in the heart and it has to be borne. Yeats felt it, Dylan Thomas, Simone de Beauvoir . . . we all feel it, bear it, hate it. Sometimes I want it back, my lovely lost past. Well, it's gone.

When I was young, I read a lot. I've continued to do so, and I will always do so, and if I'm blind I'll ask someone to read to me because books at any age are a passport to freedom. Once, in a very gloomy period of my existence, I kept sane by reading Simone de Beauvoir's series of autobiographies. I would mechanically get through my horrid day and then, clutching twenty cigarettes, get under the blanket and live a different life, a life that became more real than my own. Unhealthy, you may say, but it got me through a bad time in my life and I imagine that books will have to and will get me through more bad times. I don't have enough life left to read all that remains to be read. Apart from such old pleasures I've found new ones in middle age—gardening, listening to opera. The pleasures of the flesh? To be candid I haven't experienced them for some time but I don't think they have disimproved and I suppose everyone's life has lulls in sensuality.

Last week I saw David Shaw Smith's TV film on the life of Pauline Bewick, an artist whose work is a total celebration of womankind. In a very beautiful film, the thing that touched me most was her triumphant feeling about her future and her work now she's fifty. She looked to her future with such a shout of confidence. I would like to be like that, although I'm not.

Our friends are the most important source of pleasure. I still have the same friends that I had in my twenties, and the friendship of women is something that improves with time, because women share their sorrows, drink over them, laugh over them, grow close over them. I hope when we're old we'll be laughing more than crying.

My friends and I laughed a lot in our twenties, we got up late, looked out the window with a cup of coffee and a fag in hand and surveyed the long carefree day ahead. Then, as it was the sixties, we all got jobs we loved, and had love-lives and money and lots of crack. Then we got pregnant, and the hassles and stratagem and patchwork that are the lot of women who bring up children—especially on their own—followed. But we survived and we still enjoyed ourselves, frazzled, broke and unperceptibly ageing. We survived. What we lost with youth was freedom, the freedom, as one friend says wistfully, just to fling stuff into a rucksack and go. I was never one for rucksacks, but I know how she feels.

So I sit here at the typewriter aged forty-three and how I do feel? I think that I have not done all that I should with my life. There are moments when I feel panic-stricken and desolate: 'What if this or that happens?' 'What if it doesn't?' There are times when I trail home from work clutching the shopping and sink in front of the telly, immersed in *Hill Street Blues,* and scream silently to myself 'Is there a life out there in the world?' And yes, I know there is and I'm going out to tackle it one of these days. Perhaps I'll tackle it today. I'll put the photograph of our hopeful selves sitting on a wall in Paris in 1958 back in the album and I'll go out and confront this grey city and my life ahead.

Questions for Discussion

1. How do you feel about getting old?

2. What are the things that bother you the most about getting old? What are the things that make you feel good about ageing?

3. How does society treat older women? With respect? With indifference? With contempt? Why?

4. What relationship, if any, do younger women have with older women outside their families? Do you think that this is a source of worry for young and old?

5. Imagine yourself when you are old. What will you look like? What will you be doing? Where will you be living? With whom? How do you think you will feel?

6. Why do we try to stay 'looking young' for as long as possible? Why are we so concerned with the signs of ageing: getting grey hair, wrinkles, loose skin, etc.?

7. What effect does the menopause have on women? Do you think it is a cause of depression in women?

8. Do you think that your attitude towards sexuality will change when you're old? How?

9. What place do older women have in the women's movement? What role should they have?

10. If you are taking care of an elderly woman, how do you feel about her? How does she feel about you? Why is there so much guilt and resentment built into these relationships? What can be done about it?

Suggested Reading

Jane Barker and Rosie Graham, 'Change of Life?' *Spare Rib,* No. 51 (London: October 1976) pp. 41–3.

Colette, *Earthly Paradise: An Autobiography drawn from her lifetime writings,* Edited by Robert Phelps, (Harmondsworth: Penguin 1974).

Simone de Beauvoir, *All Said and Done* (Harmondsworth: Penguin 1977). *Old Age* (Harmondsworth: Penguin).

Barbara Macdonald with Cynthia Rich, *Look Me in the Eye: Old Women. Aging and Ageism* (London: The Women's Press 1984).

Adrienne Rich, *Of Woman Born. Motherhood as Experience and Institution* (London: Virago 1977).

Virginia Woolf, *A Room of One's Own* (Harmondsworth: Penguin 1963).

Ω

An Open Letter to the Women's Movement

by Barbara Macdonald

The following suggestions conclude a longer article entitled "An Open Letter to the Women's Movement" which deals with the widespread ageism in the women's community. The book from which this article is taken, *Look Me in the Eye,* is about women and ageing.

The following are a few suggestions to all of us for working on our ageism:

1. Don't expect that older women are there to serve you because you are younger—and *don't think the only alternative is for you to serve us.*

2. Don't continue to say "the women's movement," . . . until all the invisible women are present—all races and cultures, and *all ages* of all races and cultures.

3. Don't believe you are complimenting an old woman by letting her know that you think she is "different from" (more fun, more gutsy, more interesting than) other older women. To accept the compliment, she has to join in your rejection of old women.

4. Don't point out to an old woman how strong she is, how she is more capable in certain situations than you are. Not only is this patronizing, but the implication is that you admire the way she does not show her age, and it follows that you do not admire the ways in which she does, or soon will, show her age.

5. If an old woman talks about arthritis or cataracts, don't think old women are constantly complaining. We are just trying to get a word in edgewise while you talk and write about abortions, contraception, premenstrual syndromes, toxic shock, or turkey basters.

6. Don't feel guilty. You will then avoid us because you are afraid we might become dependent and you know you can't meet our needs. Don't burden us with *your* idea of dependency and *your* idea of obligation.

7. By the year 2000, approximately one out of every four adults will be over 50. The marketplace is ready now to present a new public image of the aging American, just as it developed an image of American youth and the "youth movement" at a time when a larger section of the population was young. Don't trust the glossy images that are about to bombard you in the media. In order to sell products to a burgeoning population of older women, they will tell you that we are all white, comfortably middle class, and able to "pass" if we just use enough creams and hair dyes. Old women are the single poorest minority group in this country. Only ageism makes us feel a need to pass.

8. Don't think that an old woman has always been old. She is in the process of discovering what 70, 80, and 90 mean. As more and more old women talk and write about the reality of this process, in a world that negates us, we will all discover how revolutionary that is.

9. Don't assume that every old woman is not ageist. Don't assume that I'm not.

10. If you have insights you can bring to bear from your racial background or ethnic culture—bring them. We need to pool all of our resources to deal with this issue. But don't talk about your grandmother as the bearer of your culture—don't objectify her. Don't make her a museum piece or a woman whose value is that she has sacrificed and continues to sacrifice on your behalf. Tell us who she is now, a woman in process. Better yet, encourage *her* to tell us. I wish you luck in your beginning. We are all beginning.

Ω

Reprinted with permission from LOOK ME IN THE EYE by Barbara Macdonald and Cynthia Rich, Spinsters/Aunt Lute Book Co., 1983. (Available from P.O. Box 410687, San Francisco, CA 94141).

The Special Plight of Older Women

by Ruth Sidel

The problems of old age in America are largely the problems of women.[1]

—*Robert N. Butler, M.D.*
Former Director
National Institute on Aging

They sit on park benches in the Bronx warming themselves in the midday sun. They walk slowly, almost apologetically, through the supermarket, choosing an apple or two and day-old bread, counting out the nickels, dimes, and pennies to pay an impatient cashier. They are lined up in wheelchairs when the television cameras visit their nursing home for the annual Christmas party. They are the fastest growing segment of the U.S. population—women over sixty-five—and nearly one out of every five lives in poverty.[2]

According to the 1980 census more than 25 million Americans, 11.3 percent of the total population, are age sixty-five and over.[3] Because of the shorter lifespan of men, women significantly out-number men in this age group; there are only sixty-eight males for every hundred females. By the year 2000, according to current projections, this ratio will be further reduced to sixty-five men for every hundred women.[4] Moreover, the number of elderly people aged seventy-five and older, often termed the "old-old," is growing rapidly. This group now comprises 38 percent of the elderly population and is expected to grow to 45 percent by the year 2000. It is estimated that two-thirds of those seventy-five and over will be women.[5] By the year 2050, according to Robert Butler, a sixty-five year-old woman can expect to live to age 85.7.[6]

The "graying of America" is no empty slogan. It is a description of our future. The census projections have enormous implications for our society—for health care, for social services, for housing, for recreation, for our productive capacity—but that is only part of the picture. The other part is that a large percentage of this rapidly growing group of older people can expect to live in poverty—many in abject poverty, many more in near poverty.

Elderly women today have a far higher rate of poverty than do elderly men. In 1984, according to the Census Bureau, 8.7 percent of men and 15.0 percent of all women age sixty-five and over had incomes below the poverty line. During the same year 13.1 percent of white women, 22.1 percent of women of Spanish origin, and an incredible 35.6 percent of black women lived in poverty.[7] Those hardest hit are single women—women who never married,

women who are widowed, separated, or divorced. It is estimated that almost 90 percent of today's elderly poor women are single.[8]

Part of the reason that women are poor in far greater numbers than men is that they survive so much longer than men do, but they also experience far higher *rates* of poverty than do men. A recent study has found that almost half of the older women in America have annual incomes of less than $5,000; fewer than one in five men have incomes that low.[9] In 1984 the median income for women sixty-five and over was $6,020, while the median income for men was $10,450.[10] Older women's incomes were on the average 58 percent of the incomes of older men, a figure strikingly similar to the 64 percent working women earn compared to the earnings of working men. This similarity is not surprising since the causes of older women's poverty are, in great measure, rooted in the expectations, roles, and work experiences of women throughout their life cycle.

Women, for the most part, work in low-paying, dead-end jobs that are mainly in the secondary labor market. Furthermore, many women work episodically and/or part-time, combining their jobs out of the home with their work inside the home. The combination of low-paying jobs, episodic work participation, and part-time work invariably means that the older woman has little in the way of savings, was probably not covered by a private pension plan, and will receive a low level of income from social security.

Moreover, the woman who wishes to find employment after age forty is often faced with discrimination because of her age, as well as her gender. There is considerable evidence that women over forty lose out on jobs both to men and to younger women. The limited job market for midlife and older women also translates into real economic loss as aging progresses. Employed women over forty-five earn even less relative to men than younger women do. But it is the woman entering the job market for the first time or reentering after an absence of many years who has the hardest time finding appropriate work.[11]

Age discrimination exists, of course, for men, too. A senior male employee may be "terminated" so that the company can hire a younger man at a significantly lower salary; older workers may be blocked for promotion or let go so that the amount companies pay out for pension plans is minimized; and the middleaged man who loses his job may well have an extremely difficult time finding another.

But entry-level age discrimination is a problem particular to women. Women are told regularly that they do not have enough experience, or that they have too much, or that they do not have the right experience. The result is that older women, compared to older men, have higher rates of unemployment and longer durations of joblessness.

Women's unemployment has exceeded men's every year from 1950 to the present; moreover, according to the U.S. Department of Labor, women make up the majority of "discouraged" workers who are not even counted in the unemployment statistics.[12]

Not only a woman's work history has a direct impact on her future financial status; her marital experience also has a significant impact as well. Most women are economically dependent in marriage; in exchange for childrearing and domestic services, the woman receives economic support. But, as one observer has noted,

Divorce severs the redistribution of income from the family bread-winner to dependent wives and children. Divorce terminates women's access (through the spouse) to resources and status available to men. . . . Men leave the marriage with their earning ability and social status intact while women lose their primary income source and encounter a gender discriminatory wage market.[13]

In fact, following divorce the woman's standard of living generally declines while the man's standard of living rises.

No-fault divorce, originally seen as a major reform of an anachronistic, hypocritical set of laws that varied markedly from state to state, is now being viewed far less favorably by those concerned with women's issues. The first no-fault statute was enacted in California in 1970. In many states the only ground necessary for divorce today is the statement of either party that the marriage is "irretrievably broken." The divorce will be granted even if the spouse is in opposition. Prior to no-fault, if the spouse objected to the divorce, he or she at least had leverage with which to bargain for a more adequate financial settlement. Now, according to a Gray Paper published by the Older Women's League, "The no-fault divorce acts have too often proved disastrous to older women."[14]

For the older woman, often without job skills, experience in the labor market, or any real assets in her own name, divorce often means more than a sharp drop in income; for some it means outright poverty. As a woman from Indiana put it: "I feel physically I've worked harder than most men I know—but what do I have to show for it? . . . I was the homemaker—the Little League Mom, Church, Roommother at school, etc. I also helped my husband pour concrete, side a house, etc. I have nothing."[15]

If there are children, the father may or, as we have seen, may well not pay child support. While the notion of alimony, or spousal support, as it is sometimes called, has lost favor among many men and women, women's childrearing and homemaking roles combined with the segregated labor market place women, particularly older women, in a most vulnerable position financially.

One of the direct results of women's work patterns is that the majority of working women are not covered by private pension plans. In 1979 about half of all wage and salary workers, approximately 30 million people, were covered by retirement plans.[16] According to the 1980 White House Miniconference on Older Women, private pensions are available, however, to only approximately 20 percent of retiring women workers.[17] Other studies indicate that while 50 percent of employed men were covered by pension plans in 1979, only 31 percent of women were covered, and that the average private pension received by a man was $4,152 a year compared to an average of $3,427 for a woman.[18] Until the recent passage of the Retirement Equity Act of 1984, women were frequently denied pension benefits they might have accrued or that their husbands might have accrued.

Under legislation sponsored in the House of Representatives by Geraldine A. Ferraro, former Congresswoman from Queens, New York, and the 1984 Democratic vice-presidential nominee, workers will be allowed to participate in pension plans at the age of twenty-one instead of twenty-five; pension plans must count the years of service from the time a person turns eighteen instead of twenty-two, as under previous legislation; employees who have worked fewer than five years may take up to five years off without losing pension credit for earlier service; and pension plans may not be permitted to count a one-year maternity or paternity leave as a break in service.[19] This legislation clearly attempts to enable women who do not fit the standard work pattern to receive retirement benefits in a more equitable fashion.

The new law also addresses the many problems women had been having vis-à-vis their husbands' pension plans. According to the Pension Rights Center, a 1978 Department of Labor study showed that approximately ten thousand widows lost their pension benefits each year because their husbands died before the retirement age set by the pension funds, usually age fifty-five, and without signing over their benefits. The 1984 legislation requires payment of benefits to the spouse of a worker who had become fully vested or who had worked the required number of years even if the worker dies before the age of fifty-five. The legislation further requires written permission of the spouse before a worker can waive benefits for a husband or wife. Many pension plans offer workers a choice between higher monthly retirement payments if the survivor option is not taken or lower monthly payments if the survivor is covered.[20] The spouse will now have a voice in that decision; and since women generally survive men, the decision becomes a critical one for them.

Ideally, income for the elderly should mean the combination of savings, private pension funds, and social security. For elderly women, however, social security is often the only source of income. Over 90 percent of all elderly women receive social security.[21] For 73 percent of nonmarried women, social security makes up 50 percent or more of their income; within that group, for 34 percent of nonmarried women, it makes up 90 percent or more of their income.[22]

In 1982, according to economist and sociologist Charlotte Muller, "The median Social Security benefit for nonmarried women was $2,830."[23] Social security benefits—tied to income—vary widely depending upon the individual's gender, work history, and marital status. Benefit levels are higher for men than for women; for individuals who are part of a two-worker couple than for those who are not; for white couples than for black couples; for white women than for black women. Benefit levels are least favorable for widows and, particularly, for divorced women.[24] It is clear that the same groups—divorced women, black women, widows, and women who never married—are at risk over and over again.

In addition to social security, the needy elderly, along with the needy blind and disabled, are covered by the Supplemental Security Income Program (SSI), which was enacted in 1972 and put into effect in 1974. While social security is based on coverage obtained through employment and is not based on need, SSI is a cash assistance, means-tested, welfare program. Approximately three-quarters of aged SSI recipients are women. As Charlotte Muller has stated, "SSI holds its recipients to a minimal standard of living."[25] As of February 1984, the maximum monthly federal SSI benefit was $314 for an individual and $472 for a couple. About two-thirds of the SSI recipients received less than the maximum amount because they had other income.[26] Only half the states supplement the federal payment and even then many people are forced to live below the poverty line.

Health, of course, is a major area of concern for older people. Since 1965 a large part of the health expenses of the elderly has been borne by Medicare. While it was meant to remove the severe burden of the cost of medical care from older people—those most likely to need care and least able to pay for it—in fact Medicare today only pays for 44 percent of the health care costs of the elderly.[27] It has been estimated that older women spend one-third of their median income on medical costs.

While programs for the elderly, including Medicare, were not affected as severely by budget cuts during the first Reagan administration as programs for children, young adults and the unemployed, reductions in other areas such as nutrition assistance, low-income energy assistance, Medicaid, and housing assistance, as well as the elimination of the CETA program, have adversely affected older people.[28]

In a telephone survey of the elderly poor of Chicago, it was found that, from 1981 to 1984, 20 percent of this group did not seek help with medical problems even though they thought they needed medical care; 17 percent were turned away from pharmacies even though they had Medicare cards; 29 percent cut down on medication and prescriptions; 15 percent did not have adequate winter clothing; 22 percent had trouble with their utilities; and 40 percent had cut down on food.[29]

The issue of dietary deficiency is a particularly important one among the elderly. It has been estimated, for example, that "approximately one-third to one-half of the health problems experienced by this group are believed to be directly or indirectly related to nutrition."[30] It is clear that the impact of the Reagan cutbacks on older Americans has been and will continue to be severe.

In addition to the direct burden of their own health expenses, older women must, if they are married, be concerned with ways of coping with a spouse's need for medical care and with ways of paying for that care. Since wives generally outlive their husbands, this is primarily a woman's problem. Not only do wives often care for their husbands at home as long as possible but they are often then required to find a way of obtaining long-term care for them.

While the emotional costs of institutionalizing a spouse may be devastating, the financial costs may be equally debilitating. As one researcher has noted:

This individual, who is usually a woman, is forced to divide one income into two parts: one portion for the payment of nursing home costs and the second for her own living expenses. This not only keeps the community-based spouse from maintaining her maximum level of functional independence, but it also increases the likelihood of her entering a nursing home. [31]

If the couple's finances simply cannot be stretched to cover long-term care, the spouse may be forced to "spend down" until Medicaid eligibility is achieved, thereby impoverishing herself. But, of course, it is not only a spouse's illness that can force an elderly person to "spend down" to the level of poverty; the individual's own illness can require the same strategy in order to be eligible for long-term care. These women, victims of their own or their husband's illness, become yet another group of the new poor, people who have lived most of their lives as part of the middle class and suddenly find themselves among the poor or the near-poor.

The elderly new poor are to be found in many communities, even in affluent ones, often struggling to remain in an area with which they are familiar; in which they have some friends, some roots. In Palo Alto, California, even the senior center looks affluent. An old firehouse, it is a white, two-story building with handsome wrought-iron decoration and huge, exotic plants inside the front door. According to Kathleen McConnell, a young social worker who works at the center, many of the women she sees were originally in the middle and upper middle classes. "They are people caught by the times, by a spouse that died and by escalating costs." Many are widows; some moved here during their retirement years, and now that their husbands have died, they can no longer afford the rents. Others, according to McConnell, "have a house, have clothes left over from when they had much more money, and may even have a car, but they have no real cash to manage day to day. Some are looking for subsidized housing; there is a waiting list of two to three years. Many spend their money on rent instead of food and some must spend their money down to the level of public assistance." But above all, she feels, "These women don't want to admit that they are needy. They look as though everything is o.k. but this image, which is good for their self-esteem, makes it very hard for them to ask for help."

Yet another problem, according to McConnell, is home care. Many of the women she sees are frail enough to need home care in order to be able to remain in their own homes. Home care in northern California costs, on the average, $8 per hour and many agencies have a four-hour minimum.

While most women do not have the extra cash to be able to pay for this service, there is also a large group whose income is not low enough for them to qualify for Medi-Cal, the California version of Medicaid. "They make do," McConnell says, "with a combination of neighbors, friends, and relatives—a patchwork. But they often continue to decline and eventually end up in a nursing home where the state has to pay." The society's reluctance, once again, to provide intermediate, preventive supports at moderate cost results in that same society eventually paying for long-term care at a far higher financial cost and at an equally high social and psychological cost to the individual. Professionals who work with the elderly—nurses, physicians, social workers, and community workers—generally agree that an elderly person who is placed in an impersonal, long-term care facility is likely to deteriorate much more rapidly than the older person who remains in his/her own environment, among familiar people and objects. The uprooting of the elderly from their environment is often a harsh, cruel act that could be prevented by earlier, less expensive, and less drastic intervention.

As one social worker who works with the elderly has pointed out:

Some sense of power—some degree of control over one's destiny—is critical to the integrity of the human personality. The new resident, by virtue of age status, pauper status, patient status, and his losses and impairments, already has experienced an erosion of his sense of autonomy or self-direction. The institution actively participates in reducing the resident to total lack of power. The fact that most often it is the place of last resort, in itself gives power to institutional management and staff. After all, where will the old person go if he does not like institutional life?[32]

And yet there are those for whom some kind of institution is the only answer; then the problem may not be how to keep them out, but how to get them into an appropriate setting. The aged black, the poor, and the hard-to-care-for are clearly discriminated against and often very difficult to place.[33] A New York City group recently completed a survey of state records and found that white patients were accepted at better nursing homes, while blacks and Hispanics were relegated to poorer ones. According to the survey, of the 153 public, voluntary, and proprietary nursing homes in New York City, "All white or virtually all-white populations were found at 54, many of which were said to offer the finest care available." The president of, the group, Friends and Relatives of the Institutional Aged, stated "Black and Hispanic aged find their final days are spent in a final segregation created by the nursing homes with the acquiescence of hospital-discharge planners and the state."[34] Many nursing homes are operated under religious auspices and are, of course, permitted to restrict admission to patients of their faith; they are not, however, permitted by law, if they admit patients of other religions, to exclude people because of their racial or ethnic background.

Potential nursing home patients are not only discriminated against on the basis of race; they are also discriminated against according to income. The nursing home industry is increasingly going after "private pay patients" rather than Medicaid patients because, as a senior vice-president of one of the leading nursing home companies has stated, that is where "the big money is." [35]

The shortage of nursing home beds, particularly for Medicaid patients, is expected to become critical by the end of this century; and not only are such homes not being built but the newest strategy is for companies to move into developing retirement communities for the affluent that guarantee "priority access" to a nearby nursing home. The deputy director of the health care statistics division in the U.S. Department of Health and Human Services has suggested that we might be moving toward a situation where "The wealthy have beds and the poor stand in line."[36]

Wherever they spend their final years, the overwhelming reality about old people in our society, particularly old women, is that they are extraneous. With American families increasingly fragmented, there is little room for the older woman within the family unit. With women of all ages working in increasing numbers, there is no one at home to care for the elderly who are often ill and cannot be left alone for long periods of time. And with rapidly changing notions about child care, many young mothers are unwilling to entrust their preschool children to the "out of date" ways of the grandmother. There are, therefore, few roles the older woman is permitted to play within the fast-paced, individual-centered family of the 1980s.

Often, after a lifetime of caring for others, elderly women are ultimately left to live in isolation. For old women are survivors in the true sense of the word. Most often they have outlived their spouses and their friends and have lost much of what made them valued in American society: their youth, their reproductive potential, their earning potential. The older woman is often devalued and ignored and is, in addition, frequently dependent on others, often strangers, for her day-to-day sustenance.

Our avoidance of the old, our reluctance to integrate them into our lives, to let them perform meaningful tasks, and to make adequate provisions for their well-being stems, in part, from our feelings about death. In avoiding the problems of old age, we attempt to avoid our old age; in turning our backs on the sick and dying, we attempt to turn our backs on our own inevitable deterioration and death. As Ernest Becker has stated with such force and clarity, "The idea of death, the fear of it, haunts the human animal like nothing else; it is a mainspring of human activity—activity designed largely to avoid the fatality of death, to overcome it by denying in some way that it is the final destiny for man."[37]

Some may be lucky enough to have a daughter or a daughter-in-law to help them—again, of course, it is women doing the caring—but these younger women are increasingly torn among their responsibilities toward their own families, their responsibilities toward the older person, and these days, a job as well. As many experts in geriatrics have pointed out, the current emphasis on alternatives to institutional care place the burden of care in the community on unpaid relatives or on low-paid health workers. Again, women are being placed in a caring role and are being exploited for fulfilling that role.

It is, of course, possible to develop alternatives to institutionalization. One such alternative is Miracle Square, a residence for elderly and disabled people in Tucson, Arizona. Established in 1982, Miracle Square is a pilot project financed partly by the residents themselves, partly through the U.S. Department of Housing and Urban Development (HUD), and partly by the local county government. It is home for nineteen residents, sixteen of whom are over sixty.

A converted motel, Miracle Square provides individual rooms for each resident and a communal area where the residents can socialize. According to Peggy McDonald, the warm, lively, gray-haired director, the goal is to provide "freedom and independence" for low-income people who do not really need to be in nursing homes but who may need a degree of caretaking. The residents are encouraged to do all they can for themselves and have their own stoves and refrigerators, but most of them also have a hot lunch provided by Meals on Wheels.

Virginia Dixon lives at Miracle Square. She is a young-looking, part-Cherokee, part-black, seventy-three-year-old mother, grandmother, and great-grandmother. Pictures of her handsome family line the walls of her comfortably furnished room. For twenty-five years she did domestic work and hairdressing in order to support herself and her daughter; her husband has been dead for forty years. Having spent her entire working life in the secondary labor market, Ms. Dixon's total income in 1983 from both social security and SSI was $302 a month, or $3,624 for the year. The poverty line for a single person in 1983 was $5,061. After paying $126.29 for rent at Miracle Square, Ms. Dixon has approximately $175 per month left for all her needs.

Virginia Dixon worked until her severe diabetes required her to be hospitalized. After discharge from the hospital, she was placed in a nursing home, where she remained for eight years. When I met her, she had been at Miracle Square for six months and said, "I am happy. I think young and I go out often—as often as I can—just about every other day. Some people go on and on about 'I'm aging and I'm dying,' but I don't like to do that or to listen to it because it's a real stress on me. It bores me."

Edith Foster, a heavy, fifty-four-year-old woman who looks many years older, also lives at Miracle Square. She is missing all her front teeth and has large elastic bandages on both knees. She lies on her bed while we talk. Foster was married to a contractor who was killed in an automobile accident twelve years before when a truck went through a stop sign. She herself had been in a severe automobile accident several years ago. "I ran into a car and I was a pedestrian," she says with a giggle. Her name had run in the obituary column of the local newspaper, but she survived. She had been in nursing homes for five years prior to coming to Miracle Square a year and a half ago.

Although she seems quite severely disabled, she manages to go shopping three times a week, goes to church every Sunday and helps another, more handicapped resident with her food preparation and with shopping. In response to my commenting about all she does for her friend, she said simply, "It makes me feel not quite such a burden."

For those older people who are relatively healthy and can live on their own, participation in community activities can make life worthwhile. Maria Ortiz, a small, extremely active sixty-seven-year-old woman, lives in the small community of Espagnola, New Mexico. She was married for over thirty-five years to a man who, among other jobs, was a uranium miner and a sheepherder. She raised three children and now has eighteen grandchildren and six great-grandchildren. Ortiz receives $228 per month from social security and $106 per month from SSI for a total annual income of $4,008. She also receives $25 worth of food stamps monthly. Out of this income she must pay all of her expenses, her rent, her food, her electricity, and her other bills.

Before Ortiz started working as a foster grandparent in the Family Learning Center in Espagnola, she suffered from severe rheumatoid arthritis, particularly severe pain in her knees. She had been in and out of the hospital and could barely walk. After she started working with the children, she found herself walking to work in the morning and home in the evening "with so much joy" that her physical problems completely went away.

Every day for four hours, she works with the children, primarily in Spanish because she and the teachers are concerned that the Spanish language and customs are fading among the Hispanic children of Espagnola. Having helped to organize the Foster Grandparent Council, she is a current member and a trainer for new foster grandparents. Maria Ortiz spoke with vigor and excitement. Her work at the center seemed to be of central importance to this vital older woman.

Ortiz's feelings of well-being that stem from her role in the community are echoed by older people all over the country. In rural North Carolina, Eva Salber, a community health physician, interviewed older people about their lives. Social supports, interconnections with others in the community, both family and friends, were found to be extremely important factors in the well-being of these older men and women.

Lillian Adams, age seventy-one, is described as a "natural helper" and "highly respected" in her community. A schoolteacher for forty-four years, she is currently active in several volunteer organizations, visits elderly shut-ins, brings friends to town for food stamps, and is generally helpful in a variety of ways. She talks about her life:

It doesn't take so much to make me happy like it does a lot of folk. If I can know that I can see people and people can come to see me, and I have something decent to wear and something to eat, and I can help people, that's about all it takes to make me happy. I do more for people now than I did when I was younger, like cooking things for people, carrying them, sharing vegetables with those who can't help themselves.[38]

Polly Williams, age seventy-five, talks about what's important to her in her day-to-day activities:

I'm not lonely. I pass the day doing a little housework, neighbors coming in, and I do a lot of visiting. . . .

The people here in the community, neighbors, we check on each other. This one can look over at that house and she can tell what's going on over there; if the shades are not up by a certain time she goes to see why. . . . Long as anybody is well and happy I pay no attention to them, but if they need my help I am there if I can get there. This woman, the second house from here, was called up to Charlotte, her sister was sick. I go over and see if everything is all right and water her flowers, and when her water went off I called her brother and let him come to see why. I check on all the people that I know in the village, if I see anything wrong, I don't have time to go to the new senior center, I'm too busy.[39]

References 1-39 are available in the original source.

Ω

The Need for Intimacy

by Jane Porcino

How long has it been since someone touched me? Twenty years? Twenty years I've been a widow, respected, smiled at, but never touched. Never held so close that loneliness was blotted out.. . . . Oh, God, I'm so lonely.

These poignant words from the poem "Minnie Remembers," by Donna Swanson, reflect one of our deepest fears about aging. No matter what our age, we each need intimacy in our lives—at least one other person with whom we can share both pleasure and pain. We hunger for someone who will accept us as delightfully different. This other person can be female or male, young or old.

Research demonstrates that babies who never are held or touched suffer psychologically and may actually wither and die. This also is true as we grow older. And yet, an increasing number of women over 65 live alone, without partners, many of them deprived of any expression of intimacy.

One reality we will face as we grow older female is that there are more women than men; we are likely to find ourselves without a male partner. In the beginning decades of this century, there were equal numbers of women and men over the age of 65. Today, there are almost 150 older women for every 100 men. Divorce after 25 to 30 years of marriage is becoming commonplace, and the average age for a widow is only 56. Complicating all of this is the fact that men who are widowed or divorced in mid- or late-life quickly remarry, most often to younger women. There are nine bridegrooms to every bride over age 65. Not only is remarriage rare for older women, but there are few social opportunities for close relationships with men. As a result, almost half of all older women live alone—many of them lonely. One woman stated the problem well when she wrote to me:

One thing unites us all—babies, adults, and grandmothers—our need for response from some living creature. Of course, tender loving care would be better, but we can survive without that luxury. What we cannot do without is some kind of reciprocal sharing of life experiences.

Are millions of us doomed to loneliness in old age? Not if we are willing to plan now for our later years, and not just let them happen to us. First, it is important to strengthen and nurture our friendships with women—indeed, glory in them. Fortunately, we were encouraged to develop close female friendships, to share trust and confidences, and to express our feelings to one another. Many of us, even many married women whose relationships with their husbands lack intimacy, presently share much of our social life with women. We seek out environments in which we can express our innermost thoughts. The coffee-klatch, PTA-days have evolved to rap groups, consciousness-raising meetings, and professional networking (the "old girls' club").

Collective living is one way to counter loneliness in our later years. Small groups of us can join together to share living space, incomes, companionship, thoughts, and tasks in a supportive environment. Women are successfully doing this throughout the country. There is a great deal that we can do together that we cannot do alone.

The seeking of intimacy could be encouraged even within nursing homes. My own mother lived out her last years in such a facility, where she developed a close friendship with another woman. They shared all the details of their daily lives, and yet to the end, these two proper women called each other "Mrs.," and rarely touched. The friendship was so deep that when one died, the other followed in a few months.

A prevailing fear of homosexuality among many heterosexual older women many prevent them from acknowledging their human need for intimacy. Some women have

Reprinted with permission of the author, from *Ms*. Magazine, January, 1982, p. 104.

shared sexual intimacy with other women most of their adult years. Even women who prefer heterosexuality are moving toward intimacy with women in their later years because of the limited choices available to them. Only a few women may find sexual gratification in their female relationships. But they will find many other kinds of intimacy. Women I know say that they enjoy the companionship of other women; many say they have no desire at all to make the accommodations that would be necessary to form new heterosexual relationships. Two wrote the following to me:

I am blessed with a few special women friendships. They are nonsexual, greatly sharing, mutually supportive "conversational love affairs."

I've a whole circle of supportive, nutritive, loving women friends. I talk over life circumstances, problems and interests with them very openly, receive a great deal of support from them, and give the same. We often have just fun together. I love them and they love me. These friendships have been the most stable thing in my life.

The upcoming generation of elderly women (those now in their late 30s and 40s—the baby-boom generation) are more open to exploring different ways to be intimate. Those of us presently in our middle or late years can learn from them. Although we have been socialized to seek only one significant other, perhaps our search should be for a few such people in our lives—people to have fun with, to share our pleasure and pain, and to give us the physical touching we need.

Love has the potential for deepening as we age. We have years of experience behind us, and now we have the time. Sensuous grandmothers abound—women like Lena Horne, Mary Calderone, and Ingrid Bergman, whose vibrant way of being in the world draws people to them. Our only limit may be a weak imagination.

Ω

The Colours of Menopause
by Margaret de Souza

In North America, books, articles and newsletters on menopause provide support and information for the health needs of the dominant white middle class woman. Unfortunately, information and support is not geared for the Black, Asian, Latin American or Aboriginal woman in our multiracial/multicultural country. In working with women from different racial backgrounds I have observed their attitudes towards the "change of life" and how for some of them, their difficulties "adjusting" to the North American environment adds to the stress of their menopausal changes. There is a difference in the needs and expectations of non-white women going through menopause.

Understanding their attitude towards menopause will help in setting up better health care strategies which are different from those required by white, middle class, and dominant culture women and which will combat the assumption that immigrant women and women of colour are not capable of understanding, choosing or acting in accordance with their own health needs.

From *Healthsharing*, Fall/Winter, 1990, pp. 14–17. Copyright © 1990 by *Healthsharing* (Canada). Reprinted by permission.

Margaret de Souza is a Ugandan-born Canadian of East Indian origin who works as the head nurse of the Family Life Program at St. Joseph's Health Centre.

I am the family life counsellor at the Women's Health Centre at St. Joseph's Health Centre and have been involved with menopausal counselling for the past five years. The women I see at the centre are from many different backgrounds including Portuguese, Italian, South Asian, Polish, Chinese, Somalian, Latin American and Canadian.

I would like to share stories of menopause from these women— stories of increasing power and status, a time of positive change and fear of aging. Their fears and strengths are largely determined by their cultural background, family and community experiences and the level of support they have as women.

Most medical literature defines menopause as a deficiency and decline—a living decay. It has been created by the medical profession as a disease needing treatment. Rarely, are women seen as a whole. A hot flash or a mood swing is viewed in isolation, ignoring other possible causes. Particularly for non-white women, how the social and political environment influences their lives must be understood and racist stereotypes dispelled.

There are also a myriad of physical and mental health problems caused by traumatic emigration experiences, cultural dislocation and loss of support systems. A 48 year old woman from El Salvador told me how she came to Canada as a torture victim and refugee with her three children a year ago. Her husband was taken as a political prisoner. She has missed her ESL (English as a Second Language) classes because of severe palpitations and chest pains. She thinks she is dying so she wants to see a cardiologist. She has had bladder infections, hot flashes, sleeplessness and sweating for the past 10 months. She used her own cultural drinks because she has no time to see a family doctor.

In "western" culture our mental, physical and spiritual health is constantly under stress. In most non-western cultures there is no concept of stress because coping techniques are built into the culture. But it is difficult to transport them into another cultural environment; they cease to work and the dominant culture determines our health.

A 49 year old Chinese woman talks of her social life being disrupted with hot flashes and heavy periods. "I cannot concentrate, my joints ache, but my twin sister, who is a Tai Chi instructor back home, does not have any of these problems."

"Western" culture glorifies youth and menopause is viewed as a period of decline. In North American menopause is viewed as an aging disease needing medical intervention—either drugs, surgery or both. Some immigrants adopt this belief, but others will seek alternative health options or traditional medicine.

A 50 year old Sikh woman from India talks about how her mother dealt with menopause differently. "My mother never dyed her hair like I do. I have to take estrogen for my sweats. My mother used to complain of a "hot fever" coming on and off with sweating. When the sweating got worse, she went to the folk doctor."

In Canada at the beginning of the century doctors hospitalized menopausal women for depression. Today, menopause continues to be treated with tranquilizers and hormones by physicians and psychiatrists.

An Italian woman describes her experience. "When I had those panic attacks my hot flashes got worse. My husband told me that this was the beginning of a nervous breakdown. He took me to a psychiatrist and I was given tranquilizers."

In dominant Canadian culture there is an emphasis on the "nuclear family." Stress due to the triple burden of the roles of wife/mother/worker can negatively effect menopausal changes.

"I could slaughter the kids!," says a 47 year old Chinese woman. "I have a bad headache, hot flashes and these palpitations. I am leaving home! I am fed up of being a taxi driver and a housekeeper."

Some cultures that are influenced by "western culture" react to menopause with a sense of loss, a loss of their ability to bear children and their youthful image. A 48 year old Polish woman describes her pain. "I am sad so sad—no more babies! These hot flashes remind me that I am getting old."

Many cultures view this midlife phase as a healthy balance because menopause liberates a woman from the fear of pregnancy, the nuisance of birth control and offers her more leisure time and privacy for love making. A 52 year old Italian woman talked about how sex was better than before. "No birth control! No babies! We have a good sex life. We spend more time getting ready."

Some cultures have a positive view of menopause. The menopause stage gives women a rise in status of power, worth and privilege. Menopausal women are seen as confidants, advisors, decision-makers and leaders of extended family and community. The Chinese, Japanese, Somalians and South Asians celebrate menopause as a triumph—women move from being powerless to being respected as wise and powerful. A Somalian woman described how her 54 year old mother is a "wise woman," who takes the young girls to initiation huts.

An Indian woman compares her menopause to that of her mother. "I am sitting at home with my hot flashes, joint pains and aches, but at my age my mother had no complaints. She became the village decision-maker and arranged prayer groups at the village temple."

Some religions and cultures view menstruation as "impure" and women are ostracized from their community, but these cultures view menopause with a positive goal. It is the end of their menstrual taboos and beginning of a new dimension.

"I can now socialize with my husband and his friends," says an Afghani woman from India. "I am free, no taboo. I can visit my friends in my community."

Accessible and culturally relevant health care for menopausal women from non-white cultures is crucial. Management of menopause depends on the total culture. The menopause experience for these women could be either a positive change or a crisis.

But Black, Asian, and Latin American women living in Canada experience linguistic and cultural barriers to health services. These women bring with them different cultural beliefs, traditions and practices which are not generally understood or respected by the medical system. This causes racist and inappropriate responses from health services.

An effective multiracial/multicultural perspective brings important insights to the area of menopausal health. Creative approaches are needed and could also help all menopausal women to deal positively with this life change.

Healthy menopausal care can be achieved through a health care system which cooperates with community-based organizations to break down cultural barriers. Instead of menopausal women being the subjects of intervention by health care professionals, these women need the tools to advocate on their own behalf.

Women going through menopause can assume responsibility for our own health care by taking control. But only if we can make choices in our health care through education, information, self-help, support and interpretation.

Black, Asian, Latin American and immigrant women need knowledge about reproductive health care and non-medical remedies such as diet, exercise and relaxation techniques in their mother tongue. This brings it closer to home and combats fear. Health information centres should be community controlled by women with a strong consumer perspective. All health information and counselling should be available in easy to understand forms in different languages.

Food patterns and dietary habits of women from different cultures must be respected. East and South Asians eat a lot of fish, sea weed, wholegrain and tofu—foods which are rich in calcium. These guard against loss of bone mass (osteoporosis) in later life. Herbal teas, herbs, licorice root, and Ginseng are used by European, Chinese African and South Asian women for hot flashes, fatigue and heavy periods which are symptoms of menopause. This optimum diet often changes through the process of emigration. Skillful health professionals can help women to avoid this change and it would be useful for all women to adopt dietary practices that prevent negative menopausal symptoms—practices that are more reliable than medical remedies.

Utilization of community based organizations and hospital resources geared to their needs will give women from diverse cultures the confidence to make choices. We will be able to choose our own doctor or health care giver who may practice holistic or traditional medicine. We will be able to take control of our own health needs by asking questions, finding options or questioning medical treatment. We will also be able to explore and possibly use non-medical remedies. Tai Chi is popular among Chinese and Philippine women, giving them vigour, flexibility and inner harmony. Relaxation techniques like yoga and medication are popular among South Asian women, helping them to calm the mind and eliminate stress. These exercises and relaxation techniques can be incorporated in community programs for immigrant women.

Some Chinese, Japanese, and African women treat joint pain, muscle spasms, and menstrual cramps with alternative methods like accupressure, shiatsu, acupuncture and massage. Sometimes these non-medical approaches are provided by the experienced wise women of their community. These wise women channel their energy through their bodies and hands to heal the ailments women experience at menopause. Women will eventually learn to combine alternative approaches with conventional remedies to their advantage.

"Self-help" is invaluable for any woman going through menopause. A self-help group can offer courage, strength and 'body' information. This support can reduce the sense of isolation as we learn the social context of our common condition. "Sex talk," for example, is taboo in many cultures, so the physiological changes of menopause cause misconceptions and misunderstanding in both men and women. Women misinterpret lack of lubrication as a sexual malfunction and men sometimes think that a longer time for sexual arousal is a sign of disinterest. Women in post-child bearing years will benefit from the knowledge on sexuality and communication they receive through participation in a self-help group.

Multicultural menopausal women can be strengthened and empowered by allowing them easy access to all resources for multicultural health care. If immigrant women are dissatisfied with their health care they can make a choice, they can shop around, thus assuming responsibility for their own health care by being in control.

Ω

The Selling of HRT:
Playing on the Fear Factor

by Nancy Worcester and Mariamne H. Whatley

Introduction

For decades, women's health activists have been critical of the medical system's lack of interest in older women's issues. Osteoporosis and heart disease were ex-

From FEMINIST REVIEW (England), No. 41, summer 1992. Copyright © 1992 by Nancy Worcester and Mariamne H. Whatley. Reprinted by permission.

cellent examples of the problematic relationship between the medical system and women who use it. These prevalent, serious, life-threatening conditions have been characterized by an almost total lack of information and research. Until quite recently, most women had never heard of osteoporosis, and cardiovascular disease was so consistently labelled as a 'men's' disease that the major studies included tens of thousands of men and *no* women.

The situation has changed dramatically in the last few years. Osteoporosis and heart disease can no longer serve as examples of neglect of older women's issues. Osteoporosis has become a household word in the United States. Most women will have seen a headline announcing 'heart disease is the number one killer of women', and the prevention of both osteoporosis and heart disease in women has become 'hot' research.

It might seem that feminist activists should be applauding this response of the medical establishment. Any woman approaching menopause is likely to receive information from her health-care practitioners on the dangers of osteoporosis and heart disease. So why are we complaining? Aren't feminists ever satisfied?

Prevention Consciousness

The sudden interest in older women's issues is directly related to the fact that the medical establishment and the drug industry have 'discovered' that healthy menopausal and postmenopausal women represent a huge market. The selling of hormones and services which promote or follow up on them fits neatly into the needs of the drug industry, as well as health-service providers and consumers. Restrictions by the government and insurance companies in the US have meant the health system cannot make enough money on sick people, and women are not having 'enough' babies; the health system has been forced to search for previously untapped markets of healthy people. Consumers may feel the health system is finally responding to their needs if services and products are marketed to play on their new-found prevention consciousness.

Contemporary US and British societies, especially the middle classes, have become highly health conscious. Advertisements in which bran cereals are pushed to prevent cancer, low cholesterol foods to reduce heart-attack risk, and exercise machines to promote 'wellness' reveal the dominance of the prevention ideology in health awareness. Sometimes the meaning gets sufficiently clouded that it seems that the appearance of health may be an end in itself rather than a means towards a higher-quality life.

The focus on prevention and self-help is part of an overall trend among consumers away from the sick-care model of the medical industry which devotes few resources to environmental and occupational issues, disease detection and control, or medical education, and instead prioritizes drugs, surgery, hospitals and high-technology equipment. This sick-care model may do an impressive job of patching up accident victims or putting a new heart into someone who has eaten the typical high-fat, low-fibre Western diet, but it does practically nothing to keep us well. The initial resistance to the medical model was often political, based, for example, on the analysis generated by the women's health movement; prevention was a way of wrestling control away from doctors and returning it to consumers.

However, it took the medical establishment and others little time to co-opt the emphasis on prevention. This consciousness has been intentionally constructed in a very individualistic, 'take care of *yourself*' (don't expect society, the government or the health system to take care of you) and victim-blaming way. In other words, 'it's the other person's fault if he chooses to live an unhealthy lifestyle'. As major consumers in the health-care system, responsible for their own health and that of other family members, women quickly got targeted as the major customers of prevention services. In her seminars on how to market women's health, Sally Rynne, consultant to for-profit women's health centres throughout the USA, notes that 18 per cent of women's medical visits are preventative, that women are the major subscribers to prevention/wellness type magazines and that the audiences at health promotion programs are predominantly women (Whatley and Worcester, 1989). Ironically, although the emphasis on prevention originated as a way to become less dependent on the medical establishment, it is now being used as a marketing technique to attract people back into the system: you cannot prevent osteoporosis or heart disease with HRT without having a doctor's prescription and surrounding services to monitor your 'progress' toward prevention!

Selling the Fear Factor

In order to maximize the market value of 'prevention', the condition to be avoided must be sufficiently serious or highly undesirable. Individuals must view the condition in question as highly prevalent or believe themselves to have a high level of personal susceptibility. Fear can become an important selling point for either true prevention or early detection tests.

As diseases become 'popular', there is a time of intense interest, during which people are inundated with media coverage of the newest plague, whether it is genital herpes, toxic shock syndrome, premenstrual tension, or chlamydia. Of course, accurate and complete information is needed about these issues; increased awareness is essential for all individuals who want to have some control over their health. However, sensational media coverage often does little besides create fear, as the AIDS panic has clearly demonstrated. Those who benefit from this popular coverage are those who offer prevention or treatment, whether they are effective or not.

The marketing of hormone products to menopausal and postmenopausal women is particularly cruel in the way that it plays on the fears of specific disabling or life-threatening conditions and also, very purposefully, on women's fear of ageing. Disabling or life-threatening conditions are frightening enough in themselves, but ones totally associated with the ageing process, growing older or *being old,* take on an increased meaning for women in an ageist society which particularly devalues older women. It is no coincidence that *Feminine Forever* was the name of the 1966 book which first popularized the notion that a wonder drug (oestrogen) could prevent the ageing process in women.

Swallowing HRT and Forgetting Its History

Feminine Forever, whose author was funded by Wyeth-Ayerst, the manufacturer of the menopausal oestrogen product Premarin, promised that oestrogen could keep women young forever and prevent the natural 'decaying' process of ageing. It is not surprising that by 1970 Premarin had become one of the top four prescription drugs in the USA (Eagen, 1989). By the mid-1970s, there were cities in the US where more than half of the menopausal women were taking oestrogen (Sloane, 1985). But, by the mid-1970s, studies were starting to show a marked increase in endometrial (lining of the uterus) cancer in women who had taken menopausal oestrogens. While Wyeth-Ayerst denied the oestrogen-endometrial cancer link and even resorted to sending 'Dear Doctor' letters to all gynaecologists in the US (Waterhouse, 1990), women became afraid of the products, doctors feared lawsuits if they prescribed it, and at least another fifteen studies proved that oestrogen use was associated with a marked increase in endometrial cancer (Sloane, 1985). By 1979, a consensus conference of the National Institutes of Health had rejected almost all claims which had been made for the physical or psychological benefits of oestrogen replacement therapy. The conference committee concluded that of all the presumed symptoms of menopause, there were only two which could be established as uniquely characteristic of menopause and uniformly relieved by oestrogen therapy. Oestrogen is only effective for controlling hot flushes (vasomotor instability) and changes in the genitals (which textbooks refer to as genital atrophy—no wonder women will resort to anything to avoid this condition).

One might think that would be the end of a product which lived up to few of its claims, in which consumers and physicians had lost confidence and which was known as a cancer-causing agent. But, drug companies had tasted the potential of marketing products to menopausal women: in the US more than 28 million prescriptions for oestrogen had been filled in 1975 (National Prescriptions Audit).

The 1980s saw two changes in the marketing of oestrogens: (1) public-relations firms were hired to promote oestrogen products in the same way that sweets, breakfast cereals or soaps are advertised; and (2) oestrogens were reintroduced on to the market in combination with progestins.

Feminist health activists have been critical of the mass marketing of oestrogen products, seeing it as irresponsible. Starting in 1985, Premarin's manufacturer, Wyeth-Ayerst, hired a public-relations firm to conduct a public-education campaign aimed at encouraging *all* women over thirty-five years to consider taking oestrogens to prevent osteoporosis instead of targeting the 25 per cent of women at high risk of suffering osteoporosis. More recently, Ciba Geigy, manufacturer of an oestrogen patch, has begun mass direct-mail solicitations promoting their patch to women throughout the US. Testifying against the mass promotion of oestrogens before the Food and Drug Administration, Cindy Pearson stated, 'The National Women's Health Network is outraged that a potentially risky drug is being promoted with the same techniques used by Publishers Clearinghouse Sweepstakes.' (This refers to the tacky but popular direct-mail selling of magazines by promising highly desirable—but seldom obtainable—prizes) (Pearson, 1991).

By the drug companies' criteria, such promotion of oestrogen products must seem phenomenally successful. In 1985, when Wyeth-Ayerst first started its 'education' campaign on osteoporosis, a survey found that 77 per cent of women had not heard of this condition (Dejanikus, 1985). Now, women have not only heard of osteoporosis, they are also frightened by the seeming inevitability of postmenopausal hip fractures or of becoming like the elderly woman with the severely bent spine they have seen in advertisements. Having dropped to approximately 15 million prescriptions per year in the US in 1979/80, oestrogen prescriptions were up to nearly 32 million in 1989. (National Prescription Audit). Premarin's annual sales alone were put at $400 million by 1989 and expected to exceed $1 billion by 1995. (Waterhouse,1990). According to federal health statistics, as many as half of all postmenopausal American women take some form of hormone 'replacement' at some time and at least 15 per cent are taking the drugs at any one time (Specter, 1989). This is probably about twice as high as the percentage of British women presently taking menopausal hormones.

Packaging as HRT or ORT

Consumers are now faced with a 'choice' of hormonal products. By the early 1980s oestrogen was often prescribed in combination with a progestin. It was believed that the progestin component would protect against the risk of endometrial cancer which was associated with oestrogen on its own.

For the rest of this paper two different terms will be used to identify the two different forms in which oestrogen is most commonly prescribed. HRT *(hormone replacement therapy)* will be used in reference to products or regimes where a woman is given *both a* oestrogen and a progestin hormone. *ORT (oestrogen replacement therapy)* will be used when a woman is given oestrogen on its own. (Note: because Americans spell oestrogen without a beginning 'o', ERT or estrogen replacement therapy is the term which is used in American publications for oestrogen on its own.) At this stage of the debate about postmenopausal hormones, it is absolutely essential that we keep track of whether we are talking about HRT or ORT.

It is accepted that ORT is related to an increase in endometrial cancer, whereas HRT is not associated with that cancer and may even have a protective effect against endometrial cancer. Any woman with a uterus (in other words women who have not had a hysterectomy) should be informed of this and offered HRT instead of ORT, if HRT is believed to fulfil the purpose for which she is considering hormones. As this paper will discuss, it is a confusing moment in history for women to be making choices about postmenopausal hormones. Most of the studies have been done with ORT, *not* HRT, but a woman with a uterus will want to take HRT. As the studies have not been done, it is simply too early to know whether the progestin component of HRT diminishes or reverses effects expected of oestrogen. As Kathleen MacPherson (1987) points out in her important article 'Osteoporosis: The New Flaw in Woman or Science?', some physicians will not prescribe the HRT combination because: (1) research on its long-term effects is scant, (2) progestins in the contraceptive pills increased the risk of hypertension and strokes, and (3) postmenopausal women may not want to have breakthrough bleeding which occurs monthly if they take the oestrogen-progestin combination.

Women who are considering taking ORT, oestrogen on its own, should be informed that in addition to the approximately five to fourteen-fold increase in endometrial cancer (National Women's Health Network, 1989), women on this regimen also increase their risk of abnormal bleeding 7.8 times, need dilation and curettage 4.9 times as often, and have hysterectomy rates 6.6 times higher, than non-users (Ettinger, 1987). Women who take oestrogens after menopause also have a two to three fold increase in their risk of gallbladder disease (National Women's Health Network, 1989).

Clearly the goal of oestrogen manufacturers is to find a way to package oestrogens so that women are willing to stay on them for their *entire postmenopausal life:*

We are still learning ways to administer estrogen and progestogen to obtain maximum effectiveness with minimum side effects. New formulations of estrogens and progestogens, new routes of administration, and improved dosage schedules should provide more convenient and acceptable long term hormone replacement, one that women can use for their entire postmenopausal life time without the inconvenience of menstrual bleeding and concern about possible side effects. (Ettinger, 1987: 36)

Hormones Dominate the System Both Physiologically and Politically

Hormones hold potential for improving quality and quantity of life for some menopausal and postmenopausal women. It will be important to come back to this point and question how feminists can better look at the potential for these hormones. Unfortunately, we seldom have the luxury of being able to do this because major forces are so persistently pushing hormones and because most information is so pro-hormones. In an effort to 'balance' the discussion, feminist health activists have often ended up as lone voices critiquing the premature, routine prescribing of these drugs of unknown safety.

Even if women have *all* the available information on postmenopausal hormones, with the present state of knowledge it is extremely difficult to weigh the potential benefits and the unknown risks. But, in fact, very few women 'choosing' to embark upon hormone treatment even know that the drugs they are taking are controversial and possibly hazardous. The information women get in the lay press is very much biased towards the use of hormones. A survey of all the articles on this topic in the magazines

most regularly read by US women found that thirty-six articles were published between 1985 and 1988. Three-quarters of the articles were clearly pro-hormones: fully half of the articles did not even mention any risks with oestrogen use (Pearson, 1991). The information women get from their doctors may be nearly as biased: a 1990 study found that over 75 per cent of US gynecologists were routinely prescribing hormones to prevent osteoporosis or heart disease in all menopausal women.

Even the smallest doses of ORT or HRT have very powerful effects on a woman's body and totally dominate her body's own regulation and production of hormones. How desirable or safe this is physiologically is a question which is still unanswered. What is known is that the way hormones are being promoted now has dangerous political implications for women and must be seen as part of a purposeful medicalization of women's lives.

Feminists have long been critical of the ways in which normal, healthy processes such as contraception, pregnancy and childbirth have been medicalized. We used to criticize the fact that real health issues such as premenstrual tension, infertility, and osteoporosis were ignored by the health system. Now that women's health issues have been 'discovered' and there are money-making drugs or technologies to offer, we see a medicalization of whole new areas of women's lives. We are already witnessing what this means. The medical profession is taking control over more aspects of women's lives, more conditions are being labelled as illness and used against the equality of women, drugs or high technology procedures have been identified as the solution to newly targeted 'problems' and, in the name of prevention, more women are being hooked into a medical system which does not meet their needs.

The medicalization of menopause means that menopause and postmenopause are defined as 'deficiency illnesses'. Even the terms 'hormone replacement therapy' and 'oestrogen replacement therapy' wrongly imply that something is missing which must be replaced. The fact that this misinformation can so easily be used as a selling point for products is a sad reflection on how little information most women have about their own bodies. As the National Women's Health Network's position paper on hormone therapy puts it, 'We object to the view of normal menopause as a deficiency disease. Menopause does not automatically require "treatment".' (National Women's Health Network, 1989: 9)

Menopause is a normal, healthy transition phase of a woman's life when her body has within it all the mechanisms necessary to gradually change from dealing with demanding reproductive cycles to meeting the different, postreproduction, physiological needs of postmenopause. The postmenopausal woman is still capable of making the oestrogens she needs: the older woman's body needs less oestrogen and makes it in a different way. During the reproductive years, a woman's ovaries will be the main producers of oestrogens and relatively high quantities of oestrogens will be produced. Menopause is the time when the ovaries gradually stop producing oestrogens and the oestrogens produced by the adrenal glands and the oestrogens produced from androgens by fat and muscle tissue become the major oestrogens in a woman's body. Menopause should be viewed as the healthy transition from premenopause to postmenopause in the same way that puberty is recognized as the time when young women make the transition from prereproduction to being capable of reproduction.

Viewing menopause as a normal, healthy transition does not imply that transition is easy for all women. Although many of the problems faced by menopausal women are social rather than physiological, women may experience symptoms such as hot flushes when or if their oestrogen levels drop rapidly (which is what happens if a woman's ovaries are surgically removed). Taking ORT or HRT works to *delay* the transition by keeping hormone levels artificially high. If a woman suddenly stops taking hormones she can experience the same or worse symptoms than the ones for which she was taking hormones. If a woman chooses to take ORT or HRT to relieve hot flushes or genital changes, to *ease* the transition she would want to take gradually reduced amounts of hormones for as short a period of time as possible for specific complaints (National Women's Health Network, 1989: 9).

The medicalization of menopause is particularly dangerous in that *all* attention has become focused on hormones as the 'answer' to whatever is identified as the menopausal/postmenopausal 'problem'. While some women may benefit from hormones, many or most women will be able to go through the transition phase and minimize osteoporosis and heart-disease risks with less hazardous measures such as a healthy diet, appropriate physical exercise, and using alternatives to hormones. Whether in determining research priorities or influencing the information the mass media should give to empower women through informed decision-making, much more attention needs to be focused on healthy alternatives to hormones. As Kathleen MacPherson (1987: 60) puts it:

To recommend widespread use of HRT as a public health measure to prevent osteoporosis without assessing the needs of individual women would be the same as recommending that everyone take antihypertensive drugs because so many people have high blood pressure. For no other condition is anything as potentially dangerous as hormones being recommended as a preventative measure.

Osteoporosis

Creating the Fear of Osteoporosis

In order to create markets for their products, both drug companies and calcium manufacturers effectively used the media to introduce people to osteoporosis, a previously ignored condition, and to scare them into buying products which promised to prevent this. Both prevention consciousness and fear of ageing contributed to the success of osteoporosis-related advertising. Many advertisements played on both of these, such as one for a calcium supplement which showed a healthy thirty-year-old transformed

to a stooped 65-year-old within thirty seconds (Giges, 1986). Such an image not only capitalizes on the fear of losing youthful attractiveness, it also draws on even deeper fears of disability leading to loss of independence. Information on hip fractures has been presented in an even more frightening way. For example, a popular guide to preventing osteoporosis states: 'The consequences of hip fractures can be devastating. Fewer than one-half of all women who suffer a hip fracture regain normal function. Fifteen percent die shortly after their injury, and nearly 30 percent die within a year' (Notelovitz and Ware, 1982: 37). The deaths are not inevitable and are related to complications such as pneumonia but they certainly serve as a useful scare tactic.

The information about complications of osteoporosis as a major 'killer' of women in their eighties and the linking of osteoporosis with menopause in such a way that osteoporosis practically becomes identified as a symptom of menopause, can be further connected to imply that menopause itself is a killer unless hormones are taken to stop this process.

In fact, osteoporosis and how it affects people, is much more complicated and unpredictable than the hormone- and calcium-promoting information suggests. Osteoporosis is not an 'all or nothing' condition, it is 'not a disease like tuberculosis that a person either has or does not have' (Parfitt, 1984). A statement like, 'It would appear inevitable that if a person lives long enough, he or she will suffer from osteoporosis.' (Kirkpatrick, 1987: 45) may help British or American women put their newly created fear of osteoporosis into perspective. However, taking a more cross-cultural approach such as, 'osteoporosis is not a natural part of ageing and does not occur all over the world, even among the elderly' (Brown, 1988) will be more useful for understanding that osteoporosis is not inevitable, is very much related to industrialized Western diets and lifestyles, and that *real* prevention has nothing to do with hormones.

Looking at cross-cultural data, we see that blaming osteoporosis on an estrogen deficiency is just a little less absurd than blaming heart attacks on a deficiency of by-pass surgery. Surgery might solve the problem for a while, but it is not a deficiency of the operation that caused the problem. (Brown, 1988: 6)

Osteoporosis often gets billed as a major health issue for all older women, when, in fact, some women are much more at risk than others. The fact that lighter complexioned women with ancestors from northern Europe or Asia are much more likely to develop osteoporosis than darker complexioned women with African, Hispanic, Mediterranean or Native American ancestry probably accounts for this condition finally receiving the attention it has. Pressing health needs of 'minority' older women as defined by the women themselves still tend to get ignored. While looking at ethnic influence on osteoporosis risk, several other points should be made. The osteoporosis risk for Jewish women seems to lie somewhere between the relatively low or relatively high risks of the above mentioned groups. The term 'Black' is used differently in American and British publications. So, while it is accurate to say Black (meaning African-American) women are less at risk than white women in the US, in the British context, it must be clarified that women of Asian descent will be at significantly higher risk than women of African ancestry. Also, just because groups have lower rates of osteoporosis, does not mean that no one in those groups is at risk. Good health information materials need to emphasize this (Partlow, 1991).

Fractures Are Not Synonymous with Osteoporosis

Similarly, the disabling or life-threatening fractures must not be seen as synonymous with osteoporosis. Not all women with osteoporosis have fractures, not all women with fractures have osteoporosis. Studies have shown that women with and without hip fractures had similar bone densities, and women in other cultures have low rates of bone fractures even with low bone density (National Women's Health Network, 1989).

Factors such as tendency to fall, muscle strength, flexibility, having to walk on icy pavements, etc., will influence the chance of fracture as much as the density of bone mass (Whatley, 1988a). Falls in the elderly are known to be significantly greater for people using antidepressants, sedative/hypnotics and vasodilators (drugs that dilate blood vessels) (Myers, 1991) and modification of medications has been shown to be an effective method of reducing falls and fractures in a nursing-home setting (Wolfe, 1991a). So in many cases, reducing rather than increasing drugs will be the key preventative issue for minimizing complications of osteoporosis in elderly women.

A more creative and caring, less profit-motivated approach might come up with some very interesting ideas about what to do about osteoporosis (Whatley, 1988a). For example, Kathleen MacPherson emphasizes that health policies must reflect the need for bold structural changes in our society instead of the usual incremental or 'bandaid' policies suggested as osteoporosis prevention (MacPherson, 1987: 61). Her recommendations are for policies 'to alleviate the feminization of poverty, a living wage, pension plans, social security benefits for homemakers, etc., and a national health care plan to provide ongoing health promotion and maintenance for all citizens.'

Although studies have shown that ORT can slow down bone loss and can reduce the risk of hip fractures, that information gets misinterpreted into inaccurate messages. ORT may slow down bone loss but it does nothing to restore bone mineral (Ettinger, 1987), but how many women with osteoporosis are informed that the most ORT can do for them is to slow down or stabilize their condition? Many women who are taking HRT are making that decision based upon what is known about ORT. A few studies have shown that HRT also helps slow down bone loss, but no study has shown a reduction in fractures in women taking HRT (National Women's Health Network, 1989).

Osteoporosis Screening

Detecting osteoporosis also gets deliberately confused with preventing the condition. In the US, osteoporosis screening has been widely promoted. Finding a noninvasive way to predict a woman's risk for fractures may seem a benefit of medical science with which few could find fault. Certainly the prevalence and potential consequences of osteoporosis are serious enough to justify screening.

However, an evaluation of bone mass measurements as a screening procedure reveals a different picture (Napoli, 1988 and Whatley and Worcester, 1989). Several techniques are currently being used to detect osteoporosis and these techniques vary in availability, cost, accuracy, reproducibility, and what they actually measure. But, there are certain problems with all of them and the most available techniques are the least reliable.

While screening can show that bone mass has been lost, screening cannot predict how rapidly someone will be losing bone and cannot predict whether or not someone is at risk from osteoporosis. Bone loss is neither constant nor predictable. Knowing someone's bone mass at one age does not help predict how fast that woman will lose bone mass; a woman with a low bone mass may end up losing at a very slow rate and a woman with a much higher bone mass might end up losing rapidly (Whatley, 1988a). Screening is even limited in its ability to identify full-blown cases of the disease. While bone density screening would be expected to differentiate between those who do and do not have osteoporosis-related hip fractures, these measurements are of little use in the most at-risk elderly population because, 'if the highest bone mass seen in patients with fractures is designated as the "fracture threshold", then nearly all women over seventy will by definition have osteoporosis' (Ott, 1986: 875).

It must be emphasized that techniques for measuring bone mass are extremely useful for research purposes. However, at this stage, unreliable but sophisticated, expensive screening has little to offer the consumer. Requiring regular monitoring of bone mass, osteoporosis screening offers enormous potential for clinics as a profitable procedure. There is also the possibility that women will be hooked into a system which has little to offer them except hormone prescriptions and the advice that weight-bearing exercises and a calcium-rich diet at an earlier age 'might have helped' (Worcester and Whatley, 1988a).

Role of Diet

Indeed, there is plenty of evidence that Western/industrialized lifestyles and diets are responsible for the prevalence of osteoporosis and the fact that it affects women much more than men. Britain and the US report much higher rates of osteoporosis than less industrialized/Westernized countries. For example, the US rate is 24 times higher than that of some other countries. People in Singapore, Hong Kong, certain parts of Yugoslavia and the Maori of New Zealand have very low rates of osteoporosis-caused fractures, and Africans and people living traditional lifestyles have been described as 'almost immune' to osteoporosis (Brown, 1988).

Osteoporosis as a male disease in Britain and the US gets very little attention (because no one has figured out how to convince men that their problems are all due to 'oestrogen deficiency'?) despite the fact that (US) men suffer one-sixth as many spinal fractures and approximately one-half as many hip fractures as women. In other parts of the world, in Hong Kong, some parts of Yugoslavia, and in the South African Bantu, it has been documented that men experience osteoporosis and fractures at the same or higher rates than women. Medical anthropologist Susan Brown (1988) gives the following explanations for the excessive development of osteoporosis in Western women: (1) as a group, women have less exposure to sunlight which helps the body make vitamin D which is essential for calcium absorption; (2) women are not encouraged to be as physically active; (3) women use more prescription drugs; (4) women are more subject to removal of the sex-hormone producing gonads, the ovaries (if the testes are removed, men also develop osteoporosis); and (5) men generally consume a higher-quality/more nutritional diet than women.

Western diets contribute to the development of osteoporosis both by not providing enough calcium in the first place, and more importantly, by 'wasting' the calcium which is ingested. The typical Western diet encourages a heavy imbalance in the ratio of phosphorus (high levels in carbonated beverages and high-protein foods, including meats) to calcium which can cause a loss of bone calcium; low levels of vitamin D and high levels of fibre, oxalates and phytates interfere with calcium absorption and high intakes of caffeine and alcohol also significantly contribute to excessive bone loss (Finn, 1987 and Brown, 1988). Instead of dealing with anything as complex as the calcium-wasting effects of our diet, or questioning reducing foods like meat which are central to our diet and economy, calcium has been promoted as something one can simply add to what one already consumes. Retail sales of calcium supplements grew from $18 million in 1980 to $166 million in 1986, a calcium-fortified sugar-free drink mix was marketed, and the sales of the diet cola, Tab, tripled when calcium was added. Jumping on the calcium bandwagon and hoping it would make people forget their cholesterol concern, the dairy industry launched a campaign with the theme 'dairy foods: calcium the way nature intended' (Giges, 1986).

It is well established that because bone mass peaks at age thirty-five years, the greatest benefit from calcium occurs in the years from birth to age thirty-five (Finn, 1987). However, it is discouraging to see how, in the push towards hormones, the role of calcium for menopausal and postmenopausal women has been ignored or discounted. In explaining why recommended intakes of calcium for older women had not been increased in the Food and Nutrition Board's latest (10th edition) *Recommendation for Daily Nutrient Allowances,* the director stated,

'because oestrogen is more effective in preventing osteoporosis than calcium'.

That answer is much too simplistic and totally ignores the risks of oestrogens and the fact that many women cannot or will not take hormones. Most importantly, such attitudes influence research and policy agendas so that the potential of calcium alone or in sufficient quantities to reduce the amounts of oestrogens needed, is not being explored despite work showing the merit of this approach. In a study believed to be the first to look at both lifelong and current calcium intake in normal postmenopausal women not taking oestrogens, researchers found a protective effect of calcium on bone density in women who reported high calcium intakes *both* throughout their lifetime and presently (Cauley, 1988). Even Bruce Ettinger, previously quoted as supporting the goal of keeping women on oestrogens for their entire postmenopausal lives, gives us reason to believe calcium deserves more attention. He states:

Although calcium given alone is incapable of maintaining skeletal mass, high intakes of calcium allow estrogen to be more effective; by simply augmenting calcium intake to 1,500 mg. per day women may be adequately protected while taking half the usual dosage of estrogen . . . It has also been suggested but not proven that very low intake of calcium—perhaps less than 300 mg. per day—can also diminish or abolish estrogen's protection (Ettinger, 1987: 33–4).

Thinking of *real* osteoporosis prevention is a useful case study of how lifelong interactions of social, economic and political issues affect women's health and how factors in a young woman's life affect her chances of being able to maximize on her full potential. With 'femininity' so closely associated with an obsession with thinness and conflicting messages given to young women about physical activity, sex-role socialization and gender identity have to be seen as causal agents of osteoporosis. The obsession with thinness and fear of fat promote osteoporosis in several different ways. First, avoiding high-calcium foods because of calorific content, dieting that results in nutritional deficiencies or nutritional imbalances, fasting and purging can be identified as behaviours which interfere with calcium absorption and contribute to low peak bone mass (Kirkpatrick, 1987). Secondly, low body weight reduces the mechanical forces applied to the skeleton by gravity and muscle contraction so there is less 'built-in' stimulation for bone formation. As a generalization, heavier people tend towards more bone mass (Goodman, 1987). Additionally, it is well established that fat tissue in a woman's body produces oestrogen and the more fat a woman has, the more oestrogen she will produce. But how many women know this or can listen to the message if they hear it? Society so consistently pushes thinness and hormones, that contradictory healthy advice like Mary Kirkpatrick's 'A Self Care Model for Osteoporosis' is seldom mentioned.

Ironically, midlife may be a good time to have a little extra weight to act as a protective mechanism against osteoporosis. If fat tissue provides more estrogen, the bone loss at menopause may be

224

slowed. Also, body weight can act as a loading factor and can produce necessary stress on the bony structure to form bone mass. (Kirkpatrick, 1987: 48–9).

Physical activity

Numerous studies have shown that exercise, particularly of the weight-bearing type, can promote bone strength in women under thirty-five and help maintain bone mass in women over thirty-five. But, how often do women, particularly young women, get useful, sensible advice about the health benefits of moderate exercise? Too often women get only one of two equally inappropriate messages: don't exercise or, do too much of it!

When tested for physical performance, girls and boys are matched up to ages ten to twelve. Thereafter, they get very different messages about what is 'ladylike' or 'masculine' and, after age twelve, boys tend to increase in strength and cardiovascular fitness more than girls who are discouraged from being physically active (Whatley, 1988b). The young women who resist the pressure to be sedentary, are often encouraged to go to the other extreme. Both the 'cosmetic athletes' who obsessively exercise to achieve 'beauty' and the serious athletes who exercise too strenuously, can delay menarche or cause amenorrhoea which can be detrimental to building bone density (Goodman, 1987).

Interestingly the relationship of 'athletic amenorrhoea' to osteoporosis started attracting quite a bit of media attention as more young women have begun to explore their athletic capabilities. Physiologically, the explanation and consequences of amenorrhoea may be the same whether caused by athletic training, ballet dancing or extreme dieting. However, as Western cultures find ballet and dieting to be ideal 'feminine' activities, the media attention has focused almost exclusively on the potential osteoporotic risks of athletic amenorrhoea. Regular, moderate, weight-bearing exercise is undoubtedly a healthier approach to osteoporosis prevention. Further research is needed to determine the type, intensity, duration and frequency of physical activity which best builds and maintains bone mass (Goodman, 1987).

When to Start Hormones?

If one believes that hormone therapy is the way to prevent osteoporosis, when should that be started?

The peak of bone mass is reached by the time a person reaches thirty-five. After that, both men and women will gradually lose minerals from their bone for the rest of their lives. Menopause gets associated with this process because women lose bone mass most rapidly during the transition years immediately before, during, and after menopause. Susan Brown (1988) explains that, 'a woman loses a full half of all the bone she will lose during her lifetime between the age of thirty-five and fifty.' Jessop McDonnell (1987: 11) states it less delicately: 'the eight to ten years following menopause may be characterized by a ravaging assault on the skeletal system.' When a woman has settled into being postmenopausal, the rate of bone loss will slow

down to being similar to the rate at which men have been losing minerals.

The years thirty-five to fifty are key years for prevention. Ettinger emphasizes:

Correct timing and adequate duration of estrogen therapy can maximize the therapy's benefits. Women should begin taking estrogen at menopause; the longer they delay, the less bone protection will be obtained. Knowing that the most rapid phase of bone loss is in the five to ten years after menopause, most experts do not recommend estrogen for postmenopausal women who have not taken estrogen during the first 10 to 15 years after the onset of menopause. (1987: 36).

Obvious problems become apparent. Many women being screened for osteoporosis *are* being started on hormones well after they would have had their most benefit. This can create a 'yo-yo' effect as the body adjusts to postmenopausal levels of oestrogen, then must readjust to artificially high levels. Not being told how hormones work, many women go on and off hormones without realizing that the 'yo-yo' effect could actually exaggerate loss of bone. Once women are on hormones, they will need to stay on them indefinitely, to keep delaying the transition which would cause loss of bone. The ramifications, of course, are that women are on hormones from premenopause for the rest of their lives and dependent upon expensive medical services to monitor how their bodies adjust to these products. A drug would have to have minimal side effects to be appropriate for continuous use for this duration of time. In fact, beginning on oestrogen during premenopausal years and continuing for many years is exactly the pattern of use which puts women most at risk for breast cancer. With that information, many women will feel that their own risk of osteoporosis does not justify the increased risk of breast cancer.

Heart Disease

Women may have become saturated with information about ORT and osteoporosis; a new angle has been necessary to raise anxiety to the point at which a new group of women will actively seek ORT prescriptions. The long overdue attention to *prevention* of heart disease in women has provided exactly the right focus for an expanded ORT market, giving physicians an additional rationale to prescribe it. The new media coverage of women and heart disease has helped generate fears and then ORT has been offered as the solution.

This contrasts with approaches in the past when very little attention had been paid to either prevention or treatment of heart disease in women, for it has traditionally been viewed as a man's disease. While men experience heart disease at younger ages and have more heart attacks than women, women account for 47 per cent of the heart-attack deaths in the United States, making it the leading cause of death for women (Winslow, 1991). In addition, women who suffer a heart attack are more likely to die than men (39 per cent vs 31 per cent) and more likely to suffer a second heart attack within four years (20 per cent vs 15 per cent) (Winslow, 1991). However, these high risks for women have not been reflected in treatment. For example, in one study of patients hospitalized for coronary heart disease, men were 28 per cent more likely to have angiography, a procedure to determine the extent of arterial blockage, and 48 per cent more likely to have bypass surgery or balloon angioplasty. In another study of men and women hospitalized for major heart attacks, men were nearly twice as likely to have angiography and bypass surgery (Winslow, 1991). This study also found that, before the heart attack, chest pains and other symptoms were more disabling for women than men. One of the authors of the latter report emphasized her concern that women who continued to have chest pains after their heart attacks still do not receive angiography (Kolata, 1991a).

These studies and others document the lack of attention by the medical profession to heart disease as a major women's health issue, but the fact that these studies exist at all is a sign that there is finally some concern. If heart disease is the leading killer of women in the United States, why has there been so little emphasis on it before? Why do so many women fear breast cancer but are apparently unaware of their risks of heart disease? Without going into reasons for past neglect, it is possible to offer some explanations for the new-found hype of heart disease as 'number 1 killer of women'. One view is that the market is fickle and there needs to be a 'disease of the month' to capture the interest of the media, consumers, practitioners, and the people (politicians included) who control research funding. However, with an old disease, only a new angle, preferably with something to sell, will generate the necessary interest. For example, there was considerable media attention when a study suggested that aspirin reduced the risk of heart attacks in men (Steering Committee of the Physicians' Health Study Group, 1989). Aspirin manufacturers must have been delighted by the press aspirin received, especially after the earlier negative publicity about Reye syndrome, a potentially fatal condition in children caused by aspirin being given during a viral infection such as flu or chicken-pox. However, the media reports rarely mentioned that the study was done on men only and could not be extrapolated to women. In response to the gap in the research, a recent study reported that women who took one to six aspirin a week experienced a 25 per cent reduction in risk of heart attack compared to women who took no aspirin (Manson, Stampfer, and Colditz, 1991). The results are hardly conclusive, however. The study, which included only nurses, was an observational one, not an experimental one (the women made their own choices about taking aspirin and reported their choices. The researchers simply looked for the effects). This leads to the strong possibility of confounding variables, for the groups may vary in much more than the factor of aspirin use (Appel and Bush, 1991).

In spite of the flaws, this study received a lot of publicity and generated more interest in women and heart disease, providing a good opening for calling attention to the role of ORT in preventing heart disease. In an apparent attempt to expand their market, Wyeth-Ayerst, the manufacturers of Premarin, the most commonly prescribed oral oestrogen, requested that the US Food and Drug Administration (FDA) allow promotion of Premarin for the prevention of heart disease, at least for women who have had hysterectomies (Rovner, 1990). The FDA Advisory Committee concluded, after listening to much conflicting testimony, that 'the cardiovascular benefits of estrogen replacement therapy with Premarin in women without a uterus may outweigh the risks, considering the individual patient's risk for various estrogen related diseases and conditions' (Rovner, 1990: 9). Dangerously, this statement, as it has been reported and repeated, has been reduced to a simple 'benefits outweigh the risks'; in addition, the distinctions between ORT and HRT are rarely clarified.

In terms of the research itself, the results are not clearcut. Generalizations are limited because almost all the subjects have been white and middle class. As with the aspirin study, these studies have been observational; the researchers did not control the choice of treatments but merely observed the results based on the women's choices. A major confounding factor is that the women who *choose* Premarin may be at reduced risk for heart attack anyway. For example, a co-author of the major lipid study cited in the FDA hearings, Elizabeth Barrett-Connor, said that women who used Premarin were also less likely to smoke, were thinner, and were better educated than non-users, all of which might have been factors in reducing risk (Rovner, 1990). One of the clearest ways to emphasize that users and non-users may represent different populations is the result of one study which found users of oestrogen had lower mortality rates, not only from heart disease, but also from accidents, suicide and homicide. As Cindy Pearson, of the National Women's Health Network, asked, when she was testifying *against* FDA approval for Premarin being promoted for the prevention of heart disease, 'Does this mean we can conclude that estrogen use protects one from being murdered?' (Rovner, 1990: 9).

No study completed to date has been without the major flaw of lack of comparability between users and non-users of ORT. This is well illustrated in a study published after the FDA hearings, which was heralded as more good news about ORT. The study of 49,000 postmenopausal women showed 44 per cent fewer heart attacks and 39 per cent reduced risk of heart-attack death in those who took ORT (Kolata, 1991b). However, the study was on nurses, 98 per cent of whom were white, who had made their own choices about use of ORT. As an example of this problem, a very heavy woman, who might be more at risk for heart attack, might also be less likely to select ORT because she would also be less likely to experience menopausal changes for which ORT is recommended. A nurse who considered herself at risk for heart disease might not have taken ORT because physicians in the 1970s were discouraging women at risk of heart disease from taking oestrogen at all (Sojourner, 1991).

Besides the studies directed at heart-attack risks, much of the support for the role of ORT in preventing heart disease comes from data on HDL (high density lipoprotein) and LDL (low density lipoprotein). *Higher* HDL and *lower* LDL are favourable to reduced risk of heart disease. A review article by Bush and colleagues (Bush *et al.,* 1988) provides a good summary of the factors affecting these lipoproteins in women. These include genetics, diet, obesity, exercise, alcohol, cigarette smoking, oral contraceptives.

The data on oral contraceptives is particularly interesting. All formulations increase LDL, the 'bad lipoprotein'. The largest increases in LDL occur with the lowest oestrogen dose and the strongest anti-oestrogenic progestin. As the potency of progestin increases, HDL, the 'good' lipoprotein, decreases. The implications from the oral contraceptive data for the use of ORT as compared to HRT are borne out by the studies on oestrogens as menopausal therapy. According to Bush and colleagues (Bush *et al.,* 1988), use of unopposed and synthetic oestrogens leads to the more favourable HDL/LDL profile. However, cyclic oestrogen-progestin therapy (HRT) has either a minimal or adverse effect on lipoproteins, depending on the progestin used. In other words, while oestrogen therapy by itself may have very positive effects, the addition of progestins completely negates those effects. HRT, therefore, in the best case, provides no benefits in terms of HDL/LDL profile, the main route by which ORT is believed to have a protective effect against heart disease. However, many women take HRT to avoid the increased risks from ORT in terms of endometrial cancer. If the progestin component protects against endometrial cancer but undoes the protective effects against heart disease, women may have to make difficult decisions about which disease they fear most.

The lipoprotein data also provides some interesting results about alcohol. Bush *et al.* (1988) state that moderate alcohol consumption is strongly related to increased HDL levels in men and women. A recent report suggested that moderate alcohol consumption has a protective effect against heart disease in men, which supports previous work finding benefits for men and women. If oestrogen manufacturers are allowed to say their products reduce heart disease, why shouldn't beer and wine companies request that the FDA allow them to promote their products as reducing risk of heart disease? Such a claim would surely be countered with the argument that the risks of alcohol consumption outweigh the benefits. But do we really know that benefits of ORT outweigh the risks?

Some of the answers about ORT and HRT may come from a new study known as PEPI, the Postmenopausal Estrogen/Progestin Interventions Trial, which is funded by the National Institutes of Health. It is a double-blinded placebo study with random assignment of women to one of five groups: oestrogen only, one of three oestrogen/progestin combinations, or placebo only. The study will measure, among other factors, cholesterol and its fractions, and blood pressure, while also studying osteoporosis and endometrial changes. When the data from this study is analysed completely, it may be appropriate to make some recommendations about HRT and ORT. Unfortunately,

the study is only for three years so only short-term consequences can be evaluated. We may know something more about short-term changes in HDL, LDL, and bone density. However, information about other risks, especially breast cancer, will not be forthcoming.

In the meantime, while we wait for the data to come in, perhaps it would be more appropriate to focus on what we do know about preventing heart disease in women and provide education about diet, exercise, smoking, and treating high blood pressure (Wolfe, 1991b).

Breast Cancer

In the attempt to reduce the risk of heart disease or osteoporosis by taking ORT or HRT, women may be replacing one disease with another. There is strong evidence that oestrogens increase the risk of breast cancer, but the issue seems to be how big a risk that really is. A Swedish study, published in 1989, showed a 10 per cent increased relative risk of breast cancer in women on oestrogens, with the risk increasing with length of treatment. After nine years of use, there was an excess risk of 70 per cent. The addition of progestins did not reduce the risk and may even have increased it slightly (Bergkvist *et al.,* 1989). The differences in the oestrogen of choice in the US and Sweden was apparently one reason why this study did not receive more press, as well as the fact that the risk was seen as only slightly increased.

A later study from the United States received more attention but also was presented as showing a slight risk. In a study that followed over 12,000 nurses for ten years, Colditz and colleagues found that women taking oestrogen were 30 to 40 per cent more likely to develop breast cancer than those who did not (Colditz *et al.,* 1990). This might be seen as a serious risk in a disease which may strike one out of nine women in the United States. However, the media coverage played down the effects as slight. For example, referring to the increased risk of 30 to 40 per cent, one article claimed, 'But this risk is considered small; it is only about half the risk a woman faces if her mother had breast cancer' (Kolata, 1990: A11). This is hardly reassuring for women considering ORT who have other risk factors, particularly the woman whose mother had breast cancer. The one note that women may actually find reassuring is that the additional risk seems to disappear a year after stopping oestrogens. However, that does not help women much who are on a long-term plan for oestrogen to maintain reduced risk of osteoporosis and heart disease.

A large number of studies on ORT and breast cancer were evaluated using meta-analysis, a statistical method to evaluate data from a number of studies, which can give a more accurate picture than a single study (Steinberg *et al.,* 1991). The data suggests an increased risk of breast cancer for women who used oestrogen for more than five years. Women with a family history of breast cancer had a markedly increased risk. A particularly interesting finding was that the studies in which oestrogen therapy was started before menopause showed a much greater increase in risk than those which included only women who started oestrogen after menopause. Because oestrogen as a prevention for osteoporosis should ideally be started *before* menopause to prevent the period of greatest bone loss, those women who follow the plan most likely to prevent osteoporosis will be at most risk for breast cancer. They will have started before menopause and they will need to continue indefinitely, because if they go off at any time the bone loss will occur quickly. The duration of oestrogen therapy is clearly related to risk and going off it seems the only way to reduce the risk. While progestins may protect these women against endometrial cancer, it will apparently do nothing to reduce breast-cancer risks.

In weighing up the risks of breast cancer versus the possibility that ORT or HRT can prevent osteoporosis or heart disease, women essentially need to decide which disease they fear the most. Dr Lynn Rosenberg, a Boston epidemiologist, says that most women decide whether to take oestrogen by a sort of fear meter, asking themselves which diseases or discomforts they most dread (Kolata, 1991c). Even more to the point, Dr Adriane Fugh-Berman (1991: 3), speaking on behalf of the National Women's Health Network puts it:

We are concerned that the concept of disease prevention may be expanded to include the concept of disease substitution.

Dr Fugh-Berman's statement was made in reference to tamoxifen, a totally different topic, but one which we mention here for the purpose of emphasizing the complications and unknowns of menopausal/postmenopausal hormones. Tamoxifen is a drug which has been recognized for its effectiveness in prolonging the disease-free interval in postmenopausal women with oestrogen receptor-positive breast cancer. However, now, tamoxifen is being experimented with in both England and the US as a way to *prevent* breast cancer in normal healthy women. In the US, the National Women's Health Network was the only organization to present testimony to the Food and Drug Administration Committee on Oncology Drugs opposing the trial. This is not the place to detail why the trial is 'premature in its assumptions, weak in its hypotheses, questionable in its ethics, and misguided in its public health ramifications' (Fugh-Berman, 1991: 3). Relevant to this paper is the fact that tamoxifen is known to be effective as breast-cancer treatment because it works as an *anti-oestrogen*: it blocks the effect of oestrogen on the breast. Researchers justify studying the effects of tamoxifen on healthy women because they feel there is sufficient evidence to suggest that blocking the effects of oestrogen on the breasts may be a way of preventing (delaying?) breast cancer.

The irony of the situation is obvious. How can it be that at this particular moment in history, in the name of 'prevention', huge numbers of women are being given oestrogen products and another group is being studied with anti-oestrogens? *All* the women taking either oestrogens or anti-oestrogens are part of massive experiments which should help us learn more about hormones but do *nothing*

to support health-promoting methods of disease prevention.

Conclusion

HRT raises large questions for individual women trying to decide whether to take it and for women's health movements which must analyse why, once again, huge numbers of women are swallowing a product of unknown safety. There are no simple answers for either individual women or for feminist health activists.

Many of the issues which individual women will want to weigh as they make their own decisions have been covered in this paper. At some level, it is a very personal decision to balance known and unknown risks with the narrow range of choices available. Each woman will want to make today's and tomorrow's decisions based on her own personal hormone history. Most of the studies which have been done have been on women for whom oral contraceptives were not available. It remains to be seen how much different formulations of oral contraceptives for different lengths of time influence issues related to ORT or HRT. Much research will be done on many aspects of hormone use in the next few years. Any woman taking, or considering, hormones should find a source of information which she trusts, such as Women's Health in England or the National Women's Health Network in North America. Excellent health check-ups, including pelvic exams, mammography and physical breast exams, pap smears, monitoring of blood lipids and blood pressure, and endometrial biopsies, must be available to all women who are or have been on hormones for any length of time.

HRT raises enormous challenges for women's health movements. Many of us have lived through the tragedies of DES daughters, the Dalkon Shield, thalidomide, and toxic shock syndrome. One of the biggest questions must be, why aren't the lessons from the immediate past more central to our present debates? Why do large numbers of women not know about, or choose to ignore, the tremendous risks involved in taking drugs whose long-term safety is not known? An even trickier question is why are so few people questioning the long-term safety of hormonal products for menopausal and postmenopausal women? A number of people who have been allies in the struggle for safer contraceptives are not involved in evaluating and critiquing the mass marketing of ORT and HRT. Is ageism a factor? Are we willing to accept a few more side effects in a product designed specifically for older women? Are we willing to lower our standards just a wee bit for products which promise to interfere with the ageing process?

The HRT debate—or more accurately, the *lack* of debate—serves as a reminder of the urgency of empowering *all* women to understand their own bodies and for them to have access to appropriate (language, reading level, relevant to own issues) information for the 'choices' they face. One of the biggest lessons in the marketing of HRT has been that many women still do not know enough about the normal healthy workings of their bodies to resist a mass manipulation of the fear factor.

ORT and HRT are valuable products. Their availability will definitely make a difference in the quality and length of life for *some* women. However, they will probably never be products which should be given to *most* women for a long length of time. If these products are as valuable as the manufacturers say, they should be available to the women who would benefit most from them. In the present situation it tends to be the healthiest groups of women with easy access to the medical system who are given hormones.

To answer any of the questions raised in this paper, long-term, controlled studies which look at multiple parameters and the interactions of many factors must be done with diverse groups of women. Without a clearer understanding of the actual value and risks of ORT and HRT, the mass marketing of these products is certainly premature. A renewed focus on *real* prevention and self-help as a way of wrestling control *for* the consumer, *away* from the medical system and makers of highly profitable products, continues to be an urgent priority for women's health movements.

Notes

The authors want to acknowledge the work of the National Women's Health Network's Hormone Education Campaign in providing the key leadership for US women in the evaluation and critique of menopausal hormones. The excellent publications and testimonies before Food and Drug Administration Committees have been extremely valuable in preparing this paper. *Taking Hormones and Women's Health* is available for $5 (+ postage) from the National Women's Health Network, 514 10th St., N.W. (Suite 400), Washington, D.C. 20004
Women's Health, 52 Featherstone Street, London, EC1Y 8RT.

References

Appel, Lawrence, J. and Bush, Trudy (1991) 'Preventing Heart Disease in Women. Another Role for Aspirin' *Journal of the American Medical Association* Vol. 266, pp. 565–6.

Bergkvist, Leif et al. (1989) 'The Risk of Breast Cancer after Estrogen and Estrogen-progestin Replacement' *The New England Journal of Medicine* Vol. 321, No. 5, pp. 293–7.

Brown, Susan (1988) 'Osteoporosis: An Anthropologist Sorts Fact from Fallacy', unpublished longer version of article which was edited and appeared as 'Osteoporosis: Sorting Fact from Fallacy' in (National Women's Health Network) *Network News* July/August, pp. 1, 5–6.

Bush, Trudy, Fried, Linda P. and Barrett-Connor, Elizabeth (1988) 'Cholesterol Lipoproteins and Coronary Heart Disease in Women' *Clinical Chemistry* Vol. 34, No. 8(B), pp. B60–B70.

Cauley, Jane, A (1988) and Gutai, James P., Kuller, Lewis H., Ledonna, Dorothea, Sandler, Rivka B., Sashin, Donald and Powell, John G. (1988) 'Endogenous Estrogen Levels and Calcium Intakes in Postmenopausal Women' *Journal of the American Medical Association* Vol. 260, No. 21, pp. 3150–5.

Cedar Rapids Gazette (1991) 'Estrogen Cuts Heart Disease Risk: Study' *Cedar Rapids (Iowa) Gazette* September 12.

Colditz, G. A., Stampfer, M. J., Willitt, W. C. et al. (1990) 'Prospective Study of Estrogen Replacement Therapy and Risk of Breast Cancer in Postmenopausal Women' *Journal of the American Medical Association* Vol. 264, pp. 2648–53.

Dejanikus, Tacie (1985)' Major Drug Manufacturer Funds Osteoporosis Education Campaign' (National Women's Health Network) *Network News* May/June, pp. 1,3.

Eagen, Andrea Boroff (1989) 'Hormone Replacement Therapy Overview' (National Women's Health Network) *Network News* May/June, pp. 1,3.

Ettinger, Bruce (1987) 'Update: Estrogen and Postmenopausal osteoporosis 1976–1986' *Health Values* Vol. 11, No. 4, pp. 31–6.

Finn, Susan (1987) 'Osteoporosis: A Nutritionist's Approach' Health Values Vol. 11, No.4, pp.20–3.

Fugh-Berman, Adriane (1991) 'Tamoxifen in Healthy Women: Preventative Health or Preventing Health?' (National Women's Health Network) *Network News* September/October, pp. 3–4.

Giges, Nancy (1986) 'Calcium Market Shrugs Off Study' *Advertising Age* Vol. 59, pp. 49,56.

Goodman, Carol E. (1987) 'Osteoporosis and Physical Activity' Health Values Vol. 11, No.4, pp. 24–30.

Kirkpatrick, Mary(1987) 'A Self Care Model for Osteoporosis' *Health Values* Vol. 11 No.4, pp.44–50.

Kolata, Gina (1990) 'Cancer Risk in Estrogen is Slight, Study Asserts' *New York Times* 28 November, p. A 11.

—(1991a) 'Women Don't Get Equal Heart Care' *New York Times* 25 July pp. A1,A9.

—(1991b) 'Estrogen After Menopause Cuts Heart Attack Risk, Study Finds' *New York Times* 12 September, pp. A1, A13.

—(1991c) 'Women Face Dilemma Over Estrogen Therapy' *New York Times* 17 September.

Macpherson, Kathleen I. (1987) 'Osteoporosis: The New Flaw in Woman or in Science?' Health Values Vol. 11, No. 4, pp. 57–61.

Manson, J. E., Stampfer, M. J., Colditz, G. A. et al. (1991) 'A Prospective Study of Aspirin Use and Primary Prevention of Cardiovascular Disease in Women' *Journal of the American Medical Association,* Vol. 266, pp. 521–7.

McDonnell, Jessop M., Lane, Joseph M, and Zimmerman, Peter A. (1987) 'Osteoporosis: Definition, Risk Factors, Etiology and Diagnosis' *Health Values* Vol. 11, No. 4, pp. 10–15.

Myers, Ann H., Baker, Susan P., Vannatta, Mark L., Abbey, Helen, and Robinson, Elizabeth G. (1991) 'Risk Factors Associated with Falls and Injuries among Elderly Institutionalized Persons' *American Journal of Epidemiology* Vol. 133, No. 11, pp. 1179–90.

Napoli, Maryann (1988) 'Screening for Osteoporosis: An Idea Whose Time Has Not Yet Come' in Worcester and Whatley (1988b) pp. 115– 19.

National Prescriptions Audit, IMS America Ltd., prepared for the National Women's Health Network (hormones and breast cancer files) by the USA Food and Drug Administration Staff, February, 1990.

National Women's Health Network (1989) *Taking Hormones and Women's Health* (available from the NWHN, 514 10th St., N.W., (Suite 400), Washington, D.C. 20004.

Notelovitz, Morris and Ware, Marsha (1982) *Stand Tall! The Informed Woman's Guide to Preventing Osteoporosis.* Gainesville, Florida: Triad.

Ott, Susan (1986) 'Should Women Get Screening Bone Mass Measurements?' *Annals of Internal Medicine* Vol. 104, No. 6, pp. 874–6.

Parfitt, M. (1984) 'Definition of Osteoporosis: Age-related Loss of Bone and its Relationship to Increased Fracture Risk', presented at the National Institutes of Health Consensus Development Conference on Osteoporosis, Bethesda, Maryland, 1–2 April, quoted in MacPherson (1987).

Partlow, Lian (1991) Personal communication.

Pearson, Cindy (1991) Testimony before the USA Food and Drug Administartion Select Committee on Ageing, Subcommittee on Housing and Consumer Interests, 30 May.

Rovner, Sandy (1990) 'Estrogen Therapy: More Data, Less Certainty' *Washington Post Health* 4 September p. 9.

Sloane, Ethel (1985) *Biology of Women* New York: John Wiley.

Sojourner (1991) 'Debating Estrogen Replacement Therapy' *Sojourner-The Women's Forum* November, pp. 13–14.

Specter, Michael (1989) 'Hormone Use in Menopause Tied to Cancer' *Washington Post* 3 August, p. 1.

Steering Committee of the Physicians' Health Study Group (1989) 'Final Report on the Aspirin Component of the On-going Physicians' Health Study' *New England Journal of Medicine* Vol. 321, pp. 129–35.

Steinberg, Karen, Thacker, Stephen, Smith, Jay et al. (1991) 'A Meta-analysis of the Effect of Estrogen Replacement Therapy on the Risk of Breast Cancer' *Journal of the American Medical Association* Vol. 265, pp. 1985–90.

Waterhouse, Mindy (1990) 'A Time Line: Premarin', National Women's Health Network Fact Sheet, prepared spring.

Whatley, Mariamne H. (1988a) 'Screening is Calculated Exploitation' (National Women's Health Network) *Network News* January/February, pp. 1,3.

—(1988b)'Women, Exercise and Physical Potential' in Worcester and Whatley (1988b).

Whatley, Mariamne H. and Worcester, Nancy (1989) The Role of Technology in the Co-optation of the Women's Health Movement: The Case Study of Osteoporosis and Breast Cancer Screening in Ratcliff, Kathryn Strother, et al., *Healing Technology—Feminist Perspectives* Ann Arbor, Michigan: University of Michigan Press, pp. 199–220.

Winslow, Ron (1991) 'Women Face Treatment Gap in Heart Disease' *Wall Street Journal* July 25, pp. B1, B4.

Wolfe, Sidney M. (1991a) editor, 'Risk Factors for Falls in the Elderly' (Public Citizens Health Research Group) *Health Letter* Vol. 7, No. 8, p. 10.

—(1991b) 'New Evidence that Menopausal Estrogens Cause Breast Cancer; Further Doubts About Prevention of Heart Disease' (Public Citizens Health Research Group) *Health Letter* June, pp. 4–6.

Worcester, Nancy and Whatley, Mariamne H. (1988a) 'The Response of the Health Care System to the Women's Health Movement: The Selling of Women's Health Centers' in Rosser, Sue V. (1988) *Feminism Within the Science and Health Care Professions: Overcoming Resistance,* Oxford: Pergamon Press, pp. 117–30.

Worcester, Nancy and Whatley, Mariamne H. (1988b) editors, *Women's Health: Readings on Social Economic and Political Issues* Dubuque, Iowa: Kendall/Hunt.

Ω

Aging, Ageism, Mid-life and Older Women's Health Issues

1. It is often hard to think about aging when we are young. However, there are many lifestyle factors throughout our lives that can have an impact on the health we experience when we get old.

   a. Examine your own health-related behaviors (nutrition, exercise, use of drugs, etc.) to see how these might affect risks for both osteoporosis and heart disease. (For men answering this question: Remember men also experience osteoporosis, but usually at a later age).

   b. What changes could you make now to decrease these risks? *Be specific!*

   c. Do you think the answers for question b will be different for a 20 year old, a 40 year old, or a 60 year old?

   d. How could health policies and health education for young people be most appropriate for maximizing on the possibility of a healthy old age?

2. Interview two older women. What are the key health issues, if any, in their lives? How secure do they feel about being able to meet their health needs in the next five years? Identify social, economic, and heredity factors which you think influence these women's lives today.

3. *ERT/HRT Summary Sheet.* On the basis of information in "The Selling of HRT" and other information, try to summarize what is and is not known which would help women evaluate and balance "choices" about the following situations:

For the "taking ERT or HRT" column, try to answer:

- would it be better to take ERT or HRT? (Would the answer be different for different women?)
- when would one start taking ERT or HRT?
- when would one stop taking ERT or HRT?
- what other specific issues would influence this "choice"?

PURPOSE	TAKING ERT/HRT	OTHER ALTERNATIVES
Easing the transition through menopause		
Reducing or coping with specific symptoms of menopause		
Reducing risks of osteoporosis		
Reducing risks of heart disease		
Reducing risks of breast cancer		
Other		

Chapter

8

Sexuality

This chapter emphasizes how social and cultural definitions of sexuality can be detrimental to our emotional and physical health. The male emphasis on vaginal intercourse as the "real thing" invalidates the experiences and preferences of many women. In "The Sex Experts Versus Ann Landers," the authors discuss the response to the famous poll that indicated that many women would rather hug than have intercourse. The question of who defines women's sexuality which is central to this chapter is next explored in terms of issues of disability. Social attitudes about women's sexuality are exaggerated and even more problematic in their impact on women with disabilities. In "Forbidden Fruit," Anne Finger examines the strong prejudice against people with disabilities in our society—the belief that they should neither be sexual nor have children.

"Invisible Women: Lesbians and Health Care" shows how a woman's sexuality often becomes a factor in the health care she receives. The article clearly demonstrates how damaging heterosexism can be to the mental and physical health of lesbians. June Jordan's essay "The New Politics of Sexuality" asserts the important points that freedom is indivisible, that the politics of sexuality are not the province of "special interest" groups, and that bisexuality gives an important perspective on the complexity of sexuality. Because feminism often focuses on the problems of heterosexuality, it is sometimes difficult for heterosexuals to be comfortable with both their sexuality and their politics. Naomi Wolf's article, "Radical Heterosexuality," explores feminist models for healthy heterosexual relationships. In response to our decision to include this article in this book, Laura McEnaney, a former teaching assistant in women's health who often speaks as a heterosexual on the sexuality panel for the class, offers her critique both of this particular article and of Wolf's recent work.

Whether identifying as heterosexual, lesbian, bisexual, or celibate, rather than just accepting male definitions of women's sexuality (and the negative consequences associated with those definitions), women have been redefining sexuality in our own terms. These redefinitions can be empowering and validating for all women.

♀

The Sex Experts Versus Ann Landers

by Barry A. Bass and Susan R. Walen

Judging from the reaction in the media of our fellow professional sex educators and therapists to the findings of an informal two-question sex survey conducted by Ann Landers, one would have thought that we had all suffered a case of collective sexual amnesia. Not since the publication of the Hite Report in 1976 can we recall such a wave of disbelief and verbal hyperbole. A return to Victorian morality and widespread sexual boredom are but two of the dire predictions made in recent days by media sex experts. All this because Ann Landers reported in her nationally syndicated column that of more than 90,000 women responding to her poll, 72% said they would be willing to forego "the act" in return for being held close and treated tenderly.

One New York sex therapist who hosts a sexual counseling television program was quoted in a Baltimore newspaper (Sex Versus Hugs, 1985) as having said that "this will get us back to the Victorian age. It's dangerous to say a high percentage of women do not expect sexual activity but only caressing." It is unclear from that statement exactly who would be in danger; the woman, the man, their relationship, the species, or the future of sex therapy?

Jim Peterson who writes the Playboy advisor for *Playboy* magazine, said the poll could give people permission to "be boring and just roll over in bed and go to sleep." Here we see quite clearly the not yet discarded sexist belief that if left to the desires of women, sex would be nothing more than a perfunctory goodnight kiss. Women refusing to perform their "conjugal duties" and widespread male sexual frustration is the scenario the enlightened editors at Playboy seem to fear, were the Landers findings to be widely disseminated.

Not withstanding the obvious methodological flaws and the bias of the sample in the Landers poll, the results should come as no surprise to the readers of this journal. At least since the publication of the first Kinsey survey we have known that for most American couples sex includes much more than the act of intercourse. Respondents to polls commissioned by *Redbook, Playboy,* and Consumers Union have consistently reported that most sexual encounters generally include sexual activities in addition to intercourse. In fact it is not unusual for sex therapists to treat individuals who are needlessly distressed over the fact that they prefer non-coital sex to "the act" itself. Thus, rather than coming as a surprise, the Landers findings only confirm what women and men have been telling us all along—that any given sexual encounter can be satisfying, with or without intercourse.

What troubles us most, however, are comments such as those of one nationally syndicated radio psychologist who was quoted as saying that she "doubts that 72% of all women would be happy without sex" ("Sex Versus Hugs," 1985). The distressing part of that quote is the implied equating of "intercourse" and "sex." If our experience is representative of other therapists, a significant proportion of therapy sessions is spent attempting to disabuse our clients of that very notion. We frequently hear ourselves telling our clients that sex is more than intercourse, more than orgasm, more than any one behavior. We believe sex to be more usefully perceived as a comprehensive term which includes but is not limited to the following concepts: body awareness, sensuality, pleasure seeking, love and caring, sex role and gender identification, cuddling, stroking, hugging, necking, petting, genital arousal, genital pleasuring, intercourse and orgasm. In fact we often begin a course of sex therapy by placing a temporary ban on intercourse, thereby forcing the couple to attend to the multitude of other behaviors available to them in a loving and sensual encounter.

Thus, we believe intercourse is only a small element of "sex" and more importantly, intercourse is not "where it's at" for most women.* Mind you, many women tell us that intercourse can be a lovely experience. When artfully and lovingly done, the woman can feel a closeness with her partner, an appreciation by her partner, a true sense of intimacy with her partner. Holding him inside her body is a very special notion indeed. Unfortunately, however, intercourse is not the best way for most women to achieve sexual release. It is probably no coincidence that in 1976, 70% of Hite's sample said they do not reach orgasm with intercourse and in 1985, 72% of Lander's sample said they could live happily without it.

It is really rather simple, we tell our clients, if only we would bother to learn our anatomy. Intercourse provides appropriate stimulation to *his* sex organ, timed to *his* rhythmic needs. *Her* sex organ, the clitoris, is usually—and quite literally—left out in the cold. She will need to teach her partner how to provide appropriate stimulation to her sex organ, or more simply, take matters into her own hands.

What is the message we wish to communicate to our fellow sex educators and therapists? Certainly we are not saying that intercourse is not or cannot be an important

---

*It is worth noting that after four decades of sex research, data on the percentage of times couples engage in loving and orgasmic sex play that does not include intercourse are not readily available. Even in our "values neutral" surveys, researchers have simply not thought to ask respondents how many of their sexual encounters do not include "the act" of intercourse.

From JOURNAL OF SEX EDUCATION AND THERAPY, Vol. 11, No. 2, Fall/Winter 1985, pp. 14–15. Copyright © 1985 by Guilford Press. Reprinted by permission.

ingredient of a satisfying sex life. What is or is not sexually satisfying for any particular woman is not the issue here. The more relevant point is that even in the mid 1980s, in the aftermath of the "sexual revolution," our fellow professionals (who frequently serve as the voice for what the rest of society is thinking) can still become irrationally upset when hearing the truth about the way things are for many women. This reaction is a more telling commentary about our sexual enlightenment than any individual finding reported by Kinsey, Masters and Johnson, Hite, or Ann Landers.

Reference

Sex versus hugs: Landers survey raises questions. *Baltimore Sun*, January 16, 1985, pp. 1b; 2b.

Ω

Forbidden Fruit

by Anne Finger

Before she became a paraplegic, Los Angeles resident DeVonna Cervantes liked to dye her pubic hair 'fun colours' —turquoise, purple, jet black. After DeVonna became disabled, a beautician friend of hers came to the rehabilitation unit and, as a Christmas present, dyed DeVonna's pubic hair a hot pink.

But there's no such thing as 'private parts' in a rehab hospital. Soon the staff, who'd seen her dye job when they were catheterizing her, sent the staff psychiatrist around to see her. Cervantes says that he told her: 'I know it is very hard to accept that you have lost your sexuality but you don't need to draw attention to it this way.' Cervantes spent the remainder of the 50-minute session arguing with him, and, in perhaps the only true medical miracle I've ever heard of, convinced him that he was wrong—that this was normal behaviour for her.

Cervantes' story not only illustrates woeful ignorance on the part of a 'medical expert'; equating genital sensation with sexuality. But it shows clearly a disabled woman's determination to define her own sexuality.

Sadly, it's not just medical experts who are guilty of ignoring the reproductive and sexual rights and needs of people with disabilities. The movements for sexual and reproductive freedom have paid little attention to disability issues. And the abortion rights movement has sometimes crudely exploited fears about 'defective fetuses' as a reason to keep abortion legal.

Because the initial focus of the women's movement was set by women who were overwhelmingly non-disabled (as well as young, white, and middle-class), the agenda of reproductive rights has tended to focus on the right to abortion as the central issue. Yet for disabled women, the right to bear and rear children is more at risk. Zoe Washburn, in her poem, 'Hannah', grieves the child she wanted to have

and the abortion she was coerced into: ' . . . so she went to the doctor, and let him suck Hannah out with a vacuum cleaner. . . . The family stroked her hair when she cried and cried because her belly was empty and Hannah was not only dead, but never born. They looked at her strange crippled-up body and thought to themselves, thank God that's over.'

Yet the disability rights movement has certainly not put sexual rights at the forefront of its agenda. Sexuality is often the source of our deepest oppression; it is also often the source of our deepest pain. It's easier for us to talk about—and formulate strategies for changing—discrimination in employment, education, and housing than to talk about our exclusion from sexuality and reproduction. Also, although it is changing, the disability rights movement in the US has tended to focus its energies on lobbying legislators and creating an image of 'the able disabled'.

Barbara Waxman and I once published an article in *Disability Rag* about the US Supreme Court's decision that states could outlaw 'unnatural' sex acts, pointing out the effect it could have on disabled people—especially those who were unable to have 'standard' intercourse. The *Rag* then received a letter asking how 'the handicapped' could ever be expected to be accepted as 'normal' when we espoused such disgusting ideas.

Because reproduction is seen as a 'women's issue', it is often relegated to the back burner. Yet it is crucial that the disability-rights movement starts to deal with it. Perhaps the most chilling situation exists in China where a number of provinces ban marriages between people with developmental and other disabilities unless the parties have been sterilized. In Gansu Province more than 5,000 people have been sterilized since 1988. Officials in Szechuan province stated: 'Couples who have serious hereditary diseases including psychosis, mental deficiency and deformity must not be allowed to bear children'. When disabled women are found to be pregnant, they are sometimes subjected to forced abortions. But despite widespread criticism of China's population policies, there was almost no public outcry following these revelations.

From *New Internatinalist*, July 1992, pp. 8–10. Copyright © 1992 by New Internatinalist. Reprinted by permission.

Anne Finger teaches English literature at Wayne State University, Detroit, US. In her book *Past Due* (Women's Press, 1990) she describes her experience of childbirth as a disabled woman.

Even in the absence of outright bans on reproduction, the attitude that disabled people should not have children is common. Disabled women and men are still sometimes subject to forced and coerced sterilizations—including hysterectomies performed without medical justification but to prevent the 'bother' of menstruation. Los Angeles newscaster Bree Walker has a genetically transmitted disability, ectrodactyly, which results in fused bones in her hands and feet. Pregnant with her second child, last year, she found her pregnancy the subject of a call-in radio show. Broadcaster Jane Norris informed listeners in a shocked and mournful tone of voice that Bree's child had a 50-percent chance of being born with the same disability. 'Is it fair to bring a child into the world knowing there's two strikes against it at birth? . . . Is it socially responsible?' When a caller objected that it was no one else's business, Norris argued, 'It's everybody's business.' And many callers agreed with Norris's viewpoint. One horrified caller said, 'It's not just her hands—it's her feet, too. She has to [dramatic pause] wear orthopaedic shoes.'

The attitude that disabled people should not have children is certainly linked with the notion that we should not even be sexual. Yet, as with society's silence about the sexuality of children, this attitude exists alongside widespread sexual abuse. Some authorities estimate that people with disabilities are twice as likely to be victims of rape and other forms of sexual abuse as the general population. While the story of rape and sexual abuse of disabled people must be told and while we must find ways to end it, the current focus on sexual exploitation of disabled people can itself become oppressive.

As Barbara Faye Waxman, the former Disability Project Director for Los Angeles Planned Parenthood states, 'The message for disabled kids is that their sexuality will be realized through their sexual victimization. . . . I don't see an idea that good things can happen, like pleasure, intimacy, like a greater understanding of ourselves, a love of our bodies.' Waxman sees a 'double whammy' effect for disabled people, for whom there are few, if any, positive models of sexuality, and virtually no social expectation that they will become sexual beings.

The attitude that we are and should be asexual seems to exist across a broad range of cultures. Ralf Hotchkiss, famous for developing wheelchairs in Third World countries, has travelled widely in Latin America and Asia. He says that while attitudes vary 'from culture to culture, from subculture to subculture,' he sees nearly everywhere he travels, 'extreme irritation [on the part of disabled people] at the stereotypical assumptions that people . . . make about their sexuality, their lack of it.' He also noted: 'In Latin American countries once they hear I'm married, the next question is always, "How old are your kids?"'

Some of these prejudices are enshrined in law. In the US, 'marital disincentives' remain a significant barrier. To explain this Byzantine system briefly: benefits (including government-funded health care) are greatly reduced and sometimes even eliminated when a disabled person marries. Tom Fambro writes of his own difficulties with the system: 'I am a 46-year-old black man with cerebral palsy. A number of years ago I met a young lady who was sexually attracted to me (a real miracle).' Fambro learned, however, that he would lose his income support and, most crucially, his medical benefits, if he married. 'People told us that we should just live together . . . but because both of us were born-again Christians that was unthinkable. . . . The Social Security Administration has the idea that disabled people are not to fall in love, get married, have sex or have a life of our own. Instead, we are to be sexual eunuchs. They are full of shit.'

Institutions—whether traditional hospitals or euphemistically named 'homes', 'schools', or newer community-care facilities— often out-and-out forbid sexual contact for their residents. Or they may outlaw gay and lesbian relationships, while allowing heterosexual ones. Disabled lesbians and gays may also find that their sexual orientation is presumed to occur by default. Restriction of access to sexual information occurs on both a legal and a social plane. The US Library of Congress, a primary source of material for blind and other print-handicapped people, was instructed by Congress in 1985 to no longer make *Playboy* available in braille or on tape. And relay services, which provide telecommunication between deaf and hearing people have sometimes refused to translate sexually explicit speech. In her poem, 'Seeing', blind poet Mary McGinnis writes of a woman being watched by sighted men while bathing nude:

. . . the guys sitting at the edge of the pond
looked at her, but she couldn't see them . . .
and whose skin, hair, shirts and belts
would remain unknown to her
because she couldn't go up to them and
say, now fair is fair, let me touch the places
on your bodies you try to hide,
it's my turn—don't draw back or sit on
your hands, let me count your rings, your
scars,
the hairs coming from your nose. . . .

I have quoted poets several times in this piece; many disability-rights activists now see that while we need changes in laws and policies, the formation of culture is a key part of winning our freedom. Disabled writers and artists are shaping work that is often powerful in both its rage and its affirmation. In Cheryl Marie Wade's 'side and belly', she writes:

He is wilty muscle sack and sharp bones fitting my gnarlypaws.
I am soft cellulite and green eyes of middle-age memory. We are
side and belly trading dreams and fantasies of able-bodied
former and not real selves: high-heel booted dancers making love
from black rooftops and naked dim doorways. . . .
. . . Contradictions in the starry night of wars within and being
not quite whole together and whole. Together in sighs we say yes
broken and fire and yes singing.

Ω

Invisible Women
Lesbians and Health Care

by Risa Denenberg

In the 1960s, when women were disclosing the intimate details of their private lives to one another in consciousness-raising groups, a body of knowledge began to emerge about women's health care experiences. The early women's health movement, which fought primarily for women's autonomy in reproduction and in opposition to medical authority, was resisted with all the force that the medical profession could muster. Despite that resistance, the women's health movement flourished and helped to usher in an era in which women have more knowledge of their bodies and a greater sense of ownership than they did in any previous generation.

As a participant in both the women's movement and the women's health movement, I know that many of the leaders were lesbians. During the years of struggling to create an autonomous movement, fighting for abortion rights, looking at our own and each other's bodies with plastic vaginal speculums, and creating feminist clinics, a mere handful of projects and programs for lesbians were developed. Our issues were subsumed within the more visible agenda for heterosexual women's rights. The women's movement both faltered and flourished. It undertook the complex task of broadening to include issues of race and class, and the single-issue battle for abortion rights became a call for prenatal and child care and against sterilization abuse. And in the 1980s, the reality of how women were being affected by AIDS became a consuming item on the women's agenda. Finally, after years of working on such crucial issues, it is still difficult for lesbians to articulate our own health care needs.

It is an even greater task to get our needs recognized by others, given the widespread view of homosexuality and lesbianism. Heterosexuality is still seen as the universal norm, and the notion persists that homosexuality, and particularly lesbianism, doesn't matter. In the right-wing, conservative view, homosexuality is sinful, and therefore matters more, but a great many liberals, and even progressives, remain doggedly blind to sexuality. This blindness comes in many forms: keeping gay concerns a low priority in progressive movements, closeting of gay leaders in such groups, and widespread discomfort with public sexuality: "That's their business, but I just wish they didn't feel such a need to flaunt it in our faces." Although the AIDS crisis

From *Health/PAC Bulletin*, Spring 1992, pp. 14–21. Copyright © 1992 by Health/PAC Bulletin. Reprinted by permission.

Risa Denenberg is a family nurse practitioner at Bronx Lebanon Hospital in New York City and a health writer.

and the gay response to it has opened the door to overcoming this invisibility and legitimizing the health needs of gay men, the attention it demands has set lesbians even further back from having our health care needs recognized—even when we have AIDS, are dying in astounding numbers from breast cancer and other cancers, and neglect our health care needs in order to care for others. And while AIDS has disproportionately affected gay men, the increase in anti-gay violence that has accompanied the epidemic affects gay men and lesbians equally.

Invisibility and Discrimination

Lesbians are like other women in their vulnerability to illness and to the damaging effect of sexism in the health care system. Lesbians also have unique concerns and experiences that must inform their health care services if individual needs are to be met. A few examples give some hint of the specific problems of discrimination that lesbians face within the health care system:

- Doris entered a therapeutic community to recover from drug and alcohol use, but she found it necessary to hide her gay life-style from the other clients and the staff.
- Evelyn was in therapy for depression for about six months when her female therapist made an overtly homophobic remark. She decided against revealing her growing sexual feelings toward a woman at her job.
- Lori was unable to find a specialist to treat her infertility and assist her with artificial insemination because she is a lesbian.
- Fran came out as a lesbian to her doctor when he was asking her about birth control. During the exam, when he was placing the speculum in her vagina, he was extremely rough, and he used a size that was uncomfortable for her. When Fran complained, he said, "I'm just trying to change your mind."
- Vivian was committed at age 15 to a psychiatric hospital by her parents when they discovered her having sex with another girl.

Although such invisibility and discrimination are not always life and death matters, they bear upon clinical practice, access to health care services, medical decision making, and the level of discomfort we all feel with wholly depersonalized, even antagonistic health care. Lesbians live in all communities and are diverse in race, ethnicity, class, and political outlook, and are not easily distinguished within health care settings. As seen in the following examples, this invisibility can thwart the receipt of decent health care:

- Sharon had a bad experience with an insensitive gynecologist when she was in her twenties. Now, at 43, she hasn't had a Pap smear in 16 years.
- Marcia was unemployed and had no health insurance when she discovered that she had a breast lump. Her lover of eight years had a job with health insurance, but couldn't place Marcia on her policy.
- Joan was given a hysterectomy at age 27 for a small fibroid tumor on her uterus. At one point her doctor mentioned doing a myomectomy—removing the tumor and saving the uterus—but after he found out that she was lesbian, he never brought it up again. He never asked her if she wanted children.
- After Sonja's surgery for breast cancer, her lover Michelle was not allowed into the recovery room. As she sat in the waiting room for three hours, Michelle noticed the nurses escorting other people in to see family members. She was afraid to complain, lest they treat Sonja badly.

Huge gaps exist in the public's and the medical establishment's understanding of lesbian culture and life-style that make it difficult to confront our invisibility. There is no standard definition of who is a lesbian. Many female couples exist in satisfying, long-term relationships without ever uttering the words lesbian or gay. Other women boldly proclaim a lesbian identity, yet at times have sexual relations with men. Lesbians live in the same unhealthy environments and engage in the same kinds of risky health behaviors as other women—drug and alcohol abuse, eating disorders, smoking, unsafe sex. Yet, lesbians are virtually unstudied as a population by any discipline.

Lesbians exhibit a wide and fluid range of attitudes, behaviors, and self-identities. One common denominator in their relationships, expression of sexuality, life-style, and experiences, however, is that they are all outsiders when it comes to getting their health needs met. When lesbians' health care needs are the same as those of other women for screening, prevention, treatment of illness, education and crisis intervention, lesbians' needs are less well met than those of heterosexuals. And when lesbians present unique problems and concerns, the medical system generally can't or won't meet them. Health care services must be evaluated to determine whether or not they are discriminatory and offensive to lesbians.

Most lesbians have heard of or personally experienced abuses within the health care system because of their sexual preference. These experiences include sexual assault, patronizing treatment, neglect, intimidation, ignorance, and discrimination. Homophobia, in the form of heterosexual presumption, is a common experience shared by all lesbians entering the health system. This is layered on top of the sexism that all women continue to meet in this arena. For lesbians of color, racism within the system adds another layer of discrimination. Poor lesbians, lesbian intravenous drug users, and lesbian mothers all face additional bias.

The collective experience of lesbians rings an alarm bell of terror for any lesbian entering the system. It is not surprising, then, that lesbians often avoid receiving health care in traditional settings as long as it is possible for them to do so. A variety of other elements and experiences help to determine lesbians' health status and relationship to the health care system, including their financial standing, work life, sexuality, reproductive life, and support systems.

Money and Work

As women, lesbians earn less money, since, according to the Census Bureau, women's earnings are only two-thirds that of men. In addition, lesbians generally have less access than other women to men's resources. Thus, a lesbian household is likely to earn less than a heterosexual household—whether single, coupled, or collective—and is likely to have fewer dollars to spend on health care services. This is compounded by discrimination against lesbians in the work world, which leads to a lack of job mobility. Lesbians may also tend to choose jobs that will not put extra stress on them if their lesbian identity is known. In addition, along with gay men and others in nontraditional families, lesbians usually cannot place a lover or a partner's children on their health insurance policy. Furthermore, lesbians may be less able to recruit support and resources from their family of origin, who often reserve such favors for their married children.

The workplace itself places enormous stress upon lesbians. In the work world one often must make the choice between being out, with the accompanying torture of gay baiting and harassment, or remaining in the closet, with the constant fear of being exposed.

Although not everyone finds pleasure in tapping into the social network in the workplace, to some extent everyone attempts to ease stress on the job by fitting in and getting along with their co-workers. It is difficult to negotiate the pressures to fit into the social networks that develop among co-workers, and camaraderie creates yet another pressure with negative effects on lesbians who must be closeted in a heterosexual world. Women often invent a "boyfriend," invert pronouns, appear falsely naive about relationships, and stay away from office parties or picnics where a male escort would be expected. For lesbians, work, however satisfying in theory, can be a stress that adversely affects self-image, mental health, household finances, and physical well-being.

Sexuality and Lesbian Relationships

Lesbians often feel isolated, especially when single, and have difficulty finding positive images of lesbian relationships and sexuality. Gay women have similar inhibitions as heterosexual women about approaching, pursuing and expressing desire to other people. The sexual or romantic isolation that a single lesbian feels may be exacerbated if her friends are competing for lovers within their small circle.

Lesbians are often singled out in medical discussion for the dubious achievement of engaging in low-risk sex. One inaccurate portrayal of lesbian sexuality is that sex is generally chaste, dry, and monogamous. This leads to the idea that lesbians are not at risk of sexually transmitted infections or HIV. It is dangerous to suggest that any category of sex is completely safe from HIV transmission. Furthermore, this stereotype contributes to the myth that lesbians don't have much sex and that this is a frequent cause of failure for lesbian relationships. Lesbian sexuality, like all sexuality, is polymorphous and diverse, and it has never been adequately described in research or literature. But clearly, sexuality is neither the only inspiration, nor the usual cause of failure for female bonding. Gay relationships are generally unsupported by families and communities, are bound by fewer legal ties, and have fewer common children to draw parties together when the relationship feels threatened from within.

Reproductive Health

Lesbians' health needs clearly differ from those of heterosexual women in the area of reproductive health. Lesbians generally have fewer pregnancies in the course of their lifetimes than other women and, hence, longer years of unrelieved menstruation. Anecdotal reports from clinicians providing care to lesbians suggest that lesbians have more complaints about menstruation and fewer about menopause. Women who have sex exclusively with women may have a lower overall incidence of sexually transmitted infections, which translates into a lower incidence of pelvic infections, ectopic pregnancies, and cervical cancer. Women who have never been pregnant have a higher incidence of breast cancer. Thus, there are a few differences that may be based on sexual preference; however, this is not the case in the incidence of most gynecological complaints: fibroid tumors, ovarian cancer, ovarian cysts, endometriosis, cystic breast disease, vaginitis, and urinary tract infections. Yet lesbians receive fewer gynecological services than other women who must seek medical care for birth control, treatment of sexually transmitted infections, and pregnancies.

While a lesbian identity does not preclude sexual activity for money or with men, lesbians often simply deny and ignore needs rather than submit to gynecologists. Often problems such as bad cramps, heavy periods, pain from endometriosis or fibroid tumors, or severe hot flashes during menopause go untreated. Lesbians skip Pap smears, breast exams, and mammograms, and, in omitting these key health care events, often receive no preventive health care services. Thus, they enter the health care system only during crisis.

Lesbians are as likely to want children as other women, but are less likely to act on these desires. External and internalized homophobic messages cast doubt on the appropriateness of raising children for all lesbians and gay

men. Both public and private adoption agencies usually bar adoption for gay couples and singles. However, many lesbians are mothers, having born children during prior relationships with men. But many of these lesbians, once out of the marriage and out of the closet, have lost custody of their children.

Mental Health and Emotional Support

In terms of emotional well-being, many gays have experienced early rejection from family, peers, and co-workers because of their sexual orientation. Many young lesbians have been confined in mental hospitals or ordered to therapy by parents for the crime of engaging in same-sex relationships. Lesbians experience the same sexist violence as other women in the form of early sexual abuse, sexual harassment on the job, and rape, and they suffer from the added abuse of homophobic assaults in all forms—comments, threats, beatings, and sexual assault—as well. Lesbians are not exempt from violence within relationships either, but they are less able to seek and receive sensitive support, refuge, and crisis intervention when battering occurs. Several studies show a higher rate of alcoholism and drug abuse among gays.

The gay community offers support to lesbians but may not be a haven. Gay and lesbian community centers—when they exist at all—often have much male and little female leadership and programming. And most towns and cities have no lesbian projects at all—no twelve-step groups, social activities, or educational programs geared for lesbians. Bars are often the only place to connect with lesbians. Rural communities often have informal social networks, but, because they are small, tend to enforce conformity. Such networks also set unrealistic expectations to provide support to group members when illness or crises occur.

Lesbians and AIDS

Lesbians have worked as activists and service workers throughout the AIDS epidemic, yet there is still controversy over whether or not AIDS is a lesbian issue. Lesbians constitute a growing segment of those who are HIV-positive. Lesbians engage in risky behaviors, including sex with those at risk (both men and women) and unsafe use of needles. Lesbian AIDS Project researchers conducted a small study of lesbian intravenous drug users in San Francisco in 1987 and found that many of these women also engaged in other high-risk behaviors such as unprotected sex with men, sex in exchange for money or drugs, and unprotected sex with other women during their periods. Similarly, a study of lesbian sexual behavior conducted by the Kinsey Institute also in 1987 revealed that 45 percent of the 262 self-identified lesbians sampled had been sexually active with men since 1980. Despite this reality, lesbians' risk of disease is overlooked because of dangerous myths about their sexual behavior.

Among groups and organizations doing work on AIDS, research, education, and outreach for lesbians is all but nonexistent. A few projects exist, created by lesbians, that deal with issues relevant to lesbians with HIV/AIDS, and there are a few support groups for HIV-positive lesbians in some communities. The Lesbians' Educational AIDS Resource Network in Tampa, Florida, has the goal of providing a forum for HIV prevention in the lesbian and female bisexual communities. Groups of lesbians working in AIDS have formed to provide support and activities for lesbians involved in advocacy and service for people with AIDS and also to specifically address lesbian HIV issues.

An important link needs to be made between HIV/AIDS issues and drug use in the lesbian communities. At present, as noted, recovery programs and twelve-step meetings specifically for lesbians are few, but such groups are an important place for lesbians to get help with drinking and drug problems.

Lesbians and Cancer

The health focus for lesbians in the 1990s appears to be cancer. The leadership and involvement of lesbians in the women's cancer movement and its projects has been significant. Composed of networks of local cancer projects, these groups reflect the community's cumulative grief and anger at too many women dying with too little being done in areas of research and meaningful prevention. In 1990, 45,000 women died of breast cancer. At least 10 percent of these were lesbian, probably more, both because the number of lesbians in the general population is usually underestimated, and because of the increased risk of breast cancer in women who have never been pregnant.

Most other cancers and chronic and life-threatening illnesses affect gay and straight women with similar frequency, but they often affect lesbians in a different way than other women. The problems lesbians often confront in dealing with the health care system—lack of health insurance, resources for health care services, and community support, the invisibility of lesbians and hostility towards the ill person's partner—all surface with particular harshness at times of immense crisis—at diagnosis, during treatment, at death. Heartbreaking stories, such as that of Sharon Kowalski (see "The Fragile Rights of Sharon Kowalski," Spring 1989 issue) are commonplace in the lesbian community.

Cancer activism is an integral part of lesbian communities throughout the country. Several projects have formed to deal exclusively with lesbian cancer issues: the Chicago Lesbian Cancer Project, the Women's Cancer Resource Center in Oakland, California, and the Mary Helen Mautner Project for Lesbians with Cancer in Washington, DC. Lesbian cancer projects organize support groups and provide services such as transportation, child care, and housekeeping for sick lesbians in addition to outreach, education, and activism. But just as gay men cannot cope with the AIDS epidemic without external supports, lesbians cannot tend to each other adequately without leadership and initiative from the medical community, the government, and the community-based organizations.

Resources

Some resources have already been created to help lesbians deal with with their health problems, although these are far too few and limited to meet the existing need. Among the published pamphlets, books, and other literature on lesbian health, the original prototype is the still-in-print *Lesbian Health Matters!* published and distributed by the Santa Cruz Women's Health Collective. *Our Bodies, Ourselves* has a chapter about lesbians, and several other books have been published by women's and gay presses (see sidebar).

Some lesbian health projects have been developed over the years by various women's and gay groups. In the 1970s, feminist-run clinics such as the Santa Cruz Women's Health Center, the several Feminist Women's Health Centers, and the Cambridge Women's Health Center commonly set aside certain nights for lesbians. Although these "lesbians nights" smacked of segregation, they allowed an unprecedented level of individual attention to the health and sexuality concerns of gay women. Most of these clinics had a majority of lesbians in leadership roles, who frequently found themselves working on heterosexual issues while complaining about "not getting to our own issues," just as lesbians now debate the virtues of fighting AIDS along with gay men while perpetually relegating lesbian issues to the back burner. Many feminist clinics have foundered altogether in the recent climate of cutbacks and anti-abortion activism, and those that continue to function have fewer resources for special programs.

Other projects were developed in the 1980s, including the Lesbian Insemination Project, the Lesbian AIDS Project, the Lesbian Health Information Project in San Francisco and Lesbian Illness Support Group in New York.

Less than a handful of lesbian health clinics currently exist. At some, including the Lyon-Martin Clinic in San Francisco and the St. Marks Women's Clinic in New York City, many straight and bisexual women also receive health care. Others are gay/lesbian clinics, such as the Community Health Project in New York, Fenway Community Health Center in Boston, and Whitman Walker in Washington, DC. Lesbians working in these projects voice concern that gay men have always been better served, and that now AIDS programming has left scant resources to serve gay women, even gay women with AIDS.

New York City has an office on lesbian and gay health concerns that functions as a liaison between the lesbian and gay communities and the health service sector. The emphasis is on providing training and education to health professionals so that they can better serve the gay community. The office also provides technical assistance and support to community organizations and co-sponsored a conference on Lesbians and Life-Altering Illness in Fall 1991.

Research

There is little research on the health of lesbians and even less that would provide evidence of the kinds of changes needed in the health care system to appropriately address lesbians' needs within the health care system. One of the few surveys of health care experiences, attitudes, and needs of lesbians was undertaken by Judith Bradford and Caitlin Ryan in 1984 through the National Lesbian and Gay Health Foundation. This ambitious 104 question survey was answered by nearly 2,000 lesbians throughout the United States. Most of the respondents were white, college-educated professionals. Some principal findings from this study include the following:

- Fifty percent of the lesbians surveyed had not had a Pap smear in the previous 12 months, and many of the respondents were not receiving any care for existing gynecological problems.
- The most common health problem reported was depression.
- Most women felt unable to disclose their sexual preference to their usual health care provider—yet 80 percent reported experiencing discrimination based on their sexual identity.
- The most frequently reported concern regarding access to health care services was insufficient money; this was the primary reason cited for not seeking health care.
- Of the women who reported the experience of rape, only one-third ever sought help.
- Stress-related illnesses, including ulcers, allergies, and hypertension, were common among the lesbians responding.

The authors conclude that the data confirm that lesbians face many obstacles in negotiating the health care system, often do not receive important health care, and have health concerns in a variety of areas. They cite the need for further research and documentation in the areas of "discrimination, physical and sexual abuse, . . . the need for mental health services and the training of providers; the impact of outness/closetness on mental health, and access to non-discriminatory and informed services."

Other research into lesbian health needs has also been conducted by the gay and lesbian community. Small-scale, unpublished, and uncompleted research exists and is passed along within small circles of lesbians involved in health politics and clinical practice. Studies of breast cancer, HIV seroprevalence, psychological needs of lesbian couples, attitudes about sexuality, sexual transmission of vaginitis between women, and incidence of environmental illnesses in lesbians all exist in various stages of completion. This type of research is severely underfunded and underreported. Nevertheless, an informal network among lesbian activists, researchers, and clinicians passes along important findings and ideas. Funding and support for this type of work would bring important information into a more public forum.

A Lesbian Health Agenda

Lesbians clearly experience health and illness differently from both gay men and heterosexual women, and their differing needs constitute a lesbian health agenda that must be articulated and made visible. The involvement and action of the health community would hasten the development and enactment of such an agenda. Identifying key issues and appropriate approaches by talking to lesbian leaders is imperative. Health planning agencies need to consult lesbian health experts to determine whether or not services are targeted to, reaching, and acceptable to lesbian clients. Slotting a seat for a lesbian on community advisory boards, medical committees, and planning boards would also be useful.

To begin work on lesbians' concerns in clinical settings, lesbians might be identified and rendered visible by asking relevant questions and using appropriate language on health forms. For example, terms such as sexual partner or significant other are non-threatening. Heterosexual presumption can be eliminated from history-taking, and lesbian-positive images and literature can be placed along with other educational materials in waiting rooms. Funding is needed immediately for lesbian programming, technical assistance, relevant educational materials, and advocacy. Among the issues on a lesbian health agenda that health professionals need to support are the following items that have already been identified.

Cancer is a serious concern of lesbians, claiming many lives and causing much disability and loss of productivity. Lesbian- informed research will continue to look for earlier detection methods and investigate both environmental and personal risk. Partners and children of lesbians who face serious illness or death need legal protection within the framework of lesbian families and relationships.

Childbearing and parenting is another primary concern for lesbians, whether single or coupled. Few sperm banks are receptive to lesbians, and discrimination hampers many lesbians' efforts to get pregnant. This often leads to informal insemination with semen from donors who are not screened for HIV and other sexually transmitted diseases. The pervasive discrimination against lesbians in custody proceedings also requires more supportive services and advocacy for lesbian families.

Drug and alcohol abuse is a high-priority issue within the lesbian community that requires research as well as community support. Lesbians and gay men cannot recover from addiction while in the closet and being bombarded with homophobic messages. Lesbians benefit tremendously from participating in lesbian recovery groups, but most communities have none.

Mental health services are a significant need in the gay community. Lesbians seek mental health services most often for depression. There is a growing body of writing and research on battering in lesbian relationships and on the effects of sexual assault and homophobic violence on lesbians. Rejection for early expression of lesbian sexuality and life-style may mark the beginning of a lifetime of alienation from family, teachers, old friends, and co-workers. The closet is a breeding ground for depression, anxiety, and physical complaints as well. Lesbians should be able to choose lesbian therapists, attend lesbian support groups, and be able to identify with a lesbian political action group.

Gynecology represents an area of dissatisfaction for almost all women. Gynecologists are still schooled in sexism. Women report being patronized, misinformed, lied to, and talked over and about in the third person. They suffer the abuses of unnecessary surgeries, sterilizations, and drug experimentation. Lesbians need lesbian-informed and sensitive obstetric and gynecological services in order to ever consider participating in the basic women's health care services.

Lesbians, like other women, are vulnerable to HIV infection and need to be rendered visible in the AIDS epidemic. A network of services, research, and support needs to be built that includes the lesbian experience of HIV/AIDS.

The time is long overdue for this agenda to be recognized and addressed by the medical community. Lesbians have contributed richly to progressive movements that have brought about changes in the health care system for heterosexual women, for gay men, and for other minority communities. We will continue to do that work, but lesbians' health needs must no longer be left off of the agenda as we fight for the changes that are so sorely needed in the health care system.

Books on Lesbian Health

The Advocate's Guide To Gay Health, Alyson Publishers 1982.

Alive and Well: A Lesbian Health Guide, by Hepburn and Gutirrez, Crossing Press, 1988.

Artificial Insemination: An Alternative Conception for the Lesbian and Gay Community, by the Lesbian Health Information Project. Order from San Francisco Women's Centers, 3548 18th Street, San Francisco, CA 94110.

Cancer as a Women's Issue, Edited by Midge Stocker, Third Side Press, 1991.

Cancer Journals, by Audre Lorde, Spinsters Ink.

Cancer in Two Voices, by Sandra Butler and Barbara Rosenblum, Spinsters Books, 1991.

Considering Parenthood: A Workbook for Lesbians, by Cheri Pies, Spinsters Books, 1985.

Lesbian Health Matters! by Santa Cruz Women's Health Collective, 1979. Write Santa Cruz Women's Health Center, 250 Locust Street, Santa Cruz, CA 95060.

Lesbian Psychologies, by Boston Lesbian Psychologies Collective, University of Illinois Press, 1987.

Lesbian Sex, by JoAnn Loulan, Spinsters Ink, 1984.

The Lesbian S/M Safety Manual, by Pat Califia, Lace Publications, 1988.

Naming the Violence: Speaking Out About Lesbian Battering, edited by Kerry Lobel, Seal Press, 1986.

The New Our Bodies, Ourselves, by the Boston Women's Book Collective, Simon and Schuster, 1992.

One in Three: Women with Cancer Confront an Epidemic, by Judith Brady, Cleis Press, 1991.

Out From Under: Sober Dykes and Their Friends, edited by Jean Swallow, Spinsters Ink, 1983.

Suzie Sexpert's Lesbian Sex World, by Suzie Bright, Cleis Press, 1990.

Ω

A New Politics of Sexuality

by June Jordan

As a young worried mother, I remember turning to Dr. Benjamin Spock's *Common Sense Book of Baby and Child Care* just about as often as I'd pick up the telephone. He was God. I was ignorant but striving to be good: a good Mother. And so it was there, in that bestseller pocketbook of do's and don't's, that I came upon this doozie of a guideline: Do not wear miniskirts or other provocative clothing because that will upset your child, especially if your child happens to be a boy. If you give your offspring "cause" to think of you as a sexual being, he will, at the least, become disturbed; you will derail the equilibrium of his notions about your possible identity and meaning in the world.

It had never occurred to me that anyone, especially my son, might look upon me as an asexual being. I had never supposed that "asexual" was some kind of positive

From *The Progressive*, July 1991, pp. 12–13. Copyright © 1991 by June Jordan. Reprinted by permission of the author.

June Jordan writes for *The Progressive* every other month. This column was adapted from her keynote address to the Bisexual, Gay, and Lesbian Student Association at Stanford University on April 29, 1991.

designation I should, so to speak, lust after. I was pretty surprised by Dr. Spock. However, I was also, by habit, a creature of obedience. For a couple of weeks I actually experimented with lusterless colors and dowdy tops and bottoms, self-consciously hoping thereby to prove myself as a lusterless and dowdy and, therefore, excellent female parent.

Years would have to pass before I could recognize the familiar, by then, absurdity of a man setting himself up as the expert on a subject that presupposed women as the primary objects for his patriarchal discourse—on motherhood, no less! Years passed before I came to perceive the perversity of dominant power assumed by men, and the perversity of self-determining power ceded to men by women.

A lot of years went by before I understood the dynamics of what anyone could summarize as the Politics of Sexuality.

I believe the Politics of Sexuality is the most ancient and probably the most profound arena for human conflict. Increasingly, it seems clear to me that deeper and more pervasive than any other oppression, than any other bitterly contested human domain, is the oppression of sexuality, the exploitation of the human domain of sexuality for power.

When I say sexuality, I mean gender: I mean male subjugation of human beings because they are female. When I say sexuality, I mean heterosexual institutionalization of rights and privileges denied to homosexual men and women. When I say sexuality I mean gay or lesbian contempt for bisexual modes of human relationship.

The Politics of Sexuality therefore subsumes all of the different ways in which some of us seek to dictate to others of us what we should do, what we should desire, what we should dream about, and how we should behave ourselves, generally, on the planet. From China to Iran, from Nigeria to Czechoslovakia, from Chile to California, the politics of sexuality—enforced by traditions of state-sanctioned violence plus religion and the law—reduces to male domination of women, heterosexist tyranny, and, among those of us who are in any case deemed despicable or deviant by the powerful, we find intolerance for those who choose a different, a more complicated—for example, an interracial or bisexual—mode of rebellion and freedom.

We must move out from the shadows of our collective subjugation—as people of color/as women/as gay/as lesbian/as bisexual human beings.

I can voice my ideas without hesitation or fear because I am speaking, finally, about myself. I am black and I am female and I am a mother and I am bisexual and I am a nationalist and I am an anti-nationalist. And I mean to be fully and freely all that I am!

Conversely, I do not accept that any white or black or Chinese man—I do not accept that, for instance, Dr. Spock—should presume to tell me, or any other woman, how to mother a child. He has no right. He is not a mother. My child is not his child. And, likewise, I do not accept

that anyone—any woman or any man who is not inextricably part of the subject he or she dares to address—should attempt to tell any of us, the objects of her or his presumptuous discourse, what we should do or what we should not do.

Recently, I have come upon gratuitous and appalling pseudoliberal pronouncements on sexuality. Too often, these utterances fall out of the mouths of men and women who first disclaim any sentiment remotely related to homophobia, but who then proceed to issue outrageous opinions like the following.

That it is blasphemous to compare the oppression of gay, lesbian, or bisexual people to the oppression, say, of black people, or of the Palestinians.

That the bottom line about gay or lesbian or bisexual identity is that you can conceal it whenever necessary and, so, therefore, why don't you do just that? Why don't you keep your deviant sexuality in the closet and let the rest of us—we who suffer oppression for reasons of our ineradicable and always visible components of our personhood such as race or gender—get on with our more necessary, our more beleaguered struggle to survive?

Well, number one: I believe I have worked as hard as I could, and then harder than that, on behalf of equality and justice—for African-Americans, for the Palestinian people, and for people of color everywhere.

And no, I do not believe it is blasphemous to compare oppressions of sexuality to oppressions of race and ethnicity: Freedom is indivisible or it is nothing at all besides sloganeering and temporary, short-sighted, and short-lived advancement for a few. Freedom is indivisible, and either we are working for freedom or you are working for the sake of your self-interests and I am working for mine.

If you can finally go to the bathroom, wherever you find one, if you can finally order a cup of coffee and drink it wherever coffee is available, but you cannot follow your heart—you cannot respect the response of your own honest body in the world—then how much of what kind of freedom does any one of us possess?

Or, conversely, if your heart and your honest body can be controlled by the state, or controlled by community taboo, are you not then, and in that case, no more than a slave ruled by outside force?

What tyranny could exceed a tyranny that dictates to the human heart, and that attempts to dictate the public career of an honest human body?

Freedom is indivisible; the Politics of Sexuality is not some optional "special-interest" concern for serious, progressive folk.

And, on another level, let me assure you: If every single gay or lesbian or bisexual man or woman active on the Left of American politics decided to stay home, there would be *no* Left left.

One of the things I want to propose is that we act on that reality: that we insistently demand reciprocal respect and concern from those who cheerfully depend upon our brains and our energies for their, and our, effective impact on the political landscape.

Last spring, at Berkeley, some students asked me to speak at a rally against racism. And I did. There were 400 or 500 people massed on Sproul Plaza, standing together against that evil. And, on the next day, on that same Plaza, there was a rally for bisexual and gay and lesbian rights, and students asked me to speak at that rally. And I did. There were fewer than seventy-five people stranded, pitiful, on that public space. And I said then what I say today: That was disgraceful! There should have been just one rally. One rally: Freedom is indivisible.

As for the second, nefarious pronouncement on sexuality that now enjoys mass-media currency: the idiot notion of keeping yourself in the closet—that is very much the same thing as the suggestion that black folks and Asian-Americans and Mexican-Americans should assimilate and become as "white" as possible—in our walk/talk/music/food/values—or else. Or else? Or else we should, deservedly, perish.

Sure enough, we have plenty of exposure to white everything so why would we opt to remain our African/Asian/Mexican selves? The answer is that suicide is absolute, and if you think you will survive by hiding who you really are, you are sadly misled: There is no such thing as partial or intermittent suicide. You can only survive if you—who you really are—do survive.

Likewise, we who are not men and we who are not heterosexist—we, sure enough, have plenty of exposure to male-dominated/heterosexist this and that.

But a struggle to survive cannot lead to suicide: Suicide is the opposite of survival. And so we must not conceal/assimilate/ integrate into the would-be dominant culture and political system that despises us. Our survival requires that we alter our environment so that we can live and so that we can hold each other's hands and so that we can kiss each other on the streets, and in the daylight of our existence, without terror and without violent and sometimes fatal reactions from the busybodies of America.

Finally, I need to speak on bisexuality. I do believe that the analogy is interracial or multiracial identity. I do believe that the analogy for bisexuality is a multicultural, multi-ethnic, multiracial world view. Bisexuality follows from such a perspective and leads to it, as well.

Just as there are many men and women in the United States whose parents have given them more than one racial, more than one ethnic identity and cultural heritage to honor; and just as these men and women must deny no given part of themselves except at the risk of self-deception and the insanities that must issue from that; and just as these men and women embody the principle of equality among races and ethnic communities; and just as these men and women falter and anguish and choose and then falter again and then anguish and then choose yet again how they will honor the irreducible complexity of their God-given human being—even so, there are many men and women, especially young men and women, who seek to embrace the complexity of their total, always-changing social and political circumstance.

They seek to embrace our increasing global complexity on the basis of the heart and on the basis of an honest human body. Not according to ideology. Not according to group pressure. Not according to anybody's concept of "correct."

This is a New Politics of Sexuality. And even as I despair of identity politics—because identity is given and principles of justice/equality/freedom cut across given gender and given racial definitions of being, and because I will call you my brother, I will call you my sister, on the basis of what you *do* for justice, what you *do* for equality, what you *do* for freedom and *not* on the basis of who you are, even so I look with admiration and respect upon the new, bisexual politics of sexuality.

This emerging movement politicizes the so-called middle ground: Bisexuality invalidates either/or formulation, either/or analysis. Bisexuality means I am free and I am as likely to want and to love a woman as I am likely to want and to love a man, and what about that? Isn't that what freedom implies?

If you are free you are not predictable and you are not controllable. To my mind, that is the keenly positive, politicizing significance of bisexual affirmation:

To insist upon complexity, to insist upon the validity of all of the components of social/sexual complexity, to insist upon the equal validity of all of the components of social/sexual complexity.

This seems to me a unifying, 1990s mandate for revolutionary Americans planning to make it into the Twenty-first Century on the basis of the heart, on the basis of an honest human body, consecrated to every struggle for justice, every struggle for equality, every struggle for freedom.

Ω

Radical Heterosexuality

by Naomi Wolf

All over the country, millions of feminists have a secret indulgence. By day they fight gender injustice; by night they sleep with men. Is this a dual life? A core contradiction? Is sleeping with a man "sleeping with the enemy"? And is razor burn from kissing inherently oppressive?

It's time to say you *can* hate sexism and love men. As the feminist movement grows more mature and our understanding of our enemies more nuanced, three terms assumed to be in contradiction—radical feminist heterosexuality—can and must be brought together.

Rules of the Relationship

But how? Andrea Dworkin and Catharine MacKinnon have pointed out that sexism limits women to such a degree that it's questionable whether the decision to live with a man can ever truly be free. If you want to use their sound, if depressing, reasoning to a brighter end, turn the thesis around: radical heterosexuality demands substituting choice for dependency.

Radical heterosexuality requires that the woman be able to support herself. This is not to belittle women who must depend financially on men; it is to recognize that when our daughters are raised with the skills that would let them leave abusers, they need not call financial dependence love.

Radical heterosexuality needs alternative institutions. As the child of a good lifetime union, I believe in them. But when I think of pledging my heart and body to a man—even the best and kindest man—within the existing institution of marriage, I feel faint. The more you learn about its legal structure, the less likely you are to call the caterers.

In the nineteenth century, when a judge ruled that a husband could not imprison and rape his wife, the London *Times* bemoaned, "One fine morning last month, marriage in England was suddenly abolished." The phrase "rule of thumb" descends from English common law that said a man could legally beat his wife with a switch "no thicker than his thumb."

If these nightmarish echoes were confined to history, I might feel more nuptial; but look at our own time. Do I want the blessing of an institution that doesn't provide adequate protection from marital rape? That gives a woman less protection from assault by her husband than by a stranger? That assigns men 70 percent of contested child custodies?

Of course I do not fear any such brutality from the man I want to marry (no bride does). But marriage means that his respectful treatment of me and our children becomes, despite our intentions, a kindness rather than a legally grounded right.

We need a heterosexual version of the marriages that gay and lesbian activists are seeking: a commitment untainted by centuries of inequality; a ritual that invites the community to rejoice in the making of a new freely chosen family.

The radical heterosexual man must yield the automatic benefits conferred by gender. I had a lover once who did not want to give up playing sports in a club that had a separate door for women. It must be tempting to imagine you can have both—great squash courts *and* the bed of a liberated woman—but in the mess hall of gender relations, there is *no such thing as a free lunch.*

Radical heterosexual women too must give up gender benefits (such as they are). I know scores of women—independent, autonomous—who avoid assuming any of the risk for a romantic or sexual approach.

I have watched myself stand complacently by while my partner wrestles with a stuck window, an intractable computer printer, maps, or locks. Sisters, I am not proud of this, and I'm working on it. But people are lazy—or at least I am—and it's easy to rationalize that the person with the penis is the one who should get out of a warm bed to fix the snow on the TV screen. After all, it's the very least owed to me *personally* in compensation for centuries of virtual enslavement.

Radical heterosexuals must try to stay conscious—at all times, I'm afraid—of their gender imprinting, and how it plays out in their erotic melodramas. My own psyche is a flagrant *son et lumière* of political incorrectness. Three of my boyfriends had motorcycles; I am easy pickings for the silent and dysfunctional. My roving eye is so taken by the oil-stained persona of the labor organizer that myopic intellectuals have gained access to my favors merely by sporting a Trotsky button.

We feminists are hard on each other for admitting to weakness. Gloria Steinem caught flak from her left-wing sisters for acknowledging in *Revolution from Within* that she was drawn to a man because he could do the things with money and power that we are taught men must do. And some were appalled when Simone de Beauvoir's letter revealed how she coddled Sartre.

But the antifeminist erotic template is *in* us. We would not be citizens of this culture if swooning damsels and

Naomi Wolf's book "The Beauty Myth" is available in Anchor Books paperback. She has written on feminist issues for "Esquire," "The New Republic," and "The Wall Street Journal," and speaks to college audiences on feminism.

abandoned vixens had not been beamed at us from our first solid food to our first vote. We can't fight it until we admit to it. And we can't identify it until we drag it, its taffeta billowing and its bosom heaving, into the light of day.

I have done embarrassing, reactionary, abject deeds out of love and sexual passion. So, no doubt, has Norman Schwarzkopf. Only when we reveal our conditioning can we tell how much of our self-abasement is neurotic femininity, and how much is the flawed but impressive human apparatus of love.

In the Bedroom

Those are the conditions for the radical heterosexual couple. What might this new creation look like in bed? It will look like something we have no words or images for—the eroticization of consent, the equal primacy of female and male desire.

We will need to tell some secrets—to map our desire for the male body and admit to our fascination with the rhythms and forces of male arousal, its uncanny counter-intuitive spell.

We will also need to face our creature qualities. Animality has for so long been used against us—bitch, fox, *Penthouse* pet—that we struggle for the merit badges of higher rationality, ambivalent about our animal nature.

The truth is that heterosexual women believe that men, on some level, are animals; as they believe that we are animals. But what does "animal" mean?

Racism and sexism have long used animal metaphors to distance and degrade the Other. Let us redefine "animal" to make room for that otherness between the genders, an otherness fierce and worthy of respect. Let us define animal as an inchoate kinship, a comradeship, that finds a language beyond our species.

I want the love of two unlikes: the look of astonishment a woman has at the sight of a male back bending. These manifestations of difference confirm in heterosexuals the beauty that similarity confirms in the lesbian or gay imagination. Difference and animality do not have to mean hierarchy.

Men We Love

What must the men be like? Obviously, they're not going to be just anyone. *Esquire* runs infantile disquisitions on "Women We Love" (suggesting, Lucky Girls!). Well, I think that the men who are loved by feminists are lucky. Here's how they qualify to join this fortunate club.

Men We Love understand that, no matter how similar our backgrounds, we are engaged in a cross-cultural (if not practically biracial) relationship. They know that we know much about their world and they but little of ours. They accept what white people must accept in relationships with people of other ethnicities: to know that they do not know.

Men We Love don't hold a baby as if it is a still-squirming, unidentifiable catch from the sea.

Men We Love don't tell women what to feel about sexism. (There's a postcard that shows a dashing young fellow, drawn Love-comix-style, saying to a woman, "Let me explicate to you the nature of your oppression.") They do not presume that there is a line in the sand called "enlightened male," and that all they need is a paperback copy of Djuna Barnes and good digital technique. They understand that unlearning gender oppressiveness means untying the very core of how we become female and male. They know this pursuit takes a lifetime at the minimum.

Sadly, men in our lives sometime come through on personal feminism but balk at it intellectually. A year ago, I had a bruising debate with my father and brother about the patriarchal nature of traditional religious and literary canons. I almost seized them by their collars, howling "Read Mary Daly! Read Toni Morrison! Take Feminism 101. *No,* I *can't* explain it to you between the entrée and dessert!"

By spring, my dad, bless his heart, had asked for a bibliography, and last week my brother sent me *Standing Again at Sinai,* a Jewish-feminist classic. Men We Love are willing, sooner or later, to read the Books We Love.

Men We Love accept that successful training in manhood makes them blind to phenomena that are fact to women. Recently, I walked down a New York City avenue with a woman friend, X, and a man friend, Y. I pointed out to Y the leers, hisses, and invitations to sit on faces. Each woman saw clearly what the other woman saw, but Y was baffled. Sexual harassers have superb timing. A passerby makes kissy-noises with his tongue while Y is scrutinizing the menu of the nearest bistro. "There, there! Look! Listen!" we cried. "What? Where? Who?" wailed poor Y, valiantly, uselessly spinning.

What if, hard as they try to see, they cannot hear? Once I was at lunch with a renowned male crusader for the First Amendment. Another Alpha male was present, and the venue was the Supreme Court lunchroom—two power factors that automatically press the "mute" button on the male ability to detect a female voice on the audioscope. The two men began to rev their motors; soon they were off and racing in a policy-wonk grand prix. I tried, once or twice, to ask questions. But the free-speech champions couldn't hear me over the testosterone roar.

Men We Love undertake half the care and cost of contraception. They realize that it's not fair to wallow in the fun without sharing the responsibility. When stocking up for long weekends, they brave the amused glances when they ask, "Do you have this in unscented?"

Men We Love know that just because we can be irrational doesn't mean we're insane. When we burst into premenstrual tears—having just realized the cosmic fragility of creation—they comfort us. Not until we feel better do they dare remind us gently that we had this same revelation exactly 28 days ago.

Men We Love must make a leap of imagination to believe in the female experience. They do not call women nags or paranoid when we embark on the arduous, often boring, nonnegotiable daily chore of drawing attention to sexism. They treat it like adults taking driving lessons: if irked in the short term at being treated like babies, they're grateful in the long term that someone is willing to teach them patiently how to move through the world without harming the pedestrians. Men We Love don't drive without their gender glasses on.

A Place for Them

It's not simple gender that pits Us against Them. In the fight against sexism, it's those who are for us versus those who are against us—of either gender.

When I was 16, my boyfriend came with me to hear Andrea Dworkin speak. While hearing great feminist oratory in a sea of furious women changed my life, it nearly ended my boyfriend's: he barely escaped being drawn and quartered.

It is time to direct our anger more acutely at the Men We Hate—like George Bush—and give the Men We Love something useful to do. Not to take over meetings, or to set agendas; not to whine, "Why can't feminists teach us how to be free?" but to add their bodies, their hearts, and their numbers, to support us.

I meet many young men who are brought to feminism by love for a woman who has been raped, or by watching

their single mothers struggle against great odds, or by simple common sense. Their most frequent question is, "What can I do to help?"

Imagine a rear battalion of committed "Men Against Violence Against Women" (or Men for Choice, or what have you)—of all races, ages, and classes. Wouldn't that be a fine sight to fix in the eyes of a five-year-old boy?

Finally, the place to make room for radical feminist heterosexuality is within our heads. If the movement that I dearly love has a flaw, it is a tendency toward orthodoxies about other women's pleasures and needs. This impulse is historically understandable: in the past, we needed to define ourselves against men if we were to define ourselves at all. But today, the most revolutionary choice we can make is to affirm other women's choices, whether lesbian or straight, bisexual or celibate.

NOW President Patricia Ireland speaks for me even though our sexual lives are not identical. Simone de Beauvoir speaks for me even though our sexual lives are not identical. Audre Lorde speaks for me even though our sexual lives are not identical. Is it the chromosomes of your lovers that establish you as a feminist? Or is it the life you make out of the love you make?

Ω

Response to Naomi Wolf's "Radical Heterosexuality"
by Laura McEnaney

I never thought about heterosexuality as anything but sexual behavior until I got to college. I took a women's studies course my freshman year, and my teacher introduced the term "sexual politics" to me. I resisted thinking about sexuality as political—I couldn't connect what I understood as "political," (elections, the presidency, etc.) with heterosexuality. And I was disturbed that my teacher had stirred up self-doubt and curiosity about something I thought was completely "natural." Now, ten years later, I cannot see sexuality as anything but political. As a graduate student, I have had the privilege of reading about heterosexuality from a historical perspective. As a teacher, I have listened to the viewpoints of many undergraduates—male and female—as they have grappled with their experiences of heterosexuality in the 1980s and 1990s. As a feminist, I have spent many hours trying to understand how feminist insights have challenged and changed this

sexual identity. And as someone who identifies as heterosexual and has been in a number of relationships with men—who have ranged from feminist to sexist to antifeminist—I have long grappled with the question posed by Naomi Wolf: "how to love a man and save your feminist soul." So, I am happy to see that Wolf has created another forum to define and debate heterosexuality as a political concept. Still, I find myself quite disturbed by her article. I have no real answers about the dilemma Wolf describes, but I am troubled by some of her depictions of feminism and by her vision of what is radical and possible for contemporary heterosexual relations.

First, I want to agree with some of Wolf's observations. I am pleased that she demands we take a more critical, less romantic look at marriage. I like the idea of celebrating freely chosen families. I agree with her argument that gender struggles do not follow neat biological categories—that women's problems cannot be explained exclusively as a battle of women versus men. The political struggles of the last twenty years have shown us that

Reprinted by permission of the author.

248

women can be anti-feminists and men can be feminists—and many other confusing variations on the political continuum. And I like her assertion that men must make a concerted effort to see sexism in all of its guises, and that they should "add their bodies, their hearts, and their numbers" to support women's causes. These are all important components of any feminist program that attempts to re-map heterosexual relations.

Yet, I am uncomfortable with many of Wolf's assertions, as well as with the overall tone of her article. First, I depart from Wolf in my understanding of what feminism has offered to women as they have struggled to find sexual identities that feel comfortable for them. Like so many other contemporary journalists, Wolf implies that the feminist movement has taken the pleasure out of heterosexual romance and ritual. She suggests that feminism has diminished women's erotic agency, and that pure "animal" sex has been replaced by political correctness. Feminism's flaw, she says, "is a tendency toward orthodoxies about other women's pleasures and needs." She uses Andrea Dworkin, in particular, as the icon of an angry, man-hating, anti-heterosexual feminism that can chew up sympathetic boyfriends at public lectures. Now that feminism has become "more mature," she says, "it's time" to challenge the ideological purity of a movement that dictated, instead of liberated, women's sexual choices.

I am confused by this. One of the chief contributions of feminist movements has been the insistence that women have a right to sexual pleasure on their own terms. Sexual liberation has always been a central tenet of second-wave women's movements. An enormous body of feminist literature has documented the diversity and variety of female sexualities. *Our Bodies, Ourselves* is the culmination of over two decades of feminist thinking and debate about sex. It is a classic feminist text that affirms women as sexual beings and offers them a very expansive, non-judgmental definition of female sexuality. Feminist movements have made women's claims to an enjoyable sex life a sign of health, not deviance, and the scores of self-help books and talk shows that encourage female pleasure attest to feminism's mainstream success in reclaiming the bedroom (and other space!) for women.

Strangely, Wolf does not acknowledge the rich history of spirited debate about sexuality within feminisms. Nor does she mention the enormous diversity of opinion about sexual politics among contemporary feminists. Instead, she suggests that feminists are a sexual monolith, disciples of a sexual-political correctness. Gloria Steinem "caught flak" from some feminists not, as Wolf says, for her sexual fantasies, but for her recent emphasis on creating "revolution from within," a frightening departure for some second-wave feminists who are still invested in fighting for equality at structural levels. I don't agree with much of what Andrea Dworkin says about sexuality, but Wolf's depiction of her (and her followers) as a force that could "draw and quarter" men is a classic stereotyping of women who speak angrily about sexism. And why does she choose Dworkin and Catharine MacKinnon as "the feminists" to

argue with? Is it because they—especially Dworkin—represent the most extreme example of female anger about the violence and powerlessness so many women have experienced in their heterosexual relationships? I wish that Wolf would have at least acknowledged some of the terrific radical thinking about heterosexuality by other feminists, such as Ellen Willis, who share Dworkin's anger about inequality, but offer different possibilities for heterosexual relations. When Wolf says, "It's time to say you *can* hate sexism and love men," she implies that she is one of the first to think through this dilemma—that as a representative of younger women who didn't fight the battles of the sixties, she can bring a fresh, more ideologically fluid perspective to this issue. She makes invisible all of the radical heterosexual women who have played key roles in women's movement activism around sexuality. And she doesn't give enough credit to feminist movements for creating the space for debate about heterosexuality. In fact, she and I wouldn't be having this printed conversation if it weren't for feminism.

I am growing weary of women like Wolf (Katie Roiphe and Karen Lehrman included) who blame feminism for ruining the romance of heterosexuality. And it worries me that this notion carries so much weight in the mainstream media. Recent episodes of "Beverly Hills 90210" and "Picket Fences," for example, have suggested that feminists have gone too far in politicizing the bedroom. I think if there are any feminist orthodoxies about sex (which I don't believe there are), they might be that women must have the right to define their own sexual identities, and that inequality between men and women makes it imperative that women understand sex as a political category. What's constricting or orthodox about this? These feminist tenets seem to *open,* not foreclose, sexual possibilities for women. Men and women do not enter a relationship as equals in society, so why shouldn't heterosexuals interested in forging equality in their relationship examine the ways in which sex, itself, is part of the larger struggle for gender equity? In fact, I think exposing how sexism shapes heterosexual relationships has the potential to make sexual relations *more,* not less, satisfying; it frees *both* men and women to challenge repressive gender expectations so that they can experience fully their relational and erotic desires. I think Wolf sometimes confuses feminist critiques of heterosexuality, which have always focused on liberation, with the mainstream media's anxious and inaccurate translation of those critiques.

I am also frustrated by the political program Wolf offers women who identify as heterosexual: out of bed, men's reeducation and making good choices; in bed, a reclaiming of the "animal." First, out of bed. Wolf is very optimistic about the possibility of raising men's consciousness about sex discrimination. Her stories of fighting with male family members, men's blindness to street harassment, and male domination of conversation are all painfully familiar to women. The story of her father and brother eventually acknowledging her feminist viewpoints tells us that men can "get it." Women and men, she argues, should be partners in the task of men's reeducation. Men shouldn't expect women to do all of the work for them, but women should direct their anger at the men they hate (nasty politicians), and "give the Men (They) Love something useful to do."

So, what's wrong with this? I'm not sure I see Wolf asking men in any concrete way to concede power. It seems like she is asking men to tolerate women more than she is demanding that they share power with them. Sharing contraception, lovingly accepting women's "irrational" premenstrual emotions, and listening to women's "often boring" chore of complaining about sexism seems to be about as radical as Wolf's vision gets. Why do women have to settle for men's understanding? Why can't women demand changes in behavior, concessions about the household division of labor, and power-sharing in and out of the bedroom? Conventional sex roles within heterosexual relationships have amazing resilience, and I think Wolf underestimates the staying power—and comfort—of those conventions. It is much easier to be angry at George Bush (what have you got to lose?) than it is to confront power differentials with the person you sleep with. Wolf suggests that men unlearn sexism, but she is unwilling to spell out exactly what that means for heterosexual relations. Who will be the tutors for these men? When a man has not yet unlearned his sexism and refuses to wear a condom, what then does his partner do? Where are the institutional and psychological supports for a man to unlearn sexism? What if "the men we love" don't change? I am all for consciousness-raising, but it can function as only one part of a much larger political movement that attacks the economic and cultural roots of men's dominance over women.

In bed, Wolf offers heterosexual women "the equal primacy of female and male desire" and a redefinition of "the animal." Well, feminism has already claimed for women the right to desire and fantasize, and I, again, state it's important for Wolf to credit feminism for this. As for her call for women to face their "creature qualities" and to "define animal as an inchoate kinship, a comradeship, that finds a language beyond our species," I am not sure I understand her meaning. What are women's "creature qualities"? Something "natural" or biologically ordained? A person's desire is shaped by the culture; there is nothing biological abut the fact that our culture finds thin blonde white women the most desirous. And how can reclaiming "our animal nature" help women? Why does Wolf accept the term "animal" for men and women at all? As she points out, this term is a by-product of racism and sexism. I think it is naive to reclaim the "animal" in a society where the term is still used so derisively against women—especially women of color. Redefining "the animal" as a program of heterosexual liberation is a political fantasy and a slippery slope. It assumes women have enough political power in society to mediate how "animal" will be redefined, and it embraces dangerous pre-feminist notions that ascribed male domination and women's supposed passionlessness to hormones. Wolf could have simply called for the continuation of feminist criticism of conventional heterosexu-

ality, emphasizing the importance of women reclaiming the erotic, however they want to define it.

I envision a different kind of radical heterosexuality than Wolf. A radical heterosexuality challenges the notion of a fixed, biologically-determined sexual identity. In other words, radical heterosexuality challenges itself. Radical heterosexuals think about heterosexuality as part of a sexual continuum that includes bisexual and homosexual fantasizing and activity. Politically, it is not enough to define radical heterosexuality as a way to reeducate a boyfriend and make sex more enjoyable for women. We need to complicate the very idea of "heterosexuality" in a way that exposes how it can reinforce conventional gender roles and foreclose opportunities for us to explore sexual aspects of ourselves that don't follow neat and supposedly biologically-determined categories of "gay" and "straight." This is controversial, I know. Some believe that sexuality is genetically determined. But radical heterosexuality should offer women a way of honestly questioning how one's sexual desires and relationships are constructed by a larger culture that is extremely uncomfortable with bi- or homosexuality.

I also think radical heterosexuality should involve an investment in building and maintaining friendships. Most of us have had the experience of either being "dropped" by a woman friend who begins a relationship, or ourselves have neglected friends as we have entered new relationships. It is a challenge to maintain friendships while we are in relationships because there is very little encouragement to do so. The contemporary notion of romantic love suggests that women (and men) can find all of their emotional fulfillment in one person—their partner/spouse. Friends are important, but are sidelined somewhat, because "the relationship" takes precedence. I think a radical heterosexuality should challenge this cultural script and blur the lines between friendship and relationship. This is not to say that relationships and friendships are or should be exactly the same; sex complicates things tremendously. But I think a radical heterosexuality should offer a better awareness about the privileging of sexual relationships at the cost of building and sustaining other friendships.

Finally, radical heterosexuality should be about, at the very least, the exposure and active challenging of heterosexual privilege. Heterosexuality is rewarded in so many invisible ways in this society—marriage and its attendant economic benefits being one of the most obvious illustrations of this. Radical heterosexuals should make themselves aware of the privileges they enjoy just for identifying as heterosexual: public displays of affection, a basic level of family approval for partner choice, and health benefits, to name only a few. This is not an exercise in liberal guilt, but an act of consciousness raising to alert people to the power they have—whether they want it or not—because of their sexual identity. Radical heterosexuality offers heterosexuals a way to openly criticize that power and a way to act against it or simply retreat from using it. It also provides an understanding of the kind of oppression that "non-heterosexuals" are bound to experience because of their sexual identities. Radical heterosexuality must always be a sexual identity engaged in fighting homophobia and heterosexual privilege, otherwise it becomes only a utopian celebration of itself

I have previously offered some of these views as a speaker on the Women's Studies 103 sexuality panel, and some students have responded by saying I am not a "real heterosexual." I can imagine some people reading my response and thinking I am overly pessimistic, bitter, and too much of a "PC-feminist." I offer these views as an optimistic contribution to the spirited debate about sexuality that has always characterized feminism. I think pushing ourselves to question every fixed category with presumed "natural" origins is liberating, not politically stifling. It frees us from gender conventions, from being suspect for knowing our desires don't follow clear, pre-determined categories, and from regulating ourselves—or being forced to live with the sexual regulation of others. No, I am not as optimistic as Wolf about the future of heterosexual relations, and I find her agenda lacking in anger, radical imagination, and concrete political meaning. But I am not pessimistic either. I think forging an equal relationship with a man is hard work, but possible. Instead of criticizing feminism for making heterosexuality less enjoyable, I credit it for creating more options for men and women in relationships. Without a feminist critique of heterosexuality, the hard work of building equality on the micro and macro level would be impossible between women and men.

Ω

Worksheet - Chapter 8
Sexuality

This worksheet should be optional. It asks personal questions which no one should be required to answer.

I. Sexual Preference

Society, parents, and friends give very clear messages about who one should relate to sexually, how and when! We are all aware that we are "breaking the rules" if we are sexually involved with someone of the "wrong" age, the "wrong" color, the "wrong" social status, or the "wrong" sex.

Heterosexism is so prevalent that most heterosexuals never think about why they relate sexually to the opposite sex. Imagine a mother asking her 18 year old daughter to explain why she is going out with men instead of women. But most lesbians and bisexuals have had to think through, question, and explain their choices.

Answer the following questions for yourself. Ask friends who would identify their sexual preference (or situation) as different from yours (lesbian — bisexual — celibate — heterosexual — virgin) to answer the same set of questions.

A. Briefly describe your present lifestyle and your sexual identify.

B. Describe how you made this choice about your sexuality. (Was it a gradual evolution or a sudden awareness? Has your sexuality changed or stayed the same since your first sexual identity? What factors have influenced this?)

C. Do you have a sexual partner or partners now? Would your sexual identity be the same if you did not have a partner/partners?

D. In what specific ways do you consciously work towards a balance of power in your relationship? How equal is your relationship sexually?

E. How does your sexual relationship/identity affect your relationships with friends, both men and women, with whom you are not having a sexual relationship?

253

F. How does your sexuality affect your choices regarding children?

G. The women's movement has emphasized that "the personal is political": the decisions we make in our personal lives and the way we live our lives are political issues. How do you see "the personal being political" relating to your sexuality and your sexual choices?

H. Do you feel there is such a thing as "heterosexual privilege"? If so, how does this affect your life?

II. Kegel Exercises

The pubococcygeus (P.C.) muscle supports the walls of the vagina, the urethra and rectum. Good, strong P.C. muscles can be important for childbirth, preventing stress incontinence (loss of urine when coughing or sneezing), and can enhance sexual enjoyment.

Kegel exercises (developed by Dr. Arnold Kegel) are designed to strengthen the P.C. muscle. Unlike most exercises, no special clothes, gyms, etc., are required. These exercises can be done anywhere and no one else will even know you are doing them.

A. Find your P.C. muscle. When you are urinating, stop the flow of urine in midstream. The muscle you do this with is your pubococcygeus muscle and is the muscle you want to strengthen.

B. Examples of Kegel Exercises:
Flicks—Do a series of contractions as rapidly as possible. It has been suggested that one does this in time to the car's turn signals.
Squeeze and hold for as long as possible, trying work up to holding for 8–10 seconds.
Take a slow, deep breath, squeezing the P.C. muscle as you are breathing in. Pretend you are slowly drawing something into your vagina.

Chapter

9

Fertility, Infertility, and Reproductive Rights and Freedom

Real reproductive rights would mean that women are able to choose when, whether, and under what conditions to have children, how many children to have, and to assume that she and her children would survive (and thrive) during pregnancy, childbirth, and the post-partum periods. What kind of health system would truly allow *all* women to have healthy babies, healthy children, and healthy families? What other societal changes need to happen for women to be able to make their own "choices" not to have children or to have the number of children they want?

Too often the media, and maybe even the movements themselves, have promoted the image that the struggle for reproductive rights is about abortion and contraceptive issues. Certainly access to affordable, safe contraception, with affordable, safe abortion as a back-up, is an essential part of women being able to control their bodies and their lives, but many other issues are also part of the bigger picture of what reproductive rights and reproductive freedom* really mean.

Building on the work of the Black Women's Health Project and African-American Women for Reproductive Rights (see *The Black Women's Health Book)*, other women of color groups have been actively organizing around and clearly articulating that an agenda for reproductive rights must be much more broadly defined to include many other issues central to their lives. The articles, "Empowerment Through Dialogue: Native American Women Hold Historic Meeting," "For Native Women Reproductive Rights Mean:" and "Latinas for Reproductive Choice" summarize more inclusive, more culturally relevant definitions of reproductive freedom and provide examples of ways Native American women and Latinas are organizing around these issues.

In working for a broader definition of reproductive rights which includes women being able to have as many children as they choose, we need to have an analysis of how the issue of infertility has been medicalized. High tech medicine certainly promises exciting possibilities for offering some women with infertility the possibility of producing a baby. In many cities, it is already routine to offer

in vitro fertilization, bypassing blocked fallopian tubes, to many heterosexual women who happen to have an extra $5000 to try it. But, health activists have questioned who benefits, who makes money, and who is determining the priorities in the rapidly growing field of infertility technology? Why is all the research emphasis on finding expensive high technological solutions instead of looking at ways to prevent infertility (safer contraceptive methods, safer work and living environments) which could benefit far more people? Which women do and do not have access to infertility investigations and infertility treatments and should it be a goal to make these resources equally available to all women? Anne Woollett's moving personal diary serves to remind us that there is much more to infertility than sophisticated medical technology: how does the health care system respond to many of the key issues of the experience of infertility (including the tests and treatments) which have to do with the effects on self-image, sexuality, relationships and dreams for the future?

We live in a reactionary climate where our access to safe, legal abortion is threatened or eroded by state decisions to restrict the availability of abortions. Working against the backlash to the few reproductive rights which we have won, often takes so much of our energy that we do not take the time to discuss controversial and contradictory issue about abortion with other reproductive rights activists. The next three articles should be thought provoking enough to stimulate some healthy debates among friends or students who usually simply pride themselves on being "pro-choice." In "Born and Unborn: The Implications of 'Choice' for People with Disabilities", Marsha Saxton, who identifies herself as a feminist who supports the pro-choice position on abortion, asks us to remember that real choice must include the choice to have a disabled child and looks at how oppressive societal attitudes about disability impact on pregnant women facing prenatal screening. We might ask ourselves what the role of prenatal screening would be in a society where many of the "handicaps" of disability had been eliminated or minimized. The article, "Menstrual Extraction: Is Self-Help Making a Comeback?" provides a history of self-help groups "for women to control *all* their reproductive processes" which existed before the 1973 Supreme Court ruling legalizing abortion. The article also initiates a debate on whether the revival of gynecological self-help is a way to ensure that lawmakers will keep abortion legal or is a "tactical error" that will play into the hands of anti-choice legislators? Connie S. Chan's "Reproductive Issues Are Essential Survival Issues for Asian American Communities" describes how she, as a middle-class, educated, bilingual Asian American, was unaware of the reproductive health issues of poor, non-English speaking immigrant women and what she learned as a translator. This article is a reminder of how easy it is not to understand what reproductive rights mean to another woman or groups of women; it begs us to think through the ramifications for poor women when health care benefits are not available to them because of their immigrant status or because Medicaid benefits will not cover abortion. At its most provocative level, this article asks us to think about the many ways the health system and society have failed a woman and her children when abortion becomes the "choice" of basic survival for the members of a family unit.

Issues about the politics of contraceptives are covered in the next three pieces. Despite the women's movements' opposition to approving new (to the USA) hormonal contraceptives of questionable longterm safety and which have a history or potential for abuse, in a climate which is increasing pro-hormones for women of all ages, the Food and Drug Administration (FDA) recently approved both Depo Provera and Norplant for American women. The National Women's Health Network's (NWHN) testimony, "Use of Depo Provera for Contraception" states many of the reasons why this organization and others opposed the approval of Depo Provera. This is the testimony which Cindy Pearson, NWHN Program Director, prepared and presented to the FDA hearings on Depo Provera. The fact that Depo Provera was approved by the FDA may be a reminder that many challenges still face

women's health movements, but the testimony can also be viewed as symbolic of the women's health movements' victories. The NWHN was founded in the early 70s as activists organized together *outside* FDA hearings to protest the fact that no consumer voices were included in the hearings about the safety of oral contraceptive pills. Now, the NWHN, a 15,000 membership organization representing consumer interests on all women's health issues, is routinely asked to give testimony *inside,* before FDA advisory committees, on almost all women's health issues! The National Latina Health Organization's "Norplant Information Sheet" summarizes some of the issues around the product's safety and particularly asks urgent questions around the actual and potential abuse of Norplant, especially for women of color. The seemingly apolitical article from the *FDA Consumer,* " 'The Pill' May Not Mix Well with Other Drugs" raises very worrying questions about the politics of information when the reader realizes that very basic information with life-changing ramifications, "certain drugs many decrease the effectiveness of your contraceptive or your contraceptive may alter the way your body responds to other medications," is not available to many women choosing to use the contraceptive pill.

Another major political question is why are "reproductive rights" so much seen as issues for women? If we lived in a more egalitarian society or if men shared equally in the responsibility for childcare, how would that affect *all* reproductive rights and health issues? Why has almost all of reproductive research focused on finding ways to interfere with a woman's body to prevent pregnancy or understanding how a pregnant woman's environment affects fetal health? Do you think we would see more articles and research like "Eight New Nonhormonal Contraceptives Methods for Men" and "Research on Birth Defects Turns to Flaws in Sperm" if more women had the power to help determine reproductive health research priorities?

---

*Loretta Ross, a long-term women's health activist, uses the term reproductive rights in connection with the more white-dominated movements which have focused very much on abortion and contraceptive issues, and the term reproductive freedom for the organizations, with women of color leadership, which have worked on a much wider range of issues related to women's reproductive lives.

Empowerment Through Dialogue:
Native American Women Hold Historic Meeting

by Donna Haukaas

Ten years ago, a young Indian woman on the Pine Ridge Indian Reservation went to the local Indian Health Service hospital and sought advice on birth control. The doctors prescribed Provera, the pill form of Depo-Provera, a drug known for its cancer-causing properties. Last year, the woman was diagnosed as having cervical cancer. She said she was never told of the drug's possible side effects by hospital staff. Ever since, this woman has blamed herself, until she went to a very important conference where she met other Indian women with similar stories and realized she was not alone.

The conference, "Empowerment Through Dialogue: Native American Women & Reproductive Rights," held in Pierre, South Dakota, was the first time ever Indian women have participated in a reproductive rights conference planned by and for Native American women. More than 30 women representing 11 tribes from South Dakota and North Dakota attended this three-day conference which was co-sponsored by the Women of Color Partnership Program of the Religious Coalition for Abortion Rights of Washington, D.C. and the Native American Women's Health Education Resource Center of Lake Andes, South Dakota.

"The purpose of the conference (is) to bring together women from across South Dakota in a collective decision-making process to recommend an agenda for Native American women's reproductive rights," said Charon Asetoyer, Executive Director of the Native American Women's Health Education Resource Center (NAWHERC). "Our reproductive rights are much broader than abortion."

Sabrae Jenkins, Director of RCAR's Women of Color Partnership Program, gave a national overview of reproductive rights and women of color. "We, as women of color, cannot afford to look at the issue of abortion in a vacuum like middle-class white women; we have too many other things to deal with," said Jenkins. "The issue of choosing when, if, where and how to have a child is tied to access to education, housing, employment, health care and child care.

"Then you bring in the issues of racism, women of color's disproportionate low-income status and sexism—we are at the bottom of the rung." she said.

Mary Louise Defender, a member of the Standing Rock Tribe of North Dakota, addressed "The Reproductive History and Tradition Within the Native American Community" from the perspective that for Indian women the past and present are tied to the future. She talked about how elders would teach the young girls about menstruation and the meaning behind it as well as child spacing. "There were ladies who would tell you how not to have a child, but this was not to be used to sleep around" she said.

"The coming generation depends on no one but we women. Our role models should be those grandmas from generations ago who took no guff. Somewhere along the way our women became a little bit shy. But we need to remember those grandmas, and think of how they were and how they would take control and do it," said Defender.

Karen Artichoker of the South Dakota Coalition for Sexual Assault and Domestic Violence spoke on "The Status of Native American Women in South Dakota." From her many travels around the state, Artichoker relayed a dismal picture to the women regarding high unemployment, the horrendous health conditions of Indian families and alcoholism.

During the second day, Charon Asetoyer discussed "Reproductive Technologies and Concerns for Native American Women" where the participants were made aware of the new technologies like RU-486 and Norplant as well as Depo Provera and forced sterilization. She also addressed "Choices After Conception" which included abortion, fetal alcohol syndrome, and prenatal care.

"In South Dakota only 37% of pregnant Indian women receive regular prenatal care compared to 64% of white women. Consequently, the South Dakota non-white population which is 90% Native American has one of the highest infant mortality rates in the country at 27.5 deaths per 1,000 live births." stated Asetoyer.

Brenda Hill closed out the second day of speakers with a frank presentation on "The Impact of Domestic Violence & Sexual Abuse on Reproductive Rights." She told the audience that the violation of reproductive rights is directly linked to sexual assault and domestic violence.

Brenda made the conference participants clearly aware of the high rates of violence which currently exist within the Indian community and why it occurs. While Native Americans only make up 6.25% of the total population of South Dakota, 50% of all domestic abuse cases occur within the Native American Community.

Donna Haukaas is a Lakota Indian and a writer for the Rosebud Reservation Newsservice. A domestic violence activist, Ms. Haukaas was a conference participant.

"We have the right to comprehensive, culturally-relevant health care that recognizes and prioritizes the safety issues of battered women and children, and that each woman has the courage to take personal responsibility to say 'violence against women is not right,'" said Tillie Black Bear of St. Francis, South Dakota and Chair of the National Coalition Against Domestic Violence.

"We have a right to come together as sisters. This includes a recognition that we are all doing the best we can at the present time, given our own oppression and internalized oppression," said Black Bear.

During the third and final day of the conference, the participants reflected on all the discussion of the previous days within small groups. Utilizing the African American Women for Reproductive Rights manifesto as a model, the women came back to the conference body with items which should be included in a reproductive rights agenda for Native American women and formed a committee to write a narrative explaining their support for reproductive rights as well as to integrate the agenda items from the small groups into one.

The participants said they were encouraged by the conference and felt inspired to pursue a broad agenda in the next year that would aid women in taking greater control over their lives. As the conference came to a close, these women discussed a specific desire to organize a coalition where the information sharing started at the conference could continue and where they could collectively fight for reproductive health care changes within their own communities.

Ω

For Native Women
Reproductive Rights Mean:
by Native Women for Reproductive Rights Coalition

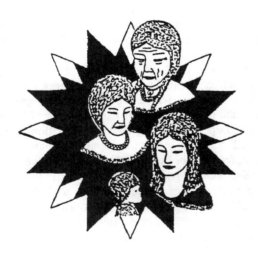

1. The right to knowledge and education for all family members concerning sexuality and reproduction that is age, culture and gender appropriate.

2. The right to all reproductive alternatives and the right to choose the size of our families.

3. The right to affordable health care, including safe deliveries within our communities.

4. The right to access safe, free, and/or affordable abortions, regardless of age, with confidentiality and free pre and post counseling.

5. The right to active involvement in the development and implementation of policies concerning reproductive issues, to include, but not limited to, pharmaceuticals and technology.

6. The right to include domestic violence, sexual assault and AIDS as reproductive rights issues.

7. The right to programs which meet the nutritional needs of women and families.

8. The right to programs to reduce the rate of infant mortality and high risk pregnancies.

9. The right to culturally specific comprehensive chemical dependency prenatal programs, including, but not limited to, prevention of Fetal Alcohol Syndrome and Effects.

10. The right to stop coerced sterilization.

11. The right to a forum for cultural/spiritual development, culturally-oriented health care, and the right to live as Native women.

12. The right to be fully informed about, and to consent to any forms of medical treatment

13. The right to determine who are members of our Nations.

14. The right to continuous, consistent and quality health care for Native People.

15. The right to reproductive rights and support for women with disabilities.

16. The right to parent our children in a non-sexist, non-racist environment.

In order to accomplish the foregoing stated rights, the Native Women for Reproductive Rights will create coalitions and alliances to network with other groups.

— Ω

Latinas for Reproductive Choice
by Latinas for Reproductive Choice

The National Latina Health Organization was co-founded by four Latinas on March 8, 1986, International Women's Day. The NLHO was formed to raise Latina consciousness about our health and health problems, so that we can begin to take control of our health and our lives. We are committed to work towards the goal of bilingual access to quality health care and the self-empowerment of Latinas through educational programs, outreach and research.

The National Latina Health Organization has been redefining reproductive issues from our very beginning. We have been actively advocating the expansion of abortion rights to include all the reproductive issues . . . family planning, prenatal care, education and information on sexuality that is culturally relevant and in our language, birth control, freedom from sterilization abuses; and above all, access to all health services. This is being done with our constituents locally and nationally.

At the beginning of 1990, the NLHO, along with other community activists, created "Latinas for Reproductive Choice", a project of the NLHO. We feel strongly that Latinas need to take a public stand on reproductive issues in the way that they affect us. We launched our project with a press conference in San Francisco on October 3, 1990, the thirteenth anniversary of the death of Rosie Jimenez. Our legislators and the general public need to become aware that we are now ready to become a very visible, public, vocal and very strong force in this historic debate that will decide the future of all women. Another very important effect of our becoming public is that other Latinas who have never openly dealt with these issues, even though they themselves may have had an abortion, will finally have the support that they need to make a

personal difference. It is very historic, that Latinas are coming together in coalition to publicly take a stand on reproductive issues.

As Latinas for Reproductive Choice we propose to:

1. Break the silence on reproductive rights issues within the Latina community and provide a platform for open discussion.

2. Debunk the myths that surround Latinas through public education.

3. Include Latinas in the national reproductive rights debate by promoting Latinas on the boards of the traditional reproductive rights groups.

4. Monitor elected officials who represent Latino communities.

5. Advocate and pressure elected officials, organizations, and individuals to support reproductive choice issues for Latinas.

We are using the following letter to bring our community together on these vital issues.

———

Dear Amiga,

Did you know. . .

. . . Latinas make up 8.4% of women 15–44 years of age in the United States, yet 13% of all abortions are performed on Latinas in that age group?

. . . the abortion rate for Latinas is 42.6 per 1,000 compared to 26.6 per 1,000 for non-Latinas aged 15–44?

. . . it is easier today for a poor Latina to be sterilized than it is for her to receive quality family planning services and obstetrical care?

. . . In some areas of the U.S., 65% of all Latina women have been sterilized?

Do you care. . .

. . . that because Latinas have been left out of the abortion debate a myth has been promulgated by others

From *National Latina Health Organization Newsletter,* Vol. 1, No. 1, 1990–91, pp. 9–10. Copyright © 1990 by the National Latina Health Organization. Reprinted by permission.

that Latinas don't have abortions (after all, we're all Roman Catholic aren't we?)

. . . that if abortion rights are restricted, Latinas will be among the first victims of illegal abortions?

. . . that a group of Latinas has banded together to address these issues and do something about them?

We are Latinas for Reproductive Choice and we will no longer stand on the sidelines and let others decide our fate. We have come together to make sure Latina voices are part of the debate and to mobilize Latinas who are as alarmed as we are at what has been happening to our hermanas across the nation.

On October 3, 1977 a poor, young Latina died because of an illegal Texas abortion. That was the year Medicaid funding for abortions was cut. The young Latina was Rosie Jimenez, the first women to die from such an operation following the cutoff of Medicaid funds for abortions. Lack of reproductive choice killed Rosie Jimenez. And we can't afford to lose any more Rosies to this kind of murder! Yet, there continue to be millions of young women just like Rosie Jimenez today. Right now, in 1990, most Latinas still do not have reproductive choice. If we do not fight to maintain access to safe and legal abortions thousands more young women like Rosie Jimenez will die needlessly.

Access to abortion is only half the issue for Latinas. Reproductive choice for us is much more than abortion—it is the ability to have healthy babies when, and if, we want. It means the freedom to choose to have one child or 10. Or even none. Reproductive choice means access to culturally-relevant, quality health care and information, education about sexuality and contraception for our daughters, and access to alternative forms of birth control, regardless of cost. Sterilization should not be our only choice simply because it is federally funded. Reproductive choice means the freedom to make informed choices about our bodies.

Reproductive health and abortion issues will dominate the 1990's. Candidates in the upcoming November election will be elected on the basis of their positions on reproductive issues. In recent months the United States Supreme Court has upheld more and more state restrictions on the right to an abortion and with the resignation of Justice William Brennan, the future is not encouraging. For the first time since the historic Roe v. Wade decision the Supreme Court appears willing to overturn a woman's right to a safe and legal abortion.

It is clear that if we do not speak for ourselves, no one else will. We need to ensure that Latina voices are heard in this historic debate because we have a unique perspective that has been ignored for too long.

This is why we have come together as Latinas for Reproductive Choice. Won't you join with us to make sure Rosie Jimenez did not die in vain? Help us provide a voice for all other Latinas who find themselves without choice. Help us speak out as Latinas on the most momentous issue of this decade. We can no longer afford to be silent. Add your name to the list of Latinas who are willing to take a stand.

Sinceramente,
LATINAS FOR REPRODUCTIVE CHOICE
PO BOX 7567
OAKLAND, CA 94601
(415) 534-1362

Ω

Discovering that You Are Infertile: One Woman's Experience
by Naomi Pfeffer and Anne Woollett

'Well,' they said, 'If you're going to have a baby you should start soon. You're not getting any younger you know.'

It took me a long time to decide that I wanted a child. I started thinking about it perhaps four years ago. I thought about it. I talked to other women. I listened to other women, to mothers and women without children. I found out about childcare arrangements. I thought about my job and how having a child would influence my work. I talked to the

Reprinted with permission from THE EXPERIENCE OF INFERTILITY by Naomi Pfeffer and Anne Woollett, Virago Press, London, 1983

man I live with about a child and the effects one might have on our lives and on our relationship. We thought about when would be a good time to have a child. A baby born in the spring or summer would fit in well with my work.

April 1978 I put my cap away.

August 1978 We go away on holiday.

September 1978 Period two days late and breasts feel very tender. Are they normally tender just before my period? I become much more sensitive to my body. I live inside myself, my centre of gravity seems to be somewhere inside my uterus. I feel full, preoccupied, pleased that I might be pregnant. Then blood. No pregnancy. No baby. Perhaps next month.

1 October 1978 Perhaps next month.

30 October 1978 Blood, period, perhaps next month.

Why am I not getting pregnant? I begin to ask questions about my body. I've been taking my temperature for several months and I know that I am ovulating. How long does it normally take to get pregnant? I had assumed it could take up to six months and we have been trying for that time.

People reassure me. Sometimes it takes a long time. I'm given advice, information, details about how other people did it. I'm consoled, never mind, you'll make it. I'm trying to grapple with the idea that perhaps I won't make it. That idea creeps into my mind and I want to discuss it. But it's not something people are willing to discuss. A friend gets pregnant. It didn't take her long. She gets bigger. We discuss home confinements, epidurals, baby clothes, names. The world seems to be full of pregnant women, in the streets, holding babies, pushing prams. I'm surrounded by pregnant women. I read up on conception and find that infertility tests begin with an examination of the man's sperm.

4 December 1978 A friend, a nurse, arranges for us to have a sperm test. She provides us with the plastic container in its brown box, complete with instructions. 'The sperm must be produced by masturbation and reach the laboratory within four hours.' So today, the alarm goes off, I get up and make a cup of tea while Paul produces the specimen (how quickly we get into the jargon) and we rush it up the road to my friend who takes it to the lab at work.

The same friend arranges for us to attend the fertility clinic attached to the birth control clinic where she works. This is the same clinic I have been attending for years. The appointment is for after Christmas. We hope that I get pregnant over Christmas so that we won't need to keep the appointment. In the meantime I read up on infertility investigations.

5 January 1979 Our first appointment. Our medical histories are taken and we are both examined physically. We are seen by the consultant separately and then he talks to us together. 'Yes, everything seems quite normal.' But we are told that the sperm count is not terribly high, about thirty million, but high enough. Conception is possible with lowish sperm counts. Paul is told to give up his Y-fronts and to wear boxer shorts. This may increase the sperm count. I'm told that from my charts it looks as though I'm ovulating. I'm to continue taking my temperature but I must use the official forms rather than bits of graph paper. We are told that the next step is the post-coital test for which I am to make an appointment after my next period has started.

In some ways I feel quite elated after this first appointment. Our problem has been recognized and something is being done for us. We go straight to Marks and Spencers to buy the shorts, feeling that things had started, that we had acquired some kind of control.

7 January 1979 Period begins. I start my new temperature chart on the official form and ring the hospital to make an appointment for a post-coital test. At this particular clinic post-coital tests are done only on Tuesday mornings.

16 January 1979 First post-coital test. Attending the clinic is a depressing experience. A feeling of heaviness comes over me as I get closer to the clinic. I walk past the Family Planning clinic which I've attended for many years, down the corridor, past the row of women waiting their turn, to the door marked 'Subfertility Clinic'. I am redefined. I am now infertile, a woman with a problem. I announce my arrival, show my card with my new number on it. When I was fertile I was E34976. Now that I'm infertile, I'm 4032.

I wait my turn, sitting by myself, getting lower and lower, trying to fight the tears, and the feelings of self-pity. It is my turn. I go in and undress, and lie on the couch as instructed. A doctor, a woman, not the one we'd seen previously, inserts a speculum and then using a long rubber tube takes a sample of my cervical mucus. While I get dressed, she goes over to the other side of the room to examine my mucus under a microscope. 'I don't like this at all,' she says. I panic. What have I done? Hadn't we followed the instructions? I feel like a naughty child and I start to cry. The tears stream down my face and they continue unabated for the rest of my appointment. It transpires that what she doesn't like is the way the sperm and the mucus are getting along. There aren't enough sperm and they don't seem to be surviving well in my mucus. The doctor suggests that Paul sprays his testicles twice a day with cold water using one of those small indoor plant sprays. I don't know how he will take to that. If this spraying is such a good idea, then why hadn't the doctor suggested it on our first visit when Paul was there. That way at least he'd have been told directly. Now it was up to me to tell him. I'd brought his sperm to them and now I was taking bad news back home. My mucus didn't meet with her approval either. It was described on my form as 'tacky.' I am given a prescription for some oestrogen tablets and told to come back next month for another post-coital test.

There are lots of questions I want to ask. But the tears are still streaming down my face and I feel far too distraught to ask them. So I fumble around for my coat and bag and leave, while the doctor talks into her tape recorder about my case.

The force of my feelings and my inability to cope with them surprises me. During the next month I think a great deal about what happened and how I might cope in the future.

8 February 1979 Period starts. I feel depressed. I've got to go back to the clinic again. I ring up to make an appointment. Tuesdays arrive this cycle either on day eight or day fifteen of my cycle. The nurse thinks that I should go for the earlier date. I take the oestrogen tablets in preparation for the appointment.

16 February 1979 Second post-coital test. This time I feel much stronger. When the doctor appears and calls my name my stomach turns over. I force it back into place and I follow her into the room. I try to attend very carefully to what she does. Both the procedure and the doctor are the same as before. 'Well, the mucus is better, but the sperm are much the same as before.' She writes this down. I confess that Paul has refused to spray his testicles. The doctor points out that this is quite important as the present emphasis is to get the balance right between my mucus and his sperm. She suggests that I douche myself with a solution of bicarbonate of soda just before intercourse during the fertile days. This may make my vagina more conducive to the survival of Paul's sperm. I tell her that I am puzzled. Should I take the oestrogen tablets for my mucus to coincide with my clinic appointments or around ovulation as the two days are a week apart? Am I undergoing tests or treatment? The doctor says that, as she has an empty slot the following Tuesday, I can return for another post-coital so she can check the sperm and the mucus nearer to ovulation and after I have been using the douche. When she'd got the mucus right, she'd move on to other things, in particular, on to checking whether my tubes were unblocked. I'm even more puzzled. Why bother spending months checking my mucus if we then discover that my tubes are blocked? Why is only one test done at a time? I suppose I'd expected the investigation to be more like an MOT, where your car is given a whole range of tests at one go, and so you know what's wrong fairly rapidly. I tell the doctor how depressed I feel and that I'm worried that the investigations might destroy the relationship into which the child would be born. But any talk of emotions is brushed aside with the comment that some people feel quite heartened to think that treatment is being offered and that some couples are willing to go to the most elaborate extremes to have a child. I take the hint and shut up.

The clinic nurse shows me how to use the douche. She is much more cheery and tries to boost me by telling me how successful the doctor is at getting women pregnant.

The visit is over. The tension gradually subsides. At least this time I didn't collapse and I did manage to ask most of my questions. Now I have to go home with my collection of bits and pieces, instructions and information and prepare us for the next appointment.

I tell Paul what the doctor said about spraying his testicles, that he must do it to improve motility. He refuses. She made it clear that this is the next step in the proceedings. If he's not prepared to do it then we've reached a stalemate. Will they be prepared to continue the investigations if he's uncooperative? I feel cross with him. I've had to go to the clinic, go through the humiliating examinations and face the doctor and now he won't do his share. Later he agrees to try. Our sex life has taken on new elements: Paul sprays his balls twice a day; just before intercourse I pop into the bathroom and spend five minutes with the douche.

20 February 1979 Third post-coital test. My mucus has remained good and the number of sperm has improved but their motility is still low. The doctor suggests I continue with the current regime of tablets, douche and spray. We now move on to other things: an X-ray of my Fallopian tubes. A form is filled in and I am told to ring the hospital's X-ray department when my next period arrives to make an appointment for day ten of my cycle. Via me, Paul is advised to see the semenologist, in six weeks' time.

26 February 1979 My fertile period is over and so the rites can cease for a while till next month. I can stop gently bullying Paul for a while, and relax. My friend has had her baby and I go to see it. I feel very thrilled for her. But after the excitement wears off I feel very sad. If I'd got pregnant quickly my baby would be almost due. I realise how much I'd stopped thinking about children and babies. My goal now is conception.

13 March 1979 Period starts. It is about three days late and I'd just begun to feel really hopeful. Yesterday I'd had moments of discomfort; and stomach ache but I'd ignored them till I saw the blood today. I feel weak and tearful. All the strength I thought I'd acquired just seems to have drained away. The discomfort serves as a reminder of my failure. So much for menstruation as a sign of femininity and the potential for motherhood. All it signifies to me is my failure.

21 March 1979 To the hospital for an HSG (X-ray of my Fallopian tubes). I had rung them beforehand to find out how long it would take and whether I would feel well enough to go back to work afterwards. I'm nervous so I've asked my friend to come with me. In the X-ray department, I undress completely and put all my clothes into a brown paper bag and cover myself with one of the hospital's green overalls. I'm shown into the X-ray room and told to sit on a long table with the equipment all around and above it. The doctor and radiographer, both men, arrive. My friend who is a nurse and works at the hospital is allowed to stay. The doctor tells me what will happen. I can watch the proceedings on a TV screen. The insertion of the dye may feel like a period pain. He inserts the dye. It is very painful and the pain gets worse. I pass out. When I come round the doctor shows me the X-ray. I try to concentrate but I can't take in what he's saying. The left tube appears to be clear but my right tube has gone into spasm. I fear there may never be a baby. I am put on to a trolley and wheeled into the corridor where I lie in pain for some time. Gradually the pain begins to ease and I am able to get dressed. My friend finds a taxi, takes me home and puts me to bed with a hot water bottle. By the evening I feel better.

The investigations seem to be taking so long. A day does not pass by without my thinking about them and my infertility. I feel I must go on with the tests, and all the pain they cause, because I need to know if I will ever be able to have a child, and because there is no other source of help for my infertility to which I can turn.

19 April 1979 Appointment with the semenologist. The appointment is at 3:40 and so at 2:30 Paul produced his sperm sample into the little plastic container provided by the hospital. We then rush to the hospital, clutching the sample. The doctor looks at some of the sperm under the microscope and sends the rest to the lab for a sperm count. He thinks that the count and motility are increased, but this will be confirmed by the laboratory test. That's it basically. It's heartening to think there's an improvement. The spraying must be working so Paul will continue with that. We fix another appointment with the semenologist to see whether the improvement has continued.

26 April 1979 I'm in contact with children who have German measles so I have a blood test to see whether I am immune to German measles.

1 May 1979 Appointment at the Infertility Clinic to hear the results of the HSG. The doctor tells me the same tale as I was told in the X-ray room. One tube is definitely clear but the result is uncertain for the other. This tube may be blocked or it might be a technical problem which made it difficult for the dye to get through. My agony is reduced to a technical hitch. If I have not conceived in three months time, I am to have a laparoscopy. This will involve a short stay in hospital. The waiting list is long so she will put my name down on it the next time I see her, in three months' time. Why do I have to wait till then? Why can't my name be put on the list now? Meanwhile, the doctor suggests I try an insemination cap. I am to return to the clinic in two days to be shown how to use it. I am to use it in the middle of the cycle and then come back to her with it in place to see if I am using it properly and to check whether it's improving the sperm's chances of survival. This calls for another new element in our sex life: I take the oestrogen tablets around the time of ovulation; then before 'intercourse' I am to spend five minutes in the bathroom with the douche after which I am to insert the insemination cap. Meanwhile Paul is masturbating into the hospital's plastic pot, with his balls nicely chilled twice daily. I am then to syringe his sperm into the tube which dangles from the insemination cap. What erotic excitement!

3 May 1979 To the hospital to learn how to use the insemination cap. It's a bit fiddly and difficult to get into place.

19 May 1979 Fourth post-coital but with insemination cap in place. The results seem exactly the same as for the test we had in February. Mucus is okay, sperm count is fine, but the motility is low. The insemination cap has not made any difference so the doctor doesn't think it's worth continuing with it. I indicate my relief at that news. We are sent back to the semenologist for a sperm-mucus compatibility test to see if my mucus is killing off Paul's sperm.

12 June 1979 Second appointment with semenologist. We go together with a sperm sample in a little container.

The semenologist examines it and pronounces his approval of both the count and motility. We then persuade him to do the sperm-mucus compatibility test which is the reason we came to see him. He seems happy with the result. I feel totally confused. One doctor says the motility is low. Another says it's fine. One tells me to douche. The other says that it's unnecessary. How am I to deal with this lack of consensus? The only response seems to be to feel cheerful. At least someone has said we're okay. I may not be pregnant but any ray of hope is to be appreciated.

1 August 1979 Appointment to see the consultant. He puts me on the list for a laparoscopy. I should have an appointment within six months. It's just a question of waiting. And because my cycle is somewhat irregular, he decides to put me on an ovulation-inducing drug. I am given one month's supply. Am I to go back each month for another prescription?

10 August 1979 We go on holiday. It is the second holiday we've taken since trying to get pregnant. Events like this remind me of time passing.

On our return from holiday, we decide to buy a house. We had been thinking for some time about where we were going to live. The flat was a bit small for a child. We had no garden and getting up and down the stairs would not have been easy with a small baby. When we first started trying to conceive, our plan had been to move out soon after the baby's birth. But as the months passed with no signs of a baby, we put this plan to one side. It just did not seem possible to make any decisions about where we were to live until we knew more about whether we were likely to have a baby. How much longer could we go on delaying plans and decision because one day there might be a baby? So many aspects of our lives were becoming controlled by our frustrated attempts to become parents. We went ahead and bought a house. It is a large house—one that gives us plenty of space for us and for children.

15 October 1979 Receive a card from the hospital telling me to fix the date for a laparoscopy in the second half of my next cycle.

7 November 1979 I enter hospital for a laparoscopy the next afternoon. I have never been in hospital before and I am nervous. It is much jollier than I expected. There are thirteen women in the ward and we quickly discover who we all are. Six of us are to be operated on tomorrow. As we have all come in for different operations, we each have different anxieties, but we are great company for one another, laughing and joking together. I realise how much more pleasant it is to have other women around you while going through tests, someone to share the worries and the news. There are two other women on the ward who are having problems in conceiving. It is good to talk to them, to compare notes about the tests and their reactions to infertility. I realise that I did not know anyone who had been through the investigations or who is infertile. While a lot of women have been very kind and listened to my tales of tests and anguish, none of them have been through similar experiences or had similar feelings. This is the first time I've spoken to women who've said, 'Yes, they did that to me,' or 'Yes, I felt like that too'. I see that I've become very careful about the people I get close to. I am only relating to close friends and relatives who know about my problem. I feel very vulnerable about stepping outside of that group into the great beyond of those who don't know.

9 November 1979 The doctor comes round to tell us all about the results of our operations. He confirms that I am ovulating and that my tubes, ovaries and uterus are okay. So I am proclaimed fit and told to report back to the consultant in six weeks' time.

I feel now as though I have done the rounds. A series of tests have revealed little that was seriously wrong with either Paul or myself. I imagined that at the next appointment I would be told that medical science had its way with us and that now it was up to us to go away, to forget the hassles we had been through, to relax and conceive.

24 November 1979 Period starts.

22 December 1979 It comes again. Another Christmas passes and I'm not pregnant.

4 January 1980 Appointment to see the consultant. This is the anniversary of my first appointment at the Infertility Clinic. The consultant looks at the report of my laparoscopy, reads all the notes and thinks. He suggests a blood test to check my progesterone level. This is fixed for 13 January as it has to be done late in my cycle. I'm also told to make an appointment for a fifth post-coital test to check that everything is still all right there.

13 January 1980 I have a blood sample taken for the progesterone test. I delay making the appointment for a fifth post-coital.

2 February 1980 We move into our new house. It requires a lot of work which the builders have started. At first I organise the rooms around a child. One room is to be a nursery. Later that same room becomes my study.

8 May 1980 I make an appointment for a post-coital test.

20 May 1980 Fifth post-coital test. I have taken the oestrogen tablets for the first time in months. I had a hard job finding them. When I arrive at the clinic, I feel that I need to explain to the nurse why I hadn't come sooner. The doctor, however, either doesn't notice or doesn't ask about the long delay. So I say nothing. I take off my knickers. I get on the couch. It's all so familiar, I feel positively light-headed. A seasoned traveller. The result seems the same as ever. The sperm are there but not very motile. So

one year and a half later, we are back where we started. The results of the progesterone test are not too encouraging. I am ovulating, but not very well. To improve my ovulation, I am given Clomid as well as oestrogen tablets. I am also sent off to have a blood test to see if I have antibodies to sperm.

I go away feeling fed-up. It seems as if a whole lot of new problems are coming up—low progesterone, sperm antibodies. If they are significant factors, why were they not looked for months ago. I've had a number of blood tests. Why hadn't these been included then? And I don't understand why the motility of Paul's sperm is a matter of differing opinions. If it is a significant factor in our infertility then why put me on Clomid? We seem to be going round in circles, backtracking over ground that I thought we'd explored. I feel like a detective story, with the doctors sniffing round for clues, going over old suspects as well as checking on esoteric possibilities. Nevertheless, I take the Clomid in my next cycle as well as the oestrogen tablets.

20 June 1980 I feel very ill.

4 July 1980 Period starts. It's fourteen days since I felt so ill so I feel sure that it was due to the Clomid. Why hadn't I been warned of the side-effects? Also, how am I to know if the Clomid is working? No tests are being done to check on my defective progesterone levels. I am depressed.

31 July 1980 Period starts. I've run out of oestrogen tablets. The hospital no longer dispenses them so I have to go to my GP. Since I moved, I haven't found a new GP. By the time I work all this out, it's too late to take Clomid this cycle.

This summer is the third since we tried to conceive. We work on the house. I find out through my friend at the hospital that the test showed that I do not have antibodies to Paul's sperm. It dawns on me that I have decided by default not to continue with the Clomid or with the tests. I feel uneasy about giving up the investigations. Having gone so far it seems silly not to continue. The next test might be the one which gives me the answer. They might just find something that works for me. But then I remember what the tests were like and I feel loathe to go back to the hospital and try again.

I feel the key question is changing slowly. I am asking less why am I infertile. Instead, I am thinking about how to reconcile myself with my infertility, and how I can move forward into a life in which children may not have a central role. I feel that this is where I prefer to put my energies, and that continuing with the tests will interfere with this. So I do not go back to the clinic.

Ω

Born and Unborn: The Implications of "Choice" for People with Disabilities

by Marsha Saxton

Some time in the first month after my conception, a disruption occurred in the growth of my lower spine, and the nerves coursing through my bladder and down to my lower legs and feet, the "perineal" tract, did not develop normally. About two out of a thousand babies are affected by this "neural tube defect" or "NTD," the second most common birth difference after cerebral palsy. The range of disability varies considerably from "spina bifida occulta" (or a slight niche in the spine which the individual my be unaware of, or experience back pain) to Myelomenigacele like mine, but sometimes characterized by paraplegia and including Hydrocephally (fluid on the brain). Some babies are born with such severe NTD they have no brain and die soon after birth.

I have been told many times how 'lucky' I am to be only moderately disabled. 'It could have been much worse,' they say, an attitude which perplexes me. I have never been told how unlucky I am to be disabled at all. At thirty-two, I have a slight limp, and somewhat skinny legs lined with pale incisions.

I have always planned and looked forward to becoming a mother. The varying statistics from doctors or books over the years about the possibility of my having a baby with my disability have not caused me to reconsider this.

As a feminist I have supported the pro-choice position on the question of abortion. I feel a woman must be able to choose motherhood or not and exert control over her own body. I view abortion as a stop-gap measure which women must maintain to counteract the oppressive forces that limit women's control over our lives, which include poor access to, and harmful birth control methods. Because of the emotional and social costs of abortion to the individual mother, fetus, and society, I cannot view abortion as another form of birth control. The debate "at what age does the fetus constitute a human life," in my estimation, can never be satisfactorily resolved. Indeed, such an argument misses the point of the true issues at hand, namely, the real resources, financial, social, and emotional of the parents and the community to welcome the child.

It is on this basis that I question the practice of systematically ending the life of a fetus *because it is disabled.* Real "choice" involves an understanding of all the options and the opportunity for flexible decision-making for the individual woman in her own situation based on an accurate assessment of her available resources. It also necessi-

tates closely scrutinizing society's view of "ablebodiedness." We need to better understand disability and our relationship to it. In particular,

1. How does society define and treat disability?
2. What are the implications of prenatal technology in relation to societal oppression of disabled persons?
3. How are disabled women affected by the new technologies and the attitudes surrounding them?
4. How can both consumers and health-care professionals more rationally consider these issues and act in humanly responsible ways?

Disability triggers much fear in our culture. Some of the recent media coverage on the topic has begun to challenge the widespread ignorance in this area, but the old attitudes persist. Perhaps from prehistoric times, disability must have appeared to humans as some mysterious force leaving many human beings with physical limitation, loss of body functions, constant pain, disfigurement, and sometimes early death. It is no wonder that we have feelings of powerlessness about disability. It forces us to confront our own vulnerability.

We, especially in the U.S., live in a culture obsessed with health and well-being. We value rugged self-reliance, athletic prowess, and rigid standards of beauty. We incessantly pursue eternal youth, and our treatment of our elders attests to an ingrained denial, fear, and even hate of our own aging and accompanying physical limitation. The disabled person in our society is the target of attitudes and behaviors from the able-bodied world ranging from gawking to avoidance, pity to resentment, or from vastly lower expectations to awe. Along with these attitudes disabled persons confront a variety of tangible barriers: architectural inaccessibility, lack of sign-language interpreters for deaf people, insufficient taped or brailled materials for blind persons. In addition, disabled persons confront less tangible barriers: discrimination in employment, second-class education, and restricted opportunities for full participation in the life of the community.

As in any kind of oppression, the attitudes are self-perpetuating, the stereotypes in the literature are reinforced in the popular media. The isolation of disabled persons limits the larger culture's exposure to their life experiences, needs, and common humanness. The child's natural curiosity and inquisitiveness in encountering the disabled person for the first time is so often met with a parent's embarrassed, "Hush, don't ask and don't stare." This child's simple wonder is thus replaced with mistrust and fear, and so handed down the generations. It is surprising

By Marsha Saxton. From *WomenWise,* Winter 1988, reprinted from Vol. 7, No. 4, Winter 1984. Copyright © 1984 by Concord Feminist Health Centers. Reprinted by permission.

to learn that as recently as the 1950's, laws remained on the books in some states prohibiting the public presence of persons "diseased, maimed, mutilated or in any way deformed so as to be an unsightly or disgusting object." The fear of vulnerability, the flight from physical limitation (perhaps from death) is at the root of such phenomena as the Eugenics Movement in the early 1900's. By 1937, 28 states had adopted Eugenics Sterilization laws aimed at persons with epilepsy, mental retardation, mental illness, and other kinds of differences where "procreation was deemed unadvisable." Such attitudes are still with us.

From the youth and beauty oriented culture we are beset with messages to buy products which hide or disguise our differences and body functions, and strive to achieve rigid standards of appearance. Such standards are particularly harsh on disabled women whose appearance or body function may be further from "acceptable."

Do we want a world of "perfect people?" I really wonder what have been the human costs of our attempts to control our differences, our vulnerability. There is tremendous pressure upon us to have "perfect babies." Where disabled persons are stigmatized, so are their parents. In some societies, including the U.S., parents have concealed the birth of disabled infants and in some cases killed or allowed the infant to die of hunger or exposure. (A contradiction to this comes from other cultures including some Native American cultures, where disabled persons are regarded as "spiritually special" and are revered and assigned specific religious or healing roles.) I have heard of cases as recently as the 1950's in Britain where Spina Bifida newborns were denied sustenance until death.

It is important to point out that physicians are to a certain extent under pressure to encourage prenatal screening and even abortion. Physicians, out of fear of malpractice suits, may lobby for enforced screening. A further concern is that women undergoing screening yet not choosing abortion would be the target of further oppression. This possibility to those of us acquainted with the mothers of disabled, particularly retarded children, does not seem so remote. They are already the target of considerable social stigma. If we are to maintain our "choice" we must include the *choice to have a disabled child.*

How do the oppressive attitudes about disability affect the woman facing prenatal screening? Very often prospective parents have never considered the issue of disability until it is raised in relation to testing. What comes to mind to most prospective parents at the mention of the term "birth defects?" Our exposure to disabled children has been so limited by their isolation that most people have only stereotyped views which include telethons, displays in drugstore counters depicting attractive "crippled" youngsters soliciting our pity and loose change. The image of a child with Down's Syndrome elicits an even more intense assumption of eternal parental burden.

The issue of the burden of a handicapped child seems to be a prominent one in the decision to abort. How much reality is there to the "burden of the disabled?"

Our assessment of the "costs" of raising a disabled child are vastly distorted by the oppressive assumptions. A common theory applied in parent counseling is that parents who gave birth to a disabled child must "grieve for the normal child they didn't have." While it is certainly helpful for parents to release feelings of sadness, shock, and so forth, this theory fails to recognize a prominent feature of this experience; parents bring a lifetime of loss, disappointment, feelings of failure, guilt, etc. to every parent-child relationship (for the most part repressed). This "grieving" point of view blames the child, but often the disabled infant is not the *cause* of the parents' grief but a *reminder* of a backlog of old pain. Very often in successful parent counseling, when parents "come to grips" with the issues in their relationship with their child, they identify previously unresolved issues from their past that were being played out in the current relationship.

Of course we cannot chastise or applaud any parent for feeling whatever one might feel about their child. Not "good" or "bad," our feelings are an expression of our history of experiences, our learning over time, and our resource to deal with past distress. But what has been confirmed for me is that one's attitude toward a disabled baby is a *point of view, a relative position.*

Related to this issue is the fact that the oppression of women as the sole and often isolated caretakers of children affect the resources of many mothers in caring for their disabled children, an issue which deserves considerably more attention. The oppression of disabled persons falls upon the parents who may be limited in obtaining needed compensatory aids, medical assistance, and respite care. Many factors in the culture, such as the weakening of the extended family, contribute to the isolation and feelings of overwhelm by the mother. Such issues are typically ignored, again placing the blame of "burden" on the disabled child.

Another of the myths affecting prospective mothers is about the "suffering" of the disabled.

There is no doubt that there are disabled people who "suffer" from their physical conditions. There are even those who may choose to end their lives rather than continue in pain or with severe limitations, but is this not obviously as true for nondisabled people who suffer from emotional pain and limitation of resource? As a group, people with disabilities do not "suffer" any more than any other group or category of humans. Our limitations may be more outwardly visible, our need for help more apparent, but like anybody else, the "suffering" we may experience is a result of not enough human caring, acceptance, and respect. The discriminatory attitudes and thoughtless behaviors, that's what makes life difficult. This is the source of the real limits: the oppression, the architectural barriers,the pitying stares or frightened avoidance, the unaware assumptions that you couldn't do the job, couldn't order for yourself in a restaurant, couldn't find a mate or direct your own life.

How Women Typically Learn About Their Options About Pre-natal Testing

"Choice" requires that information be presented in an unbiased way. Most physicians will indicate their intention to adhere to a "nondirective" philosophy where decisions are left up to the patient. However, not just in my childhood, but recently when I have mentioned to medical professionals my intention to get pregnant, I have encountered a wide array of emotional responses. An orthopedic surgeon to whom I indicated a desire to minimize the use of X-ray while I was trying to conceive blurted out, "You're going to get pregnant? I hope you'll get an amniocentesis."

The standard philosophy in relation to amniocentesis for women particularly over thirty-five years of age is that given the low risk to the fetus, why not go ahead and do it? Very often women are encouraged to have an amniocentesis without reconsideration to what action the parents might take if an abnormality is discovered. This attitude is not derived from careful individualized consideration of the parent's values and decision options, including an appraisal of the risks and consequences of miscarriage for *these particular individuals* is irresponsible, needlessly expensive, and ultimately hurtful to the parent, child, and society.

Medical services consumers tend to put considerable faith in their physicians and assume that physicians are acting in their best interest. Few consumers are made aware that while some medical procedures may be necessary and life sustaining, many are also in the financial interest of the health care industry. Ninety-five percent of all amniocenteses performed indicate no anomaly, and thus function only to reassure parents that their baby is fine. The real value of such an invasive, risky, and expensive procedure must be questioned. As my genetics counselor stated, screening is "sometimes used as a substitute for thinking." On this basis the American College of Obstetrics and Gynecology, and the American Academy of Pediatrics oppose routine Alpha-feto protein screening.

The biggest challenge to health care workers who are counseling both disabled and nondisabled prospective parents about options and the use of reproductive technologies is in presenting the information in understandable and nonbiased ways.

Almost every health care professional is motivated by a deep sense of human caring, and yet is as subject to confusion and prejudice as anyone. While health care professionals have a responsibility to present information in as unbiased a way as possible, blaming them for not doing so does not advance the cause of the consumer. Regarding ourselves as hapless victims of an oppressive profit-motivated health care system does nothing to enhance our power or to challenge the institutionalized patterns of the health care industry. We as women consumers have to regard ourselves as powerful and assert this power in the face of others' possible confusion and prejudice.

We must regard ourselves as the directors of our own needs. Health care professionals are available to us as educators and consultants, but we must be the ones to make the decisions. To do this we must take responsibility for obtaining the necessary information and we must trust our own thinking. We, more than any other, know of our own life circumstances, goals, and capabilities. Disabled women, in our more frequent encounters with the medical system, are particularly vulnerable to feelings of powerlessness to challenge stereotyped and hurtful interactions with unaware professionals. An important goal for us as women and mothers is to make our decisions based on clarity about our values, adequate knowledge of the issues, and an accurate appraisal of our own resources. One avenue toward obtaining that needed confidence is through meeting and sharing with other women where we can gain safety, clarity, and strength. Peer groups are an excellent place to begin discussion about the issues raised here. (Saxton, 1981)

What would I ask or tell another woman considering an amniocentesis with intent to abort a disabled fetus? Was she satisfied that she had sufficient knowledge about disability, an awareness of her own feelings, that she could make a rational choice? Did she personally know any disabled adults or children? What was she taught about disability by adults when she was young? Was she aware of the distorted picture of the lives of disabled people presented by the posters, telethons, and stereotyped characters in the literature and media? I would also ask her to consider the personal and emotional cost that abortion could take. Was the elimination of a disabled fetus worth that cost?

Do I think all disabled fetuses should be born to this world as it is now? Do I think parents should be forced to accept and care for a baby born disabled? No, I don't. I feel our priority should be to assess our current capabilities, determine the realities of the situation, and make decisions that are workable for all concerned.

The questioning by disabled activists of abortion of disabled fetuses has been criticized by some feminists as "too much like Right to Life." I can understand this fear, for the control over our lives as women that access to abortion has provided is currently so tentative that any challenge to abortion may feel threatening. But I feel that it's important to point out that the basis for choosing to abort a disabled fetus is the same basis for choosing to abort a fetus *because it is female,* a practice clearly denounced by the Women's Movement. But regardless of the logic of our current views as activists, we have a responsibility to persistently re-evaluate the implications of our position and examine how they apply to individuals and specific populations.

At this point, if I became aware that the fetus I was carrying would be disabled, I would not choose to abort it. These are my reasons: I hope for and look forward to a time when all children can be welcomed to a world without oppression. I would like to exercise this view if only in my own personal world.

Marsha Saxton's article is an edited excerpt from a paper which appears in Test-Tube Women, *1984, Pandora Press (Routledge & Kegan Paul) and is reprinted with their permission.*

Ω

Menstrual Extraction:
Is Self Help Making a Comeback?

by Rebecca Salstrom

Five Los Angeles women formed a gynecological self-help group in 1971 with the goal of organizing women to work for abortion rights. A short time later, one of the women observed a doctor performing an abortion and brought back to the group the device he had used. It consisted of a Karman cannula (a flexible tube named for its inventor) attached directly to a syringe. With this device as a prototype, they developed a technique for extracting menstrual fluid from a woman's uterus.

The idea wasn't new. Planned Parenthood International and the U.S. Agency for International Development had trained lay women and midwives in Third World countries to use similar techniques—variously called menstrual regulation, endometrial extraction, or menstrual induction—as a means of population control.

The Los Angeles self-helpers didn't set out to design an early abortion technique; they merely wanted to learn about and take control of their own bodies. Menstrual extraction (or ME, as they called their procedure) could be performed as soon as a woman began or missed her regular menstrual period. It was usually done as one of a series of monthly extractions. ME gave a woman control over the timing of her menstrual flow and eliminated the nuisance of menstrual periods. It relieved cramps and backache. But it also proved to be a way for women to control *all* of their reproductive processes (menstruation, conception, and birthing) before the Supreme Court affirmed—temporarily, at least—that right.

Lorraine Rothman, a school teacher and one of the founding members of the L.A. self-help group, invented a menstrual-extraction device she called the Del-Em—a Mason jar with two pieces of flexible aquarium tubing protruding from its two-hole rubber stopper, one tube leading to a 4-millimeter cannula and the other to a 50-cubic-centimeter syringe. A one-way bypass valve at the tip of the syringe prevented air from entering the uterus and causing a potentially fatal embolism.

From *WomenWise*, Vol. 15, No. 1, Spring 1992, pp. 6,9. Copyright © 1992 by Concord Feminist Health Centers.

Learning the Technique

ME was performed at the group's regular meeting place or at the home of the woman undergoing the procedure. Generally, three women participated: the woman having ME, a woman monitoring the equipment for proper functioning, and another woman to insert and manipulate the cannula. Other group members watched to learn the technique.

The first step was to sterilize the equipment. Then the woman having ME would make herself comfortable, insert her own speculum, and examine her cervix. She and the others would note the location, size, and shape of her uterus and ovaries.

If the woman suspected she might be pregnant, she would discuss her gynecological history, including the date of her last period and probable date of conception, and extra care would be taken to completely remove the uterine lining and any microscopic-sized products of conception (POC) that might exist.

Next, one woman would don sterile surgical gloves and insert the cannula through the cervical os. The woman having ME would create suction in her uterus by pumping the syringe, and the woman manipulating the cannula would gently and continuously turn it, causing the lining of the uterus to slough off and flow through the tubing into the collection jar.

Although the procedure caused cramping—sometimes severe but usually of brief duration—the woman having ME was always in control and could pause at any time if she became uncomfortable.

Potential Complications

The self-helpers maintained close telephone contact for several days following the procedure in case there were any complications. Chances of an incomplete abortion proved to be the same as for a first-trimester abortion: once in every 500 cases. The women learned to recognize symptoms of infection, such as a rise in temperature to 100.5 degrees F. or higher for eight or more hours; pain or cramping in the lower abdomen; passing of clots or tissue;

268

or profuse bleeding. If the woman exhibited these symptoms, she would see a physician immediately and obtain antibiotics. (Infection could occur due to faulty sterilization of equipment; more likely, it would be due to a pre-existing condition such as chlamydia.)

One important aspect of ME was that it could be performed in a private home with other women present for assistance and support. In fact, ME was and still is taught by its proponents *only* as a group experience; it is *not* a solo, do-it-yourself technique. In a self-help group, novices observe as more experienced women perform MEs, and a woman always undergoes the procedure before attempting to assist someone else.

Although the Supreme Court's 1973 ruling in *Roe v. Wade* legalized abortion, some women continued to learn and practice ME because they considered it to be a safer method of birth control than oral contraceptives or intrauterine devices (IUDs). Feminists have long viewed gynecologic self help as important political tools for empowering women. In an article for *Quest,* (Vol. IV, No. 3, Summer 1978) Laura Punnet wrote: "In contrast to patriarchal medicine, self help is a positive experience for women, affirming our experiences, our bodies, and our ability to act concretely to fulfill our own needs."

Promoting Self Help

After the 1989 Supreme Court decision in *Webster v. Reproductive Health Services,* state governments began to restrict abortion services, and women again began to worry about their reproductive rights. Proponents of self help want women to examine their options in case *Roe* is eviscerated. At a recent meeting of the American Public Health Association, the National Women's Health Network sponsored a panel discussion on integrating the self-help approach into community health programs. Carol Downer of the Federation of Feminist Women's Health Centers told the group: "Self help starts with women's own experience as its base, and validates women." (*Network News,* January/February 1992).

The Federation disseminates books and pamphlets on gynecologic self help; sponsors a speakers bureau; offers self-help tours for groups interested in learning ME; and promotes a video, *No Going Back,* that demonstrates ME. *When Birth Control Fails,* a 1979 book by Suzann Gage, was recently reprinted. It relates the self-help group theory and information on birth control, abortion, and ME. (To learn more about gynecologic self help, contact the Federation of Feminist Women's Health Centers, 1690 N. Vine Street, Suite 1005, Los Angeles, CA 90028, 213-957-4062.)

U.S. courts and the medical establishment view any procedure with the potential to terminate a pregnancy as a medical procedure properly (read "legally") performed only by a licensed physician. The unwillingness of the medical field to recognize women's right to control their own bodies is a familiar story. American physicians wrested the birthing process away from women in the 18th Century by denouncing midwives as untrained and untrainable, excluding them from medical schools, and then refusing to license them because they weren't "trained."

Legal and Medical Objections

Dr. Grant Bagley, co-founder of the Utah Women's Health Center, addressed the legal issue in an article for *In Health* (November 1991). Comparing ME to other procedures, such as enemas, circumcisions, and insulin injections, Bagley wrote: "No one has been particularly alarmed that we're exporting this technology to Third World Countries. But somehow, if women in the U.S. are going to be using the same techniques, it's dangerous."

Planned Parenthood Federation of America (PPFA) now advises against gynecologic self help. Its literature states that "so-called 'self-help' procedures (very early abortions done at home) are not advised by Planned Parenthood because they are riskier than dilation/suction abortions performed in a medical setting by trained medical professionals."

Many physicians object to ME on the grounds that if a woman is not pregnant the procedure is "unnecessary." Others note that because pregnancy is difficult to detect in the first few weeks, a woman having ME may have an incomplete abortion without knowing it. Proponents count as a bonus the fact that a woman can use ME as soon as she has missed a period and not have to confront the issue of pregnancy.

Some choice activists view the revival of gynecologic self help as a tactical error and say that the issue could be seen by anti-choice legislators as a taunt: "Go ahead and make abortion illegal; we'll take care of it." Supporters of self help interpret the message differently: "Women will no longer accept outside control, so lawmakers might as well keep abortion legal."

Women already involved in self help say that meeting in sunlit rooms to support and assist their sisters is a positive experience. Speculums are transformed—from mysterious tools of the gynecologist to instruments of women's empowerment.

[The views expressed in the preceding article are not an endorsement of menstrual extraction by CFHC. Menstrual extraction should not be attempted by anyone not trained in the technique. –Ed.]

Ω

♀

Reproductive Issues are Essential Survival Issues for Asian American Communities

by Connie S. Chan

When the Asian-American communities in the U.S. list their priorities for political action and organizing, several issues concerning basic survival are usually included: access to bi-lingual education, housing, health, and child care, among others. Yet the essential survival issue of access to reproductive counseling, education, and abortion is frequently missing. Why are reproductive issues perceived as unimportant to the Asian-American communities? I think there are several reasons—ignorance, classism, sexism, and language barriers. Of course, these issues are interrelated, and I'll try to make the connections between them.

First, let me state that I am not an "expert" on the topic of reproductive issues in Asian-American communities, but that I have some firsthand experiences which have given me some insight into the problems. Several years ago, I was a staff psychologist at a local community health center serving the greater Boston Asian population. Most of our patients were recent immigrants from China, Vietnam, Cambodia, Laos, and Hong Kong. Almost all of these new immigrants understood little or no English. With few resources (financial or otherwise) many newcomers struggled to make sense of life in America and to survive in whatever fashion they could.

At the health center, the staff tried to help by providing information and advocacy in getting through our confusing system. I thought we did a pretty good job until I found out that neither our health education department nor our ob/gyn department provided *any* counseling or information about birth control or abortion services. The medical department had interpreted our federal funding regulations as prohibiting not only the performance of abortions on-site, but prohibiting the dissemination of information which might lead to, or help patients to obtain an abortion.

Needless to say, as a feminist and as an activist, I was horrified. When I found out that pregnant women who inquired about abortions were given only a name of a white, English speaking ob/gyn doctor and sent out alone, this practice seemed morally and ethically neglectful. One of the nurse-midwives agreed with me and suggested that I could serve as an interpreter/advocate for pregnant women who needed to have abortions or at least wanted to

discuss the option with the English-speaking ob/gyn doctor. The only catch was that I would have to do it on my own time, that I could not claim any affiliation with the health center, and that I could not suggest follow-up care at the health center.

Not fully knowing the nature of what I was volunteering for, I agreed to interpret and advocate for Cantonese-speaking pregnant women at their appointments with the obstetrician. It turned out that over the course of three years I interpreted during at least a hundred abortions for Asian immigrant women who spoke no English. After the first few abortions, the obstetrician realized how essential it was to have an interpreter present, and began to require that all non-English speaking women have an interpreter during the abortion procedure.

As a middle-class, educated, bi-lingual Asian-American woman, I was aware of the importance of having the choice to have an abortion, and the necessity to fight for the right to choose for myself, but I had been unaware of how the right to have an abortion is also a right to survival in this country if you are a poor, uneducated, non-English speaking immigrant.

The women I interpreted for were for the most part not young. Nor were they single. They ranged in age from 25–45, with a majority in their late twenties and early thirties. Almost all of the women were married and had two or more children. Some had as many as five or six children. They needed to have an abortion because they had been unlucky enough to have gotten pregnant after arriving in this country. Their families were barely surviving on the low wages that many new immigrant workers earned as restaurant workers, garment factory workers, or as domestic help.

Almost all of the women worked full-time: the ones who had young children left them with older retired family members or did piecework at home; those with older children worked in the factories or hotels. Without fail, each woman would tell me that each needed to have an abortion because her family could not afford another mouth to feed, that they could not afford to lose her salary contribution, not even for a few months, to care for an infant. In some ways, one could not even say that these women were *choosing* to have abortions. The choice had already been made for them and it was a choice of basic survival for the members of their family unit.

Kai was one of the women for whom I interpreted. A 35-year old mother of four children, ages 2 to 7, she and her husband emigrated to the U.S. from Vietnam. They had no choice in their immigration, either, they were refugees

From *Common Ground—Different Planes*, July 1990, pp. 6, 12. Copyright © 1990 by The Women of Color Partnership Program of the Religious Coalition for Reproductive Choice.

Connie Chan is a native Hawaiian. An activist and feminist, Ms. Chan is an Associate Professor of Human Service at the University of Massachusetts in Boston.

whose village had been destroyed, and felt fortunate to escape with their lives and all four of their children. Life in the U.S. was difficult, but they were scraping by, living with another family in a small apartment where their entire family slept in one room. Their hope was that their children would receive an education and make it in American society: They lived with the day-to-day hope of that deferred dream for the next generation.

When Kai found out that she was pregnant she felt desperate. Because she and her husband love children and live for their children, they wanted desperately to keep the child, this one that would be born in America and be an American citizen from birth. Yet they sadly realized that they could not afford another child, they could not survive on just one salary, they could not feed another one. Their commitment was to the children they already had, and keeping their family together.

When I accompanied Kai to her abortion, she was saddened, but resigned to what she had to do. The $300 that she brought to the clinic represented almost a month of wages for her, she had borrowed the money from family and friends. She would pay it back, she said, by working weekends for the next ten weeks. Her major regret was that she would not be able to buy any new clothes for her children this year because of this unexpected expense.

Kai spoke very little English. She did not understand why she had to go to a white American doctor for her abortion, instead of receiving services from her Asian doctor at the health center. She had no understanding, really, of reproductive rights issues, of *Roe v. Wade,* or why there were demonstrators waving pictures of fetuses and yelling at her as we entered the clinic. Mercifully, she did not understand the questions they shouted at her in English, and she did not ask me what they said, remarking only that they (the protestors) seemed very angry at someone. She felt sure, I think, that they were not angry at *her*.

She had done nothing to provoke anyone's anger. She was merely trying to survive in this country under this country's rules.

It is a moral crime and an injustice that Kai could not receive counseling in her language by her doctors at the Asian neighborhood health center. It is an injustice that she had to borrow $300 to pay for her own abortion, because her Medicaid benefits did not pay for it. It is a grave injustice that she had to have me, a stranger, interpreting for her during her abortion because her own doctor could not perform the procedure at her clinic . Again, it was not a matter of choice for her to abort her pregnancy, but a matter of basic survival.

Kai will probably never attend a march or rally for choice. She will not sign any petitions. She might not even vote. But it is for her and the countless thousands of immigrant women like her that we need to continue the struggle for reproductive rights. Within the Asian American community, the immigrant women who are most affected by the lack of access to abortions have the least power. They do not speak English, they do not demand equal access to health care; their needs as easily overlooked.

Thus it is up to us who are bi-lingual, those of us who can speak English and who can speak to these issues, to do so. We need to insure that the issue of reproductive rights is an essential one in the Asian American political agenda. It is not a woman's issue; it is a community issue.

We must speak for the Kais, for their children, for their right to survive as a family. We must, as activists, make the connection between the issues of oppression based upon gender, race, national origin, sexual orientation, class or language. We can, and must lead the Asian American community to recognize the importance of the essential issue of reproductive rights for the community's survival.

Ω

Use of Depo Provera for Contraception
Testimony by Cindy Pearson

Food and Drug Administration
Fertility and Maternal Health Drugs Advisory Committee

Paper by Cindy Pearson on the testimony on the Use of Depo Provera for Contaception, June 19, 1992, Food and Drug Administration, Fertility and Maternal Health Drugs Advisory Committee Hearings. Reprinted by permission of the author and the National Women's Health Network.

The National Women's Health Network is opposed to the approval of Depo Provera for contraceptive use. Depo Provera is a questionable drug contained within a problematic delivery system. American women may need more contraceptive choices, but they need safe choices which remain under their control throughout the entire duration of use.

The primary reason the NWHN opposes the approval of Depo Provera is the risk of irreversible long-term effects, specifically cancer and bone loss. These conditions are both of urgent concern to women in this country, where the incidences are already high.

Our gravest concern is the association of Depo Provera with breast cancer. The members of this Committee are well aware of the ever-increasing numbers of women in the US who are diagnosed with breast cancer. What is most important for our discussion today is the rise in the number of young women diagnosed with breast cancer in the last decade. These premenopausal breast cancers are the most devastating because their prognosis is so poor. It is important for the Committee to keep in mind the public health imperative of avoiding any further increase in what is already an unacceptable number of women with cancer.

When the FDA was last asked to consider approval of Depo Provera, there were uncertainties as to the relationship of progestogens to breast cancer. There now exist three case control studies of Depo Provera use and breast cancer in women. All three studies point in the same direction, that of increased risk for at least some women.

The Costa Rican study conducted by Dr. Lee found a relative risk of 2.6 in women who had ever used Depo Provera.[1] Although the researchers were not able to interview a significant number of cases, nor control for some of the known risk factors for breast cancer, this positive finding should not be dismissed out of hand.

In 1989, a second case control study again found an increased risk of breast cancer in Depo Provera users.[2] Conducted in New Zealand, this study did not find an increased risk for all users, but found significantly increased risks (between two and four times that of controls) in women whose use began under age twenty five and lasted for two years or more, and for all women who used the drug between the ages of twenty five and thirty four. The highest risk of breast cancer was found in women who used Depo Provera for more than six years between ages twenty five and thirty four, although this group was small.

The most recent study, conducted by the World Health Organization, again found an increased risk of breast cancer in young women using Depo Provera.[3] In the first four years after their initial use, the risk of breast cancer doubled.

We believe that the proper reaction to these studies is to neither dismiss the increased risk identified consistently for young women, nor to assume that the lack of risk found for older users is conclusively demonstrated. Each of these studies, with the exception of New Zealand, was conducted in countries with breast cancer rates less than half that of the United States. A study done in a low incidence country requires much greater numbers to have the power to find an association.

The risks that have been found in these studies may also be understated. If one of the reasons American women experience higher breast cancer rates is because of greater exposure to carcinogenic initiators, then the cancer promoting effects of Depo Provera could result in an even higher relative risk of breast cancer that those reported to date.

In sum, there has been a failure by Upjohn to collect the data necessary to reassure us that Depo Provera does not increase the risk of breast cancer. In fact, a recent review article, paid for by Upjohn itself, concluded that "there is need for further study, particularly of patients in potentially high-risk groups. . . ".[4] Even Upjohn recognizes the need for more studies before the breast cancer risk of Depo Provera can be conclusively determined.

These results in women are also troubling to us because they are supported by basic science which has demonstrated in at least three species that progestogens are mitogenic for breast epithelium.[5] Some researchers have described the potential effects of progestogens on breast cancer by saying that progestogens are to the breast what estrogens are to the endometrium. This concept is not new to the Advisory Committee. It has been raised in a number of the hearings that have been held on various issues related to the postmenopausal use of estrogen and progestogens. The Committee has heard preliminary data from the ongoing breast cancer study in Los Angeles which has found that women using estrogen plus a progestogen have a significantly higher risk of breast cancer than women on estrogen alone.[6]

Cervical cancer has been reported to be associated with Depo Provera use, as well.[7] The sponsor dismisses these reports with the often cited explanation that it is not possible to control for other factors associated with cervical cancer, such as number of heterosexual partners. Women have heard this tired excuse long enough. Surely someone, somewhere, can design a careful interview form for cases and controls and ferret out a conclusive answer. Until then, the Network believes that the FDA should consider Depo Provera to be possibly associated with cervical cancer. Given the rising rates of cervical cancer among some groups of women, it is important for the FDA to be cautious on this matter.

Why would this Committee consider approving Depo Provera for contraception when troublesome data suggest its relationship to cancer in young women? I believe that you will be presented arguments on behalf of the sponsor that this breast cancer risk is no greater than the risk of breast cancer experienced by young women who use oral contraceptives for five or more years before their first full-term pregnancy. The sponsor may plan to argue that if the breast cancer risk of Depo Provera is no greater than the breast cancer risk of oral contraceptives, which are already approved, then Depo Provera should be approved as well. The NWHN completely disagrees with this argument. You can't have it both ways. As virtually all of the current Committee members will remember, in January, 1989, this Committee declined to recommend changes in oral contraceptive labelling to indicate a breast cancer risk associated with early, long-term use. If you are now persuaded that the evidence of the oral contraceptive link to breast cancer is conclusive, please act immediately to inform the women of this country. If you are not convinced that long-term use of oral contraceptives increases the risk of breast cancer, then you must respond to the sponsor that Depo Provera is more risky than other contraceptives currently marketed and should not be approved.

In addition, there is another reason for rejecting Upjohn's argument. These disturbing data are emerging from much smaller groups of women than was the case with oral contraceptives. The oral contraceptive/breast cancer link took a lot of digging to find, and many large studies to confirm. Only three epidemiologic studies have been done on Depo Provera and breast cancer and all three raise a red flag. When we find an association with breast cancer in the relatively small groups in low incidence countries studied so far, we can not conclude that the actual effect is comparable to that seen in multiple, larger studies of oc users.

At the time of the last FDA hearings on Depo Provera, questions existed as to progestogens effect on bone strength. We now have direct data for the first time on osteoporosis, and it is not reassuring. Very recent data suggest a link between Depo Provera and loss of bone mass.[8] This is not surprising, as some Depo Provera users have low estradiol levels. Upjohn, in its materials submitted to the Committee, tries to explain the findings away by saying that the study was not well designed. Why hasn't Upjohn done better? A prospective bone density study with an appropriate concurrent control group would not be technically difficult to conduct. Given the serious nature of osteoporosis, we believe that more information on this question should be gathered and evaluated before approval is granted. Since many potential Depo Provera users would be women who need to avoid estrogen use, it could be unwise to recommend estrogen therapy as a means of avoiding bone loss in these women.

You will be asked to consider other arguments in favor of approving Depo Provera. Some in the family planning community believe that Depo Provera's unique features as a short-term long acting method could outweigh its risks, at least for some women. It does not require a subsequent removal procedure. It is highly effective while avoiding the use of estrogen. And for those women who do not experience significant short-term side effects, it is very convenient. The NWHN does not believe that the Committee should recommend approval based on these arguments.

A significant minority of women experience very troubling acute side effects for which there is no safe antidote. During the late 1970s and 1980s, both the National Women's Health Network and the National Black Women's Health Project were contacted by hundreds of American women who described their experiences with Depo Provera use. Depression and loss of libido were reported by a significant proportion of women. These effects of Depo Provera sometimes take weeks and even months to wear off, since, unlike other progestogen-only contraceptives (like the mini pill and Norplant) Depo

Provera is an injectable method that cannot be made immediately and safely reversible. There is no antidote to Depo Provera. Moreover, because the initial progesterone blood levels are much higher in Depo Provera users than in Norplant users, problems such as depression, which can be life threatening, tend to be more common and more severe among Depo Provera users.

Weight gain is also reported by the sponsor as an effect of Depo Provera use. In a group of 2200 Depo Provera users in the US, sixteen percent had gained more than ten pounds in the first six months of use. The weight gain increased steadily over time in this study, and by four years, the average weight gain was nearly fourteen pounds. The sponsor states that the only necessary reaction to this is for health practitioners to counsel women to expect to gain weight. The Network believes that it is more important for this Committee to consider the adverse effects of being overweight and its association with increased rates of other medical problems such as diabetes and hypertension.

If the Committee disregards our advice, and votes to recommend approval of Depo Provera, we would like to offer some suggestions to minimize the possible harm that could occur with premature approval. First, a registry should be mandated by the FDA, similar to the registry that has begun for women receiving silicone breast implants. If the FDA allows Upjohn to market Depo Provera in the US, there will be no incentive for the company to conduct the kind of epidemiologic studies that are necessary. A registry would enable researchers to identify adverse long-term effects more rapidly, thus avoiding harming greater numbers of women.

We are also concerned that Depo Provera, if it is approved for use as a contraceptive in the United States, will be selectively offered, that women with the least power in our society will be encouraged and possibly coerced into using this potentially harmful drug. The women's health movement has already documented many cases of coercion even while Depo Provera was not approved as a contraceptive. It is likely that these practices will continue after approval. In France, where Depo Provera is approved for use as a contraceptive, one study documented a highly disproportionate pattern of use. Only four percent of contracepting French-born women used Depo Provera, compared to fifteen percent of Algerian women living in France and twenty percent of sub-Saharan African women.[9] These results can not be explained as merely the "choice" of the women involved. A review of the records revealed that African women initially requested a method other than Depo Provera more than twice as often as French women.

Given the less than admirable track record the United States medical and scientific community has with providing informed consent, especially to communities of color, low income, institutionalized, and otherwise disenfranchised people, we believe that this Committee has a moral duty to make strong recommendations to the FDA regarding written informed consent for Depo Provera.

Because this drug is administered by a health care practitioner, and not obtained from a pharmacist, the Network believes that the FDA should encourage Upjohn to require health care providers to agree in writing that written consent forms provided by the manufacturer will be used with each woman requesting Depo Provera. The content of the written consent form should be approved by the FDA. It should include thorough information about the long-term irreversible risks, including cancer and possible bone loss. It should also include information about the short term side effects. It should spell out clearly that there is no immediate antidote, and undesirable acute effects can persist for six to ten months after the injection. It is important that the informed consent document advise women that Depo Provera does not protect against sexually transmitted diseases. The consent form should stress the importance of regular Pap smears because of the possible increased risk of cervical cancer.

We would like to remind the Committee that there are already in the contraceptive development pipeline alternative short-term long acting contraceptives such as microspheres that reduce the initial surge of progestogens. These would reduce the problems reported by a significant minority of Depo Provera users in the US. Given that there are other progestogen-only methods that allow for immediate reversal, and given that we have no adequate short-term recourse for the women who are adversely affected by Depo Provera, we believe that approval is not warranted.

Notes

1. Lee, NC, Rosero-Bixby L, Oberle MW, et al. A case-control study of breast cancer and hormonal contraception in Costa Rica. JNCI 1987; 97: 1247–54.
2. Paul, C, Skegg DCG, Spears GFS. Depot medroxyprogesterone (Depo Provera) and risk of breast cancer. Br Med J 1989; 299: 759–62.
3. WHO Collaborative Study of Neoplasia and Steroid Contraceptives. Breast cancer and depot-medroxyprogesterone acetate: a multinational study. Lancet 1991; 338: 833–38.
4. Staffa, JA, Newschaffer, CJ, Jones, JK, et al. Progestins and breast cancer: an epidemiologic review. Fertility and Sterility 1992; 57: 473–91.
5. Horwitz, KB. THe molecular biology of RU 486. Is there a role for antiprogestins in the treatment of breast cancer? Endocrine Reviews 1992; 13: 146–
6. Mack, TM. Risk benefit analysis of ERT vs HRT. Fertility and Maternal Health Drugs Advisory Committee hearing June 21, 1991.
7. WHO Collaborative Study of Neoplasia and Steroid Contraceptives. Depot-medroxyprogesterone acetate (DMPA) and risk of invasive squamous cell cervical cancer. Contraception 1992, 45: 299–312.
8. Cundy, T, Evans, M, Roberts, H, et al. Bone density in women receiving depot medroxyprogesterone acetate for contraception. Br Med J 1991; 303: 13–6.
9. Bretin, H, Job-Spira, Piet, E, et al. Contraceptive prescribing practices of family planning centers in Ile-de-France. Eur J Pub Health 1991; 1: 79–85.

Norplant Information Sheet
by National Latina Health Organization

The National Latina Health Organization (NLHO) is committed to work toward the goal of bilingual access to quality health care and the empowerment of Latinas through culturally sensitive educational programs, health advocacy, outreach, research and the development of public policy.

The NLHO would like to break some myths and set the record straight... Latinas do believe in reproductive rights, do use birth control, do get abortions, and do believe passionately that women should be able to make their own reproductive decisions without any political, social or religious interference. An eighty-four year-old Mexican Catholic woman sums it up very neatly: "If women don't have that (right), what do they have?"

Norplant. . . is it the answer to a woman's prayers? Or is it a form of social control that will be used to control the reproduction of particular groups of women? Is it a safe form of birth control?

The National Latina Health Organization (NLHO) is very concerned with its safety. The NLHO does not feel that there has been sufficient research done. We are not convinced that twenty years of research is enough to give us information on long-term effects and generational effects. No research or testing has been conducted on women under eighteen years of age so we don't know the short or long-term effects on them. Federal Drug Administration (FDA) requirements and criteria and the FDA seal of approval do not guarantee the complete safety of Norplant. We are still living with the results of the Dalkon Shield, Depo-Provera and silicone breast implants.

We are concerned that actual and possible side-effects and the degree of their seriousness have been down-played by many health practitioners. Irregular bleeding occurs in 80% of all women. This can mean bleeding two weeks out of the month or not having periods at all. We are concerned that irregular bleeding, an early symptom of uterine cancer is not being dealt with. Once women are implanted, how will they know whether the irregular bleeding is due to Norplant or an actual symptom of cancer? There is no set protocol on how soon a woman should be examined after Norplant insertion. Will those women who do not have access to regular health care but have been implanted with Norplant, have the regular exams that they need?

Side effects also include headaches, mood changes and acne. The so-called 'experts' are saying that women with high-blood pressure and smokers don't have any special concerns. But the Office of Family Planning Policy Statement Guidelines of California and the Wyeth "Norplant System Patient Labeling" make a point of this. To quote, "Women who use the oral contraceptives should not smoke as it greatly increases the risk of serious adverse effects on the heart and blood vessels; therefore, it is likely that it may be a problem with Norplant use." There is no consensus in the medical field that side effects and conditions that are specific to estrogen-based oral contraceptives need not be considered with Norplant.

We are concerned with how quickly Norplant and funding was made available in all fifty states and the District of Columbia. So quickly that there wasn't adequate or language appropriate information available so women could truly be able to make an informed decision. In February of 1992, the state of California made $5 million dollars available to provide Norplant to women eligible for the Office of Family Planning and Medi-Cal services. How much of this money is being used to target and inform specific or particular groups of women, i.e. women on welfare, Immigrant women or women of color? This has never been done before for any other type of birth control. Hundreds of health personnel have been trained to implant Norplant, but they have not all been trained to remove it.

We are not being paranoid when we question the ethics of Norplant. We have been victims of selective reproductive control before. The forced sterilization of Latinas and other women of color was blatant and widespread until the class action suit against U.S.C.-Los Angeles County Medical Center in 1975. Approximately twelve Chicanas had undergone forced sterilization, in some instances, without their knowledge. One of the results of this case is that sterilization consent forms are now multilingual. Yet these abuses continue to happen, sometimes in very subtle ways. . . doctors will not give all information necessary so women can make their own decisions; or they will give their 'medical opinion' for what they think is 'best'.

The overt and covert coercion of the 'Norping' of women is our biggest concern. When women go to their clinics for birth control, is Norplant the only birth control method available at their clinic? Is it low-cost or free? Are other forms of birth control equally available, equally recommended, and equally funded? Are appointments for other forms of birth control difficult to schedule? Once Norplant is implanted, will there be trained personnel available to remove it at the end of five years? If a woman wants it removed before the fifth year, will it be difficult to schedule an appointment for its removal? Will her request be granted? Will she be encouraged to keep it in another few months? Will it be removed regardless of whether she can afford the removal fee that can be as high as $300?

Obviously this is the real issue. Norplant is NOT WOMAN CONTROLLED. So whose control is it under?

What is most alarming about Norplant is the immediate potential for, and actual abuse. Norplant was approved by the FDA in late December, 1990. By January 5th, 1991, Judge Broadman in Visalia, California ordered a woman to have Norplant implanted as a condition of her probation. Seven states have introduced legislative bills involving Norplant since then. One type links the use of Norplant and public assistance benefits, either by providing financial incentives to encourage women who receive financial assistance to use Norplant; or by requiring Norplant use as a condition for receiving public assistance. The second mandates that women convicted of particular crimes, usually child abuse, child neglect or drug use, be required to have Norplant implanted. Assemblyman Murry in the 56th District of California attempted to pass a bill that linked AFDC benefits to Norplant. Fortunately this bill no longer exists in any recognizable form because of the NLHO involvement at the state level.

We are hearing from Latinas that they are being pressured into using Norplant rather than other contraceptives. We know that some clinics have Spanish language Norplant pamphlets in their waiting rooms, but none in English. We know that Native American women on reservations are being 'Norped'. On a reservation in Montana, a large majority of the young teens, have been 'Norped', yet nowhere on the reservation are there condoms available. A woman from another state came to an Oakland clinic during the summer of 1992 to have Norplant removed after a judge in her home state had ordered her implanted. The clinic did not remove the Norplant until they had called a meeting of their medical board. Why wasn't it removed on demand?

We know that there are very unethical practices being used when training health providers to implant Norplant. A woman in Southern California complained that after being recruited to have Norplant implanted free of charge, her calls were not returned when she requested that Norplant be removed because of the side effects. When her call was finally returned, she was told that it would cost her $300 to have it removed. We alerted "Street Stories", a television program in New York that was preparing a story on Norplant. With the permission of the young woman, a "Street Stories" reporter contacted the clinic. The Clinic providers were very upset, and couldn't understand why the young woman thought she could not have it removed. Why must we go through these extraordinary efforts?

The Baltimore School is now making Norplant available through their school clinic. It is extremely important to note that the Norplant 'consent forms' state that the removal of Norplant may not be available through their clinic and that one may have to go to another clinic for removal at the individual's own expense. In addition, when the Health Department Director and the clinic director were questioned about the sex education that was provided for their students, they admitted that students only get a few hours of sex education during their entire junior high and high school career.

A clinic provider (who wishes to remain anonymous) in Savannah, Georgia, claims that young adolescent women are being encouraged to accept Norplant. The Norplant 'consent form' states that if the individual wants it removed, she will have to go to a local hospital for the procedure; and that it is up to the hospital to decide whether it will be removed or not.

Clinics in South Dakota are adopting the policy of not removing Norplant unless it is 'medically indicated'. A woman cannot have it removed simply because she requests it for whatever reason. If side-effects are intolerable to her, it is still up to the provider to decide whether it should be removed.

A social worker in New Jersey has counseled a young mother that cut the Norplant out of her own arm because her clinic providers refused to remove it.

After having Norplant implanted, a young black adolescent in Atlanta complained about irregular bleeding to her provider. The provider prescribed oral contraceptives to regulate her menstrual cycle. Now this young women has two systemic hormonal contraceptives coursing through her body.

A clinic in San Francisco at first refused to accept young Asian women in their clinic because they were prostitutes. They were told that they did not accept "their kind of people", that they served middle-class white women. Once an advocate intervened so that the women could be taken care of, the clinic provider kept encouraging the use of Norplant and would not offer another method.

These are the stories we are hearing; there are hundreds more untold stories that have not reached us yet. The women of Color Coalition for Reproductive Health Rights, along with other organizations, has been meeting with David Kessler, Commissioner of the FDA and his staff; and Patsy Fleming and Dennis Hayashi of Donna Shalala's office to discuss our deep concerns regarding the abuse of Norplant. We must keep telling these stories and advocating for and intervening for women that have no other recourse.

The National Latina Health Organization believes that women should have all reproductive options available. . . culturally relevant quality health care and information; education about sexuality; alternative forms of woman-controlled birth control that are safe and affordable; prenatal care so that we can have healthy babies; fertility services; safe and legal abortions; and freedom from reproductive abuses. The NLHO also believes that all forms of birth control be developed with the purpose of giving safe, affordable choices to women of all ages so that they can control their own reproductive lives. This is not an unreasonable expectation. It is a very sane and logical expectation.

Ω

'The Pill' May Not Mix Well with Other Drugs

by Judith Willis

A young newlywed had been taking birth control pills several months in the early 1970s when she developed a bladder infection. She consulted her doctor, who prescribed an antibiotic. The infection cleared up quickly. But nine months later she gave birth to her first child.

Today, with proper communication between physician and patient, the inadvertent pregnancy in this mythical example would be far less likely to occur. Many interactions between oral contraceptives (OC's) containing both estrogen and progestogen and other drugs are now well-known and included in both the physician and patient labeling of the pill.

Such interactions can not only diminish the contraceptive's effectiveness, but also increase or decrease the potency of the other drug. Both those who take oral contraceptives and those who don't may find it interesting to look at what is known about the how and why of such OC-drug interactions.

Some drugs decrease contraceptive effectiveness apparently because they increase the metabolism of the contraceptives. This means that the liver breaks down the hormones in the contraceptive faster, and they are

From *FDA Consumer*, March, 1987, Government Printing Office, by the U.S. Department of Health and Human Services.

Judith Willis is editor of the *FDA Drug Bulletin*, a publication for health professionals.

eliminated from the body more quickly. Thus, the levels of estrogen and progestogen are reduced, sometimes so much that they no longer suppress ovulation. Breakthrough bleeding is often a symptom of this reduced effectiveness. This type of interaction is of even more concern with the very-low-dose contraceptives, since the level of hormones they contain is already low.

The first drug with which that type of OC interaction was reported was rifampicin, used to treat tuberculosis. In the early 1970s, medical journals reported breakthrough bleeding and contraceptive failure in OC users taking rifampicin. Alerted to this effect with one drug, physicians over the next few years noted the possibility of this type of decreased effectiveness with many different drugs. They include:

- antibiotics such as isoniazid, ampicillin, neomycin, penicillin V, tetracycline, chloramphenicol, sulfonamides, nitrofurantoin, and griseofulvin,
- barbiturates,
- anticonvulsants such as phenytoin and primidone, and
- the anti-inflammatory phenylbutazone.

Also, some analgesics, tranquilizers and anti-migraine preparations may have this type of interaction. OC users taking such drugs are advised *to use an additional form of contraception until they discontinue therapy with the second drug*.

When it comes to the other side of the coin—OC's affecting the potency of other drugs—knowledge about such interactions is more limited. But again, the how and why seem to be tied to the way the drug is metabolized; that is, changed into a form that can be eliminated from the body.

Some drugs are metabolized in the liver primarily by oxidation, and thus are excreted through the kidneys rather than the bowels. These drugs appear to be metabolized more slowly in OC users, according to research by a group of scientists headed by Darrell Abernathy, M.D., Ph.D., and reported in the April 1, 1982, *New England Journal of Medicine*. The researchers reported that long-term use of low-dose estrogen-containing OC's may cause diazepam (Valium), a benzodiazepine anti-anxiety drug, to stay in the body longer. This means that OC users may require lower dosages of diazepam and other drugs that are metabolized in the same way. However, since not all people metabolize drugs in the same way, the patient should be monitored by her physician to see if the dose should be adjusted. Other drugs that may stay in the body longer because of OC's include: other benzodiazepines such as chlordiazepoxide (Librium); hydrocortisone; antipyrine; phenothiazines; and some tricyclic antidepressants.

In contrast, some drugs that are excreted mainly through the bowels (and at times partly through the kidneys) may be eliminated more quickly in OC users. Even though the metabolism of some benzodiazepines may be slowed by OC's, there are other benzodiazepines (such as lorazepam, oxazepam and tamazepam) whose metabolism may be enhanced, so they may be excreted more quickly in women taking birth control pills. However, information

on exactly how such drugs interact with OC's is scarce. In an article in the September 1982 issue of *Obstetrics & Gynecology*, Abernathy reported that, in women using low-dose OC's containing estrogen for more than three months, acetaminophen (Tylenol) was eliminated more quickly than in non-OC users. The authors theorized that this increase in the speed at which the drug is eliminated from the body might offer some protection against liver toxicity in cases of acetaminophen overdose.

But OC users taking only the recommended dosages of acetaminophen might need a higher dosage than non-OC users. Again, because response to medication is so individual and because different combinations and dosages of estrogen and progestogen may have different effects, OC users should consult their physicians about any deviation from recommended dosages.

OC users taking other drugs may need to have the dosage monitored and possibly adjusted for a variety of reasons. Some epileptics may need a change in the dosage of an anticonvulsant drug they are taking, depending on the type of OC they're using. But other women taking the same combination may not need the dosage changed. The exact reason for this "iffiness" is not known, but it may be because OC-related changes in fluid retention could influence the frequency of seizures. Because of these difficulties, many doctors recommend that women taking anticonvulsants rely on another contraceptive than birth control pills.

A similar recommendation is often made for diabetics, because OC's may cause blood sugar levels to rise. If a diabetic does take birth control pills, she should be closely monitored to see if there needs to be a change in her diabetes medication.

Hypertension can be a problem in women on birth control pills, and elevated blood pressure has been known to occur in women not hypertensive before taking OC's. To complicate matters further, some of the medications used to control high blood pressure do not work the same way in those on The Pill as in non-OC users. In particular, the blood pressure drug guanethidine often does not adequately control hypertension in OC users. OC users taking blood pressure drugs need to be more carefully monitored.

In addition to interactions with drugs, OC's may also interact with certain vitamins. Labeling for birth control pills notes that OC users may have disturbances in the metabolism of tryptophan, an amino acid. Although such a disturbance is not considered cause for undue concern, it may result in a deficiency of pyridoxine (vitamin B6). Whether that is a cause for concern is not known. Also, in rare cases, megaloblastic anemia, a certain type of anemia due to insufficient pyridoxine, has been reported in OC users. In addition, levels of folic acid—one of the B vitamins—may be lower in women on The Pill.

Preliminary studies have shown that vitamin C may increase the bio-availability of estrogens. This means that women using birth control pills who take large doses of vitamin C may be risking increased side effects from the pill's estrogen. For this reason, some experts suggest that OC users take no more than 1,000 milligrams of vitamin C daily.

Some laboratory test results can be altered by OC use. The pathologist or other lab personnel should be informed when a woman undergoing lab tests is taking birth control pills so that this can be taken into consideration when evaluating the tests. Tests that are altered by OC use include those measuring: liver function, coagulation (clotting), thyroid function, blood triglycerides and phospholipid (fats) concentrations, serum folate, glucose tolerance, and plasma levels of some trace minerals.

In most young, healthy women, the effects of taking other drugs while using oral contraceptives are no cause for alarm and should not keep women who can benefit from the contraceptive effectiveness of OC's from taking them. The effects of OC-drug interactions may vary greatly from woman to woman. Yet women should be aware of the possibility of such interactions and tell their doctor if they are taking birth control pills so that other therapy can be properly coordinated.

Ω

Eight New Nonhormonal Contraceptive Methods for Men
by Elaine Lissner

Can you think of a male contraceptive other than the condom and vasectomy? Probably not, and for good reason: though more than eight new methods exist, some of them ready to use, none have been publicized. The methods range from simpler, safer, less surgical vasectomy to ancient "folk" methods which have performed well under scientific scrutiny. They are:

#1 No-scalpel vasectomy. According to Dr. Douglas Huber, recent medical director of the Association for Voluntary Surgical Contraception, "The no-scalpel vasectomy technique is the way all vasectomies should be done. If a vasectomy can be accomplished with this minimal surgery, then any surgeon doing more surgery should justify why more is necessary."

No-scalpel vasectomy, which has been performed for 4-8 million men in China and more than 1500 men in the rest of the world, involves gently poking and stretching a small opening in the scrotal skin rather than cutting the skin. Each vas deferens (sperm duct) is then blocked just as in a standard vasectomy. No-scalpel vasectomies bleed less and heal faster than standard vasectomies; they also eliminate the need for stitches. A list of U.S. physicians who perform no-scalpel vasectomy can be obtained from the Association for Voluntary Surgical Contraception at (212) 561-8000.

From CHANGING MEN, issue 24, Summer/Fall 1992, pp. 24–25. Copyright © 1992 by Elaine Lissner. Reprinted by permission of the author.

Elaine Lissner has been studying nonhormonal male contraception for the past several years. She recently established the Male Contraception Information Project, a national effort to publicize the methods. This article is based on her work, "Frontiers in Nonhormonal Male Contraceptive Research," which can be obtained (along with more information) by writing to Elaine Lissner, P.O. Box 3674, Stanford, CA 94309. Please include 75 cents in postage stamps.

#2 Permanent contraception by injection. In this experimental method, an injection of chemicals is used to close off the vas deferens, rather than cutting it surgically.

#3 Potentially reversible contraception by injectible vas deferens plug. Tests in China in over 512,000 men have shown a 98% effectiveness rate, and all the men who have had their plugs removed for at least a year have regained fertility. Encouraged by these results, the World Health Organization recently started tests in ten men. Continued success will reportedly lead to a trial in 3500 men around the world (and availability in some parts of the world within two years).

#4 Potentially reversible contraception by surgically implanted vas deferens plug. Here, a soft silicone plug, or "Shug," is implanted in the vas deferens in an operation similar to vasectomy. The Shug's main advantage over injectible plugs is its two-plugs-in-one design, which gives it the potential to be more leak-free. Any sperm which leak past the first plug are likely to stay in the space between the plugs rather than continuing on their course. Currently being studied on men in the Chicago area, the Shug is proceeding slowly but steadily.

#5 Temporary injectible contraception. The interior of the vas deferens is coated with a sperm-killing solution that keeps its effects for up to five years and can be reversed before then with a simple injection. Fertility can be restored at any time. This method has been completely safe and effective in ten years of animal trials. Human trials are beginning in India, but testing in the United States is stalled partly because the necessary polymer has not been sent to the National Institutes of Health.

#6 Wet Heat method. The deleterious effect of heat on male fertility has been known since the time of Hippocrates. Much as aspirin was "discovered" in the

1800s from a bark that Native Americans had long been accustomed to chewing to relieve pain, heat methods are now being "discovered" as a new form of male contraception. In this method, the testes are bathed in hot water every night for three weeks. Effectiveness goes up with increased temperature (hot tub temperature is not enough). At the recommended temperature, 116 degrees Fahrenheit, forty-five minutes per day provides contraceptive effect for six months. Although 116 degrees may sound very hot, one man has reported that this temperature is actually more comfortable on the testes than on any other part of the body.

Heat methods should be used in conjunction with sperm count checks (unless, for example, the heat method is just being used to enhance another method such as condoms or diaphragms). Sperm count can be checked easily at a doctor's or urologist's office.

#7 Artificial Cryptorchidism ("Jockey Method").
Special jockey shorts are worn during the day to hold the testes inside the inguinal canal (the same tube to which the testes retract naturally during cold or dangerous conditions.) This raises the testes to body temperature, thereby achieving the heat effect. Men appear to be about equally divided between those who find it a strange feeling and those who wouldn't mind it. Some men have expressed concern that this method would cause "jock itch," but this problem has not arisen for volunteers.

#8 Ultrasound method.
Ultra-short sound waves (the same type used by physical therapists to heal injuries) are applied to the testes for ten minutes once every six months, efficiently achieving the heat effect. Ultrasound should be used only after knowing all the details, as it may also be a permanent method in much greater doses.

All of these methods are nonhormonal (and thus not as prone to complicated side effects). Two of the methods (artificial cryptorchidism and wet heat) require little or no doctor intervention and could be put to use almost immediately. In addition to providing self-determination to men, any of these methods would improve the health, economic status and survival rates of women in countries (including the United States) where inadequate medical care makes many female methods unsafe or unavailable.

Do you wonder why you've never heard of these? In addition to the hurdles which face all contraceptive development, research bias has played a large part. In the past, funding agencies have found reasons not to fund research on male contraceptives, such as claiming that men are not committed to contraception (even though vasectomy makes up 12% of the world's contraceptive use) and that new male methods shouldn't be developed because they don't prevent the spread of HIV (even though new female methods such as Norplant don't either). Simple methods with low profit-margins have received even less support. With funding levels so low, even supportive researchers couldn't accomplish much.

According to a 1990 committee convened by the Institute of Medicine/National Research Council, "Unless immediate steps are taken to change public policy, the choice of contraceptives in the United States in the next century will not differ appreciably from what it is today." However, many researchers and policymakers believe men don't care about contraception.

How can this be changed? Read up on the subject and make it one of your priorities, since research will increase only when public pressure is strong enough to provide incentive. Think about these methods, talk about them, and share this article with a friend. Bias is already fading, and with eight new methods in the wings, men and women don't need to wait any longer.

If You Want to Use These Methods

The only methods which are "ready to go" are wet heat, artificial cryptorchidism and no-scalpel vasectomy.

No-scalpel vasectomy is a small improvement on vasectomy. However, if you or someone you know is considering a vasectomy, this is the way to do it. To get a list of physicians who perform no-scalpel vasectomies, call the Association for Voluntary Surgical Contraception's general number at (212) 561-8000. No-scalpel vasectomy is even safer and less invasive than the already safe vasectomy procedure.

Wet-Heat method and artificial cryptorchidism ("jockey method") are in some sense ready to use—if you are willing to be your own researcher, method user, doctor and critical thinker all rolled into one. Neither of these methods is in widespread use or well-known to doctors. Hopefully, in the near future men will be able to go to their doctors for an ultrasound treatment or for a "do's and don'ts" manual for using the other heat methods. However, until that time men and women who use these methods must take full responsibility for reading up, knowing what they're doing and making a fully informed choice.

If you are interested, start by reading the original paper, **"Frontiers in Nonhormonal Male Contraceptive Research."** Then go to a medical library and photocopy all the references in that citation on heat methods in general and the specific method you're interested in. Be certain to read the Kandeel and Swerdloff paper, even though it is very technical. **Contact the Male Contraception Information Project if you need more information.**

If you decide to use the wet heat method you'll have to experiment a bit to find a way to keep the water hot. Be creative. For example, modified old-style baby bottle warmers might work. If you come up with a good idea, let us know so we can pass it on. Regarding the use of hot tubs, you should know that it would take hours of hot-tubbing every day to produce contraceptive effect. That is why the wet heat method involves testes-only bathing at higher temperatures.

—Elaine Lissner
Male Contraception Information Project

Ω

Research on Birth Defects Turns to Flaws in Sperm

by Sandra Blakeslee

After three decades of efforts to discover how a pregnant woman's environment can affect the health of her fetus, researchers are turning their attention to events before conception, in particular to fathers and the sperm's vulnerability to toxins. The new research, much of it in early stages, suggests that certain substances can cause genetic mutations or other alterations in sperm that can lead to permanent defects in children.

These include familiar birth defects like heart abnormalities and mental retardation as well as less familiar ones like childhood cancer and learning disorders.

The new findings may force health authorities and occupational safety experts to rethink or expand regulations intended to prevent birth defects that have limited women, but not men, from jobs considered hazardous to the fetus.

Each year in the United States, at least 250,000 babies are born with physical birth defects while thousands more develop behavioral and learning defects that appear to have a genetic component. The cause of 60 to 80 percent of birth defects is not known, although many scientists suspect that environmental toxins play a role in a sizable number of them. The male contribution may be substantial, researchers now say.

Society has focused on the mother and fetus because they are easier to study, said Dr. Devra Lee Davis, a scholar in residence at the National Academy of Sciences who edited a recent book on biological markers in reproductive toxicology.

Since thalidomide vividly demonstrated that drugs a woman takes during pregnancy can harm her fetus, scientists have discovered more than 30 drugs, viruses, chemicals and other substances that can cross the placenta and cause structural damage to the fetus. Researchers estimate that another 900 chemicals are toxic to human development.

As a result, some American companies have developed fetal protection policies that banish women of child-bearing age from the factory floor, even if they do not intend to have children.

Animal experiments and human epidemiological research had previously linked men's exposures to certain substances with birth defects in their children, said Dr. Donald R. Mattison, dean of the School of Public Health at the University of Pittsburgh. Most of the earlier research has been ignored, he said, because scientists could not identify any possible biological mechanism to explain its findings.

Scientists also held to what some refer to as a "macho sperm theory of conception," the idea that only the fittest sperm were hardy enough to go the distance necessary to fertilize an egg. In fact research now shows that tiny hairs in the female reproductive tract move sperm along whether they are healthy or defective.

"You don't have to be Sigmund Freud to figure out there are cultural factors to say why we have paid so much attention to the female and so little to the male," Dr. Davis said.

The tools of molecular biology are now pointing to plausible mechanisms in which damage to sperm could lead to birth defects, said Dr. Marvin Legator, a genetic toxicologist at the University of Texas Health Sciences Center in Galveston. Scientists can pluck single diseased genes from cells, examine the hundreds of newly discovered proteins in sperm, place special markers on sperm to follow their development and watch how chemicals interact with sperm proteins and DNA.

Vulnerability of Sperm

Researchers have found several childhood cancers that primarily arise from new mutations traced to sperm, never to eggs.

They believe defects may originate during the division of the cells that generate sperm cells. Cells are most vulnerable to genetic damage when they divide because they are more likely to absorb and metabolize toxic substances than are quiescent cells.

Eggs do not divide; all the eggs a woman has are present before birth.

By contrast, next to the cells in the developing fetus the stem cells that produce sperm are among the most rapidly dividing cells in the human body. Moreover, researchers now realize that the barrier between blood vessels and tissue in the testes is very thin, allowing many toxic substances to enter testicular structures and seminal fluid.

Animal studies have identified more than 100 chemicals that produce spontaneous abortion or birth defects in offspring fathered by exposed males, said Dr. Mattison. Among them are alcohol, opiates like heroin and methadone, gases used in hospital operating rooms, lead, solvents, pesticides and a variety of industrial chemicals.

In some instances, litter size is greatly reduced or the offspring are deformed. In other cases, the young animals appear healthy but cannot negotiate mazes as well as control animals.

One case pending before the United States Supreme Court involves restrictive work rules intended to protect women of childbearing age from exposure to lead, which can cause neurological defects. But in one recent study, Dr. Ellen Silbergeld, a toxicologist at the University of Maryland in Baltimore, exposed male rats to relatively low levels of lead, equivalent to amounts encountered by many factory workers. The male rats' offspring showed defects in brain development, even if the female rats were not exposed to lead at all, Dr. Silbergeld said.

Other scientists have conducted scores of epidemiological studies looking for links between a father's occupation and birth defects in children. They have found numerous associations:

Wives of men exposed to vinyl chloride and waste water treatment chemicals have more miscarriages. Welders who breathe toxic metal fumes develop abnormal sperm, even after exposure stops for three weeks. Firemen who are exposed to toxic smoke have an increased risk of producing children with heart defects. Several studies have found that fathers who take two or more alcoholic drinks a day have smaller than average infants.

A British study recently found that men exposed to low levels of radiation at a single nuclear power plant had a higher than expected number of children with leukemia. The greater the exposure, the greater the risk. Some American investigators claim to have found a link between fathers' exposure to the defoliant Agent Orange in Vietnam and a variety of birth defects in their children. Both studies are controversial, and large Government-sponsored studies on Agent Orange have failed to confirm the link.

A spate of new research is finding that some rare forms of childhood cancer are closely linked with the father's genes and occupations. Garage mechanics, auto body workers and other men exposed to hydrocarbons, solvents, metals, oils and paints have a four to eightfold increased risk of having children with Wilm's tumor, a kidney cancer. Fathers who work with lead have an almost fourfold increased risk of producing such children.

An abnormal gene associated with a rare eye cancer, retinoblastoma, can be inherited from a parent who already carries it, or it can arise as a spontaneous mutation in the parent's egg or sperm. Researchers are finding that the spontaneous form seems to always stem from a mutation in the father's sperm, said Dr. Merlin Butler, pediatrician and genetics expert at Vanderbilt University in Atlanta.

Pinpointing Cause

Similarly, a genetic disorder called Prader Willi syndrome stems from errors found in the father's chromosomes, said Dr. Butler. The syndrome has been linked to children of men who work with solvents and hydrocarbons.

But epidemiological studies cannot prove cause and effect, said Dr. John Peters, an epidemiologist at the University of Southern California. In real life, people are exposed sporadically to combinations of substances that might interact, he said. A child can encounter toxic chemicals by contact with the father's clothing.

Unlike the case of thalidomide, in which the association was unmistakable, the findings linking a father's occupation and birth defects are statistically significant but not dramatic, Dr. Peters said. He said at least a dozen of the recent studies are particularly well done and "strongly suggest" that fathers contribute to birth defects, including childhood cancers. To show more dramatic associations, he said, scientists would need to study hundreds of thousands of people over many years, research that would be too expensive and too difficult to carry out.

Sperm: Not So Simple

Molecular biologists are conducting experiments that may explain the mechanisms involved, said Dr. Andrew J. Wyrobek, a researcher at the Lawrence Livermore Laboratory in Livermore, Calif. Methods are being developed to detect sperm with missing or extra chromosomes, study chromosome regions that tend to get shuffled around in the presence of chemicals, locate single gene mutations and identify how chemicals might attach themselves to proteins or DNA within sperm.

Ultimately it will be possible to follow sperm from their earliest formation through fertilization, explaining how and where damage occurs, the researchers said. For example if the stem cells that give rise to sperm suffer permanent genetic mutations, errors would always be present in a significant number of sperm. It should be possible to pinpoint such mutations.

If toxins are drawn to specific regulatory genes because of a chemical affinity, then specific patterns of genetic damage could result. For example, a solvent might attach itself to a master gene that determines the fate of many subsequent cells in heart tissue. Heart defects would be a common outcome of exposure to the chemical. Other chemicals could affect sites that determine whether genes are expressed. Yet others could induce transposable elements in chromosomes—regions that naturally jump around—to break or form harmful combinations.

In another case, which has been shown to happen in laboratory experiments, a chemical attaches itself to a protein within the sperm head. Upon fertilization the chemical is carried into the egg where it could exert an effect on the earliest stages of embryo growth.

Researchers used to think of sperm as being relatively simple, stripped-down vehicles for carrying male DNA into an egg, said Dr. Anthony Bellve, a Columbia University urologist who is a leading expert on sperm genetics. But new research shows that each sperm head contains 300 to 400 novel proteins. Each sperm membrane contains another 300 to 400 proteins. It is entirely possible, said Dr. Bellve, that these proteins exert powerful influences on early embryogenesis. If they sustain chemical damage, a fetus could suffer.

According to Dr. Silbergeld, lead could have such an effect by attaching itself to zinc binding proteins found in sperm, fetuses and adults. Tiny amounts of lead in an early embryo, she said, could alter zinc pathways and affect brain development.

While scientists explore such mechanisms, people should not panic, Dr. Mattison said. But it may make sense to clean up the work place for fathers as well as for mothers.

Ω

Fertility, Infertility, and Reproductive Rights/Freedom

1. Three situations are described below. Make a list of all possible contraceptives which are options in the situations and briefly comment on the pros and cons for each.

Linda and Larry

Linda and Larry are 22. They have been married for one year and want a family someday. Linda feels it is very important that she does not get pregnant now while she is supporting both of them because Larry (a scientist) is unemployed. Because of their shared religious beliefs, Larry is not happy about Linda using birth control and both feel very strongly against abortion. Linda does not feel comfortable with her own body and does not have much understanding of the menstrual cycle or the process of fertilization.

Betsy and Bob

Betsy and Bob are 22. They have been married for one year and want a family someday, but want to wait until they are older. Betsy and Bob are working towards equality in their relationship so both are working half time and going to school half time. Although Betsy and Bob hope to prevent an unplanned pregnancy, they have the money and "attitude" which would permit abortion as back-up to failed contraception. Both Betsy and Bob feel pretty comfortable with their bodies and both recently got A's in a women's health course.

Susie and Sam

Susie and Sam are 22. Susie identifies as bisexual. She is mostly sexually active with women, but once in awhile she is still sexually active with her old boyfriend, Sam. Both Susie and Sam are responsible and well informed about sexual relationships. Both Susie and Sam feel strongly that their infrequent sexual encounters should not result in a pregnancy.

2. We get very used to thinking about ways a woman can control her fertility to limit the number of children she has. As reflected in the articles in this chapter, true reproductive freedom means being able to have as many or as few children as desired. List a wide range of factors which would enable women to have as *many* children as they wish:

3. After reading "Born and Unborn: The Implications of 'Choice' for People with Disabilities," identify some of the ramifications of routine prenatal genetic testing.

    a. Give a reason why a woman might choose to have prenatal genetic testing even if she knew she would not choose to have an abortion.

    b. What could our society do to make it easier for women to choose to have a child with a disability?

Chapter

10

Childbearing

Many of the problems in the relationship between women and the health care system are clearly visible in the area of childbearing. The paternalism, the reliance on technology, and the performance of unnecessary surgery characterizing the medical profession in the United States are all evident. On a positive note, this is also an area in which organized movements by women have had an impact in improving care for women and their babies and increasing the options available. It is an area of continuing struggle, in which apparent victories may sometimes actually weaken the movement for more fundamental changes. For example, in some cases, "birthing centers" are merely hospital rooms decorated to look like home, with families allowed to be present for the birth, sometimes with a nurse midwife attending, but with the same medical interventions and little change in who is making the decisions. However, such birthing centers may "pacify" some women who would otherwise work for more major changes.

Doris Haire's classic paper "The Cultural Warping of Childbirth," was first published in the *International Childbirth Education Association News* in 1972. It was a very influential article, comparing the experience and mortality of childbirth in the US with that of other countries. It identified common pathologically orientated obstetrical practices throughout the entire pregnancy and post-partum period which "served to warp and distort the childbearing experience in the United States." The specific issues de-

fined in this paper became many of the key issues around which childbirth activists organized for the next twenty years. "Hot off the press" (literally arriving as this book goes to press) is an excerpt from the new booklet "Childbearing Policy Within a National Health Program: An Evolving Consensus for New Directions" which is in many ways remarkably similar to the Doris Haire classic. More than twenty years later, the need for redefining childbirth as a natural healthy process with midwives as the appropriate caretaker for most childbearing women, instead of viewing childbirth as a medical event requiring maximum technological intervention, seems as urgent as ever. The childbearing policy paper serves as an excellent representation of a collaborative effort of a number of women's health organizations, trying to make sure that women's voices and women's issues are core to the national debates on health reform.

The meanings of mothering are central to the experiences of pregnancy and birthing. Debbie Field's "The Mother Myth—A Feminist Analysis of Post-Partum Depression" not only summarizes what is known about post-partum depression but also uses post-partum depression as a metaphor of women's oppression as mothers. The author identifies the need for revolutionary changes from the ways that women are expected to parent in isolating circumstances.

The Cultural Warping of Childbirth

by Doris Haire

While Sweden and the Netherlands compete for the honor of having the lowest incidence of infant deaths per one thousand live births, the United States continues to find itself outranked by fourteen other developed countries.[1] A spokesman for the National Foundation March of Dimes recently stated that according to the most recent data, the United States leads all developed countries in the rate of infant deaths due to birth injury and respiratory distress such as postnatal asphyxia and atelectasis. According to the National Association for Retarded Children there are now six million retarded children and adults in the United States with a predicted annual increase of over 100,000 a year. The number of children and adults with behavioral difficulties or perceptual dysfunction resulting from minimal brain damage is an ever growing challenge to society and to the economy.

While it may be easier on the conscience to blame such numbing facts solely on socioeconomic factors and birth defects, recent research makes it evident that obstetrical medication can play a role in our staggering incidence of neurological impairment. It may be convenient to blame our relatively poor infant outcome on a lack of facilities or inadequate government funding, but it is obvious from the research being carried out that we could effect an immediate improvement in infant outcome by changing the pattern of obstetrical care in the United States. It is time that we take a good look at the overall experience of childbirth in this country and begin to recognize how our culture has warped this experience for the majority of American mothers and their newborn infants.

As an officer of the International Childbirth Education Association, I have visited hundreds of maternity hospitals throughout the world—in Great Britain, Western Europe, Russia, Asia, Australia, New Zealand, the South Pacific, the Americas, and Africa. During my visits I was privileged to observe obstetric techniques and procedures and to interview physicians, professional midwives, and parents in the various countries. My companion on many of my visits was Dorothea Lang, C.N.M. (Certified Nurse-Midwife), Director of Nurse-Midwifery for New York City. Miss Lang's experience as both a nurse-midwife and a former head nurse of the labor and delivery unit of the New York-Cornell Medical Center made her a particularly well-qualified observer and companion. As we traveled from country to country certain patterns of care soon became evident. For one, in those countries that enjoy an incidence of infant mortality and birth trauma significantly lower than that of the of the United States, highly trained professional midwives are an important source of obstetrical care and family planning services for normal women, whether the births take place in the hospital or in the home. In these countries the expertise of the physician is called upon only when the expectant mother is ill during pregnancy, or when labor or birth is anticipated to be, or is found to be, abnormal. Under this system, the high-risk mother—the one who is most likely to bear an impaired or stillborn child—has a better opportunity to obtain in-depth medical attention than is possible under our existing American system of obstetrical care where the obstetrician is also called upon to play the role of midwife.

Deprivation, birth defects, prematurity, and low birth weight are not unique to the United States. While it is tempting to blame our comparatively high incidence of infant mortality solely on a lack of available prenatal care and on socioeconomic factors, our observations indicate that, comparatively, the prenatal care we offer most clinic patients in the United States is not grossly inferior to that available in other developed countries. Furthermore, the diet and standard of living in many countries which have a lower incidence of infant mortality than ours would be considered inadequate by American standards.

As an example, when one compares the availability of prenatal care, the incidence of premature births, the average diet of various economic groups, and the equipment available to aid in newborn-infant survival in two such diverse countries as the United States and Japan, there are no major differences between the two countries. The differences lie in (a) our frequent use of prenatal and obstetrical medication, (b) our pathologically oriented management of pregnancy, labor, birth, and postpartum, and (c) the predominance of artificial feeding in the United States, in contrast to Japan.

If present statistics follow the trend of recent years, an infant born in the United States is more than four times more likely to die in the first day of life than an infant born in Japan. But a survival of the birth process should not be our singular goal. For every American newborn infant who dies there are likely to be several who are neurologically damaged.

Unfortunately, the American tendency to warp the birth experience, distorting it into a pathological event rather than a physiological one for the normal childbearing woman, is no longer peculiar to just the United States. In my visits to hospitals in various countries I was distressed to find that some physicians, anxious to impress their colleagues with their "Americanized" techniques, have

Abridged version of an article that originally appeared in the International Childbirth Education Association *News* (Spring 1972). Copyright © 1972 by ICEA. Reprinted by permission of Doris Haire. Unabridged version available from ICEA, Box 20048, Minneapolis, MN 55420.

unfortunately adopted many of our obstetrical practices without stopping to question their scientific or social merit.

Few American babies are born today as nature intended them to be.

It is not unlikely that unnecessary alterations in the normal fetal environment may play a role in the incidence of neurological impairment and infant mortality in the United States. Infant resuscitation, other than routine suctioning, is rarely needed in countries such as Sweden, the Netherlands, and Japan, where the skillful psychological management of labor usually precludes the need for obstetrical medication. In contrast, in those European countries, such as Belgium, where the overall pattern of obstetrical care is similar to our own, the incidence of infant mortality also approaches our own.

Obviously there will always be medical indications which dictate the use of various obstetrical procedures, but to apply the following American practices and procedures routinely to the vast majority of mothers who are capable of giving birth without complication is to create added stress which is not in the best interests of either the mother or her newborn infant.

Let us take a close look at some of our common obstetrical practices from early pregnancy to postpartum which have served to warp and distort the childbearing experience in the United States. While not all of the practices below affect infant mortality, it is equally apparent that they do not contribute to the reduction of infant morbidity or mortality and therefore should be reevaluated.

Withholding information on the disadvantages of obstetrical medication. Ignorance of the possible hazards of obstetrical medication appears to encourage the misuse and abuse of obstetrical medication, for in those countries where mothers are not told routinely of the possible disadvantages of obstetrical medication to themselves or to their babies the use of such medication is on the increase.

There is no research or evidence which indicates that mothers will be emotionally damaged if they are advised, prior to birth, that obstetrical medication may be to the disadvantage of their newborn infants.

Requiring all normal women to give birth in the hospital. While ICEA does not encourage home births, there is ample evidence in the Netherlands and in Chicago (Chicago Maternity Center) to demonstrate that normal women who have received adequate prenatal care can safely give birth at home if a proper system is developed for home deliveries. Over half of the mothers in the Netherlands give birth at home with the assistance of a professional midwife and a maternity aide. The comparatively low incidence of infant deaths and birth trauma in the Netherlands, a country of diverse ethnic composition and intermarriage, is evidence of the comparative safety of a properly developed home delivery service.

Dutch obstetricians point out that when the labor of a normal woman is unhurried and allowed to progress normally, unexpected emergencies rarely occur. They also point out that the small risk involved in a Dutch home delivery is more than offset by the increased hazards resulting from the use of obstetrical medication and obstetrical tampering which are more likely to occur in a hospital environment, especially in countries where professionals have had little or no exposure to normal labor and birth in a home environment during their training.

Elective induction of labor. The elective induction of labor (where there is no clear medical indication) appears to be an American idiosyncrasy which is frowned upon in other developed countries.

The elective induction of labor has been found almost to double the incidence of fetomaternal transfusion and its attendant hazards.[2] But perhaps the least appreciated problem of elective induction is the fact that the abrupt onset of artificially induced labor tends to make it extremely difficult for even the well-prepared mother to tolerate the discomfort of the intensified contractions without the aid of obstetrical medication. When the onset of labor occurs spontaneously, the normal, gradual increase in contraction length and intensity appears to provoke in the mother an accompanying tolerance for discomfort or pain.

Since the British Perinatal Hazards Study found no increase in perinatal mortality or impairment of learning ability at age seven among full-term infants unless gestation had extended beyond forty-one weeks,[3] there would appear to be no medical justification for subjecting a mother or her baby to the possible hazards of elective induction in order to terminate the pregnancy prior to forty-one weeks' gestation.

Separating the mother from familial support during labor and birth. Research indicates that fear adversely affects uterine motility and blood flow,[4] and yet many American mothers are routinely separated from a family member or close friend at this time of emotional crisis.

In most developed countries, other than the United States and the Eastern European countries, mothers are encouraged to walk about or to sit and chat with a family member or supportive person in what is called an "early labor lounge." This lounge is usually located near but outside the labor-delivery area in order to provide a more relaxed atmosphere during much of labor. The mother is taken to the labor-delivery area to be checked periodically, then allowed to return to the labor lounge for as long as she likes or until her membranes have ruptured.

Confining the normal laboring woman to bed. In virtually all countries except the United States, a woman in labor is routinely encouraged to walk about during labor for as long as she wishes or until her membranes have ruptured. Such activity is considered to facilitate labor by distracting the mother's attention from the discomfort or pain of her contractions and to encourage a more rapid engagement of the fetal head. In America, where drugs are frequently administered either orally or parenterally to laboring mothers, such ambulation is discouraged—not only for the patient's safety but also to avoid possible legal complications in the event of an accident.

Shaving the birth area. Research involving 7,600 mothers has demonstrated that the practice of shaving the perineum and pubis does not reduce the incidence of infection. In fact, the incidence of infection was slightly higher among those mothers who were shaved.[5] Yet this procedure, which tends to create apprehension in laboring women, is still carried out routinely in most American hospitals. Clipping the perineal or pudendal hair closely with surgical scissors is far less disturbing to the mother and is less likely to result in infection caused by razor abrasions.

Professional dependence on technology and pharmacological methods of pain relief. Most of the world's mothers receive little or no drugs during pregnancy, labor, or birth. The constant emotional support provided the laboring woman in other countries by the nurse-midwife, and often by her husband, appears greatly to improve the mother's tolerance for discomfort. In contrast, the American labor room nurse is frequently assigned to look after several women in labor, all or most of whom have had no preparation to cope with the discomfort or pain of childbearing. Under the circumstances, drugs, rather than skillful emotional support, are employed to relieve the mother's apprehension and discomfort (and perhaps to assuage the harried labor attendant's feeling of inadequacy).

Routine Electronic Fetal Monitoring. The wisdom of depending on an experienced nurse using a stethoscope to monitor accurately the effects of obstetrical medication on the well-being of the fetus has been demonstrated by Haverkamp.[6] No one knows the long-term or delayed consequences of ultrasonic fetal monitoring on subsequent human development. The fact that some electronic fetal monitoring devices require that a mother's membranes be ruptured and the electrode be screwed into the skin of the fetal scalp creates hazards of its own. Current research indicates that obstetrical management which reduces the need for such monitoring is advisable.

Chemical stimulation of labor. Oxytocic agents are frequently administered to American mothers in order to intensify artificially the frequency or the strength of the mother's contractions, as a means of shortening the mother's labor. While chemical stimulation is sometimes medically indicated, often it is undertaken to satisfy the American propensity for efficiency and speed. Hon suggests that the overenthusiastic use of oxytocic stimulants sometimes results in alterations in the normal fetal heart rate.[7] Fields points out that the possible hazards inherent in elective induction are also possible in artificially stimulated labor unless the mother and fetus are carefully monitored.[8]

Shortening the phases of normal labor when there is no sign of fetal distress has not been shown to improve infant outcome. Little is known of the long-term effects of artificially stimulating labor contractions. During a contraction the unborn child normally receives less oxygen. The gradual buildup of intensity, which occurs when the onset of labor is allowed to occur spontaneously and to proceed without chemical stimulation, appears likely to be a protective mechanism that is best left unaltered unless there is a clear medical indication for the artificial stimulation of labor.

Delaying birth until the physician arrives. Because of the increased likelihood of resultant brain damage to the infant the practice of delaying birth by anesthesia or physical restraint until the physician arrives to deliver the infant is frowned upon in most countries. Yet the practice still occurs occasionally in the United States and in countries where hospital-assigned midwives do not routinely manage the labor and delivery of normal mothers.

Requiring the mother to assume the lithotomy position for birth. There is gathering scientific evidence that the unphysiological lithotomy position (back flat, with knees drawn up and spread wide apart by "stirrups"), which is preferred by most American physicians because it is more convenient for the *accoucheur,* tends to alter the normal fetal environment and obstruct the normal process of childbearing, making spontaneous birth more difficult or impossible.

The lithotomy and dorsal positions tend to:

1. Adversely affect the mother's blood pressure, cardiac return, and pulmonary ventilation.[9]

2. Decrease the normal intensity of the contractions.[10]

3. Inhibit the mother's voluntary efforts to push her baby out spontaneously[11] which, in turn, increases the need for fundal pressure or forceps and increases the traction necessary for a forceps extraction.

4. Inhibit the spontaneous expulsion of the placenta[12] which, in turn, increases the need for cord traction, forced expression, or manual removal of the placenta[13]— procedures which significantly increase the incidence of fetomaternal hemorrhage.[14]

5. Increase the need for episiotomy because of the increased tension on the pelvic floor and the stretching of the perineal tissue.[15]

Australian, Russian, and American research bears out the clinical experience of European physicians and midwives—that when mothers are supported to a semisitting position for birth, with their feet supported by the lower section of the labor-delivery bed, mothers tend to push more effectively, appear to need less pain relief, are more likely to want to be conscious for birth, and are less likely to need an episiotomy.[16]

The increased efficiency of the semisitting position, combined with a minimum use of medication for birth, is evidenced by the fact that the combined use of both forceps and the vacuum extractor rarely exceeds 4 percent to 5 percent of all births in the Netherlands, as compared to an incidence of 65 percent in many American hospitals. (Cesarean section occurs in approximately 1. 5 percent of all Dutch births.)

The routine use of regional or general anesthesia for delivery. In light of the current shortage of qualified anesthetists and anesthesiologists and the frequent scientific papers now being published on the possible hazards resulting from the use of regional and general anesthesia, it would seem prudent to make every effort to prepare the mother physically and mentally to cope with the sensations and discomfort of birth in order to avoid the use of such medicaments. Regional and general anesthesia not only tend adversely to affect fetal environment pharmacologically, which has been discussed previously herein, but their use also increases the need for obstetrical intervention in the normal process of birth, since both types of anesthesia tend to prolong labor.[17] Johnson points out that peridural and spinal anesthesia significantly increase the incidence of midforceps delivery and its attendant hazards.[18] Pudendal block anesthesia not only tends to interfere with the mother's ability effectively to push her baby down the birth canal due to the blocking of the afferent path of the pushing reflex, but also appears to interfere with the mother's normal protective reflexes, thus making "an explosive" birth and perineal damage more likely to occur.

The routine use of forceps for delivery. There is no scientific justification for the routine application of forceps for delivery.[19] The incidence of delivery by forceps and vacuum extractor, combined, rarely rises above 5 percent in countries where mothers actively participate in the births of their babies. In contrast, as mentioned previously, the incidence of forceps extraction frequently rises to as high as 65 percent in some American hospitals.

Routine episiotomy. There is no research or evidence to indicate that routine episiotomy (a surgical incision to enlarge the vaginal orifice) reduces the incidence of pelvic relaxation (structural damage to the pelvic floor musculature) in the mother. Nor is there any research or evidence that routine episiotomy reduces neurological impairment in the child who has shown no signs of fetal distress or that the procedure helps to maintain subsequent male or female sexual response.

The incidence of pelvic floor relaxation appears to be on the decline throughout the world, even in those countries where episiotomy is still comparatively rare. The contention that the modern washing machine has been more effective in reducing pelvic relaxation among American mothers than has routine episiotomy is given some credence by the fact that in areas of the United States where life is still hard for the woman pelvic relaxation appears in white women who have never borne children.

In developed countries where episiotomy is comparatively rare the physiotherapist is considered an important member of the obstetrical team—before as well as after birth. The physiotherapist is responsible for seeing that each mother begins exercises the day following birth which will help to restore the normal elasticity and tone of the mother's perineal and abdominal muscles. In countries where every effort is made to avoid the need for an episiotomy, interviews with both parents and professionals indi-

cate that an intact perineum which is strengthened by postpartum exercises is more apt to result in both male and female sexual satisfaction than is a perineum that has been incised and reconstructed.

Why then, is there such an emotional attachment among professionals to routine episiotomy? A prominent European professor of obstetrics and gynecology recently made the following comment on the American penchant for routine episiotomy, "Since all the physician can really do to affect the course of childbirth for the 95 percent of mothers who are capable of giving birth without complication is to offer the mother pharmacological relief from discomfort or pain and to perform an episiotomy, there is probably an unconscious tendency for many professionals to see these practices as indispensable."

Interviews with obstetrician-gynecologists in many countries indicate that they tend to agree that a superficial, first degree tear is less traumatic to the perineal tissue than an incision which requires several sutures for reconstruction. There is no research which would indicate otherwise.

Early clamping or "milking" of the umbilical cord. Several years ago De Marsh stated that the placental blood normally belongs to the infant and his or her failure to get this blood is equivalent to submitting him or her to a rather severe hemorrhage. Despite the fact that placental transfusion normally occurs in every corner of the world without adverse consequences, there is still a great effort in the United States and Canada to deprecate the practice. One must read the literature carefully to find that placental transfusion has not been demonstrated to increase the incidence of morbidity or mortality in the placentally transfused infant.[20]

Delaying the first breast-feeding. The common American practice of routinely delaying the time of the first breast-feeding has not been shown to be in the best interest of either the conscious mother or her newborn infant. Clinical experience with the early feeding of newborn infants has shown this practice to be safe.[21] If the mother feels well enough and the infant is capable of suckling while they are still in the delivery room then it would seem more cautious, in the event of tracheoesophageal abnormality, to permit the infant to suckle for the first time under the watchful eye of the physician or nurse-midwife rather than delay the feeding for several hours when the expertise of the professional may not be immediately available.

In light of the many protective antibodies contained in colostrum it would seem likely that the earlier the infant's intake of species specific colostrum, the sooner the antibodies can be accrued by the infant.

Offering water and formula to the breast-fed newborn infant. The common American practice of giving water or formula to a newborn infant prior to the first breast-feeding or as a supplement during the first days of life has not been shown to be in the best interests of the infant. There are now indications that these practices may, in fact, be harmful. Glucose water, once the standby in every Ameri-

American hospital, has now been designated a potential hazard if aspirated by the newborn infant, yet it is still used in many American hospitals.

Restricting newborn infants to a four-hour feeding schedule and withholding nightime feedings. Although widely spaced infant feedings may be more convenient for hospital personnel, the practice of feeding a newborn infant only every four hours and not permitting the infant to breast-feed at all during the night cannot be justified on any scientific grounds. Such a regimen restricts the suckling stimulation necessary to bring about the normally rapid onset and adequate production of the mother's milk. In countries where custom permits the infant to suckle immediately after birth and on demand from that time, first-time mothers frequently begin to produce breast milk for their babies within twenty-four hours after birth. In contrast, in countries where hospital routines prevent normal demand feeding from birth, mothers frequently do not produce breast milk for their babies until the third day following birth.

Overdistention of the breast or engorgement is a hospital acquired condition which does not occur to any comparable degree in cultures where mothers are permitted to breast-feed their babies on demand from birth.[22]

Preventing early father-child contact. Permitting fathers to hold their newborn infants immediately following birth and during the postpartum hospital stay has not been shown by research or clinical experience to increase the incidence of infection among newborns, even when those infants are returned to a regular or central nursery. Yet only in the Eastern European countries is the father permitted less involvement in the immediate postpartum period than in the United States.

Research has consistently confirmed the fact that the greatest sources of infection to the newborn infant are the nursery and nursery personnel.[23] One has only to observe a mother holding her newborn infant against her bathrobe, which has probably been exposed to abundant hospital-borne bacteria, to realize the fallacy of preventing a father from holding his baby during the hospital stay.

Restricting intermittent rooming-in to specific room requirements. Throughout the world great effort is made to keep mothers and babies together in the hospital, no matter how inconvenient the accommodations. There is no research or evidence which indicates that intermittent rooming-in should be restricted to private rooms or to rooms which have a sink, or which provide at least eighty square feet for mother and baby. Such requirements are based on conjecture and not on controlled evaluation.

Restricting sibling visitation. The common American practice of prohibiting toddlers and children from visiting their mothers during the hospital stay is an emotional hardship on both the mothers and their children and is unsupported by scientific research or evidence. Experience in other countries and in several hospitals here in the United States suggests that where sibling visitation is permitted, a short explanation as to the importance of not bringing suspect illnesses into the hospital seems to be effective in controlling infection.

Summary

As mentioned previously, most of the practices discussed above have developed not from a lack of concern for the well-being of the mother and baby but from a lack of awareness as to the problems which can arise from each progressive digression from the normal childbearing experience. Like a snowball rolling down hill, as one unphysiological practice is employed, for one reason or another, another frequently becomes necessary to counteract some of the disadvantages, large or small, inherent in the previous procedure.

The higher incidence of fetal, neonatal, and maternal deaths occurring in our large urban hospitals, as opposed to our smaller community hospitals,[24] is undoubtedly due, in part, to the greater proportion of high-risk mothers in the urban areas. But we in the United States must stop looking for scapegoats and face up to the fact that by individualizing the care offered to maternity patients, much can be done immediately to improve infant outcome without the slightest outlay of capital.

There is currently an increasing emphasis on consolidating maternity facilities. However, we in ICEA do not see the consolidation of community obstetrical facilities as being always in the best interest of the vast majority of mothers who are capable of giving birth without complications. There should, of course, be centers where those mothers who have had no prenatal care or who are anticipated to be obstetrical risks can be properly cared for. But to insist that every healthy mother must go to a major maternity facility which is unnecessary for her needs and inconvenient for her family, and where she is very apt to be "lost in the crowd," will only spur the growing trend in the United States toward professionally unattended home births.

Throughout the United States the current inclination of many expectant parents is to seek out, to "shop around" for the type of physician and hospital they feel they need in order to have the type of childbearing experience they want. They not only want a doctor who will support them in their efforts to have a prepared, natural birth, with a minimum of or no medication; they also want a hospital which offers education for childbearing and a supportive family-centered atmosphere. These expectant mothers appreciate the availability of such facilities as an early labor lounge, a dual purpose labor-delivery room, a mother-baby recovery room, and a children's visiting room if they have older children. But most of all they want a supportive atmosphere in which they can share the childbearing experience to the extent that they desire, and one which makes an effort to meet the individual needs of the mother, the father, and their newborn baby as they form their family bonds during the hospital stay.

NOTES

1. H. Chase, "Ranking Countries by Infant Mortality Rates," *Public Health Reports* 84 (1969): 19–27; M. Wegman, "Annual Summary of Vital Statistics—1969," *Pediatrics* 47 (1971): 461–64.
2. A. Beer, "Fetal Erythrocytes in Maternal Circulation of 155 Rh-Negative Women," *Obstet. & Gynec.* 34 (1969): 143–50.
3. N. Butler, "A National Long-Term Study of Perinatal Hazards," Sixth World Congress of the Federation of International Gynecology & Obstetrics, 1970.
4. J. Kelly, "Effect of Fear Upon Uterine Motility," *Am. J. Obstet. & Gynec.* 83 (1962): 576–81.
5. R. Burchell, "Predelivery Removal of Pubic Hair," *Obstet. & Gynec.* 24 (1964): 272–73; H. Kantor et al., "Value of Shaving the Pudendal-Perineal Area in Delivery Preparation," *Obstet. & Gynec.* 25 (1965) 509–12.
6. Haverkamp, A. D., Thompson, H. E., McFee, J. G. et al., "The Evaluation of Continuous Fetal-Heart Monitoring for High Risk Pregnancies." *Am. J. Obstet. & Gynec.* 125, no. 3 (June 1, 1926): 310–20.
7. E. Hon, "Direct Monitoring of the Fetal Heart," *Hospital Practice* (September 1970): 91–97.
8. H. Fields, "Complications of Elective Induction" *Obstet. & Gynec.* 15 (1960): 476–80; H. Fields, "Induction of Labor: Methods, Hazards, Complications, and Contraindications," *Hospital Topics* (December 1968): 63–68.
9. C. Flowers, *Obstetric Analgesia and Anesthesia* (New York: Hoeber, Harper & Row, 1967); L. S. James, "The Effects of Pain Relief for Labor and Delivery on the Fetus and Newborn," *Anesthesiology* 21 (1960): 405–30; A. Blankfield, "The Optimum Position for Childbirth," *Med. J. Australia* 2 (1965): 666–68.
10. Blankfield, "The Optimum Position for Childbirth"; F. H. Howard, "Delivery in the Physiologic Position," *Obstet. & Gynec.* 11 (1958): 318–22; I. Gritsiuk, "Position in Labor," *Ob-Gyn Observer* (September 1968).
11. Blankfield, "The Optimum Position for Childbirth"; Howard, "Delivery in the Physiologic Position"; N. Newton and M. Newton "The Propped Position for the Second Stage of Labor," *Obstet. & Gynec.* 15 (1960): 28–34.
12. Newton and Newton, "The Propped Position for the Second Stage of Labor."
13. M. Botha, "The Management of the Umbilical Cord in Labour," *S. Afr. J. Obstet.* 6, no. 2 (1968): 30–33.
14. Beer, "Fetal Erythrocytes in Maternal Circulation of 155 Rh-Negative Women."
15. Blankfield, "The Optimum Position for Childbirth."
16. Ibid.; Newton and Newton, "The Propped Position for the Second Stage of Labor."
17. L. Hellman and J. Pritchard, *Williams Obstetrics,* 14th ed. (New York: Appleton-Century-Crofts, 1971).
18. W. Johnson, "Regionals Can Prolong Labor," *Medical World News,* October 15, 1971.
19. Butler, "A National Long-Term Study of Perinatal Hazards."
20. S. Saigal et al., "Placental Transfusion and Hyperbilirubinemia in the Premature," *Pediatrics* 49 (1972): 406–19.
21. H. Eppink, "Time of Initial Breast Feeding Surveyed in Michigan Hospitals," *Hospital Topics* (June 1968): 116–17.
22. M. Newton and N. Newton, "Postpartum Engorgement of the Breast," *Am. J. Obstet. & Gynec.* 61 (1951): 664–67.
23. H. Gezon et al., "Some Controversial Aspects in the Epidemiology of Hospital Nursery Staphylococcal Infections," *Amer. J. of Public Health* 50 (1960): 473–84; R. Ravenholt and G. LaVeck, "Staphylococcal Disease—An Obstetric, Pediatric & Community Problem," *Amer. J. of Public Health* 46 (1956): 1287–96.
24. E. Bishop, "The National Study of Maternity Care." *Obstet. & Gynec.* (1971): 745–50.

Ω

Excerpts from *Childbearing Policy Within a National Health Program: An Evolving Consensus for New Directions.*

A collaborative paper by:
Boston Women's Health Book Collective
National Black Woman's Health Project
National Women's Health Network
Women's Institute for Childbearing Policy

Note from the collaborating organizations: The following selection is excerpted from a large booklet. In addition to the material that appears here, the booklet contains acknowledgments, a summary, an opening section on "The Failure of the Present System to Meet Needs of Childbearing Women and Families" with extensive supporting documentation, eight appendices presenting a broad range of information and additional support for the positions taken in the paper, and information about the four collaborating organizations. The complete document may be obtained for $10 postpaid (checks made out to Women's Institute for Childbearing Policy) from: Jane Pincus, WICP, PO Box 72, Roxbury, VT 05669. The collaborative paper is a project of the Women's Institute for Childbearing Policy. We are grateful to the Midwifery Communication and Accountability Project for support that enabled the creation of the revised and expanded 1994 edition.

The Value of Women's Health and Public Health Perspectives

The solution to current problems lies in a shift from the present emphasis on a medical approach to an approach that combines women's health and public health perspectives. *From a women's health perspective, the needs of women and children are central.*[18] *In the best public health tradition, in this country as well as Europe, clinical services are only one component of a broader approach; moreover, these clinical services give priority to primary care.* Many advocates of reform speak of a National *Health* Program, when what they really mean is a National *Medical Care* Program. Our challenge is to develop and implement a genuine National Health Program that includes the conditions of daily life that influence health, provides universal access to prevention-oriented health care services, and insures medical services when necessary.

Childbearing policies that reflect women's health and public health perspectives would promote healthful living conditions. As the National Association for Public Health Policy asserts, the campaign for a national program of clinical services "must be part of an overall movement for full employment, higher wages, improved working conditions, decent housing, better education, and affirmative action to end discrimination in all areas of our national life" (1989). Public policies must assure: access to adequate family leave and social supports; availability of adequate housing and nourishing food; control of environmental hazards; and freedom from the havoc of violence and of alcohol, tobacco, cocaine and other drugs. *Social and economic conditions, and the presence or lack of social supports, are directly linked to the quality of birth outcomes* (Barrera et al. 1992; Terris 1990a, 1990b; Elbourne et al. 1989; Ottawa Charter for Health Promotion 1986).

Maternity care services based upon women's and public health perspectives would be provided routinely by primary caregivers who are trained to understand, promote and sustain health. These caregivers would recognize the importance of nutritional, educational, social, psychological, and cultural factors. They would pay vigilant attention to mothers and babies, consult and refer when appropriate, and provide continuous, individualized care and a range of basic services. They would develop a trusting relationship with the woman and her support network. Care would be given in small-scale, community-based settings that give priority to community participation, employ community residents, and provide convenient and coherent services. All women would be able to give birth in the location of their choice, including freestanding birth centers and homes. Consultative and specialist back-up services would always be readily available.[19]

On a small scale within this country, and on a large scale in Europe and other nations, midwives most consistently offer this optimal care for women and newborns. We call for a national health program that recognizes that midwives' philosophy, education and standards of practice make them the most effective and optimal front-line caregivers for the great majority of childbearing women.[20] The Core Values segment of the "Statement of Values and Ethics" of the Midwives Alliance of North America reflects many of the distinctive elements of midwifery care and underscores the sharp contrast between prevailing medical approaches and midwifery approaches to maternity care.[21]

It is important to note that obstetricians and family practitioners can, and occasionally do, provide midwifery care as we describe it below. Unfortunately, however, the limitations of medical education and practice and the potential for restrictive and punitive behavior by colleagues severely limit the ability of physicians to deviate from medical standards.[22]

Similarly, we call for a national health program that recognizes that freestanding birth centers and homes are the most appropriate and enabling settings for Primary Maternity Care. These community-based sites enhance the likelihood that care will be non-bureaucratic; individualized; woman- and family-oriented; protected from unnecessary medicalization and interventions; and physically, culturally and psychologically accessible.

In advocating such care, we do not mean the mere substitution of one type of practitioner and site of practice for another, but the *substitution of one system and philosophy of care for another.* It is critical that the reconfiguration of maternity care addresses appropriate type of front-line caregiver, settings for care, and content and philosophy of care. Addressing only one or two of these dimensions will not assure necessary change in the maternity care system

Benefits of a Primary Maternity Care System

1. Primary Maternity Care involves education, health promotion, social support, clinical assessment, and continuity of care. Midwifery care is primary care at its best. Midwives have regularly demonstrated a commitment to understanding and maintaining normal birth and the health of women and infants. Basic preventive practices, such as offering information and advice on diet and breastfeeding, and enhancing the integrity of the childbearing family, are the foundation of midwifery practice. Midwives address social, cultural, psychological, ethical, and political aspects of pregnancy, birth, and parenthood. They recognize and affirm the meaning and importance of childbearing in the lives of women and their families. They work to build a trusting, close relationship with women, which tends to be the cornerstone of their practice. Many midwives choose to work in community-based settings. Within this framework, they offer prenatal care that is rich, contextual, multifaceted, accessible and acceptable to women and that promotes the health of mothers and babies.[23]

2. Primary Maternity Care is safe. Numerous studies, some of which have been controlled, have shown that the maternity care provided by nurse-midwives and other mid-wives in hospitals, birth centers and homes result in birth-weights, mortality rates, and other health indicators that are similar to, or better than, those obtained by specialists in acute medical settings (Durand 1992; Mayes et al. 1987; Feldman and Hurst 1987; Scupholme et al. 1986; Piechnik and Corbett 1985; Baruffi et al. 1984a; Beal 1984; Mehl et al. 1980; Slome et al. 1976). In the United States, most of the published studies describe the practice of certified nurse-midwives. However, extensive data from European studies demonstrate the excellent record of non-nurse-midwives working in many settings.[24]

Investigators of the large multi-site National Birth Center Study similarly conclude that freestanding "birth centers offer a safe and acceptable alternative to hospital confinement" (Rooks et al. 1989). The absence of maternal mortality and low intrapartum and neonatal mortality experiences in this study compare favorably with mortality rates of low-risk women using hospitals (Rooks et al. 1992c). [25] Despite the widespread belief in the U.S. that home birth involves greater risk than hospital birth, the hospital has never been shown to be safer than home or birth center births (Hughes 1992; Campbell and MacFarlane 1986; Institute of Medicine 1982). On a large scale in the Netherlands and on a smaller scale in the United States, the United Kingdom and other nations, birth at home has involved very low mortality rates (Hughes 1992; Treffers et al. 1990; Campbell and MacFarlane 1986; Treffers and Laan 1986; van Alten 1989). In a meta-analysis pooling data from U.S. studies and considering international data, Hughes concludes, "Currently available research suggests that home birth, in the presence of qualified and appropriately equipped attendants, is ... at least as safe as hospital birth" (1992). This finding is echoed both by the Oxford Database of Perinatal Trials project, whose organizers conclude that policies for "universal institutional confinement" should be abandoned in light of available data (Chalmers et al. 1989b), and by a recent House of Commons report that supports the choice of home birth (Great Britain 1992).

Several studies suggest that healthy women using more technology-intensive birth settings experience greater morbidity than those in less intensive sites (Campbell and MacFarlane 1986; Baruffi et al. 1984a, 1984b; Mehl and Peterson 1981). These diverse and consistent studies, and the vital statistics of several European nations (Miller 1987; Wagner 1988), thus contradict the prevalent belief that healthy women inevitably experience excess morbidity and mortality when *not* attended by specialists in acute care settings.

3. Primary Maternity Care enhances access. Midwives have been honored to serve women of all social groups and to work in diverse community-based settings. They have provided effective, sensitive, respectful, empowering, community-oriented services to women who have often been rejected by physicians by virtue of their insurance status, economic class, race, ethnicity, foreign birth or

geographical location. They have worked disproportionately in underserved areas, with underserved populations, and with women lacking private insurance (Scupholme et al. 1992; Declercq 1992; U.S. Department of Health and Human Services 1984; Langwell et al. 1980).[26] In addition to their willingness to care for the underserved, the sensitive *way* midwives have regularly been found to care for all types of women, and the cost effectiveness of their care, enhance access. The increased access has been associated with significant, and dramatic, improvements in health status indicators of more vulnerable women and infants (e.g., Levy et al. 1971; Montgomery 1969).

Attributes of freestanding birth centers similarly enhance access to maternity care. They can be situated in communities and oriented toward the needs of communities, creating a sense of ownership, belonging and familiarity. They avoid the barriers of large-scale, bureaucratic institutions, which can be alienating and difficult and time-consuming to negotiate (see Institute of Medicine 1988). These centers may thus have a major role to play in improving the care of more vulnerable childbearing families who now rely extensively upon services in tertiary hospitals. Because freestanding birth centers can operate in rural areas that do not have hospital obstetrics departments (Rooks et al. 1989), they also can play a major role in bringing access to the many rural areas that now lack adequate maternity services (see Lewis-Idema 1989).

4. Primary Maternity Care offers special benefits for virtually all childbearing women. With their commitment to education, prevention, providing social support and individualized care, and developing a close relationship with the childbearing woman and her family, midwives provide excellent and particularly appropriate care to women who are often considered "high-risk" (Reedy 1979). Their approach is well-suited, for example, to providing support for pregnant adolescents, helping women with gestational diabetes maintain a healthy diet, and working with women who are HIV-positive or are addicted to drugs. (When indicated by medical conditions, midwives and physicians collaborate in the care of childbearing women.) So-called high-risk women who receive midwifery care consistently attain excellent outcomes, which are typically more favorable than those of the general population. Midwifery care is also ideally suited for the special needs and interests of many other women, including single mothers, lesbian mothers, childbearing women who are older, childbearing women with disabilities, and those who wish to incorporate personal or cultural rituals into their unique childbearing experiences. Women in the United States from every kind of social and economic background have sought out and benefited from this care.

In a similar fashion, freestanding birth centers and homes offer possibilities for personal and individualized care and the fulfillment of diverse wishes and expectations of childbearing families that are difficult or impossible to provide in clinic and hospital settings. They also offer these families greater amounts of privacy and greater opportunities for control of the care environment.[27]

5. Primary Maternity Care involves judicious use of technology. In a system of Primary Maternity Care, technological interventions are used only when needed to promote the health and well-being of mother and baby, and not as routine interventions or substitutes for social support, education, attentiveness, patience or preventive measures. Controlled studies repeatedly show that, relative to standard medical care, midwifery care involves significantly less use of such interventions as anesthesia, intravenous hydration, electronic fetal monitoring, artificial augmentation of labor, episiotomy, forceps and cesarean birth (Feldman and Hurst 1987; Scupholme et al. 1986; Baruffi et al. 1984b; Beal 1984).

Primary Maternity Care sites have also been associated with relatively low rates of interventions. For example, relatively few women participating in the National Birth Center Study experienced continuous electronic fetal monitoring (8%), artificial augmentation of labor (2%), and cesarean section (4%) (Rooks et al. 1992b). Many obstetrical technologies are simply unavailable in home settings. Those who provide care in home settings tend to work to avoid interventions or to use lower technology interventions.[28]

The differences in rates of procedures between Primary Maternity Care and conventional maternity care can be quite substantial. For example, a comparison of a group of women who began their labors at home with independent midwives and a similar group using conventional care found that the former had 91% fewer cesarean births (1.5% vs.16.5% cesarean rates) (Durand 1992). These studies find that the reduced use of technology does not compromise outcome; in fact, women receiving such care benefit by avoiding the risks, discomfort and disruption that these procedures impose.[29]

6. Primary Maternity Care is associated with a highly favorable liability record. In 1987 surveys, 10% of nurse-midwives had been named in one or more liability claims, as opposed to 71% of obstetrician-gynecologists (Adams 1989; Opinion Research Corporation 1988). This comparison is not adjusted for years of practice, severity of caseload and other factors that could influence experience with claims. However, the size of the difference strongly suggests that it is real. Aspects of midwifery care and freestanding birth center and home care settings that have been associated with favorable liability experiences include avoiding unnecessary procedures, developing a personal and trusting relationship, and carefully observing principles of informed consent (Relman 1989; O'Reilly et al. 1986; Gilfix 1984; Shearer et al. 1976). In accord with their philosophy and values, midwives usually provide more satisfactory communication and greater continuity of care than obstetricians; spend more time with women prenatally, during labor and following birth; and show greater care and respect to women. These practices are likely to contribute to their more favorable liability expe-

rience. Physicians in hospital settings may be sued more often because of their tendency to have brief prenatal visits, to have relatively limited contact during labor and birth, to use as birth attendants on-call physicians whom women do not know, to work in settings that emphasize efficiency and focus excessively on progress in labor, and to prefer hierarchical relationships that inhibit satisfactory communication. LoCicero identifies a variety of ways that medical maternity care thwarts common expectations of childbearing women (1993). Such a mismatch may help to explain why obstetricians' liability experiences are disproportionately unfavorable relative to nearly all other medical specialties.[30]

7. Primary Maternity Care is well-received by women. As women, we value patient, personalized, respectful, non-hierarchical care that addresses many dimensions of our lives and helps us to take responsibility for our health. We have regularly welcomed midwives' commitment to principles of informed choice and the opportunity for genuine participation in decisions about our care. We often feel especially comfortable with caregivers who are women and who are often themselves experienced mothers (Kelly-McCormick 1989; Lazarus 1988b; Wellish and Root 1987).[31]

Women participating in the National Birth Center Study also reported high rates of satisfaction with their care. Ninety-nine percent of those giving birth in the centers said that they would recommend the center to friends and 94% said they would use the center in a subsequent pregnancy. Of those who were transferred to hospitals for their birth, 97% said they would recommend the center and 83% would use it again (Rooks et al. 1989, 1992c).

Interestingly, it is difficult to find informative studies on women's satisfaction with home birth. Since home birth is actively sought out and women continue to choose home birth in spite of cultural, economic and institutional obstacles to this choice, it seems clear that they are highly satisfied with their experiences. Women choosing home birth have been very articulate about their experiences, describing them, as well as the reasons for their choices, in great detail in magazines, journals and books (e.g., *Birth Gazette; C/SEC Newsletter, The Clarion;* Gaskin 1990; Kitzinger 1988; Wellish and Root 1987; Ashford 1984).

8. Primary Maternity Care is highly cost-effective. Studies of midwifery care, both in and out of hospitals, show major cost savings relative to dominant medicalized maternity care (e.g., Krumlauf et al. 1988; Seiner and Lairson 1985; Cherry and Foster 1982; Reid and Morris 1979). Midwifery fees tend to be lower than physician fees despite the fact that midwives spend considerably more time with women and offer services that may otherwise be provided by an entire team. Other aspects of midwifery care that involve significant cost savings relative to the present reliance upon front-line physician care include the considerably lower costs to educate midwives, their much more favorable experience with legal claims and suits, the lower rates of intervention associated with their care, the shorter length of hospital or birth center stay of midwifery clients (e.g., Baruffi et al. 1984a; Cherry and Foster 1982), and midwives' greater willingness to work in non-hospital settings.[32]

Primary Maternity Care sites have similar cost advantages. Charges of freestanding birth centers have consistently been found to be well below those of hospitals. In 1989, for example, the average cost of birth center care, including prenatal and postpartum visits, was about one-half of the average cost of a vaginal birth in the hospital and about two-thirds of a one-day hospital maternity stay (Health Insurance Association of America 1989).[33] Birth at home eliminates facility expenses entirely and involves modest expenses for supplies and equipment.

The system we are proposing has important precedents. At the present time and on a national scale, the Netherlands has the most exemplary system of Primary Maternity Care in the world and there is much we can learn and adapt from it. We must be aware, however, that the Dutch system is experiencing various types of pressure to become more medicalized and technology intensive. Presently, to give citizens the benefits of primary care, facilitate use of appropriate levels of care, and contain costs, Dutch government policies strongly support home births, midwives and the avoidance of unnecessary obstetrical procedures (World Health Organization 1986). Structural incentives contribute to the maintenance of this system of Primary Maternity Care. For example, maternity care costs for healthy women are only covered in full if such women use midwifery services (where available) and give birth at home or in short-stay "polyclinic" settings. At present, midwives attend about 43% of births and about 35% occur at home (Treffers et al. 1990). A large proportion of the institutional births are polyclinic births of less than 36 hours (Hingstman and Boon 1988). Other administrative and organizational features help sustain this primary care system. Midwives are educated to function as independent practitioners with the authority to screen and refer.

Although the Netherlands has a socio-demographic profile similar to the U.S., with a diverse immigrant and indigenous population, the Dutch infant mortality rate has consistently been among the lowest in the world. In 1989, it ranked 4th compared to 19th for the U.S. (Rosenbaum et al. 1991). Another distinctive feature of this system is the social support available through its postpartum home care program. Women are entitled to eight days of assistance by trained maternity home aides who care for them and their babies, assist with breastfeeding, care for older children, and perform housekeeping tasks. The health promoting primary care system in the Netherlands is associated with low rates of obstetrical intervention, and the standards of midwifery home care have a restraining influence on interventive patterns of obstetrical care. In 1985, for example, when the U.S. cesarean rate was 22.7%, the Dutch rate was 6.6%.[34]

Policy Proposals:
Improved Standards of Living and Systematic Transition to a Primary Maternity Care System

We intend to work with other groups to develop the following proposals about childbearing policy in a national health program.[35]

1. As a society, we should work to enhance the conditions of everyday life that influence the health of women and their infants. Favorable conditions include: economic security, high-quality education, the availability of adequate family leave provisions and other social supports, the elimination of occupational and environmental hazards, the availability of safe housing and nourishing food, and the eradication of harmful drugs and violence. Short-term policies should specifically address the effect of these areas on childbearing women and their infants, while long-term policies should be developed to improve the conditions of everyday life for all citizens. We must implement a true National Health Program that addresses these primary determinants of health. While neither national health care policy nor a National Health Care Program in themselves can create the kind of social change we describe, policy makers can build coalitions with groups working on these issues and stress the critical nature of such efforts to their own work.

2. We who are taking the leadership for a national health program should establish a task force to investigate and propose guidelines for systematic transition to a system of Primary Maternity Care. This task force should reflect appropriate racial and economic diversity and be composed of leaders who represent the following perspectives: women's health, childbirth reform, midwifery, and public health, as well as other health and medical professionals and community representatives who are engaged in health planning and decision making, committed to a primary care model and knowledgeable about the distinctive record of midwifery care, freestanding birth centers and home birth.

This task force should carefully consider past and present exemplary models of Primary Maternity Care. In the U.S., these include the Frontier Nursing Service in rural Kentucky; Boston's Traditional Childbearing Group; the Maternity Center Association's Childbearing Center in New York; the Childbearing Center of Morris Heights; other members of the National Association of Childbearing Centers; and midwives who have traditionally served women in our African American, Latino, Native American and Asian American communities (Rooks et al. 1992a, 1992b, 1992c; Sakala 1989; Holmes 1986; Branca et al. 1984; Lubic and Ernst 1978; and Breckinridge 1952).

The task force should take into account the growing data affirming the relative safety of home birth in the U.S., data which are supported by the home birth experience in the Netherlands and research conducted on out-of-hospital births in the United Kingdom (Hughes 1992; Campbell and MacFarlane 1986; Great Britain 1992; Tew and Damstra-Wigmenga 1991; Mehl 1981). On an international level, the task force should study the Dutch maternity care model and strengthen and adapt it to conditions in the U.S.

In addition, the task force should critically appraise medical education, the training of midwives and nurses, the scope and standards of practice of various practitioners, approaches to regulation, mechanisms for integrating current midwives, and projected need for primary and specialist maternity caregivers and primary and acute maternity care settings. Utilizing all this information, the task force should develop related policy recommendations leading to a strong system of Primary Maternity Care that gives priority to the interests of childbearing families and resists cooptation involving acute and other medical settings and specialist and other medical caregivers.[36]

3. We should greatly expand opportunities to educate midwives, the most appropriate providers of Primary Maternity Care. Midwifery can and should be an autonomous profession. This position is supported by the boards of the Midwives Alliance of North America and the American College of Nurse-Midwives. Both nurses and those with other backgrounds should be welcomed into midwifery education programs and, on demonstrating proficiency in midwifery knowledge and skills, be recognized as fully competent midwives. The International Confederation of Midwives and the International Federation of Gynecologists and Obstetricians recognize multiple routes of entry into the practice of midwifery. Many states legally recognize well-educated and well-trained community midwives (also known as direct-entry, independent, empirical, traditional, or lay midwives), who have a strong record throughout the country and have begun to receive Medicaid reimbursement in various state programs. Similarly, European nations have had outstanding experiences with midwives from many backgrounds.[37]

U.S. training programs should make special efforts to recruit and educate women of color, low-income women and women from rural areas, many of whom will choose and be most qualified to provide services within their own communities. Although the Clinton proposal includes midwives, it fails to address the systemic issues related to site and content of care addressed in this paper, fails to recognize multiple routes to midwifery practice, and fails to acknowledge the barriers faced by currently practicing midwives.

4. We should greatly expand opportunities for women to give birth in freestanding birth centers and at home, if they choose. Community-based freestanding birth centers, are, in our judgment, highly appropriate maternity care sites. They are the most feasible sites for Primary Maternity Care from social, psychological, organizational, political, and economic perspectives.[38] These centers should provide a broad range of formal and informal health and support services for childbearing women and their infants and should also help involve fathers in the childbearing process and in parenting. Women who wish to give birth at home must be supported in this choice as a covered

service and by hospitals and medical caregivers providing full cooperative back-up. Of all sites, home tends to be the most demedicalized, to involve the least high-tech interventions, and to offer women and their families the greatest freedom of choice.[39]

5. We should emphasize and develop small-scale community-based and -oriented services. This goal should be a priority when recruiting caregivers, establishing the location of maternity services, and determining the type of care provided. Women who use the services should have substantial input into the development of policies and programs through participatory processes for resource allocation and other decisions.[40] We should give special attention to the development of supportive client-oriented services for women who have limited social supports and negative, stressful life circumstances.[41]

6. We should develop effective policies that commit our national health program to a system of Primary Maternity Care. These policies should ensure that midwives are autonomous practitioners and that specialist and tertiary care back-up are readily available for any medical problems. Women should have ready access to midwifery, home birth and freestanding birth center services in their communities and should be free to choose their caregiver and the place where they receive maternity care and give birth; policies should ensure that all women receive accurate and detailed information about these choices. Adequate funds should be available for widespread public education about the benefits of Primary Maternity Care, for Primary Maternity Caregiver education and training programs, and for all Primary Maternity Care services. Present difficulties in securing reimbursement for these services should be eliminated. Primary Maternity Care services, as well as any necessary medical care, should be covered in full, with no co-payments or other out-of-pocket expenses. Finally, ongoing mechanisms of accountability must be established to apply research findings and ensure that maternity practices are safe, effective, and conducive to a positive quality of life.

7. We should regulate Primary Maternity Care through independent boards. In order to assure public accountability, these boards should be composed predominantly of public members; they should also include midwives and other health professionals who are knowledgeable about and respect the primary care model. Board composition should reflect the diversity of community women, including women of color and women of various economic backgrounds.

8. We should establish a major research program to support Primary Maternity Care. Research on normal childbearing and prevention of complications should be given priority. Childbearing technology assessment should address many dimensions, including positive and negative impact on physical, psychological and social well-being (both short- and long-term); political and ethical issues; and economic implications. Sensitive morbidity measures should be developed to address the period from pregnancy through the child's first year, and data on these measures should be regularly collected. All aspects of the Primary Maternity Care system should be thoroughly evaluated, with systematic mechanisms for incorporation of relevant findings into future programs.

———————

As women's health advocates, we support childbearing policies and programs that are in the best interests of women and infants. We must ensure that a national health program addresses healthy living conditions as the major determinants of health. Clinical services can never compensate for inadequate social supports, and high-cost, high-tech medical approaches do not solve economic and social problems. With respect to maternity care services, the optimal form of care is a system that gives priority to Primary Maternity Care and utilizes midwives and free-standing birth centers as recommended forms of care for most childbearing women. It is our conviction that this best form of care for mothers and babies will also be of great interest to policy makers: it is safe, of high quality, cost-effective, and greatly appreciated by women. The solution to many of our pressing childbearing problems is within our reach.

Notes

18. A women's health perspective addresses not just the health status of women but how women relate to the system, are treated by it and are workers within it. This approach looks at the needs of women beyond medical needs and addresses the way gender differences, ways of knowing, psychosocial development and power differentials within the culture affect maternity care (Jordan 1987). In an article addressing the non-medical factors that contribute to high rates of intervention, LoCicero (1993) considers contemporary theories of gender and psychosocial development. Her analysis concerns gender difference (in cognition, moral development, sense of self, empathy and helpfulness, and power), gender role expectations, and gender identity. She concludes that in each of these dimensions prevailing medical approaches are compatible with conventional masculine standards and fundamentally incompatible with the needs and expectations of most women, and are likely to have a negative effect on women's ability to labor effectively. Midwifery care, she proposes, is far more compatible with women's needs in these respects.

19. In their summary of the longitudinal Oxford Database of Perinatal Trials project, which identifies and synthesizes thousands of perinatal trials, Enkin and colleagues endorse the primary care concept:

.... it is inherently unwise, and perhaps unsafe, for women with normal pregnancies to be cared for by obstetric specialists ...

Midwives and general practitioners, on the other hand, are primarily oriented to the care of women with normal pregnancies, and are likely to have more detailed knowledge of the particular circumstances of individual women. The care that they can give to the majority of women whose pregnancies are not affected by any major illness or serious complication will often be more responsive to their needs than that given by specialist obstetricians.

Optimal care can only occur when both primary and secondary caregivers recognize their complementary roles. There is no place for rivalry or competition between those whose expertise is in the supervision of health and the detection of disease, and those whose specialty is the management of disease and the restoration of health. [1989]

The authors also state that policies supporting "universal institutional confinement" should be abandoned in light of existing evidence (1989).

20. Obstetrician-gynecologists serve as the first contact with the medical care system for many women. The usual care that these surgeon-specialists provide, however, *cannot be considered to be primary care* (see Burkons and Willson [1975] and accompanying discussion). The most appropriate role for the obstetrical specialist is (1) as direct caregiver for women who are at high medical risk or have developed serious medical complications and (2) as consultant and back-up to midwives who serve as Primary Maternity Caregivers to all other women.

We are not optimistic about the use of family physicians for Primary Maternity Care. Although we respect and applaud their primary care philosophy, we regret that in their provision of maternity services, the great majority of family practitioners have been obliged to emulate and practice the specialist model (Brody and Thompson 1981). Additional constraints are provided by the challenge of incorporating maternity services and of supporting maternity liability premiums within a general practice. We also respect the primary care philosophy of nurse-practitioners and their work with childbearing women. We cannot, however, recommend that they have a major role in a Primary Maternity Care system because they cannot provide continuity of care during the critical period of labor, birth and early postpartum.

21. The ethics statement was the result of a two-year consensus-building process that involved hundreds of practicing midwives.

A focus on life and health pervades this statement. Sakala (1993d) summarizes the values articulated in this statement:

The midwives emphasize that pregnancy and birth are intrinsically normal life processes, and that it is desirable to enhance this normalcy ... and to help women with complications move toward greater well-being... The statement places childbearing within the context of the totality of women's lives.... It asserts that physical, emotional, mental, psychological, and spiritual dimensions of life experiences are interrelated and cannot be viewed in isolation. . . . Pregnancy and birth are simultaneously personal, intimate, sexual, and social events; these experiences in turn influence women's self-esteem, health, ability to nurture, and personal growth.

The midwives also give priority to respect for the mother. . . and the baby and the integrity of their relationship. . . . They enhance childbearing by respecting women's capabilities,. . . empowering women to be confident and strong. . . and identifying other sources of support. . . They value honesty and communication. . . and honor women's right to self determination. They value the diversity of women's experiences and needs, and individualized care. . . .

22. For examples of physicians who have adopted a frame of reference and attitudes compatible with midwifery see Odent (1984) and Sagov et al. (1984). For examples of impediments that physicians place before reformist colleagues, see Savage (1986) and Harrison (1983). On the effectiveness of medical education in socializing physicians into medical approaches to care, see Davis-Floyd (1992).

23. Descriptions of midwifery care include Rothman (1989), Sullivan and Weitz (1988) and Annandale (1988). Kitzinger (1988) provides a comparison, in their own words, of the position of midwives in the medical systems of different nations. She sees midwives as the greatest challenge world-wide to high-technology, conveyer-belt obstetrics. On how midwives see themselves, their practice and education, see Gaskin (1990), Steiger (1987), Varney (1987) and Davis (1987).

Roger A. Rosenblatt points to an important policy benefit of such a broad and continuous view of maternal and child health. This view involves "longitudinal responsibility for a series of intertwined clinical interventions," and provides incentives to emphasize prevention and minimize use of costly, disruptive and ethically complex salvage technologies. He argues that we should encourage this perspective by capitating caregivers for the entire period from conception through the neonatal period, in contrast to our present policies of economic and service fragmentation (1989). The recent Public Health Service report on prenatal care strongly recommends that the prevailing emphasis on medical concerns be balanced by greatly increased attention to social, psychological and educational concerns (United States Department of Health and Human Services 1989).

Rates of breastfeeding might be considered to be a measure of midwives' commitment to and effectiveness with health-promoting care. Reported rates of early postpartum breastfeeding by women who have received midwifery care are consistently higher than rates in the general population, ranging from 78% to 99% (Nichols 1985; Baruffi et al. 1984a; Bennetts and Lubic 1982; Mann 1981; Hewitt and Hangsleben 1981; and Gaskin and Gaskin 1979). These reports describe women of many social and economic backgrounds, including women using clinic services. By contrast, the Public Health Service reports

that in 1988 54% of women in the U.S. were breastfeeding in the early postpartum period. This figure drops to 32% for low-income mothers and 25% for Black mothers (United States Department of Health and Human Services 1991).

24. While there is a growing body of research suggesting that care provided by independent (non-nurse) midwives is as safe, effective and desirable as that provided by nurse-midwives (e.g., Durand 1992; Hinds et al. 1985; Sullivan and Beeman 1983; Burnett et al. 1980; McCallum 1979), most research in the United States has been conducted on nurse-midwives and has focused on assessing the care they provide. Institutional support and funding as well as the presence of nurse-midwifery training programs in academic settings have fostered this research. Independent midwives place high value on knowledge, experience, and the refinement of skills (Davis 1981; Steiger 1987). These are acquired in a variety of ways, including study groups, apprenticeships, classes, and highly structured programs such as the Seattle Midwifery School. The Pilot Data Collection Project of the Midwives Alliance of North America (MANA), which includes both independent midwives and nurse-midwives, has been designed to gather information needed for further research, both quantitative and qualitative, on independent midwifery practice and home birth. This information will complement the data from the Netherlands and throughout Europe (Miller 1987) that reveal the excellent record of non-nurse midwives practicing in many settings. See also note 34.

25. The National Birth Center Study involved nearly 12,000 women who received care during labor and birth at 84 centers throughout the nation (Rooks et al. 1992a, 1992b, 1992c, 1989). For a summary of birth center outcome research and a report of consistent and favorable outcome data from a similar study of over 3,400 women receiving this same care at 25 California birth centers, see Eakins (1989).

26. A 1991 national survey found that 34% of clients of active certified nurse-midwives reside in low-income inner-city areas and 22% in rural areas. Eighty percent of respondents described their practices as including women from at least five of the following eight vulnerable groups: adolescents, African Americans, Native Americans, Asian Americans, Latinas, low income individuals, migrant workers, and people without insurance (Scupholme et al. 1992). A small areas analysis indicates that U.S. counties with the highest ratios of nurse-midwives per 100,000 15- to 44-year-old women are low-income areas with small populations, few hospital beds and high birth rates (Langwell et al. 1980). Nationally, about 40% of reimbursement for services of certified nurse-midwives is from Medicaid (Scupholme et al. 1992), whereas the average obstetrician receives not more than 8% from that program (Schappert 1993).

On studies assessing the effectiveness of midwives working with low-income or otherwise disadvantaged women and their infants, see note 27.

27. Midwifery programs for historically vulnerable women have regularly been associated with physical outcomes superior to those in the local area, state and/or nation. These programs have served many rural and urban areas in the country and have provided care in hospitals, freestanding birth centers and homes. See Cavero et al. (1991), Haire and Elsberry (1991), Brucker and Muellner (1985), Mann (1981), Haire (1981), Burnett et al. (1980), Reid and Morris (1979), Browne and Isaacs (1976), Murdaugh (1976), Meglen (1972), Levy et al. (1971), Montgomery (1969), Metropolitan Life Insurance Company (1960) and Laird (1955). One study found similar or better physical outcomes among higher-risk women receiving midwifery care in a maternity center when compared to matched women receiving usual care, that is, dominant medical care, in a tertiary teaching hospital (Baruffi et al. 1984a). Whether analyzed by education, age, parity, race, or place of birth, national birthweight data from 1978 are consistent with the favorable evaluations of individual midwifery programs: in every group the percentage of low birthweight babies is lower for midwives than for all hospital births, physician- attended out-of-hospital births, and other categories (Declercq 1984).

The repeated finding that women who historically have experienced high rates of adverse physical outcomes experience rates more favorable than the mean for the general population when using midwifery care suggests that lack of access to appropriate services is a major and common risk factor for vulnerable women and their infants. Unfortunately, this risk factor has not been considered in the many studies examining risk factors for mothers and infants (e.g., Nersesian 1988).

Lisbeth Schorr has written an important book on the distinguishing characteristics of successful intervention programs for vulnerable children. *Within Our Reach* identifies general qualities that precisely describe midwifery care and the kind of care that is regularly and readily provided in freestanding birth centers and homes. She argues that successful programs: offer a broad spectrum of services that transcend conventional professional and bureaucratic boundaries, maintain flexibility and continuity, offer coherent services that are easy to use, consider people in the context of their broader life circumstances, and convey a sense of respect and trustworthiness. These programs, Schorr argues, fundamentally "take their shape from the needs of those they serve rather than from the precepts, demands, and boundaries set by professionalism and bureaucracies" (1988). Similarly, these forms of Primary Maternity Care have much in common with the recommendations that came out of the World Health Organization conferences on appropriate technology and childbearing.

28. Research reports comparing midwifery and medical approaches to common indications for cesarean birth and to pain suggest that midwives tend to understand these situations in different ways and to address them with a wide range of techniques that tend to be relatively simple, inexpensive and noninvasive. Their knowledge and practice are to a great extent derived from and oriented toward women's childbearing experience (Sakala 1993c, 1988).

Nurse-midwives in acute settings are more interventive than those who practice in childbearing centers (Fullerton and Severino 1992). Similarly, California childbearing centers with obstetricians as sole provider use a range of interventions and technology not used in centers with nurse-midwives as sole providers. Nationally, centers where physicians attend any or all births tend to be more technologically intensive than those with only midwives (Eakins 1989).

It is important to note that midwives are inevitably vulnerable to medicalization when they are educated in and/or practice in medical environments. These environments (including clinics, hospitals or nursing schools) influence how midwives practice, how they think and the language they use. For example, women receiving care in hospitals tend to become "patients," regardless of their health status, with all the associations of illness, passivity and impaired ability. When midwives adopt the language of obstetrics, they tend to adopt the values and limitations of obstetrics, in ways of which they may not be aware.

29. Two carefully matched studies comparing midwifery care to usual care found significant excess morbidity among low-risk women in the usual care group. Authors of these reports hypothesize that this finding is attributable to risks associated with more extensive use of procedures in the usual care groups. See Baruffi et al. (1984a) and Mehl et al. (1980).

30. The Department of Professional Liability of the American College of Obstetricians and Gynecologists publishes a series of risk management circulars for the association's membership. These guidelines emphasize such routine attributes of midwifery care as commitment to good communication and rapport, provision of fully informed consent, and acknowledgment of the possibility of undesirable outcomes, all of which are in conflict with the time constraints and professional training of medical specialists (1983).

31. A greater-than-sixfold increase in the number of births attended by midwives from 1975, when this figure first became available, to 1991 (National Center for Health Statistics 1993; U.S. Department of Health and Human Services 1984) strongly suggests the degree to which women appreciate midwifery care.

In a randomized controlled trial, Flint (1988) found that women working with midwives perceived their experience of mothering to be easier than those working with obstetricians. This suggests that the care received, and the birth experience facilitated by the midwives, increase women's self-esteem and sense of competence as parents. Similarly, a randomized controlled trial considering the impact of a supportive companion throughout labor found differences favoring the supported group in many "psychosocial" areas in the day, weeks, and/or months after birth. These include the mothers': anxiety level, impression of how well their labors and births had gone, experience of discomfort, sense that the transition to motherhood had been easy, sense they were doing a good job of mothering, report of exclusive breastfeeding, report of their babies' appetites, report that breastfeeding had primarily been discontinued due to insufficiency of milk, report of how long it had taken them to establish a relationship with the baby, report of number of hours per week spent apart from the baby, and depression scores (Trotter et al. 1992; Klaus et al. 1992; Hofmeyr et al. 1991). This line of inquiry warrants a major systematic research program to identify the range and duration of differences in psychosocial effects of different forms of care. A series of randomized controlled trials throughout the world have similarly documented consistently favorable experiences with the course of labor, interventions during labor and birth, and physical outcomes through use of supportive labor companions (Klaus et al 1992).

32. The Health Insurance Association of America reports that the average physician's fee for vaginal birth in 1989 was $1,492, in contrast to $994 for the average fee of midwives (1989). The Office of Technology Assessment compares the estimated cost of training a physician in 1985 —$86,100—to the estimated cost of obtaining a nurse-midwifery certificate and master's degree—$16,800 (United States Congress 1986). Saving associated with differences in interventions may be considerable. As noted above, for example, midwifery care has been associated with up to 91% fewer caesareans than medical care of similar women, with no apparent compromise in safety. Nearly one million caesareans are performed annually in the U.S., and on the average a cesarean birth cost $2,852 more than a vaginal birth in 1989 (Health Insurance Association of America 1989).

33. In 1989, the average hospital stay for a vaginal birth cost $4,334, and a one-day hospital stay averaged $3,233; by contrast, a one-day birth center stay averaged $2,111. The latter charge includes laboratory tests, childbirth education, home visits, prenatal visits and postpartum visits (Health Insurance Association of America 1989).

34. On general health policies of the Netherlands, see World Health Organization (1986) and Tiddens et al. (1984). On the Dutch maternity care system, see Treffers et al. (1990), Smulders (1989), Smulders and Limburg (1988), Miller (1987), Hingstman and Boon (1988), Phaff (1986), Ris (1986), and Verbrugge (1968). Tew and Damstra-Wijimenga (1991), Treffers et al. (1990), van Alten et al. (1989), van Alten (1986), and Ris (1986) offer data on the relative safety of that system. On international cesarean trends, see Notzon (1990) and Notzon et al. (1987).

35. We are aware that these proposals often conflict with the interests of many groups, including physicians and other medical personnel, hospitals and medical and insurance industries. These groups have had the power to shape both knowledge and practice, including what ideas are respected and what is done to women in childbirth. They have been able to maintain their positions in a society that has little faith in women's ability to give birth and great faith in technology and the authority of powerful professions and institutions. In addition, marketing strategies have led much of the public to believe that significant change has already taken place. These strategies have also led many women to believe they are receiving the highest quality of care.

While most women and infants emerge from this system in a physically healthy state, we believe the changes we advocate will improve the pregnancy and birth experiences for large numbers of women and make important contributions to disadvantaged and minority women. They will also reduce the rate of cesarean sections and of many other procedures and tests and, combined with increased social supports and improved economic and social conditions, reduce the infant mortality and low birthweight rates for disadvantaged women. There is also the possibility, increasingly suggested in the research literature, that the kind of care we describe will contribute to the self-esteem of many childbearing women and their sense of competence as individuals, caregivers and parents, and will decrease postpartum depression, improve family relationships, increase participation of fathers in caretaking, and so forth (e.g., Mutryn 1993; Trotter et al. 1992; Hofmeyr et al. 1991). Extensive research needs to be done in this direction.

36. The recent report and other activities of the Task Force on the Implementation of Midwifery in Ontario can serve as an important model for this work (Task Force on the Implementation of Midwifery in Ontario, 1987), as can the British Health Committee Report on Maternity Services from the House of Commons (Great Britain 1992).

37. On a small scale in the United States and on a larger scale in other nations, independent midwives have a strong record with respect to access, quality and cost (Durand 1992; Tew and Damstra-Wijimenga 1991; van Alten et al. 1989; Ris 1986; Hinds et al. 1985; Sullivan and Beeman 1883; Burnett et al. 1980; Mehl et al. 1980; McCallum 1979).

38. Approximately one hundred and thirty freestanding childbearing centers are operating presently in the United States, and the National Association for Childbearing Centers has about 55 Developing Birth Center members (Ernst 1992). Important mechanisms to support birth center development are in place and the Commission for the Accreditation of Freestanding Birth Centers has been active since 1985. Reports of the National Birth Center Study (Rooks et al. 1989; Rooks et al. 1992a, 1992b, 1992c), and additional studies using that data-base (Fullerton and Severino 1992) demonstrate advantages of this form of care. The National Birth Center Study provides data from

84 childbearing centers and summarizes the experience of 18,000 women using these centers. A study of 25 California birth centers produced similar findings (Eakins 1989). Branca et al. (1984) project that freestanding birth centers have the potential to offer high quality care with major cost savings to a large proportion of childbearing women and infants in the United States.

A study done by Scupholme and Kamons (1987) sheds an interesting light on consumer preference. This study involved a group of women who were assigned involuntarily to a birth center due to hospital overcrowding. It found that these women had positive experiences and that their outcomes were comparable to women who had chosen to use that site. Significantly, these women tended to choose the birth center for subsequent births and to refer family members and friends to the center.

Most people do not know that facilities and procedures for birth in U.S. hospitals were modeled on arrangements for industrial production, including operations research techniques designed for efficient production of weapons during World War II (Lindheim 1981; see also Martin 1987). Emphasis on standardization and rapid processing of childbearing women disregards physiologic patterns of labor, involves unnecessarily high rates of interventions, and dehumanizes participants. Simply put, hospitals are not healthy places for childbearing women or practitioners who want to function as primary care providers, and support and facilitate normal birth. Medical clinics similarly involve inappropriate medical values, beliefs, and practices and impose these on women and infants who have no medical problems.

Social science research has consistently identified the great degree to which hospital and clinic routines and provider interests take precedence over the pregnant and birthing woman's own situation and preferences in determining the type of care she receives. See Sakala (1993a, 1993d), Davis-Floyd (1992), Lichtman (1988), Danziger (1986, 1980), Rothman (1983), Scully (1980), Shaw (1974), Kovit (1972), and Rosengram and Devault (1963).

39. Hughes (1992) used meta-analytic techniques to pool data from U.S. studies and looked at studies of home birth from other nations. She concludes that available research finds planned home birth to be as safe as hospital birth. Anderson and Greener (1991) did a descriptive analysis of home births attended by CNMs in two nurse-midwifery services. The British House of Commons Report (Great Britain 1992) gives strong support for the availability of home birth services for women who choose them and underscores the value and appropriateness of the style of care that occurs at home. Even on a small scale, birth at home clarifies that childbirth is not inherently a medical matter, but is fundamentally related to the life and well-being of women, infants and families. Demedicalized birth is also the best way for practitioners and researchers to understand normal birth and the most effective ways to support it (Rothman 1983).

40. The distribution of knowledge and power is influenced by the social environment in which care takes place. Low-technology birth settings—i.e., freestanding birth centers and homes—that rely primarily on everyday materials and language involve a far more equal balance of knowledge and power than acute and other medical settings. In low-technology settings, caretakers tend to show greater respect for the individual woman's self-knowledge and capabilities and encourage and allow for greater involvement in decision-making. Care marked by this kind of respect and mutuality empowers women and families in their early parenting and postpartum adaptation (Hofmeyr et al. 1991), and in ways that may have long-term effects. In hierarchical hospital settings, where information is tied to sophisticated technology, only highly trained professionals are considered competent to interpret and apply it to the situation (Jordan 1987). This applies equally to midwives, family physicians and obstetricians. The degree of knowledge and power sharing appears to be linked to the kind and amount of intervention in the birth process that takes place. Refer back to notes 28 and 29.

41. The director of one center, located in the South Bronx, reports that activities such as these have helped a community of women who live under difficult circumstances to come together and support one another. Individual women in these groups have made significant changes in their lives such as returning to school and finding employment. Community women have also been empowered by serving on the birth center's advisory committee and by learning new skills through their employment at the center (Sanders 1992; Dohrn, interview with Gaskin 1991).

Ω

The Mother Myth

by Debbie Field

When I planned to have children, it never occurred to me that I would experience anything but the greatest joy after giving birth. In fact, I felt pity and extreme disassociation from women who were distressed in their post partum (after birth) period. So, along with the other almost unbearable feelings I had after the birth of both my children—depression, anxiety, insomnia, despair and fear of suicide—I was shocked and ashamed. How could I feel anything negative? Both children were healthy and wonderful and I was in a loving and long-standing relationship with my partner.

I write this article to deal with that shame, to publicly empathize with the hell that post partum depression is, even though I had the great luck to pass through the worst of it within six months of my children's births. I write for myself in the ongoing process of understanding what happened to me and to reach out to those who are currently experiencing it. I write to argue for a change in the social definition of what acceptable feelings are in motherhood, to de-stigmatise and help alleviate the pain of post partum depressed women. And since post partum depression is a metaphor of women's oppression as mothers, I write to ask some crucial questions about the problems that isolated nuclear family parenting poses for women.

Had I not been so deeply shaken by the rawness of my feelings after my children were born, I would have continued to believe that parenting should always feel positive, that any ambiguous feelings towards the children had to be repressed. Like other depressions, post partum can become a valuable gift, filled with insights into ourselves and the contradictions of loving anyone, particularly children.

Few extensive studies exist on why post partum depression occurs, how many women experience it, how long it lasts or what the best options are for alleviating it.

Both the medical profession and the self-help movement use three classifications. During the first three weeks of their baby's life, somewhere between 60 and 75 per cent of women experience a day or a week of the "baby blues," with wild mood swings, unexplained rages and inconsolable tears.

At the other end of the spectrum is post partum "psychosis," affecting one in 1,000 new mothers. These women have a complete breakdown with extreme suicidal or homicidal feelings, hallucinations and reality shifts. They are usually hospitalized and/or heavily medicated.

Somewhere between these two, one in 10 women are estimated to have strong feelings of depression, anxiety and fear of homicide or suicide for six months to a year. Though they remain capable of functioning, they are often terrified that forced hospitalization, medication and potential loss of their children are right around the corner.

The creation of these categories tends to hide the fact that all three conditions bear similarities with each other *and* with the feelings of mothers who are generally happy in their post partum. Because post partum depression relates to the role of mothering, most women will find minutes or hours reminiscent of post partum depression long past the end of the first year when the crisis has passed.

The classifications, with their apparent clinical basis, serve to make post partum depression into a medical condition. Instead of seeing isolated motherhood as the cause of a woman's anxiety, the medical profession defines post partum depression as an illness requiring medical intervention. The most common treatment is anti-depressants. Though extreme cases may require drugs, the majority of women need counseling and strong, consistent family/ community support.

Extreme anxiety, not depression, is the most common symptom. Hildi Wolfish, a Toronto therapist with a specialty in post partum, suggests that pre-parenting anxiety is a more accurate term to describe post partum depression.

The anxiety takes different forms. Some women, overwhelmed with concern over the child's health, will run into the baby's room every few minutes to see if she is still breathing. Others, so concerned about cleanliness and germs, do not leave their houses.

For others, the anxiety is not about the child's safety, but their ability to effectively mother. Previously self-contained women become incapacitated with insecurities and doubts about their ability to parent. Eventually she may come to doubt her ability to love the child and this feeds her shame in talking about her anxiety and depression.

Some women experience free floating anxiety—one moment they are calm and content, the next they have broken into a cold sweat, heart pounding, knots in their stomach. This often comes in the night, keeping a woman from sleeping, even when the baby does. Inability to sleep becomes another example of their failure as a person and mother. Rather than situating their insomnia in the reality of a pattern of sleep deprivation and disruption, never being sure whether the next baby's cries will be in 20 minutes or two hours, the woman blames herself.

From *Healthsharing,* Winter 1989, pp. 17–21. Copyright © 1989 by Healthsharing. Reprinted by permission.

Debbie Field works as an assistant to a Metro Toronto Councillor and has years of experience as an activist in the women's, union and solidarity movements.

All new mothers will recognize these anxieties. The difference is in their degree, and the mother's ability to keep the anxiety from taking over. A generally happy mother may feel anxious for a short time, but it passes. Another woman's anxieties may last for months as she loses all sense of herself, caught in a maze of fears.

For all the focus on the desirability of men sharing child-rearing, most women continue to take major responsibility, whether as single mothers or in a couple. Women's special claim to post partum depression is an indicator of how strongly we continue to internalize the responsibility of being the primary parent. Planning and worrying, two important components of parenting, become the basis for acute post partum anxiety. Likewise, women's ability to put the child's need before their own, particularly in the early period, leaves them vulnerable to a degree of self sacrifice that borders on self destruction.

Babies are simultaneously wonderful, beautiful balls of love and affection and totally frustrating creatures of need. What person in her right mind could blame a defenceless, loveable little baby for her problems? For the anxious mother it becomes necessary to blame herself, and internalise feelings of anger and frustration triggered by the immense responsibility and sheer physical exhaustion of taking care of a child.

Not letting herself feel anger at the baby, at her sense of deep isolation, the new mother becomes depressed. Her mother, siblings and other relatives, in most cases, live far away and are unavailable for daily support. She knows no one on her street. The few other new mothers she meets, at stores, the park, post natal classes, seem to be having a fantastic time.

She is angry at her friends who are never around when she needs them, and say things which make her feel more like a pariah. She represses all negative feelings towards the others, and tells herself she should be happy, should be making good use of the time off work, should be appreciative of all the love of those around her towards the baby.

The massive energy spent repressing so many real feelings results in full blown depression. She fears she will never return to her energetic, productive self. Everything seems completely bleak. She finds it harder and harder to feel any love for the baby, her companion, her family and friends. A terrifying tower of suicidal feelings develops from the building blocks of more understandable feelings. Placing exhaustion on top of inexperience, guilt, insecurity and fear of being alone, she comes to feel totally trapped.

Some women turn their negative feelings outward, fantasizing hurting or killing the baby. All parents will recognize these feelings, usually in milder forms. Alone all day with a child, it is hard for an adult not to become frustrated and lose patience. The generally happy mother will snap out of her anger while the post partum depressed mother becomes fixated on the idea that she is going to harm the child.

Both the woman who is depressed and suicidal, and the one so anxious and fearful of abusing her child, could be helped. If the social supports were there, for example, if there was someone she trusted to hand the baby to, her depression, anxiety and fear would never get out of control.

The symptoms and diagnosis of post partum depression vary widely. In my reading and through discussions with close to two dozen women of varying sexual orientation, countries of origin, races and classes, I have identified four common characteristics. They are not a formula, but a series of *potential* indicators.

First and foremost, post partum sufferers are isolated from their extended families, either geographically or emotionally. At no time in history have women been expected to raise children in such a private and isolated fashion. In the majority of third world countries today, as in most pre-industrial societies, new mothers are surrounded and supported by the women of their community. In the 1950s, during the growth of North America's suburban communities, new mothers enjoyed extended support systems based on close proximity of neighbours who were likewise full-time mothers. From the coffee klatch to the car pool, these women shared many aspects of day-to-day mothering.

Now, most women living in "western" capitalist countries raise children alone in their apartment or house, far away from friends or family. Without experienced mothers to guide and assist new mothers, it is harder to learn to become one.

Second, post partum depressed women are usually accomplished, highly productive and in control of their daily lives. This affects women who have been in the work force for years, used to the social recognition of paid work, as well as women who have worked only in the home. All of a sudden it is impossible to get a meal cooked, let alone finish a sewing project or a letter. This role dislocation can be extremely jarring to a woman's identity.

Most post partum depressed heterosexual women report anger that the life of their male companion remains relatively undisturbed while their life has been completely transformed. Often this anger translates into struggles over when the companion is coming home and when the woman can get a few hours off. A woman, married for years, living a relatively equal life with her spouse, each working and sharing domestic chores, now finds it a shock to be a full-time mom and housewife.

One of the many questions which needs to be researched is whether single mothers or lesbian mothers involved in co-parenting with another woman, face the same incidence of post partum depression. What effect does the absence of struggle with a male partner over domestic division of labour have on the experience of single and lesbian mothers?

Third, post partum depressed women seem to have had problems getting their own most basic needs met when they were babies. This can have different roots—the death of a parent, their parents' preoccupation with economic survival or other siblings. Whatever the reasons, post partum depressed women have often experienced abandonment as children. As a result they have negative feelings about how they were mothered, which leads them to feel inadequate as mothers.

If feelings of childhood abandonment are unresolved it is difficult to be around a needy child. Faced with a crying baby, the adult is reduced to her own past neediness.

The final indicator relates to hormonal imbalances. All women take a hormonal roller coaster ride after birth. But no one knows whether this is stronger for post partum depressed women. They will tell you that their depressions and anxieties feel as if they have a physiological logic beyond any emotional explanation they can muster. Until research is done, we don't know to what extent post partum depression is hormonal.

Much of the current medical treatment for post partum depression rests on the assumption that some women's hormones just go "snaky" and they need drugs to adjust them. But if the problem is hormonal why are anti-depressants rather than hormones the remedy? Drugs numb depression and anxiety and hide them behind a veil of sedated feelings instead of producing insights and changes in a woman's life.

The medical profession has done virtually nothing to uncover the causes and develop an appropriate therapeutic strategy for post partum sufferers. What stands out is the same shallow, pseudo-scientific response which is characteristic of the approach to so many "women's problems." Though doctors may legitimately be trying to stop a woman's pain and save her life, drugs are prescribed above all to conceal and suppress the symptoms of a larger social problem.

For me, time healed the hormonal disruptions, while psychotherapy brought insights into my childhood feelings of abandonment. I needed to hear that I would survive and return to my old self and the only advice that consistently worked for me was that my depression, like others, would pass. Returning to paid work affirmed my identity outside of the mothering role. And discussions with my partner clarified his willingness and need to share childrearing equally after the initial period of breast feeding. Exercise was important, enabling me to regularly get out of my head, into my body, helping me to sleep better.

If there is any advice I would give to women in the midst of a difficult post partum period, it is to make sure you are talking, especially to those who can identify with your experience. Through counseling, self-help groups, discussions with friends, family and former post partum sufferers, you can reduce your risk and alleviate the anxiety.

An effective post partum support network would include: a 24-hour hot-line staffed, if possible, by women who have been post partum depressed; affordable therapists to see a woman often, even daily, during her worst periods; a drop-in location, with childcare, exercise facilities, kitchen or restaurant; and availability of alternate treatments such as acupuncture, chiropractic treatments, nutritional therapy and massage.

Women who can't get out of the house need someone to come to them, to talk, cook and clean and take care of the child (or children), whatever the social cost and organizational difficulties of providing such a service.

Since there is no one solution, doctors with expertise in post partum drugs should be part of the support network. Anti-depressants, as a way of getting through the worst, can be very effective, as can the selective use of sleeping pills to break insomnia. If a woman is stuck and drugs work, no one should moralise about how drugs aren't the best way.

As we envision an effective post partum support system, we come up against the major problem facing post partum depressed women—the reality of isolated mothering.

As women, so many of our battles have been about our right to equal employment, equal pay, equal education, equal status in the world outside the home. And though we continue to make substantially less than men, more of us work in the paid workforce than ever before.

But while we have entered the public world, we have been expected to continue our primary role in raising children. The few concessions we have been able to wrest from the system, such as childcare, come nowhere close to being substantive social supports for our child rearing efforts.

And so we are caught, wanting it all, being expected to do it all. Post partum depression is a flag, letting us know that a very large number of us, can't in fact manage it all.

Grappling with the contradictions between women's increased activity in the public arena, and her continued responsibility for the private one, theoreticians in the women's and socialist movements have demanded that children become the responsibility of society. Elaborate collective child-rearing was tried, and then given up, in the Soviet Union after the 1917 revolution. A more lengthy experiment occurred during the 1950s and 60s in the Israeli kibbutz, where extensive reorganization of child-rearing was attempted. In order to allow women to fully participate in production, children were raised from their earliest months in same age groups, surrounded by consistent and loving staff. Parents and children would spend a few hours a day together, but the great part of their daily maintenance was considered a shared community responsibility. Besides freeing women, the kibbutz system attempted to free children from negative nuclear family patterns.

After the birth of my children, I could see why there was a movement away from collective child-rearing as a model. Cosy and warm in my nuclear family, in love with my babies, I could identify with the strong parental feelings which defeated alternative arrangements.

Now I find myself returning to earlier views on childrearing. It may be that Soviet and kibbutz models were too rigid, with insufficient time allotted for parents and children.

But as long as we continue to isolate what has for centuries been a collective task—the raising of children, we will continue to have serious problems. To the devastation caused by sexual and physical abuse within the nuclear family, we can now add the anguish faced by a large percentage of women who find isolated mothering too difficult.

Ultimately, post partum depression will not be eliminated as a widespread condition that debilitates and sometimes destroys women until we provide some fundamental social supports for women and men who are parenting. This may involve collective arrangements such as past experiments. Other plans which more accurately reflect the cultural preferences of today's society might be more successful, such as a reduced work week which would enable mothers and fathers or perhaps a larger extended family team of adults to raise children. In demanding broader community involvement in child-rearing, we not only save women from shouldering too much responsibility, but we also humanize our society, providing more adults with the opportunity to experience the immense satisfaction of parenting.

While we await a revolution in child-rearing, parents can arm ourselves against the worst effects of the nuclear family. Support systems such as daycare, links with other adults raising children and the incorporation into our extended family units of adults who do not have children, all help to break down isolation. Most importantly mothers can remember that what we experience through the sieve of our personal anguish is often the contradictions of current mothering structures.

Ω

Childbearing

1. Doris Haire's "The Cultural Warping of Childbirth" identified many common obstetrical practices from early pregnancy to post partum which "served to warp and distort the childbearing experience in the U.S." List ten of the practices Haire identified. For each practice, identify how you think the situation has or has not changed since 1972:

      + =   totally improved, issue no longer an issue for activists

      = =   remains a problem

      x =   situation is even more exaggerated today than it was in 1972

      ? =   not known

  new =   new technology/changed situation impacts on this issue

Practices	Changed?
1	
2	
3	
4	
5	
6	
7	
8	
9	
10	

2. Interview two women who have given birth or interview a woman who has given birth at least twice. (If you have given birth, you are encouraged to ask yourself these questions.) Ask the following questions about each pregnancy and birth.

   a. How was she treated in pregnancy by health providers and others? Was she healthy during the pregnancy? Did she have access to regular pre-natal care? During her pregnancy, did she have strong ideas of what she wanted the childbirth experience to be?

      birth 1   birth 2

   b. For the birth event, where was the birth, who assisted in the delivery, and what kind of birth was it (natural childbirth, some intervention, cesarean section) ?

      birth 1   birth 2

   c. Did the woman feel she had control in the process and did she have the childbirth experience she had hoped for?

      birth 1   birth 2

3. For the two pregnancy and birth experiences described above, identify social and economic factors which you think influenced similarities and differences in the two childbirths.

11

The Politics of Disease

The politics of disease can be seen in the decisions made by government agencies, pharmaceutical companies, and the health care industry regarding priorities in funding, research, and education. Another aspect of the politics of disease is how women interact as both consumers and practitioners with these systems to fight for the priorities we identify. The first section focuses on breast cancer, which it is estimated one out of eight women in the United States will develop. Currently, there is a network of breast cancer activists around the country pushing for changes in research and the health care system. The chapter begins with an excerpt from *The Cancer Journals* by Audre Lorde, an extraordinary writer who recently died of breast cancer (also see her essays in this book: "There Is No Hierarchy of Oppressions" and "Age, Race, and Sex: Women Redefining Difference"). The excerpt examines from a very personal and political perspective the complexities around her decision not to use a prosthesis after mastectomy. Following this is an article on Dr. Susan Love, a surgeon who specializes in breast cancer, who can serve as a model of what women should be able to expect from a physician when dealing with breast cancer diagnosis and treatment. The article also touches on some of the controversies around breast cancer—such as the value of mammography for women under age 50. The third article, "Breast cancer: The Environmental Connection," turns to the issue of true prevention, that is, keeping women from developing cancer, not merely detecting it early. After examining the roles of radiation, pesticides, and other forms of pollution in causing cancer, the authors call for a grass-roots movement that will push for change in governmental priorities towards the elimination of environmental causes of cancer. Following up on the importance of consumer activism, "Ten Years of Self Help Achievement" is an interview with a co-founder of the Endometriosis Association. This group has been able to influence the health care system by providing information about endometriosis, as learned from the women who experience this disease, as well as providing support and information for those women.

Because the next section focuses on two diseases involving the immune system, we begin with a clear explanation of the immune system by Susan Elliott. "The ABCs

of Immunology" is a helpful reference in trying to understand both AIDS and Chronic Fatigue Syndrome (CFS), which is also known as Chronic Fatigue Immune Dysfunction Syndrome (CFIDS). Andrea Rudner's article about CFS, besides explaining what is known about this disease, shows how this issue can illustrate much about women's health issues: the way these issues are often trivialized or assumed to be "all in her head," as well as the role of activism and self-help movements in pushing for a more appropriate response from the health care system.

The chapter concludes with several articles on AIDS, a disease that was once incorrectly considered a man's disease. However, it is now recognized that women comprise the fastest growing segment of the population with AIDS. Because most of the early cases of AIDS in the U.S. were men, the definitions of the disease were based on the opportunistic infections that men experienced. A person who was HIV+ (had antibodies to HIV, the virus that causes AIDS) and had specific symptoms was given the diagnosis of AIDS. Because women do not get the same opportunistic infections as men (women may have pelvic inflammatory disease, invasive cervical cancer, persistent and severe vaginal yeast infection, for example), HIV+ women were not being diagnosed with AIDS. However, in 1993, the Centers for Disease Control (CDC) changed the definitions to be more inclusive, especially of women. Some may ask why a woman who is HIV+ would *want* to be defined as having AIDS and there are several answers to that question. One is that the Social Security Administration uses the CDC definitions to determine if someone who is HIV+ would be eligible for disability benefits (See Sharon Lerner's "The Dysfunctional Definition of Disability" in *Health/PAC Bulletin*, Spring, 1992, pp. 40-41). In addition, these definitions have caused an underestimation of the prevalence of women with AIDS, thereby leading to inappropriate distribution of resources, misdirected education, and a false sense of security. When reading any of the articles written before 1993, it is important to remember that the number of women with AIDS would be under-reported.

The lead-off article in this section, "HIV: The National Scandal," gives an excellent overview of the impact of the AIDS epidemic on women, placing this health crisis in the broader context of the politics of women's health. This lack of attention to women's issues can be seen in the next article, which summarizes a survey that indicates how little attention has been paid through out the nation to developing policies specifically addressing women and AIDS. Together these two articles emphasize the problems of leaving women out of the picture when approaching prevention, education, and policy development.

The last two articles examine issues around preventing transmission of HIV and other sexually transmitted diseases (STDs). First, Jane Juffer, in "Spermicides, Virucides, and HIV," examines what is known about options in addition to condoms for preventing HIV transmission, emphasizing the need for women-controlled methods. Next, Carol Camlin presents the debates about safer sex for lesbians. Although focusing on lesbian issues, the article is a presentation of explicit and concrete information that may be useful to anyone who is sexually active with one or more partners. She gives practical advice about reducing risk while putting that risk in clear perspective.

Together the articles in this chapter illustrate the need for input by women—both as consumers and practitioners—into the decisions that are made about research priorities, policies, and the information/education about diseases that can affect our lives.

Breast Cancer: Power vs. Prosthesis

by Audre Lorde

On Labor Day, 1978, during my regular monthly self-examination, I discovered a lump in my right breast which later proved to be malignant. During my following hospitalization, my mastectomy and its aftermath, I passed through many stages of pain, despair, fury, sadness and growth. I moved through these stages, sometimes feeling as if I had no choice, other times recognizing that I could choose oblivion—or a passivity that is very close to oblivion—but did not want to. As I slowly began to feel more equal to processing and examining the different parts of this experience, I also began to feel that in the process of losing a breast I had become a more whole person.

After a mastectomy, for many women including myself, there is a feeling of wanting to go back, of not wanting to persevere through this experience to whatever enlightenment might be at the core of it. And it is this feeling, this nostalgia, which is encouraged by most of the post-surgical counselling for women with breast cancer. This regressive tie to the past is emphasised by the concentration upon breast cancer as a cosmetic problem, one which can be solved by a prosthetic pretence. The American Cancer Society's Reach for Recovery Program, while doing a valuable service in contacting women immediately after surgery and letting them know they are not alone, nonetheless encourages this false and dangerous nostalgia in the mistaken belief that women are too weak to deal directly and courageously with the realities of our lives.

The woman from Reach for Recovery who came to see me in the hospital, while quite admirable and even impressive in her own right, certainly did not speak to my experience nor my concerns. As a 44-year-old Black lesbian feminist, I knew there were very few role models around for me in this situation, but my primary concerns two days after mastectomy were hardly about what man I could capture in the future, whether or not my old boyfriend would still find me attractive enough, and even less about whether my two children would be embarrassed by me around their friends.

My concerns were about my chances for survival, the effects of a possibly shortened life upon my work and my priorities. Could this cancer have been prevented, and what could I do in the future to prevent its recurrence? Would I be able to maintain the control over my life that I had always taken for granted? A lifetime of loving women had taught me that when women love each other, physical change does not alter that love. It did not occur to me that anyone who really loved me would love me any less because I had one breast instead of two, although it did occur to me to wonder if they would be able to love and deal with the new me.

In the critical and vulnerable period following surgery, self-examination and self-evaluation are positive steps. To imply to a woman that yes, she can be the 'same' as before surgery, with the skillful application of a little puff of lambswool, and/or silicone gel, is to place an emphasis upon prosthesis which encourages her not to deal with herself as physically and emotionally real, even though altered and traumatised. This emphasis upon the cosmetic after surgery reinforces this society's stereotype of women, that we are only what we look or appear, so this is the only aspect of our existence we need to address. Any woman who has had a breast removed because of cancer knows she does not feel the same. But we are allowed no psychic time or space to examine what our true feelings are, to make them our own.

Ten days after having my breast removed, I went to my doctor's office to have the stitches taken out. This was my first journey out since coming home from the hospital, and I was truly looking forward to it. A friend had washed my hair for me and it was black and shining, with my new grey hairs glistening in the sun. Colour was starting to come back into my face and around my eyes, I wore the most opalescent of my moonstones, and a single floating bird dangling from my right ear in the name of grand asymmetry. With an African kentecloth tunic and new leather boots, I knew I looked fine, with that brave new-born security of a beautiful woman having come through a very hard time and being very glad to be alive.

The doctor's nurse, a charmingly bright and steady woman of about my own age who had always given me a feeling of quiet no-nonsense support on my other visits, called me into the examining room. On the way, she asked me how I was feeling.

'Pretty good,' I said, half-expecting her to make some comment about how good I looked.

'You're not wearing a prosthesis,' she said, a little anxiously, and not at all like a question.

'No,' I said, thrown off my guard for a minute. 'It really doesn't feel right,' referring to the lambswool puff given to me by the Reach For Recovery volunteer in the hospital.

Usually supportive and understanding, the nurse now looked at me urgently and disapprovingly as she told me that even if it didn't look exactly right, it was 'better than nothing,' and that as soon as my stitches were out I could be fitted for a 'real form'.

'You will feel so much better with it on,' she said. 'And besides, we really like you to wear something, at least when you come in. Otherwise it's bad for the morale of the office.'

I could hardly believe my ears! I was too outraged to speak then, but this was to be only the first such assault on my right to define and to claim my own body.

A woman who is attempting to come to terms with her changed landscape and changed timetable of life and with her own body and pain and beauty and strength, that woman is seen as a threat to the 'morale' of a breast surgeon's office!

Yet when Moishe Dayan, the Prime Minister of Israel, stands up in front of parliament or on TV with an eye patch over his empty eye socket, nobody tells him to go get a glass eye, or that he is bad for the morale of the office. The world sees him as a warrior with an honourable wound, and a loss of a piece of himself which he has marked, and mourned, and moved beyond. And if you have trouble dealing with Moishe Dayan's empty eye-socket, everyone recognises that it is your problem to solve, not his.

Well, women with breast cancer are warriors, also. I have been to war, and still am. So has every women who had had one or both breasts amputated because of the cancer that is becoming the primary physical scourge of our time. For me, my scars are an honorable reminder that I may be a casualty in the cosmic war against radiation, animal fat, air pollution, McDonald's hamburgers and Red Dye no. 2, but the fight is still going on, and I am still a part of it. I refuse to have my scars hidden or trivialised behind lambswool or silicone gel. I refuse to be reduced in my own eyes or in the eyes of others from warrior to mere victim, simply because it might render me a fraction more acceptable or less dangerous to the still complacent, those who believe if you cover up a problem it ceases to exist. I refuse to hide my body simply because it might make a woman-phobic world more comfortable.

Prosthesis offers the empty comfort of 'nobody will know the difference'. But it is that very difference which I wish to affirm, because I had lived it, and survived it, and wish to share that strength with other women. If we are to translate the silence surrounding breast cancer into language and action against this scourge, then the first step is that women with mastectomies must become visible to each other. For silence and invisibility go hand in hand with powerlessness. By accepting the mask or prosthesis, one-breasted women proclaim ourselves as insufficients dependent upon pretence.

In addition, we withhold that visibility and support from one another which is such an aid to perspective and self-acceptance.

As women, we cannot afford to look the other way, nor to consider the incidence of breast cancer as a private or secret personal problem. It is no secret that breast cancer is on the increase among women in America. According to the American Cancer Society's own statistics on breast cancer survival, of women stricken, only 50% are still alive after three years. This figure drops to 30% if you are poor, or Black, or in any other way part of the underside of this society. We cannot ignore these facts, nor their implications, nor their effect upon our lives, individually and collectively. Early detection and early treatment is crucial in the management of breast cancer if those sorry statistics of survival are to improve. But for the incidence of early detection and early treatment to increase, American women must become free enough from social stereotypes concerning their appearance to realize that losing a breast is infinitely preferable to losing one's life (or one's eyes, or one's hands . . .).

Although breast self-examination does not reduce the incidence of breast cancer, it does markedly reduce the rate of mortality, since most early tumours are found by women themselves. I discovered my own tumour upon a monthly breast exam, and so report most of the other women I know with a good prognosis for survival. With our alert awareness making such a difference in the survival rate for breast cancer, women need to face the possibility and the actuality of breast cancer as a reality rather than a myth, or retribution, or terror in the night, or a bad dream that will disappear if ignored. After surgery, there is a need for women to be aware of the possibility of bilateral recurrence, with vigilance rather than terror. This is not a spread of cancer, but a new occurrence in the other breast. Each woman must be aware that an honest acquaintanceship with and evaluation of her own body is the best tool of detection.

The greatest incidence of breast cancer in American women appears between the ages of 40 to 55. These are the very years when women are portrayed in the popular media as fading and desexualised figures. Contrary to the media picture, I find myself as a woman of insight ascending into my highest powers, my greatest psychic strengths, and my fullest satisfactions. I am freer of the constraints and fears and indecisions of my younger years, and survival throughout these years has taught me how to value my own beauty, and how to look closely into the beauty of others.

There is nothing wrong, *per se*, with the use of prostheses, if they can be chosen freely, for whatever reason, after a woman has had a chance to accept her new body. But usually prostheses serve a real function, to approximate the performance of a missing physical part. In other amputations and with other prosthetic devices, function is the main point of their existence. Artificial limbs perform specific tasks, allowing us to manipulate or to walk. Dentures allow us to chew our food. Only false breasts are designed for appearance only, as if the only real function of women's breasts were to appear in a certain shape and size and symmetry to onlookers, or to yield to external pressure. For no woman wearing a prosthesis can even for one moment believe it is her own breast, any more than a woman wearing falsies can.

Attitudes towards the necessity for prostheses after breast surgery are merely a reflection of those attitudes within our society towards women in general as objectified and depersonalised sexual conveniences. Women have been programmed to view our bodies only in terms of how they look and feel to others, rather than how they feel to ourselves, and how we wish to use them. As women, we fight this depersonalisation every day, this pressure towards the conversion of one's own self-image into a media expectation of what might satisfy male demand. The insistence upon breast prosthesis as 'decent' rather than functional is an additional example of that wipe-out of self in which women are constantly encouraged to take part. I am personally affronted by the message that I am only acceptable if I look 'right' or 'normal', where those norms have nothing to do with my own perceptions of who I am. Where 'normal' means the 'right' colour, shape, size, or number of breasts, a woman's perception of her own body and the strengths that come from that perception are discouraged, trivialised, and ignored.

Every woman has a right to define her own desires, make her own choices. But prostheses are often chosen, not from desire, but in default. Some women complain it is too much effort to fight the concerted pressure exerted by the fashion industry. Being one-breasted does not mean being unfashionable; it means giving some time and energy to choosing or constructing the proper clothes. In some cases, it means making or remaking clothing or jewellry. The fact that the fashion needs of one-breasted women are not currently being met doesn't mean that the concerted pressure of our demands cannot change that.

Some women believe that a breast prosthesis is necessary to preserve correct posture and physical balance. But the weight of each breast is never the same to begin with, nor is the human body ever exactly the same on both sides. With a minimum of exercises to develop the habit of straight posture, the body can accommodate to one-breastedness quite easily, even when the breasts were quite heavy.

Women in public and private employment have reported the loss of jobs and promotions upon their return to work after a mastectomy, without regard to whether or not they wore prostheses. The social and economic discrimination practised against women who have breast cancer is not diminished by pretending that mastectomies do not exist. Where a woman's job is at risk because of her health history, employment discrimination cannot be fought with a sack of silicone gel, nor with the constant fear and anxiety to which such subterfuge gives rise. Suggesting prosthesis as a solution to employment discrimination is like saying that the way to fight prejudice is for Black people to pretend to be white. Employment discrimination against post-mastectomy women can only be fought in the open, with head-on attacks by strong and self-accepting women who refuse to be relegated to an inferior position, or to cower in a corner because they have one breast.

Within the framework of superficiality and pretence, the next logical step of a depersonalising and woman-devaluating culture is the advent of the atrocity euphemistically called 'breast reconstruction'. It should be noted that research being done on this potentially life-threatening practice represents time and research money spent—not on how to prevent the cancers that cost us our breasts and our lives—but rather upon how to pretend that our breasts are not gone, nor we as women at risk with our lives.

Any information about the prevention or treatment of breast cancer which might possibly threaten the vested interests of the American medical establishment is difficult to acquire in the country. Only through continuing scrutiny of various non-mainstream sources of information, such as alternative and women's presses, can a picture of new possibilities for prevention and treatment of breast cancer emerge.

The mortality for breast cancer treated by conventional therapies has not decreased in over 40 years (Rose Kushner, *Breast Cancer*, Harcourt, Brace & Jovanovitch, 1975, p. 161). Since the American medical establishment and the ACS are determined to suppress any cancer information not dependent upon western medical bias, whether this information is ultimately useful or not, we must pierce this silence ourselves and aggressively seek answers to these questions about new therapies. We must also heed the unavoidable evidence pointing towards the nutritional and environmental aspects of cancer prevention.

Cancer is not just another degenerative and unavoidable disease of the ageing process. It has distinct and identifiable causes, and these are mainly exposures to chemical or physical agents in the environment. In the medical literature, there is mounting evidence that breast cancer is a chronic systemic disease. Post-mastectomy women must be vigilantly aware that, contrary to the 'lightning strikes' theory, we are the most likely of all women to develop cancer somewhere else in the body.

Every woman has a militant responsibility to involve herself actively with her own health. We owe ourselves the protection of all the information we can acquire about the treatment of cancer and its causes, as well as about the recent findings concerning immunology, nutrition, environment and stress. And we owe ourselves this information *before* we may have a reason to use it.

It was very important for me, after my mastectomy, to develop and encourage my own internal sense of power. At all times, it felt crucial to me that I make a conscious commitment to survival. It is physically important for me to be loving my life rather than to be mourning my breast. I believe it is this love of my life and myself, and the careful tending of that love which was done by women who love and support me, which has been largely responsible for my strong and healthy recovery from the effects of my mastectomy. But a clear distinction must be made between this affirmation of self and the superficial farce of 'looking on the bright side of things'.

Last week I read a letter from a doctor in a medical magazine which said that no truly happy person ever gets cancer. Despite my knowing better, and despite my having dealt with this blame-the-victim thinking for years, for a moment this letter hit my guilt button. Had I really been guilty of the crime of not being happy in this best of all possible infernos?

The idea that the cancer patient should be made to feel guilty about having had cancer, as if in some way it were all her fault for not having been in the right psychological frame of mind at all times to prevent cancer, is a monstrous distortion of the idea that we can use our psychic strengths to help heal ourselves. This guilt trip which many cancer patients have been led into (you see, it *is* a shameful thing because you could have prevented it if only you had been more . . .) is an extension of the blame-the-victim syndrome. It does nothing to encourage the mobilisation of our psychic defenses against the very real forms of death which surround us. It is easier to demand happiness than to clean up the environment. The acceptance of illusion and appearance as reality is another symptom of this same refusal to examine the realities of our lives. Let us seek 'joy' rather than real food and clean air and a saner future on a liveable earth! As if happiness alone can protect us from the results of profit-madness.

Was I wrong to be working so hard against the oppressions afflicting women and Black people? Was I in error to be speaking out against our silent passivity and the cynicism of a mechanized and inhuman civilisation that is destroying our earth and those who live upon it? Was I really fighting the spread of radiation, racism, woman-slaughter, chemical invasion of our food, pollution of our environment, the abuse and psychic destruction of our young, merely to avoid dealing with my first and greatest responsibility—to be happy?

The only really happy people I have ever met are those of us who work against these deaths with all the energy of our living, recognising the deep and fundamental unhappiness with which we are surrounded, at the same time as we fight to keep from being submerged by it. The idea that happiness can insulate us against the results of our environmental madness is a rumour circulated by our enemies to destroy us. And what Woman of Colour in America over the age of 15 does not live with the knowledge that our daily lives are stitched with violence and with hatred, and to naively ignore that reality can mean destruction? We are equally destroyed by false happiness and false breasts, and the passive acceptance of false values which corrupt our lives and distort our experience.

The idea of having a breast removed was much more traumatic for me before my mastectomy than after the fact, but it certainly took time and the loving support of other women before I could once again look at and love my altered body with the warmth I had done before. But I did.

Right after surgery I had a sense that I would never be able to bear missing that great well of sexual pleasure that I connected with my right breast. That sense has completely passed away, as I have come to realise that that well of feeling was within me. I alone own my feelings. I can never lose that feeling because I own it, because it comes out of myself. I can attach it anywhere I want to, because my feelings are a part of me, my sorrow and my joy.

I would never have chosen this path, but I am very glad to be who I am, here.

30 March 1979

Ω

Dr. Susan Love: Making Patients Medical Partners
by Sue Frederick

On a warm March day in Boston, surgical oncologist Dr. Susan Love, wearing a pin that reads "Keep ABreast: Get A Second Opinion," is seven hours into her 12-hour day at the Faulkner Breast Centre, examining yet another patient after a morning spent performing a lumpectomy.

Love sits patiently with the frightened woman, explaining cancer, how it spreads, and the pros and cons of treatment options. Love adds gently, "It's not going to hurt anything if you wait a few weeks to consider your options."

Then the room is quiet, almost like a confessional, as the woman whispers her fears and questions to the doctor. After answering all of them, Love sits calmly, willing to talk some more. And suddenly, to hear her patients tell it, breast cancer just isn't such a big deal.

Indeed, that's Love's intention: To help women face the trauma of a disease that the American Cancer Society estimates will strike one of every 10 women in their lifetime. She goes about it in a uniquely feminine—some say feminist—way by arming her patients with knowledge, which she considers the antidote to fear.

She isn't afraid to speak her mind. According to Love:
- Breast self-exams, invented by men, are taught wrongly, and that may be why nobody does them.
- Fibrocystic disease is a "garbage" term.
- Most women aren't given enough time and information to make a wise treatment decision when it comes to breast cancer.

But to hear her patients tell it, this outspoken woman is the doctor to see after a breast cancer diagnosis. As one woman says of Love, "She makes me feel at ease. She treats me like an intelligent human being."

From *Cope*, July 1988, pp. 27–32. Copyright © 1988 by Pulse Publications, Inc. Reprinted by permission.

Elaine Ullian, president of Boston's Faulkner Hospital where Love is director of the Breast Centre, is another admirer.

"I made up my mind to recruit her here before I'd even met her," she recalls. "Her reputation is incredible, not only in the medical community. Every woman I'd ever heard of who had breast disease was beating a path to Dr. Love's office."

Indeed, Love, who's also an assistant surgery professor at the Harvard Medical School and a surgical oncologist in the breast-evaluation center at Boston's Dana-Farber Institute, has impressive credentials and a growing reputation as a top-notch breast-cancer specialist. Yet, not all medical experts are enamored with her, a fact Love is quite aware of.

"My reputation is that I'm outspoken, that I speak my mind. And that's good and bad," she admits. "It's blocked off some avenues for my career."

Dr. Robert Goldwyn, head of the plastic surgery division at Beth Israel Hospital and another surgery professor at the Harvard Medical School, is quite familiar with Love's reputation.

"I think she's done a lot for medicine and for patients. She's done a lot for us here at Beth Israel," he says. "It's certainly not a dull experience working with her.

"But there are people, and I'm not one of them, who think she's rather extreme and champions a philosophy that might be detrimental to patients in the long run. But they don't want to speak out against her because she's a feminist and it would look like they were speaking out against feminism. People don't want to attack feminism."

Yet Love's honesty and directness, which may cause her problems in the medical world, are traits that pay off well in the examining room. That's where she kicks into gear, often seeming more a teacher than a surgeon, what with her charts and X-rays and detailed explanations of cancer.

"This isn't so bad," she says softly to a patient who has tears in her eyes. "Breast cancer is scary business. But we still cure 80 percent of all early breast cancers. Most people don't hear about those survivors. You hear about the ones who go downhill fast. You don't hear about those who go on quietly with their lives."

As Ullian puts it: "She has the wonderful combination of being an excellent surgeon and also having an incredible ability to talk to her patients. These women get a difficult diagnosis from one doctor that leaves them feeling utterly destroyed, and they go see Dr. Love, who gives them the same diagnosis. But the women walk out of her office feeling hopeful and not powerless anymore."

"I feel like I'm a teacher with these women," Love says. "My job is to educate the woman so she understands what's going on, so together we can come up with the best plan for her care. Teaching is very important."

Indeed, those who appear in her office face a challenge. This year, the American Cancer Society estimates some 135,000 women will be diagnosed with breast cancer in the United States, and 42,000 will die from it. But Love is used to tackling challenges, a necessary skill for a woman fighting her way up the ranks of a male-dominated system. When she entered medical school in 1971, only 8% of the physicians in this country were women; the figure now stands at around 15%.

Along the way, Love has collected quite a few stories about being a woman in medicine.

When she applied for a residency at Columbia University in 1974, they asked her what type of birth control she used, and if she planned to have children—"standard questions back then," remembers Love, who ended up doing her residency at Beth Israel Hospital in Boston, where she spent seven years as breast-clinic director.

She has since become somewhat infamous in her medical circles for her professional, as well as personal, style.

She is 40 years old, unmarried, and plans to raise her three-month-old girl, Katy, with her female companion. In her examining room, there are buttons with feminist observations that not all men find amusing, slogans like, "On the seventh day, when God created man, she made a mistake."

However, Love's opinion of men is not as extreme as it would initially seem. For one, her mentor is Dr. William Silen, the chief of surgery at Beth Israel.

"I truly respect Dr. Silen," Love says. "He's been a real role model for me in terms of taking patients seriously. And he's somebody who knows how you can still be caring and compassionate and still be a very good surgeon."

But her opinions about breast cancer do raise eyebrows—opinions that would be controversial even if they weren't coming from a woman. For example, she calls fibrocystic disease a "garbage term."

"It doesn't mean anything," she says flatly. "It means lumpy, painful breasts that don't have anything to do with cancer. To pathologists, it covers 15 different pathological entities common in all breasts, yet none causes lumps or pain. And on a mammogram, it's a term used for dense breasts.

"So they're all talking about a different thing, which would be okay except that some doctors say it increases your chance of getting breast cancer, which it doesn't. We need to get rid of the term and call them lumpy breasts or painful breasts."

Dr. Norman Sadowsky, chief of radiology at Faulkner Hospital and director of the diagnostic branch of the Faulkner Breast Centre, agrees.

"Most people know fibrocystic disease is a waste-basket term, but people still tell their patients they have it, and the patient thinks something is wrong with them.

"It's normal to have nodular breasts and painful breasts at certain times of the month, and there's nothing wrong with you if you have that. Love is mainly responsible for populating the idea that that's not a disease. She's had a big effect on doctors' thinking. They won't use the term now without thinking about it a little more."

But Dr. Ezra Greenspan, a clinical professor of medicine and the associate chief of the oncology division at

New York's Mount Sinai School of Medicine, sees it differently.

"What she [Love] says about fibrocystic disease is a gross overstatement," he declares. "True, it is a 'dump' term covering several different conditions, but some of those conditions are not normal. And studies have shown that 30 percent of women with breast cancer have fibrocystic disease.

"And there are dozens of papers showing these women with fibrocystic disease do have a slightly higher incidence of cancer. So she's not quite accurate there."

Love says it can be argued both ways: "[Greenspan] is right in a way. In its broadest sense, fibrocystic disease covers a precancerous condition called atypia hyperplasia, which is not common and doesn't cause lumps or pain, but is under the broad pathological umbrella of the term fibrocystic disease."

The controversies continue.

Love was one of the few doctors to criticize Nancy Reagan's decision to go immediately from biopsy to surgery after the first lady was diagnosed with breast cancer last year.

"That really put us back," says Love. "Not that she chose to have a mastectomy, but that she didn't explore the options. She said she did before the biopsy, but you can't know the options before the biopsy.

"I think her choice is fine, but doing it in one stick is what I don't agree with. She should've taken the time to get a second opinion."

Indeed, Love encourages her own patients to take the time to make good treatment decisions: "Basically, the old theory was that breast cancer would go up the lymph nodes and get out into the body fast. So women went straight to surgery from the biopsy. But now, we know it takes 90 days for one cancer cell to become two cells.

"And most cancers are present 8 to 10 years before we feel the lump or see it on the mammogram. So if it wanted to get out, it's gotten out already, and it's a question then of how well your immune system has taken care of it. But the idea of it getting out tomorrow is baloney."

Love believes that when a woman is diagnosed with breast cancer, she goes into a temporary state of shock, which isn't a good state of mind in which to make decisions that will affect the rest of her life. As she says, "It is much safer to take a deep breath and wait a day or two, or a week or two, and get a second opinion and figure out the best treatment for you. If you rush in, you can't change things later."

Perhaps because of this outspokenness, or perhaps because she is a successful female surgical oncologist with a six month backlog of patients waiting to see her, Love has suddenly, quite to her own surprise, become a public figure. Recently, she was featured on the Public Broadcasting System's *Nova* series, as well as on ABC's *20/20*. And *The New York Times Magazine* shot her photo for a story on women surgeons.

"My success has surprised me, but it shows there's an enormous demand for physicians who will spend time talking to patients," she explains. "My success is not based on my skills in the O.R., which are okay, but it's based on the time I take to talk to women.

"If you can take a very scary crisis situation and explain it to someone clearly, and explain the unknown, you can empower them."

Love does know how to put women at ease. Her earthy honesty, her confident voice and her clear explanations are a salve to the women who seek her out. In fact, Love often puts women at ease with a subject few doctors are willing to sway from the party-line about: breast self-exams.

At least once a day, Love finds herself talking to a woman who feels terribly guilty and scared because she doesn't perform BSE's the way they're described in the American Cancer Society pamphlets. To that, Love says, "Stop feeling guilty. Nobody's doing them."

To her, these elaborate exams where a woman carefully searches her breasts for hidden lumps were born out of a male perspective on a female problem.

"These were invented by a man and nobody does them, but everybody feels guilty about it," she says. "Doing it like the ads say, in front of the mirror, is too much of a deal. You don't do it. You feel little things everywhere and don't know what they are. You don't know what you're looking for, so you get anxious and stop doing it. Then you feel guilty for not doing it. It's another example of blame the patient."

But Dr. Arthur Holleb, the former senior vice president of medical affairs for the American Cancer Society, has long believed in the value of thorough BSE's in early cancer detection.

"If a woman is terrified of doing the self-exam and has nodular breasts, I'd say come to me every three months, and I'll do the exam for you and won't charge you. I did this in my practice," he explains.

Silen at Beth Israel sides with Love.

"I don't disagree with her about self-exams," he explains. "They've never really taken hold. Studies suggest they aren't making a huge difference. Women don't follow the routine taught by the ACS anyhow."

Indeed, a recent Oregon Medical Association survey of 618 Oregon women with breast cancer showed that many women never perform the technique. In fact, only 63% of that group detected their lumps either by self-exam or accidental discovery. The reason they cited for avoiding the technique: Their breasts were lumpy anyway.

Even the New York-based National Alliance of Breast Cancer Organizations acknowledges that the elaborate procedure intimidates some women. NABCO estimates that only 30% of women who know about BSE's regularly practice the procedure. Says a NABCO spokesperson: "We encourage women to examine their breasts in any way they can, however they're comfortable doing it. It's better than not doing it at all."

Holleb says doctors should be teaching the procedure to women: "We recommend the doctor teach the technique to the woman when he examines her. The advantage of the BSE is that the woman can do it every month, and the more frequently you do the BSE, the better your chance of finding an early cancer."

Holleb's main contention with Love's approach is that a large number of women in this country can't afford to visit a doctor for regular check-ups; often, they can't afford mammograms, either.

"If we discard BSE's, we're doing a great disservice to these women especially . . . and, really, to all women," Holleb says. "In the past, there were few rewards for doing the BSE and finding an early cancer. The reward then was a radical mastectomy. But nowadays, if you find it early, you can often save the breast and have a much better chance of survival."

But Love contends that, "There are no studies that show breast self-exams increase the survival rate of breast-cancer patients.

"Cancer can't be felt when it's a little bee-bee, so the little lumps she finds aren't usually cancer. And by the time a woman finds a cancerous lump, it's pretty advanced.

"These exams were invented at a time when women never touched themselves 'down there.' Now, women do run their hands over their bodies and are acquainted with their breasts."

Her recommendation: "Once a month in the shower when you're soaped up, run your hands over your body and get acquainted with your breasts, not looking for anything. Don't focus on anything. And you'll notice a change if there is one."

Love agrees with the ACS, however, that mammograms are the best way to detect cancer since they can find a malignancy in an early stage when it's far too small to be detected by hand.

But Love isn't crazy about their use in women under 40: "When they first came out, the doctors thought, 'Hey this is great. We'll do mammograms every year.' And they discovered they'd cause as many cancers as they cured if they did that.

"So, the answer is somewhere in between. The radiation risk is greater in younger women than older women. So if you're over 50, there's no question that mammograms improve the cure rate of breast cancer. From 40 to 50, it doesn't seem to have as much impact. The breasts are denser. Things are harder to see."

Nevertheless, Love says women over 40 should probably have them done every year, but she doesn't recommend them for women 35 to 40: "We need to get rid of the idea of a baseline mammogram. That idea comes from tuberculosis. The chest doesn't change every year, but breasts do change every year. So it's not a good comparison point. To compare one mammogram to another from one year to the next is false information."

Dr. Paul Stomper, a radiologist at the Dana-Farber Cancer Center and an assistant professor of radiology at the Harvard Medical School, disagrees.

"There's no data to back up her comments," he says. "As someone who takes mammograms everyday, I know that a woman's breast doesn't change that much on a mammogram from age 35 to 40. And studies have shown that the cut-off for radiation risks at low doses is at age 30. It stops being dangerous to have a mammogram at age 30. The risk then is negligible if at all . . .

"Mammograms are the only way to beat breast cancer, and physicians must be responsible and explain both sides of the issue to their patients. It's a very complex area."

Love's next patient of the day is 31-year-old Luz Landrau, who has just had a lumpectomy after six months of chemotherapy. Love examines the woman's breasts, asks about her energy since the surgery, and then makes her raise her left arm. Landrau raises the limb halfway and winces. Love says "good, great," and they laugh together.

Landrau is grateful to Love for getting her through what she calls the "toughest year of my life." After being diagnosed and starting her chemotherapy regimen, Landrau decided that treatment wasn't for her and she stopped it. She told Love she wanted to cure herself "the natural way" with diet and vitamins.

Love was patient, continuing to see Landrau for checkups. "She made me reason with her logically," Landrau recalls. "The tumor grew when I stopped chemo and she showed it to me on the mammogram. So after two months, I went back to chemo."

But that wasn't the end of Landrau's struggles. After completing the rigorous chemotherapy regimen, Love scheduled her for a lumpectomy. The night before the operation, Landrau called and said she was too afraid to go through with the surgery.

"Dr. Love said okay and gave me two weeks to get ready. She calmly helped me through my fears. She's a very special doctor," says Landrau.

Love says she's not angered by patients who want to try alternative therapies: "There's no question there's a real mind-body connection. The danger is using any one therapy to the exclusion of all others.

"With surgery, radiation therapy and chemo, we're trying to get rid of the large number of cancer cells, so the immune system can take care of itself. Many alternative therapies boost the immune system, so it makes sense to combine the two methods. And the macrobiotic diet is not well-tested, but it makes sense that a diet low in animal fat could improve the treatment of cancer. But it should be combined with conventional treatment.

"I tell patients the important thing is to make a package deal that combines the methods they like, and to be sure to include everything: prayer is probably as viable as diet or anything else."

Landrau's choice of a lumpectomy over a mastectomy is a common one in Love's office.

"Ninety percent of my patients have lumpectomy and radiation, and if they choose mastectomy, they often have immediate reconstruction," Love explains.

However, NABCO cites a 1985 study conducted by Dr. Bernard Fisher of the University of Pittsburgh School of Medicine who determined that, nationwide, only 30% of the women eligible for lumpectomies choose that procedure over mastectomies.

Says a NABCO spokesperson: "Dr. Sue Love's experience is very unusual. It shows she's in a very sophisticated medical community."

Love points to an Italian study that showed no difference in survival rates between patients with lumpectomies and those with mastectomies.

"But the American doctors didn't believe it," she says. "Now there's been an American study that shows the same thing—no difference in survival between lumpectomies with radiation versus radical mastectomies. Now the question is, 'Do you always have to use radiation?'"

Love is currently conducting a study with Boston's Joint Center for Radiation Therapy on the use of lumpectomy without radiation in negative-lymph-node women. It's an ongoing study with 50 patients so far, but many more are needed. They plan to follow these patients for some 15 to 20 years and won't have preliminary results for five years.

Silen at Beth Israel agrees with Love about the benefits of lumpectomies:

"The doctors can twist it anyway they want with body English and the way they explain the options. There are still physicians who believe the gold-standard treatment is a radical mastectomy, yet no studies have confirmed that."

But then again, Love is always pushing the boundaries of "standard treatments"—asking why and why not at every turn. It was these types of questions that first drew her into science as a child, when she took biology and physiology courses.

Her strong character may have been molded by her unusual childhood that began in New Jersey, where she was the oldest of five children. Her father, who worked for a large corporation, was transferred to Puerto Rico when Love was in the seventh grade. And due to another family move, Love spent her high school years in Mexico.

"I think there's a real advantage to growing up in other parts of the world. You realize that there's not only one way to live, and you realize what it's like to be in the minority," she says. "It makes you strong in a way, especially to do that during your high school years. My parents never really pushed us or anything, but all of us have turned out to be independent."

Indeed, it was Love's natural sense of adventure and her love of science and teaching that led her to study medicine. When she spent time in college working for the Red Cross in Latin America, it became clear to her that she would become a doctor.

However, Love didn't intend to specialize in breast surgery. She began her career as a general surgeon until she realized that women with breast cancer wanted to be treated by women doctors: "I found I made the most difference in breast surgery. Women liked women doctors—felt they had more sensitivity. So I saw lots of women. At Dana-Farber, I was seeing 90% breast cases and got more interested in it.

"It seems to me that women think differently from men. It's hard for a man to understand breast lumps and what it's like to face a mastectomy. I think that's where I can make a difference.

Later, walking down the hall to see her next patient, Love says: "If you can explain things, it takes away fear. Women are better at explaining these things than men are, because I think women spend more time empathizing and are socialized to talk more openly. And lots of men don't want to take the time."

Love says she has a male physician friend who's always able to take new patients immediately, rather than have them wait months, and who sees several more patients a day than Love can ever fit in.

"I asked him how he does it, how he could be seeing so many patients. And he said, 'Susan, you talk to the patients too much.'"

Leona Mendelbaum and her husband are sitting in the waiting room. "I've come to Dr. Love to get a second opinion," she says quietly. "I'm not happy with what my physician in New York told me, and I did some checking and Dr. Love has an excellent reputation."

Her doctor in New York told her she had a precancerous condition and recommended a mastectomy as a preventive measure; another doctor told her to do nothing. Mendelbaum says there must be an alternative.

In the examining room, Mendelbaum tells Love she was having strange discomfort in her breasts before she went for an exam. Her doctor found a cyst, aspirated it, found atypical cells, and called it lobular carcinoma *in situ*.

Love says, "We don't consider that cancer. And later I'll explain everything you ever wanted to know about lobular carcinoma *in situ*."

She gets a history from Mendelbaum, about the births of her four children. Then, she asks the patient to put her hands on her hips, her arms up, her arms together, and to lean forward. "You have a nice matched set of ribs," she says, making Mendelbaum laugh. "Look, you know what you have here. Feel that line, that dimple. It's an irritated vein. That's not bad at all. Just interesting."

She stands facing Mendelbaum, puts her hands on the woman's shoulders, looks her in the eyes, and says, "It's nothing to worry about."

Mendelbaum smiles gratefully and the exam is over. Back in the office, Mendelbaum confesses that she's very worried about having cancer. Love begins her lecture, the one she gives to all new patients. She holds up Mendelbaum's mammogram film and explains, "The breast is a milk gland with two parts to it: lobules and ducts that carry the milk. Everything that happens in the breast happens in the ducts or the lobules . . .

"Lobular carcinoma *in situ* is too many cells in these lobules. It doesn't cause lumps, and it's not detected on mammograms, either. What this is is just a marker that says this woman has a 1% higher chance of getting cancer each year, or 30% in 30 years. It's the same as if your mom had it, and now we should watch you carefully."

At these moments, Love is a teacher, clear and succinct in her explanations: "And there's two school of thoughts about how to treat it. At Sloan-Kettering, they see this and say, 'Take both breasts off to prevent it from turning into cancer.' But if only 30% of women will get cancer, this means you'll take the breasts off of 70% of the women for no reason.

"But over at Columbia, the doctors say, 'Just watch these women. They don't need a mastectomy.' A researcher there says that of the patients he's followed with this condition, no one ever died of breast cancer.

"So the choices are either take off both the breasts to be 100% sure you never get breast cancer, or wait and watch it. And if it appears, find it early, and do a lumpectomy.

And there is a 1 percent chance you'll get a cancer so aggressive we wouldn't find it in time. But that's the same chance any woman has of getting cancer."

Love says gently, "I think you'll be fine. I can follow you here, or you can go back to your first doctor, whatever you're comfortable doing."

Mendelbaum pauses, takes a long deep breath and smiles at the doctor.

"I feel very comfortable with you. You're a woman and can offer me a woman's perspective. I'd rather come to you."

Ω

Breast Cancer: The Environmental Connection
by Rita Arditti and Tatiana Schreiber

Today in the United States, we live in the midst of a cancer epidemic. One out of every three people will get some form of cancer and one out of four will die from it. Cancer is currently the second leading cause of death; by the year 2000, it will likely have become the primary cause of death. It is now more than two decades since the National Cancer Act was signed, yet the treatments offered to cancer patients are the same as those offered 50 years ago: surgery, radiation, and chemotherapy (or slash, burn, and poison, as they are called bitterly by both patients and increasingly disappointed professionals). And in spite of sporadic optimistic pronouncements from the cancer establishment, survival rates for the three main cancer killers—lung, breast, and colo-rectal cancer—have remained virtually unchanged.

In the '60s and '70s, environmental activists and a few scientists emphasized that cancer was linked to environmental contamination, and their concerns began to have an impact on public understanding of the disease. In the '80s and '90s, however, with an increasingly conservative political climate and concerted efforts on the part of industry to play down the importance of chemicals as a cause of cancer, we are presented with a new image of cancer. Now it is portrayed as an individual problem that can only be overcome with the help of experts and, then, only if one

has the money and know-how to recruit them for one's personal survival efforts. This emphasis on personal responsibility and lifestyle factors has reached absurd proportions. People with cancer are asked why they "brought this disease on themselves" and why they don't work harder at "getting well."

While people with cancer should be encouraged not to fall into victim roles and to do everything possible to strengthen their immune systems (our primary line of defense against cancer), it seems that the sociopolitical and economic dimensions of cancer have been pushed completely out of the picture. "Blaming the victim" is a convenient way to avoid looking at the larger environmental and social issues that form individual experiences. Here we want to talk about environmental links to cancer in general and to breast cancer in particular, the kinds of research that should be going on, why they're not happening, and the political strategies needed to turn things around.

Extensive evidence exists to indicate that cancer *is* an environmental disease. Even the most conservative scientists agree that approximately 80 percent of all cancers are in some way related to environmental factors. Support for this view relies on four lines of evidence: (1) dramatic differences in the incidences of cancer between communities—incidences of cancer among people of a given age in different parts of the world can vary by a factor of ten to a hundred; (2) changes in the incidence of cancer (either lower or higher rates) in groups that migrate to a new country; (3) changes in the incidence of particular types of cancer with the passage of time; and (4) the actual identification of the specific causes of certain cancers (such as the case of beta-naphthylamine, responsible for an

From *Sojourner: The Women's Forum*, (December, 1992). Copyright © 1992 by Sojourner, Inc. Reprinted by permission.

Rita Arditti is a biologist, a woman with breast cancer, and a founding member of the Project. She is also an editor of *Issues in Reproductive and Genetic Engineering—A Journal of International Feminist Analysis*.
Tatiana Schreiber is the editor of the *Resist* newsletter and a freelance journalist.

epidemic of bladder cancer among dye workers employed at du Pont factories). Other well-known environmentally linked cancers are lung cancer, linked to asbestos, arsenic, chromium, bischloromethyl ether, mustard gas, ionizing radiation, nickel, polycyclic hydrocarbons in soot, tar, oil, and of course, smoking; endometrial cancer, linked to estrogen use; thyroid cancer, often the result of childhood irradiation; and liver cancer, linked to exposure to vinyl chloride.

The inescapable conclusion is that if cancer is largely environmental in origin, it is largely preventable.

Our Environment Is a Health Hazard

"Environment" as we use it here includes not only air, water, and soil, but also our diets, medical procedures, and living and working conditions. That means that the food we eat, the water we drink, the air we breathe, the radiation to which we are exposed, where we live, what kind of work we do, and the stress that we suffer—these are responsible for at least 80 percent of all cancers. For instance, under current EPA regulations as many as 60 cancer-causing pesticides can legally be used to grow the most commonly eaten foods. Some of these foods are allowed to contain 20 or more carcinogens, making it impossible to measure how much of each substance a person actually consumes. As Rachel Carson wrote in Silent Spring in 1962, "This piling up of chemicals from many different sources creates a total exposure that cannot be measured. It is meaningless, therefore, to talk about the 'safety' of any specific amount of residues." In other words, our everyday food is an environmental hazard to our health.

Recently, a study on the trends in cancer mortality in industrialized countries has revealed that while stomach cancer has been steadily declining, brain and other central-nervous- system cancers, breast cancer, multiple myeloma, kidney cancer, non-Hodgkin's lymphoma, and melanoma have increased in persons aged 55 and older. Given this context, it is not extreme to suspect that breast cancer, which has reached epidemic proportions in the United States, may be linked to environmental ills. This year, estimates are that 180,000 women will develop breast cancer and 46,000 will die from it. In other words, in the coming year, nearly as many women will die from breast cancer as there were American lives lost in the entire Vietnam War. Cancer is the leading cause of death among women aged 35 to 54, with about a third of these deaths due to breast cancer. Breast cancer incidence data meet three of the four lines of reasoning linking it to the environment: (1) the incidence of breast cancer between communities can vary by a factor of seven; (2) the risk for breast cancer among populations that have migrated becomes that of their new residence within a generation, as is the case for Japanese women who have migrated to the United States; and (3) the incidence of breast cancer in the United States has swelled from one in twenty in 1940 to one in eight in the '90s.

A number of factors have been linked to breast cancer; a first blood relative with the disease, early onset of menstruation, late age at first full-term pregnancy, higher socioeconomic status, late menopause, being Jewish, etc. However, for the overwhelming majority (70 to 80 percent) of breast cancer patients, their illness is not clearly linked to any of these factors. Research suggests that the development of breast cancer probably depends on a complex interplay among environmental exposures, genetic predisposition to the disease, and hormonal activity.

Research on the actual identification of causal factors, however, is given low priority and proceeds at a snail's pace. We still don't know, for example, the effects of birth control pills and the hormone replacement therapy routinely offered to menopausal women. Hormonal treatments are fast becoming the method of choice for the treatment of infertility, while we know nothing about their long-range effects. And the standard addition of hormones in animal feed means that all women (and men) are exposed to hormone residues in meat. Since there is general consensus that estrogen somehow plays a role in the development of breast cancer, hormonal interventions (through food or drugs) are particularly worrisome.

A startling example of the lack of interest in the prevention of breast cancer is the saga of the proposed study on the supposed link between high-fat diets and breast cancer. The "Women's Health Trial," a fifteen-year study designed to provide conclusive data about the high fat-cancer link, was denied funding by the National Cancer Advisory Board despite having been revised to answer previous criticisms and despite feasibility studies indicating that a full-scale trial was worth launching. Fortunately, it now appears that the study will be part of the Women's Health Initiative, a $500-million effort that will look at women's health issues. This success story is a direct result of women's activism and pressures from women's health groups across the country.

But even if the high fat-breast cancer correlation is established, it is unlikely to fully explain how breast cancer develops. The breast is rich in adipose cells, and carcinogens that accumulate in these fat tissues may be responsible for inducing cancer rather than the fat itself or the fat alone. Environmental contamination of human breast milk with PCBs, PBBs and DDE (a metabolite of the pesticide DDT) is a widely acknowledged phenomenon. These fat-soluble substances are poorly metabolized and have a long half-life in human tissue. They may also interact with one another, creating an additive toxic effect, and they may carry what are called "incidental contaminants": compounds like dibenzofurans, dioxins, etc., each with its own toxic properties.

Among the established effects of these substances are: liver dysfunction, skin abnormalities, neurological and behavioral abnormalities, immunological aberrations, thyroid dysfunction, gastrointestinal disturbances, reproductive dysfunction, tumor growth, and enzyme induction. Serious concerns have been raised about the risks that this contamination entails for infants who are breast-fed. But what is outrageous in the discussion about human breast-milk poisoning is that little or no mention is made of the possible effects on the women themselves, particularly since it is known that most of these substances have *estrogenic* properties (that is, they behave like estrogen in the body). It is as if the women, whose breasts contain these carcinogens, do not exist. We witness the paradox of women being made invisible, even while their toxic breasts are put under the microscope.

The Pesticide Studies

Very recently, some scientists have at last begun to look at the chemical-breast cancer connection. In 1990, two Israeli scientists from Hebrew University's Hadassah School of Medicine, Elihu Richter and Jerry Westin, reported a surprising statistic. They found that Israel was the only country among 28 countries surveyed that registered a real drop in breast cancer mortality in the decade 1976 to 1986. This happened in the face of a worsening of all known risk factors, such as fat intake and age at first pregnancy. As Westin noted, "All and all, we expected a rise in breast cancer mortality of approximately 20 percent overall, and what we found was that there was an 8 percent drop, and in the youngest age group, the drop was 34 percent, as opposed to an expected 20 percent rise, so, if we put those two together, we are talking about a difference of about 50 percent, which is enormous."

Westin and Richter could not account for the drop solely in terms of demographic changes or improved medical intervention. Instead, they suspected it might have been related to a 1978 ban on three carcinogenic pesticides (benzene hexachloride, lindane, and DDT) that heavily contaminated milk and milk products in Israel. Prior to 1978, Westin said, "at least one of them [the three pesticides] was found in the milk here at a rate 100 times greater than it was in the U.S. in the same period, and in the worst case, nearly a thousand times greater." This observation led Westin and Richter to hypothesize that there might be a connection between the decrease in exposure following the ban and the decrease in breast cancer mortality. They believed the pesticides could have promoted enzymes that in turn increased the virulence of breast cancer in women. When the pesticides were removed from the diet, Westin and Richter speculated, there was a situation of much less virulent cancer and the mortality from breast cancer fell.

Westin and Richter are convinced that there is a critical need to increase awareness about environmental conditions and cancer. Health care clinicians, for example, could play an important role in the detection of potential exposures to toxic chemicals that might be missed in large studies. This is a refreshing view since it encourages individual physicians to ask questions about work environments, living quarters, and diet, the answers to which could provide important clues about the cancer–environment connection.

In the United States, only one study we know of has directly measured chemical residues in women who have breast cancer compared to those who do not. Dr. Mary Wolff, a chemist at New York's Mount Sinai School of Medicine, recently conducted a pilot study with Dr. Frank Falck (then at Hartford Hospital in Hartford, Connecticut) that was published in *The Archives of Environmental Health*. In this case-controlled study, Falck and Wolff found that several chemical residues from pesticides and PCBs were elevated in cases of malignant disease as compared to nonmalignant cases.

The study involved 25 women with breast cancer and the same number of women who had biopsies but did not have breast cancer. The results showed differences significant enough to interest the National Institute for Environmental Health Sciences, which will fund a larger study to look at the level of DDT and its metabolites in the blood samples of 15,000 women attending a breast cancer screening clinic in New York. A recent report just released by Greenpeace, entitled "Breast Cancer and the Environment: The Chlorine Connection," provides further evidence linking industrial chemicals to breast cancer.

In the United States, levels of pesticide residues in adipose tissue have been decreasing since the 1970s (following the banning of DDT and decreased use of other carcinogenic pesticides) while the breast cancer rate continues to rise. This observation would seem to contradict the pesticide hypothesis. However, it is important to remember that the chemicals could act differently at different exposure levels, they are unlikely to act alone, and the time of exposure may be important. For example, if a child is exposed during early adolescence, when breast tissue is growing rapidly, the result may be different than exposure later in life.

Radiation and Mammography

Another area that demands urgent investigation is the role of radiation in the development of breast cancer. It is widely accepted that ionizing radiation at high doses causes breast cancer, but low doses are generally regarded as safe. Questions remain, however, regarding the shape of the dose-response curve, the length of the latency period, and the importance of age at time of exposure. These questions are of great importance to women because of the emphasis on mammography for early detection. There is evidence that mammography screening reduces death from breast cancer in women aged 50 or older. However, Dr. Rosalie Bertell (director of the International Institute of Concern for Public Health, author of *No Immediate Danger: Prognosis for a Radioactive World* [1985] and well-known critic of the nuclear establishment) raises serious questions about mammography screening. In a paper entitled "Comments on Ontario Mammography Program," Bertell criticized a breast cancer screening program planned by the Ontario Health Minister in 1989. Bertell argued that the program, which would potentially screen

300,000 women, was a plan to "reduce breast cancer death by increasing breast cancer incidence."

Bertell's critique of mammography suggests that the majority of cancers that would have occurred in the group could have been detected by other means. A recent Canadian mammography study on 90,000 women looked at cancer rates between 1980 and 1988. Preliminary results show that for women aged 40 to 49, mammograms have no benefits and may indeed harm them: 44 deaths were found in the group that received mammograms and 29 in the control group. The study also suggests that for women aged 50 to 69, many of the benefits attributed to mammography in earlier studies "may have been provided by the manual breast exams that accompanied the procedure and not by the mammography," as Bertell noted in her paper. Not surprisingly, the study has been mired in controversy. As study director Dr. Anthony Miller remarked, "I've come up with an answer that people are not prepared to accept."

According to Bertell, the present breast cancer epidemic is a direct result of "above ground weapons testing" done in Nevada between 1951 and 1963, when 200 nuclear bombs were set off and the fallout dispersed across the country. Because the latency period for breast cancer peaks at about 40 years, this is an entirely reasonable hypothesis.

Other studies have looked at the effect of "low-level" radiation on cancer development. A study investigating the incidence of leukemia in southeastern Massachusetts found a positive association with radiation released from the Pilgrim nuclear power plant. (The study was limited to cases first diagnosed between 1978 and 1986.) In adult cases diagnosed before 1984, the risk of leukemia was almost four times higher for individuals with the greatest potential for exposure to the emissions of the plant. Other types of cancer take a greater number of years to develop, and there is no reason to assume that excessive radiation emission was limited to the 1978-to-1986 time frame. In other words, as follow-up studies continue, other cancers (including breast cancer) may also show higher rates.

The Surveillance Theory

Current theory supports the concept that cancerous mutations are a common phenomenon in the body of normal individuals and that the immune system intervenes before mutated cells can multiply. Known as the "surveillance" theory of cancer, the basic premise is that cancer can develop when the immune system fails to eliminate mutant cells. Carcinogenic mutations can be induced by radiation or chemicals, for instance, and if immunological competence is reduced at a critical time, the mutated cells can thrive and grow.

Given the apparent importance of the immune system in protecting us from cancer, we ought to be concerned not only with eliminating carcinogens in our environment but also with making certain that our immune systems are not under attack. Recent evidence that ultraviolet radiation depresses the immune system is therefore particularly

ominous. At a hearing on "Global Change Research: Ozone Depletion and Its Impacts," held in November 1991 by the Senate Committee on Commerce, Science, and Transportation, a panel of scientists reported that ozone depletion is even more serious than previously thought. According to the data, the ozone layer over the United States is thinning at a rate of 3 to 5 percent per decade, resulting in increased ultraviolet radiation that "will reduce the quantity and quality of crops, increase skin cancer, *suppress the immune system,* and disrupt marine ecosystems" [our emphasis]. (The report also states that a 10 percent decrease in ozone will lead to approximately 1.7 million additional cases of cataracts world-wide per year and at least 250,000 additional cases of skin cancer.) As the writers make chillingly clear, since this is happening literally over our heads, there is no place for us to run.

In addition, dioxin (an extremely toxic substance that has been building up steadily in the environment since the growth of the chlorinated-chemical industry following World War II) can produce alterations that disrupt the immune system. "Free radicals" created by exposure to low-level radiation can cause immune system abnormalities. In other words, our basic mechanisms of defense against cancer are being weakened by the chemical soup in which we are immersed.

It follows that an intelligent and long-range cancer-prevention strategy would make a clean environment its number one priority. Prevention, however, is given low priority in our national cancer agenda. In 1992, out of an almost $2 billion National Cancer Institute (NCI) budget, $132.7 million was spent on breast cancer research but only about 15 percent of that was for preventive research. Moreover, research on the cellular mechanism of cancer development, toward which much of the "prevention" effort goes, does not easily get translated into actual prevention strategies.

In his 1989 exposé of the cancer establishment, *The Cancer Industry,* Ralph Moss writes that until the late '60s, the cancer establishment presented the view that "cancer is … widely believed to consist of a hereditable, and therefore genetic," problem. That line of thinking is still with us but with added emphasis on the personal responsibility we each have for our cancers (smoking and diet) and little or no acknowledgement of the larger environmental context. In a chapter appropriately titled "Preventing Prevention," Moss provides an inkling of why this is so.

The close ties between industry and two of the most influential groups determining our national cancer agenda—the National Cancer Advisory Board and the President's Cancer Panel—are revealing. The chair of the President's Cancer Panel throughout most of the '80s, for example, was Armand Hammer, head of Occidental International Corporation. Among its subsidiaries is Hooker Chemical Company, implicated in the environmental disaster in Love Canal. In addition, Moss, formerly assistant director of public affairs at Memorial Sloan-Kettering Cancer Center (MSKCC), outlines the structure and affiliations of that institution's leadership. MSKCC is the world's largest private cancer center, and the picture that emerges borders on the surreal: in 1988, 32.7 percent of its board of overseers were tied to the oil, chemical and automobile industries; 34.6 percent were professional investors (bankers, stockbrokers, venture capitalists). Board members included top officials of drug companies—Squibb, Bristol-Myers, Merck—and influential members of the media—CBS, the *New York Times*, Warner's Communications, and *Reader's Digest*—as well as leaders of the $55-billion cigarette industry.

Moss's research leaves little doubt about the allegiances of the cancer establishment. Actual cancer prevention would require a massive reorganization of industry, hardly in the interest of the industrial and financial elites. Instead of preventing the generation of chemical and toxic waste, the strategy adopted by industry and government has been one of "management." But as Barry Commoner, director of the Center for the Biology of Natural Systems at Queens College in Brooklyn, New York, put it rather succinctly, "The best way to stop toxic chemicals from entering the environment is to not produce them."

Instead, the latest "prevention" strategy for breast cancer moves in a completely different direction. A trial has been approved that will test the effect of a breast cancer drug (an antiestrogen, tamoxifen) in a healthy population, with the hope that it will have a preventive effect. The trial will involve 16,000 women considered at high risk for breast cancer and will be divided into a control group and a tamoxifen group. The National Women's Health Network (a national public-interest organization dedicated solely to women and health) is unequivocal in its criticism of the trial. Adriane Fugh-Berman, a member of the Network board, wrote in its September/October 1991 newsletter, "In our view the trial is premature in its assumptions, weak in its hypothesis, questionable in its ethics and misguided in its public health ramifications." The criticisms center on the fact that tamoxifen causes liver cancer in rats and liver changes in all species tested and that a number of endometrial cancers have been reported among tamoxifen users. Fugh-Berman points out that approving the testing of a potent, hormonal drug in healthy women and calling that "prevention" sets a dangerous precedent. This drug-oriented trial symbolizes, in a nutshell, the paradoxes of short-sighted cancer-prevention strategies: more drugs are used to counteract the effect of previous exposures to drugs, chemicals or other carcinogenic agents. It is a vicious circle and one that will not be easily broken.

Cancer, Poverty, Politics

Though it is often said that affluent women are at higher risk for breast cancer, this disease is actually on the rise (both incidence and mortality) among African-American women, hardly an "affluent" population overall. The African-American Breast Cancer Alliance of Minnesota, organized in October 1990, has noted this steady increase and the limited efforts that have been made to reach African Americans with information and prevention strategies. People of color often live in the most polluted areas of this country, where factories, incinerators, garbage, and toxic waste are part of the landscape. Native American nations are particularly targeted by waste-management companies that try to take advantage of the fact that "because of the sovereign relationship many reservations have with the federal government, they are not bound by the same environmental laws as the states around them."

Poverty and pollution go hand in hand. The 1988 Greenpeace report *Mortality and Toxics Along the Mississippi River* showed that the "total mortality rates and cancer mortality rates in the counties along the Mississippi River were significantly higher than in the rest of the nation's counties" and that "the areas of the river in which public health statistics are most troubling have populations which are disproportionately poor and black." These are also the areas that have the greatest number of toxic discharges. Louisiana has the dubious distinction of being the state with the most reported toxic releases—741.2 million pounds a year. Cancer rates in the Louisiana section of the "Chemical Corridor" (the highly industrialized stretch of river between Baton Rouge and New Orleans) are among the highest in the nation. Use of the Mississippi River as a drinking-water source has been linked to higher than average rates of cancer in Louisiana. The rates of cancer of the colon, bladder, kidney, rectum, and lung all exceed national averages. Louisiana Attorney General William J. Guste, Jr., has criticized state officials who claimed that people of color and the poor *naturally* have higher cancer rates. You can't "point out race and poverty as cancer factors," said Guste, "without asking if poor people or blacks … reside in less desirable areas more heavily impacted by industrial emissions."

It follows that African-American women, living in the most contaminated areas of this country, would indeed be showing a disproportionate increase in breast cancer incidence. However, widespread epidemiological studies to chart such a correlation have not been undertaken. For instance, given the evidence implicating pesticides in the development of breast cancer, studies of migrant (and other) farm workers who have been exposed to such chemicals would seem imperative.

Women's groups around the country have started organizing to fight the breast cancer epidemic. A National Breast Cancer Coalition was founded in 1991. Its agenda is threefold: to increase the funding for research, to organize, and to educate. All of the recently organized groups consider prevention a priority, and one of their tasks will undoubtedly entail defining what effective prevention really means. In Massachusetts, the Women's Community Cancer Project, which defines itself as a "grassroots organization created to facilitate changes in the current medical, social, and political approaches to cancer, particularly as they affect women," has developed a Women's Cancer Agenda to be presented to the federal government and the NCI. Several demands of the agenda address prevention and identification of the causes of cancer. The group has received endorsements of its agenda from over 50 organizations and individuals working in the areas of environmental health, women's rights, and health care reform and is continuing to gather support. This effort will provide a networking and organizing tool, bringing together different constituencies in an all-out effort to stop the cancer epidemic.

Cancer *is* and needs to be seen as a political issue. The women's health movement of the '70s made that strikingly clear and gave us a road map to the politics of women's health. In the '80s, AIDS activists have shown the power of direct action to influence research priorities and treatment deliveries. In the '90s, an effective cancer-prevention strategy demands that we challenge the present industrial practices of the corporate world, based solely on economic gains for the already powerful, and that we insist on an end to the toxic discharges that the government sanctions under the guise of "protecting our security." According to Lenny Siegel, research director of the Military Toxic Network, the Pentagon has produced more toxic waste in recent years—between 400,000 tons and 500,000 tons annually—than the five largest multinational chemical companies combined.

Indeed, if we want to stop not only breast cancer but all cancers, we need to think in global terms and to build a movement that will link together groups that previously worked at a respectful distance. At a worldwide level, the Women's World Congress for a Healthy Planet (attended by over 1500 women from 92 countries from many different backgrounds and perspectives) presented a position paper, Agenda 21, at the 1992 United Nations Earth Summit conference in Brazil. The paper articulates a women's position on the environment and sustainable development that stresses pollution prevention, economic justice, and an end to conflict resolution through war and weapons production, probably the greatest force in destroying the environment.

On February 4, 1992, a group of 65 scientists released a statement at a press conference in Washington, D.C., entitled "Losing the 'War against Cancer'—Need for Public Policy Reforms," which calls for an amendment to the National Cancer Act that would "re-orient the mission and priorities of the NCI to cancer causes and prevention." The seeds of this movement have been sown. It is now our challenge to nourish this movement with grassroots research, with demonstrations, and with demands that our society as a whole take responsibility for the environmental contamination that is killing us.

Author's note: Many thanks to the women of the Women's Community Cancer Project in Cambridge, Massachusetts, for their help and support. A longer version of this article with complete footnotes and references appeared in the Resist *newsletter (May/June 1992). Copies of the issue (which includes the Women's Cancer Agenda) are available from: Resist, One Summer St., Somerville, MA 02143. Send $1.00 for handling.*

Ω

♀

Ten Years of Self-Help Achievement

Interview with Mary Lou Ballweg,
President and Co-founder Endometriosis Association

by Carolyn Keith

The Endometriosis Association, headquartered in Milwaukee, WI, started 10 years ago with its first support group meeting of eight women with endometriosis. From that base, a highly successful self-help women's health organization has grown. The Association now has almost ten thousand paid members, chapters and support groups all across North America, a unique research registry and research program, and highly acclaimed educational materials.

CK: How is the concept of self-help expressed currently in the Association?

ML: This organization , which has grown immensely, is run by a majority of women with endometriosis at every level. From top to bottom, the organization is run by women with the disease. Every chapter is run by women with the disease and the groups are started by women with the disease. Every so often a physician will want to start a chapter, but we will always get it started by women and then connect them to the supportive physician.

From *The Network News,* (March/April 1990). Copyright © 1990 by National Women's Health Network. Reprinted by permission.

Carolyn Keith was Health Education Coordinator at Bread & Roses Women's Health Clinic in 1980 when she and Mary Lou Ballweg started the Association. Carolyn is now involved in geriatric health concerns.

The research program includes a data registry (the only data registry in the world on endometriosis) that relies on reports from women. A rather radical thing that we've done is to take information from "patients" and compile solid data that serve as the basis for our work and for articles published in scientific journals. Through the Association, women have made a difference in the research and in what's known about the disease. The medical establishment has accepted this information because we have been very professional about how we've presented it. But it is really rather radical to have that kind of information and research come from lay people and we faced a lot of questioning about that when we started.

Another aspect of self help that is critical is by having a disease *in* you, you can put it all together in a way that no physician can—you *feel* it, you have the motivation, you have all the information and experience all in one body.

Modern medicine is so super-specialized. Particularly for endometriosis, I don't think we're going to get answers unless we cross specialties. *We* don't have territory to protect if it relates to the disease. I think one of the best examples of this is the work we did linking endometriosis and candidiasis (systemic yeast infection). That linkage points to the immune system. Now a few of the research studies on endometriosis are starting to evolve from the immunological side of it, a process that is starting to tie it together a little. The women experiencing these problems aren't tied to the professional "Bibles" that say this is the only way it can be. They commit medical heresy every day. And medical heresy is what's needed to break through some of these walls. Also, lay people can sometimes do things that medical people can't do.

CK: Such as?

ML: Well, for example, Dr. Billy Crook, who wrote THE YEAST CONNECTION, was at headquarters recently. He was talking about how to get the information about candidiasis out and how to get medical credibility. We were talking about what he could do, what doctors could do, what lay people could do. I really pushed him to help start lay groups. Lay groups can form a national, regional or local network and either create business or take business away from physicians. The medical establishment may pay lip service to science, but they live day-to-day with their business and their pocketbooks.

We've seen it in city after city where we get groups going—the physicians really start to treat women with endo a lot better. It's consumer power. When they start listening, they learn, and it just moves everything along a lot faster. Then you start to see a few of the little breakthrough research studies. For endometriosis, the studies really are just beginning, but at least it's starting to happen and it wouldn't have happened without the Association. The medical establishment would have been more than happy to do another 30 years of hormones and surgeries; drug companies could make millions and millions on new hormonal drugs that shut down the system, but that wouldn't get us anywhere. With the Association, we can force a direction. We can also benefit from some of the millions that are made by those drug companies if we can propose projects that we need to get done that we don't have money for and say, "Look drug company, you're making millions on women with endo, will you help us do this outreach?" This, I know, is a controversial point.

CK: It's like accepting *Playboy* money.

ML: It's not like *Playboy* money because I think *Playboy* money is dirty money made off the backs of women by hurting women. In contrast, the pharmaceutical companies have indeed made life tolerable. Danazol, when it first came out, scared the wits out of all of us. But danazol forestalled hysterectomy for so many thousands of women that, while it's not the answer or the cure, it's better than what we had before. Now the new GnRH (gonadotropin-releasing hormone) drugs will help a lot of women by buying more time to keep them from hysterectomy and surgical castration. So, I think it's ok money. They made their money on the drug, but I like to see some of it go back to help women.

FDA Approves Synarel

In mid-February, 1990, the FDA approved Synarel for treatment of endometriosis. It is the first GnRH drug approved for this condition. Synarel, which is administered as a nasal spray, acts to stop production of the hormones of the menstrual cycle. Although Synarel is not a cure for endometriosis, the Endometriosis Association welcomes FDA approval of the drug because it gives women another treatment option.

CK: So you've helped them to do that.

ML: Yes, I've helped them to do that. I was amazed when I added up the cost involved in our 1987 advertising campaign that was funded by a drug company. We advertised in 20 national magazines using full-page ads and several insertions. We reached many hundred thousand women and obviously educated many on endometriosis. That campaign alone cost more than all the funds that we've raised in the Association's operating budget in 10 years, over $1.3 million. So do we hurt women by taking that million plus? The project didn't mention their drug or their company, except for one line I added to the ad so that people wouldn't think that *we* had that kind of money because we depend on donations for other programs. I think it would have been really sad to miss that tremendous opportunity to educate all those women about the symptoms and maybe they'd get diagnosed earlier and they'd find the Association. But there are some people that would say, no, don't take any money like that.

CK: What do you see as the difference?

ML: First, our main operating budget comes from women with the disease and always has—over 80% from membership dues, literature sales, and donations from members. We use corporate contributions for special projects outside the main annual operating budget. Second, *we* propose projects, so these are things we want to do. Third, we maintain total control over the project and make that clear to the potential donor from the outset. In fact, I see us with far more control over our special projects than many nonprofits have after they've bent themselves to fit philanthropic proposal guidelines.

For instance, now we really have our hearts set on programs to reach black women and teen women with endo. We are just really tired of what's happening to these 15- and 16-year-olds with severe problems. They need help and nobody is helping them. It's going to take some fairly serious money. A drug company can see that a 15-year-old with endometriosis is perhaps their future market. That's the kind of project that we don't have the money for now, but maybe we can get. And it's *our* project. So if somebody has the money to give, and the money might even have been made from women with endometriosis, my word, why not use it.

While you're being pure, somebody else out there right now is screaming in pain or crawling to the bathroom. I think that's part of what makes a difference—that the Association is real women with real pain with real disease. We become practical.

CK: This started out as a support group—a self-help support group—wow, when did we do that?

ML: January 1980. Eight women met on January 14. By summer, I think we were up to 50 or 60 women. In August we got the yellow brochure ["What is Endometriosis?"] out. Then, we helped the women who found us by word-of-mouth or through feminist publications. Then they asked, "How do we do it out here in San Francisco or New York?" You sent out materials for starting chapters and then

we had to develop guidelines for who's officially affiliated with us, how do we handle dues, etc. Pretty soon there was too much work and we had to get more staff, and more staff . . .

The need for the Association will probably continue for a long time, even if we are lucky enough to find a cure (which I don't think is going to be soon . . .). But even if we were that lucky, we'd have to work through the Association or with women who have a serious vested interest in this disease of the most female of functions. What's really at the heart of endometriosis and the awful attitudes about it and toward women with it are cultural taboos about menstruation and female sexuality and infertility and what it means to be a female.

Those kinds of attitudes come out every single day in the Association. Today on the way home I was reading a letter from a woman who has severe throbbing pain in her clitoris from the endometriosis. She has been insulted time and time again by physicians who, of course, have said kind of what you would expect: "It's because you don't have a sexually fulfilling relationship," or "You're hung up," or whatever. Endo is those kinds of experiences. The attitudes of people are really appalling. Men who think the only kind of sex is intercourse; women who think they're not women because they can't have babies; the reluctance to talk about *normal* menstruation, much less painful menstruation. A woman with endometriosis has to deal with all of this because her life often eventually comes to a screeching halt because of the disease. This woman is at the forefront and the cutting edge of changing attitudes. It's also critical to all women who don't have the disease that we do what we're doing because we're out here saying, "Look, to be female is not to have pain. To have pain with your periods is a disease." I think our medical establishment and main culture tell us that our normal bodily functions are goofed up just because we're female.

Ω

A B Cs of Immunology
by Susan Elliott

We are all familiar with the symptoms of the 'flu—fever, aches and pains, exhaustion, a general feeling of being 'under the weather.' Most of us don't give the causes of all this misery a second thought. We just want to feel better.

From *Healthsharing*, Spring 1989, pp. 17–19. Copyright © 1989 by Healthsharing. Reprinted by permission.

Susan Elliott worked for a number of years in immunology research and is a member of Women Healthsharing.

What many of us don't know is that these symptoms are the signs of a competently functioning immune system working to rid our body of an infectious agent. The fact that we feel bad now probably means that we will feel better soon.

Our immune system has been getting a lot of press lately. AIDS, increasing numbers of immunological disorders and diseases like 'Total Allergy Syndrome' or 20th Century Disease are all in the news. Other diseases like multiple sclerosis, arthritis and diabetes in which our immune systems attack our own bodies also seem to be more prevalent. And a chronic illness which occurs after infection with the Epstein-Barr virus is so common now that it has been termed the 'Yuppie flu.' To understand what our immune system is and how it functions, we need to become familiar with the language of immunology and the processes that occur when we are exposed to infection.

Our Immune System

Our immune system is a complex organization of cells and organs located throughout our bodies, connected by chemical messengers that travel in our blood and other body fluids. Unlike other body systems, our immune system does not reside in specific organs. Instead, it is made up of a diffuse network of white blood cells and chemical messengers. In a very general sense, our immune system can be divided into two distinct components—humoral immunity and cellular immunity.

Humoral immunity refers to antibacterial substances known as antibodies in the 'humors' as the ancient Greeks called the bloodstream. Circulating antibodies are our first line of defence against infection. They attach themselves to the infective agent, either killing it outright or making it possible for white blood cells to kill it. However, there are so many different infective agents that we cannot possibly have enough types of antibody to destroy every potential infection. When our bodies identify a new virus or bacteria or a foreign protein, in the case of an organ transplant, other components of the immune system are alerted and kick in to make new antibodies that are specifically directed against this particular threat to our health.

Cellular immunity refers to the different kinds of white blood cells that become involved as the second line of defense against infection. Some of them can destroy the infection immediately, others pass the word on to even more potent cells that rapidly reproduce themselves and flock to the site of the infection.

Communication between defense cells is essential to orchestrate a response to an infection. Our immune cells communicate by means of chemicals called lymphokines that are produced by some of them and recognized by all the others.

Defense Cells

Our blood is composed of red blood cells or erythrocytes (which carry oxygen to our tissues), platelets (which aid in clotting) and white blood cells or leukocytes (which are our defense cells). Leukocytes include a variety of cells: macrophages, lymphocytes, neutrophils, eosinophils and basophils. One of the symptoms of an infection is often an increase in the total number of white blood cells in the blood or leukocytosis. When there is a reduction in the number, as in AIDS, it is termed leukopenia.

The macrophages or 'cell-eaters' are the largest of the leukocytes. They make up only about eight per cent of the total number of leukocytes but are extremely important nonetheless. Some of them congregate in the liver and the spleen where they eat up old red blood cells, viruses or chemical pollutants. Others remain in the blood ready to engulf any invader. When macrophages spot an infection such as a virus particle, they send out a lymphokine called interleukin-1 which alerts other defense cells to spring into action. Interleukin-1 causes the body temperature to rise giving us a fever. This further stimulates the immune system since all the cells work more effectively at a slightly higher than normal body temperature. Interleukin-1 also breaks down muscle fibres to release needed nutrients, resulting in aching muscles and fatigue.

The smallest of the immune cells but the most diversified is the lymphocyte. Lymphocytes comprise about 25 per cent of the total number of leukocytes. There are two types of these cells, B-lymphocytes and T-lymphocytes.

B-lymphocytes (also referred to as B-cells) are formed in the bone marrow. When they have matured, they move out and live in the blood or in one of the areas of lymphatic tissue (like the tonsils) scattered around the body. They produce antibodies 'on demand' against infections. Once a B-cell receives information about what kind of antibody to produce, it churns out quantities of that particular antibody. It is now specialized and cannot make any other kind of antibody. As soon as the infection is destroyed this group of B-cells retires since their special antibody is no longer needed. A few stay on in the body serving as 'memory' cells, ready to reproduce themselves if that same infective agent shows up again. This process is termed 'acquired immunity' and explains why a person who has had the virus causing chicken pox as a child will probably never get it again even if exposed to someone with the infection.

T-lymphocytes (also called T-cells) are named because they migrate from the bone marrow when newly formed to the thymus, an organ located behind the breastbone, above the heart. There they mature and specialize into the more than 10 types now recognized. They are identified by protein markers that appear on their surfaces, and which have been given numbers to distinguish them, hence the name 'T-4 lymphocytes' which have been featured in press reports about AIDS. T-lymphocytes have the ability to recognize hundreds of millions of different invaders, each one identifiable by its characteristic biochemical markers. T-lymphocytes are critical to the immune system because even if there are great numbers of B-lymphocytes around, without properly functioning T-cells our body can't mount an effective immune response and we will catch infections like pneumonia. Three of the more important T-cells are the 'Killer T-cells,' the 'Helper T-cells' and the 'Suppressor T-cells.'

Killer T-cells are activated by lymphokines to reproduce themselves and rush to the site of the infection. Their methods are different than the macrophages which engulf the invader and 'digest' it. Killer T-cells latch on to the invading cell and kill it by causing it to split open.

Helper T-cells direct other T-cells. When they come into contact with an invader or receive a chemical message from a macrophage, they stimulate other elements of the immune system to gear up. One helper cell can activate hundreds of other cells by releasing a lymphokine called interleukin-2. Interleukin-2 is thought to work by de-activating Suppressor T-cells which normally keep everything on hold and turn off the immune response once the infection is cleared up. By de-activating these cells, our immune process is set in motion and all the elements work together to destroy the infective agent. Helper T-cells of the T-4 category (the ones involved in AIDS) also produce chemicals called interferons which also work to regulate the immune response. Some interferons keep macrophages at the site of infection, others enhance killer cell activity and still others stimulate B-lymphocyte antibody production.

Suppressor T-cells turn off the defense cells as soon as the infection is cleared, to prevent the immune response from getting out of control. These are the cells that are thought to be defective in people with auto-immune disorders such as rheumatoid arthritis where a continuous immune response against the lining of the joints causes pain, swelling and eventual deformity.

Medium-sized cells called neutrophils make up 50 to 75 per cent of the leukocytes in our blood at any one time. Although capable of traveling throughout the body, neutrophils tend to remain in the blood. They migrate to areas of infection, exude chemicals that attract other cells and cause symptoms of inflammation such as swelling and pus formation. Like macrophages they can also engulf foreign matter but will only destroy it if it is packaged in a particular way. Neutrophils will only accept particles, for example, that have been attacked and surrounded by antibodies.

Cells responsible for allergic reactions normally make up only four percent or less of the total leukocytes. They are called eosinophils. They secrete chemicals called histamines which cause blood vessels to dilate, allowing other immune cells to get the area of infection quickly. Excess histamines are released when a person comes into contact with something she is allergic to. The result is often a runny nose and eyes and a constriction of bronchial smooth muscle in the lungs making breathing difficult. People with allergies have a higher count of eosinophils in their blood.

The least numerous of the leukocytes are the basophils. They make up less than .5 per cent of the total leukocytes. They also produce histamines and are found in increased numbers in certain infections like chicken pox, smallpox and chronic sinus congestion. Although they constitute only .5 per cent of the leukocytes, their total number in an average person with six litres of blood is approximately 200 million.

Antigens and Antibodies

An antigen is any substance either from outside our body ('foreign') or part of our body ('self') that triggers an immune response. Examples of foreign antigens are viruses, bacteria or pollen. Self antigens are portions of our own bodies like the joint lining that is attacked in rheumatoid arthritis.

An antibody is a Y-shaped chain protein made by B-lymphocytes to match each antigen. B-lymphocyte antibodies are manufactured as a response to an invading organism. For example, when a virus enters the body, B-lymphocytes go into high gear and produce custom-made antibodies which are only able to bind to that particular strain of the virus. Sometimes antibodies can inactivate an infection themselves, but more commonly they attach to the infective agent and make it 'visible' to other cells like macrophages or killer T-cells which then destroy it.

Antibodies travel in the blood and other body fluids when not attaching themselves to antigens. They are transferred to the fetus during gestation giving the baby a temporary 'passive immunity' against diseases the mother has been exposed to in the past. Unfortunately this type of immunity is short-lived and by the time the child is about six months old she must begin to depend on her own developing immune system which produces antibodies as she is exposed to infections. If a very young or premature infant develops a serious infection, it is sometimes possible to boost the child's immunity by giving an injection of gamma globulin, an antibody which has been separated from the blood and purified.

Organs of the Immune System

Even though there is no one 'immune organ,' a number of organs are important to the immune system. These are the bone marrow, the thymus, the spleen and the lymph nodes.

Blood cells are formed in the bone marrow which is the spongy substance found in the centre of our bones. Leukocytes destined to become T-lymphocytes travel from here to the thymus where they mature and specialize. The thymus also releases hormones into the body which affect the cells of the immune system. The thymus itself is very sensitive to stress hormones released by other organs in our bodies. When we are under a lot of stress our thymus can shrink and thus leave us vulnerable to infections.

The spleen is located behind our lower ribs on the left side of the body. It is normally the size of a fist but in certain immune disorders it enlarges dramatically. Before birth, blood cells are formed in the spleen, but after birth the site of production moves to the bone marrow and the spleen is no longer essential for life. Vast numbers of leukocytes congregate in the millions of tiny blood vessels of the spleen. They are on alert for any infection in the blood that passes by. They also get rid of old unwanted red blood cells and debris. Occasionally they become overzealous and start destroying healthy red blood cells causing anemia. When this happens the spleen is often surgically removed. People who have had a 'splenectomy' for this reason or because their spleen was badly damaged in an accident may be slightly more susceptible to infection, but for the most part they live normal lives since immune cells are found in so many other parts of our bodies.

Lymph nodes are small dense structures up to an inch in length, found all over our bodies. There are a number of them in the armpit and along the chest, all interconnected. They contain large numbers of lymphocytes which trap infections present in body fluids other than the blood. Because they are interconnected, cancer cells can often spread quickly through them which is why the ones on the chest wall and in the armpit are sometimes removed during mastectomy. Like the spleen, they are a part of a larger system and are not essential to life.

Even though our understanding of the immune system is rapidly increasing, there is still a great deal that is unknown. As researchers uncover more of the mysteries of the immune system we can only marvel at the design and functioning of one of the most intricate and vital parts of our bodies.

Ω

Chronic Fatigue Syndrome
Searching for the Answers
by Andrea Rudner

California, March 1984: Jan Montgomery set off down Interstate 80 for a business meeting in Marin County. But before she could complete her mile-long journey, a sudden feverishness and weakness overcame her, making driving impossible. She pulled over and called a friend to rescue her.

For the next few years intense muscle pains, vertigo, light sensitivity, swollen glands, severe fatigue, and low-grade fevers would be a constant part of her life. "Sometimes, I would be so weak I had difficulty moving the muscles in my chest to breathe," she says. She had to quit her job, and then the ultimate frustration: she couldn't find a doctor who would believe her. "I must have gone to ten. When my lymph glands were swollen, one said, 'Maybe you're wearing the wrong bra size.' Another said, 'Maybe you are allergic to your pillow.'"

Her story is typical of those who suffer from the misunderstood malady—chronic fatigue syndrome (CFS). The illness, previously known as chronic Epstein-Barr virus (EBV) or chronic mononucleosis, not only causes unrelenting fatigue, but often brings on an array of incapacitating neurological and cognitive symptoms. Heated debate revolves around its cause—viral, genetic, or environmental—and whether it is one disease or many. But there is agreement that the body's immune system is involved. The hostility, disbelief, accusations of malingering, and insistent referrals for psychiatric care encountered by CFS sufferers have spawned a growing network of support and advocacy groups that are publicizing the message that CFS is a social, economic, and political issue; at the heart is society's attitude toward chronic illness, women, and women's health.

But what exactly is this illness? Does being tired mean you have chronic fatigue syndrome?

Not necessarily. There are numerous causes of fatigue. Many exhausted women sorely need support, relief, and time to themselves, but this is a societal problem, not an illness. Fatigue is one of the most common reasons people visit a health professional, and CFS is not usually the culprit. Many other conditions, such as cardiovascular disease, cancer, and multiple sclerosis, also cause fatigue. Actually, fatigue is only one of a constellation of symptoms that make up CFS. They include a flu-like malaise, and cognitive and neurologic abnormalities. To complicate the diagnosis, not everyone has the most severe form of the illness—an almost complete incapacitation with constant physical pain. Some people have mild symptoms that require only a reduction in activity level, not complete bed rest. (See box on next page.)

Even the use of the word "fatigue" in the name is a source of controversy. Doctors working with the federal Centers for Disease Control (CDC) initially saw fatigue as a common denominator, but activists have renamed the condition chronic fatigue immune dysfunction syndrome (CFIDS). The CDC name is akin to "calling diabetes chronic thirst syndrome," says Marya Grambs, the co-director, with Jan Montgomery, of the CFIDS Foundation in San Francisco. "'CFS' is a terrible name," agrees Dr. Walter Gunn, principal CFS investigator at the CDC until last year. "Put the words 'chronic' and 'fatigue' together, and you have a truly demeaning label."

From *Ms. Magazine,* May/June 1992, pp. 33–36. Copyright © 1992 by Ms. Magazine. Reprinted by permission.

Andrea Rudner is a science, health, and technology writer and political activist living in New York City.

Women are not the only sufferers—though they do make up the vast majority (and of these, many diagnosed with CFS are middle-class European Americans). Men constitute about 20 percent of the adult cases in the U.S.; the caseload of Dr. David Bell of Cambridge, Massachusetts, who specializes in pediatric CFS, is equally split between girls and boys. Still, many cases may be missed, and poor people who rely on local emergency rooms may never be properly diagnosed. Public concern about the syndrome is mounting; the CFIDS Association in North Carolina, the country's largest support group, logs about 7,000 calls per month on its information lines.

The syndrome has been identified in several countries. Researchers across the globe believe it has been cropping up for years in different guises: "febricula" and "neurasthenia," terms used to describe "nervous disorders" afflicting nineteenth-century women; a postpolio viral epidemic in 1934 (the "cure" was hysterectomy—it didn't work); "Iceland Disease," striking 6 percent of the population in a region of Iceland in 1948; "Royal Free Disease" in England, where CFS is now known as myalgic encephalomyelitis; and "Soldiers Disease" among troops at war.

The high proportion of women among people with CFS—and their mistreatment by the medical system—has led many to view CFS as a political issue. Over the last decade most physicians consulted by women experiencing the puzzling CFS symptoms assigned the disorder to the realm of women's imaginary illnesses. "Because my body didn't respond to their treatments, they became extremely short-tempered and implied that *I* was doing something wrong," relates Yvonne Eastman, a single mother of two who was initially misdiagnosed with pneumonia.

Members of other marginalized groups can experience special difficulties when dealing with the medical establishment. "Lesbians cannot afford any medical ambiguity because it will immediately be used as a sign of emotional deviance, even in this day," says Joan Nestle, co-founder of the Lesbian Herstory Archives in New York City who was "ambushed" with CFS in the late 1970s. And women aren't the only ones being disbelieved, according to Dr. Bell: "Kids are told they're just school phobic."

But in 1984 a turning point occurred. At Incline Village, Nevada, and two nearby towns, hundreds of people became ill with the same set of mysterious symptoms. Chronic fatigue syndrome finally made the news. In 1988 the CDC began to research CFS. CDC funding and the National Institutes of Health's (NIH) formation of three new cooperative research centers last year brings total federal allocation to CFS research to $4.7 million. Critics charge that public funding is inappropriately low for what may be a widespread and growing problem.

Naomi Weisstein, a research psychologist, writer, and longtime feminist activist who has been sick with CFS for 12 years, attributes some of the foot-dragging to the fact that CFS has primarily affected women. "The medical profession assumes women are just a kind of permanently sick people, and there's no reason to study anything as trivial as women being tired, because allegedly they want attention and don't want to do housework."

* * *

So what is going on in the bodies of people with CFS? Immunologists have theorized that the immune systems of people with CFS are in a state of constant excitement, or "up-regulation." Normally, the body orchestrates the demise of viral and bacterial intruders by deploying cellular and chemical protection: macrophages, natural killer cells, B cells, T cells, and cytokines. The chemical cytokines cause the flu symptoms that make people feel sick. But when the virus is vanquished, the body sends out a cut signal. People with CFS have abnormally high levels of cytokines, which would explain the constant flu symptoms. For them, it could be that the crucial turnoff signal never arrives.

The cause of all this activity is yet to be discovered. Virologists are hot on the trails of several viral culprits. "There's a big search on for *the* virus, but I would caution that we shouldn't be narrowing down to a single virus theory," says Nancy Klimas, an immunologist who has studied CFS for several years. Most controversial has been Dr. Elaine DeFreitas' reports of retrovirus-fragment sightings; AIDS is also thought to be caused by a retrovirus, prompting unfounded speculation about a possible connection.

Other intriguing theories are emerging from research labs. Reports out of Ann Arbor, Michigan, hint at something awry with a complex brain-adrenal hormone feedback loop. In January, researchers used magnetic resonance imaging (MRI) and discovered brain abnormalities in 78 percent of CFS patients studied. But MRI scans aren't recommended as a diagnostic tool until further studies are completed. Toxins and pollutants in the environment have been blamed for autoimmune diseases; they may also play a role in CFS.

Yet another group of researchers—a minority—steadfastly maintains that the cause of chronic fatigue syndrome is not fundamentally physical, noting what they say is the high incidence of psychiatric illness among people with the disorder. But CFS advocates don't buy it and charge the researchers with confusing cause and effect. "I have never been a depressed person ever, except after I developed severe CFS," says New Hampshire resident Lisa Millimet, who had CFS for 17 years and has recovered. Indeed, studies comparing blood, immunologic, and psychological profiles of clinically depressed people to those of people with CFS don't match. Also, only 50 percent of CFS patients display any evidence of depression, and most of that can be seen as a normal response to a severe illness. "An absolute requirement in the diagnosis of clinical depression is loss of interest in surroundings," says Paul Cheney, one of the Nevada doctors who originally helped bring the syndrome to national attention. "I see that relatively rarely in this disease. In fact, the opposite is the case."

Some CFS investigators go for a unified theory involving a range of viral, environmental, and genetic triggers. A California psychotherapist is currently investigating the incidence of CFS among survivors of child sexual abuse, theorizing that there may be a link. Another concern is whether the disease can be passed from one person to another. The San Francisco-based CFIDS Foundation suspects transmission, but at a low rate, and tells people with the syndrome to behave as if they had a cold and not to share food or eating utensils.

* * *

If you suspect that you or someone you know may have CFS, the first important thing to do is to find a health professional who is familiar with the disease. If that isn't financially or geographically feasible, the resource groups can supply articles for your health care provider (see page 332). Once CFS is diagnosed, the issue becomes treatment. Unfortunately, medical care remains stopgap and limited to an assortment of "anti" drugs—antipain medications, antifungal preparations, anti-depressants, and anti-inflammatories.

Only two drugs have received full clinical trials in the U.S., and one of them, acyclovir, had no effect. Ampligen, an antiviral drug used for people with AIDS, made an appearance on the CFS treatment scene through a chance encounter on a plane. The husband of a woman with CFS overheard a discussion about ampligen and AIDS, and guessed that it might be beneficial for people with CFS. After several patients received ampligen on an experimental "compassionate care" basis, they improved drastically. Their remarkable progress spurred a full clinically controlled study of the drug.

In the study, ampligen caused a significant abatement of symptoms in a subset of patients who had brain abnormalities combined with a sudden onset of the disorder. This research has been eagerly received in the chronic fatigue syndrome community, but the FDA still considers the drug experimental; though it was approved for "compassionate care" cases, the drug is almost impossible to obtain.

But patients reluctant to wait are exploring other options. Kudipressin, a liver extract, may have an antiviral effect, according to *CFIDS Treatment News*, of the CFIDS Foundation. Gamma globulin (a blood component that contains antibodies) injections are in common use and are moderately successful. Other medications being tried in the U.S. include Coenzyme Q-10 for muscle weakness and cardiac problems; vitamin B_{12} shots and magnesium injections for relief of general symptoms; and Klonopin and Zantac for sleep disorders and cognitive difficulties.

Many women have spent years sampling an assortment of traditional and nontraditional remedies. Millimet recalls thinking her condition was low blood sugar. She tried yoga and a macrobiotic diet, but didn't notice any significant improvement until she started taking spirulina, a kind of algae, "Maybe I was just in the right place to get better, but I started to have an interest in things again and my mind came back."

Not everyone can take these medications. New Yorker Kathleen Doherty was extraordinarily sensitive to most of the usual Western and non-Western treatments. "I had a dramatic negative reaction to acupuncture; it stimulated all my symptoms and it took about a year for me to recover," she says. "Meditation has turned out to be the most beneficial treatment for me." Others have found acupuncture to be helpful in alleviating sleep disorders, headaches, and muscle pain.

But these medications can run to hundreds of dollars a month, and health insurance policies don't cover experimental treatments. Chiropractic, massage, shiatsu, and kinesiology—body-based treatments—alleviate symptoms for some people. In Japan, CFS has been treated with some success using LEM and lentinan, derivatives of extracts from shiitake mushrooms.

There is danger here, though. Desperately ill people make excellent customers for unethical health practitioners and manufacturers. Homeopathy, the use of pills containing an infinitesimal dosage of various substances, is one controversial treatment. Some CFS patients say they've been helped, but others attribute any curative results to a placebo effect. Silver amalgam replacement is another disputed practice. Most of the reports of treatment success and failure are anecdotal—none but ampligen and acyclovir have been tested against a control group of people receiving a placebo. But it pays to be informed. "If you're playing chemistry set with your body, the treatment may be worse than the illness," warns Orvalene Prewitt, president of the National CFS Association in Kansas City.

Coping on a day-to-day basis is a continuing emotional and financial challenge. The help given by well-meaning friends and family can dwindle after years of the same old illness. Insurance companies, predictably, have created difficulties by routinely denying medical benefits, and disability compensation has been hard to come by. That's improved since the CDC published its case definition in 1988, but the companies still resist. "How can women, especially, afford it?" asks author Phyllis Chesler, who has CFS. "I keep writing checks and I hope they don't take me to debtors' prison." For those without resources, the U.S. is a particularly grim place to have CFS. The CFIDS Foundation is hoping to open a clinic in San Francisco modeled on a successful Seattle CFIDS clinic. But the foundation suspects that the symptoms, together with the growing public fear of contagion, are leading to homelessness and institutionalization.

Children, adolescents, and college students with the condition face the same isolation and disbelief from school boards and universities reluctant to provide the extra services that are legally mandated for disabled students. Last September, a graduate student committed suicide after having CFS for more than three years. In a note she left, she said, "Every day I hung on the edge, maybe today will be tolerable. That's all I asked for. That's what my expectations had been chiseled down to—tolerable. Maybe the pain in my eyes, head, back, legs, feet, knees, hips, and the nerve pain all over . . . maybe I'll be able to tolerate it all today."

Her roommate, Cindy Schifman Bookbinder, who also has CFS, says her friend tried every traditional and non-traditional medication she could find, but none helped the pain for long. "For people who have severe forms of this, it's like having multiple sclerosis, rheumatoid arthritis, and Alzheimer's all together."

Some feminist activists are disappointed with the women's community's response to the illness. "I don't in any way want to be competitive with people who have AIDS. People who have AIDS are dying," says one woman with CFS. "But it does need to be said that there has been much more concern about AIDS than there has been about this disease, that the women's community has not been as fast as it should have been to respond to this."

Despite some disappointments, the community response can be heartening. As public awareness of the illness heightens, this may improve further. In Jan Montgomery's case, her friends got organized. "When I was first quite ill all my friends got together and raised over $1,000 and started the CFIDS Foundation," she says.

Although Montgomery is still ill, she sees some improvement over the years. She still has serious relapses but her remissions are stronger. "From the beginning we thought of this as a political disease, and it does seem CFIDS is finally getting some serious scientific scrutiny. When I compare it to diseases like lupus and multiple sclerosis that also affect mainly women, we're really moving pretty fast."

Resources

These groups offer information on treatments, how to live with the disorder, names of doctors, and other references.

Center for Medical Consumers
(Reference library available on walk-in
 basis only)
237 Thompson Street
New York, NY 10012
(212) 674-7105

Centers for Disease Control
(Recorded information on CFS and
other diseases)
(404) 332-4555

CFIDS Association
P.O. Box 220398
Charlotte, NC 28222
Toll-free: (800) 44-CFIDS
Recorded information:
(900) 988-CFID

CFIDS Foundation
965 Mission Street, Suite 425
San Francisco, CA 94103
(415) 882-9986

Lesbian Herstory Archives
(Resource on CFS and lesbians)
P.O. Box 1258
New York, NY 10116
(212) 874-7232

Massachusetts CFIDS Association
(Information about children and adolescents)
808 Main Street
Waltham, Mass. 02154
(617) 893-4415

National CFS Association
3521 Broadway, Suite 222
Kansas City, Mo. 64111
(816) 931-4777

Ω

HIV: The National Scandal

by Peg Byron

Harlem Hospital's HIV outpatient clinic was emptying into the gray afternoon and Wilda Correa was still waiting to see the doctor. Nervous but trying to be cooperative, she had already waited three months for the appointment since taking the blood test for HIV, the human immunodeficiency virus responsible for AIDS. Inside the crowded clinic, Correa, a 43-year-old mother of three, knew it would take a lot to keep the once-silent virus from totally destroying her immune system.

In many ways, Correa epitomizes the people who are at great risk yet are most ignored in the U.S. AIDS epidemic: poor women of color and IV drug users, who, because of sex, race, and class, are viewed as the "throwaways" of society. But Harlem is not the only place in the U.S. where women must wait too long to get HIV care. And delays mean deterioration as the infection destroys the immune system and spirals into devastating diseases and, often, death.

AIDS might be described most accurately as a late stage of HIV disease. There are some long-term AIDS survivors, but the outlook for most women is bleak. One small New Jersey survey found that women diagnosed with AIDS live an average of barely four *months*, while white gay men with AIDS live 1.3 to 1.7 *years;* studies conducted in New York and San Francisco corroborate the differential. African American women in 1988 died at nine times the rate of European American women. Does this reflect the difference in the quality of health care available to these groups? Is HIV affecting women in different ways? Are different epidemics striking different communities? Experts say they don't know.

They don't know because these questions remain unexplored. But the lack of interest and the high death rate for women are two sides of the same crime: women are being ignored in the AIDS epidemic.

Women continue to get the attention of most AIDS researchers only as possible infectors of children and men. It is as if HIV-infected women are viewed solely as carriers of disease. Seen as pregnancy risks and troublesome with their child care and transportation problems, women also are widely excluded from experimental drug trials—making up only 7 percent of the enrollment in AIDS treatment research. Yet such drug trials are usually the only sources of potentially crucial medicine for this as yet incurable condition.

More often than men, women with HIV/AIDS suffer from lack of money or insurance for basic care. Yet without the data to define how they get sick with HIV differently from men, many women are denied desperately needed disability benefits.

Still, no major research has addressed the question of whether women may experience any symptoms different from men's. Dr. Daniel Hoth, AIDS division director for the National Institute of Allergy and Infectious Diseases (NIAID), a man who controls millions of research dollars, reluctantly concedes he has sponsored no studies about women's health. And the situation is the same at the National Cancer Institute; together, the two institutes get the bulk of U.S. AIDS research dollars, but neither has gotten around to asking what AIDS looks like in women.

According to Dr. Kathryn Anastos, director of HIV primary care services at Bronx-Lebanon Hospital Center in New York, one third to one half of all HIV-infected women have gynecological complications before the appearance of any other symptoms, except possibly fatigue; 32 percent to 86 percent of HIV-infected women have abnormal Pap smears and are at risk for cervical cancer; there is some evidence that pelvic inflammatory disease (PID) is more aggressive and caused by a wider array of organisms; irregular periods and infertility have been reported, suggesting unknown hormonal effects.

For at least three years, reports in medical journals have warned about severe, hard-to-treat gynecological infections linked to HIV (see *Ms.*, July 1988). But not a single female genital complication is included in the federal guidelines set by the Centers for Disease Control (CDC) for AIDS diagnoses or even as signs of HIV infection.

"It's a major problem," said Dr. Mardge Cohen, who is director of the Women and Children with AIDS Project at Cook County Hospital in Chicago. "It would make more sense to consider gynecological manifestations as representative of the clinical spectrum of AIDS. If it's not AIDS by the official definition, we see women who are desperate for those benefits."

The very definition of AIDS, as set forth by the federal government, excludes women. The CDC has characterized AIDS based on what government scientists knew when clusters of gay men were stricken in the early 1980s. Originally called GRID, for Gay-Related Immune Deficiency, AIDS was gradually defined. If many women or intravenous drug users were dying in similar ways then, they were not noticed and their particular symptoms were not included in the AIDS definition. The human cost of that exclusion continues today each time a woman confronts her HIV problems.

"HIV: The National Scandal" by Peg Byron from *Ms. Magazine*, Jan./Feb. 1991, pp. 24–29.

Peg Byron is a United Press International reporter based in New York. She recently completed a Knight Journalism Fellowship in medicine and writes on health and public policy issues.

"Look at my hands," Correa says, still waiting for her clinic appointment. They are covered with strange, reddish-brown spots, a few of which faintly scatter her cheek. "It feels like something crawling up my face. They itch." The spots appeared during the summer when Correa first got sick and lost 30 pounds with a severe bout of diarrhea.

She saw a doctor about fatigue and shortness of breath just two years earlier. He did not suggest an HIV test, though intravenous drug use accounts for over 50 percent of all U.S. women who have been diagnosed with AIDS and he knew she had a ten-year-long heroin habit. He diagnosed an enlarged heart and warned her to clean up her lifestyle. Since then, she's been off both heroin and methadone.

Dr. Wafaa El-Sadr calls Correa into one of the clinic's examining rooms and decides to hospitalize her to get her heart and blood pressure under control before starting HIV treatment. Chief of the hospital's infectious disease department, El-Sadr says Correa does not have what is officially AIDS. She will try an antibacterial ointment on Correa's rash, which she says is not Kaposi's sarcoma lesions (common among gay men with AIDS but almost never seen on others diagnosed with AIDS).

Did Correa have any unusual gynecological symptoms? The doctor says she doesn't know. While the city-run clinic supplies at no cost an expensive regimen of drugs, it does not have the equipment to do pelvic exams. The examining tables don't even have stirrups.

The doctor describes the clinic's almost 600 patients as "desperately poor," many of them homeless. Women make up 30 percent of her AIDS caseload—triple the national AIDS rate for women. The Egyptian-born El-Sadr says the high percentage of women she treats are the leading edge of the epidemic. "We're seeing the evolution of the epidemic."

Women throughout the country are the fastest growing part of the AIDS epidemic. Several years ago, they made up 7 percent of all those who were diagnosed. Now, women with AIDS number about 15,000; of these, 72 percent are African American or Latina. "If AIDS has done anything for us, it has magnified the other social and health problems that exist for women of color," said Dàzon Dixon, executive director of SISTERLOVE, an affiliate of the National Black Women's Health Project.

By 1993, women will make up 15 percent of the people with AIDS in the U.S., according to the CDC; several AIDS researchers argue that the CDC's figures on women are at least 40 percent too low, in part because of its failure to count many of women's HIV-induced illnesses as AIDS.

Even when examining tables have stirrups, most researchers aren't interested in the woman, but in the fetus she is bearing.

For a new national AZT study called protocol 076, 700 pregnant women are being sought to determine if the drug reduces the chance of an infected woman transmitting the virus to the baby. The protocol, still under review, as recently as last March included no evaluation of the women's health or the drug's impact on the mothers. A letter from NIAID's Hoth explained that protocol 076 "was not designed to be a study of pregnant women, although this topic is most important. . . ." NIAID has since revised the study to include a maternal health component, but it is not for purposes of the woman's health.

Hoth said an interview, "As we move on in our thinking, we realize we have two patients to account for in pregnancy studies." This startling revelation is a chilling reminder of the history of interference with women's reproductive choices, from forced sterilizations and denial of abortions to the current concern for fetal rights.

For a woman with HIV, pregnancy poses a dilemma: if she wants to deliver (the odds of having a healthy baby are estimated to be 70 percent), she may be pressured to end the pregnancy. But if she chooses to abort, many clinics refuse to assist anyone who has HIV, and 37 states do not allow Medicaid or other public funds to be used for abortion.

In the limited studies that do involve pelvic exams, abnormal cervical Pap smears have been detected at rates five to eight times greater than in non-HIV women in the same communities. Other studies suggest a dangerous synergy between HIV and a common virus that causes genital warts, called the human papillomavirus, or HPV. Women with both HIV and HPV infections are 29 times more likely than non-HIV women to have cervical cancer, one study found.

"HPV is a ubiquitous virus. It is found in the inner cities, the upper classes. Some studies suggest that it is found in a third of all adolescents in the inner cities and a quarter of all women," said Dr. Sten Vermund, chief of epidemiology for NIAID. He warns that once HIV infected women start reaching the same life expectancy as HIV-infected men, an epidemic in cervical cancer may emerge due to the HIV-HPV combination.

Doctors who treat many women with HIV infections (in clinics with properly equipped examining tables) say they already see higher rates of abnormal cervical conditions rapidly progressing to invasive cancers.

Advanced HPV with HIV, argues Vermund, should be considered one of the opportunistic infections that define AIDS—making many more women count in both the AIDS toll and benefit programs. "I'm having trouble getting people's attention on this matter. I have had a paper about it in review at the *American Journal of Obstetrics and Gynecology* for a god-awful long time," said Vermund.

Dr. Mathilde Krim of the American Foundation for AIDS Research (AmFAR) says how women are counted "matters a lot when it comes to entitlement to disability payments or Medicare. The rest of the government relies on this definition. And where women are left out of the system, the lack of treatment can shorten their lives."

There are conflicts over the hierarchy of AIDS illnesses, which not only affects who qualifies for limited disability benefits but how the shape and scope of the epidemic is defined. And that affects how both public and private agencies must respond.

The battles pit the sick against the dying in a fight over money. Scientists and doctors, for example, are in a fierce competition for limited research funding: the scientists are focused on long- range goals to stop HIV with the development of antiviral drugs and a vaccine, while doctors are desperate for ways to treat people already infected. But President Bush and the Congress—which will spend a projected $800 billion on the S&L crisis and $2.2 billion a month in the Persian Gulf—have capped NIAID's AIDS research funding at $432.6 million and NCI's at $161 million for fiscal year 1991.

AIDS activist Maxine Wolfe, who demonstrated and sat in at CDC and NIAID offices as part of the Women's Caucus of AIDS Coalition to Unleash Power (ACT UP), says: "The whole size of the epidemic is being squashed. Can you imagine if they added TB with HIV, or vaginal thrush with HIV, or PID or syphilis with HIV? The number of cases out there would be enormous. By not having that number, they [the feds] justify so little government money for research and treatment."

Following pressure from activists as well as the Congressional Caucus for Women's Issues, NIAID sponsored a special conference on women and HIV in December to help prioritize women's needs. At another meeting at NIAID last year, Wolfe, a professor at the City University of New York Graduate Center, and other ACT UP activists confronted NIAID chief Dr. Anthony Fauci, Hoth, and other officials to demand that "women be treated as women and not as fetus-bearers." Even Fauci had to concede that there had been few women included in AIDS drug trials.

Not surprisingly, the blind sexism of the NIH establishment is also reflected in the institute's attitudes toward women researchers. According to Dr. Deborah Cotton, an assistant professor of medicine at Harvard Medical School who chaired the session on women in clinical trials at NIAID's December conference, condescension was the typical response to criticisms from her and other women of the Food and Drug Administration committee reviewing protocol 076.

"As a woman, part of the problem in talking about clinical trials in women is that people don't listen," said Cotton. "They consider it a political statement . . . as if we are overstating what the scientific issues are." Pressure from women's advocates has helped, she said. "I think it did take that kind of advocacy to put women at the top of the agenda."

Legal pressure may also help. A class-action lawsuit has been filed against Health and Human Services Secretary Louis Sullivan, who oversees the Social Security Administration as well as CDC, NIH, and NCI. The suit seeks to grant disability benefits for a broader range of HIV diseases, including HIV-induced gynecological diseases. Legal services attorney Theresa McGovern filed the case from her cramped New York City office after hearing from dozens of people like S.P., a 23-year-old with two children in foster care.

S.P. said she can't have her name published because she must keep her HIV condition a secret from her father, with whom she shares a tiny, dilapidated apartment. She can't afford her own apartment unless she receives Social Security Disability insurance and Supplemental Security Income benefits. Without adequate housing, she has been unable to convince the family court to return her children.

"I get headaches, throw up a lot. I've got a lot of pain in my side," S.P. said. She has outbreaks of painful pelvic inflammatory disease for which she has been hospitalized. Her immune system is nearly depleted.

The benefits would mean a monthly grant of $472 instead of the $113 she gets from local assistance programs. Despite her own doctor's testimony at a hearing last fall that she is unable to work, an administrative law judge deemed the rail-thin woman's testimony "not credible" and denied her claim. The class-action suit, in U.S. District Court in Manhattan, could affect thousands of women as well as male IV drug users.

"This should have been a national class action but we just didn't have the money to do it," McGovern says. Other nonprofit legal service groups joined in the suit, including the gay-rights oriented Lambda Legal Defense and Education Fund. But McGovern said that support from major AIDS groups has been slower in coming.

McGovern's lawsuit—like the Women's AIDS Network in San Francisco and the handful of other such efforts for women—has been run on a shoestring. These groups get little of the money that flows, for example, to New York's Gay Men's Health Crisis (GMHC), the country's biggest AIDS service group. GMHC, for its part, did not join the lawsuit, though it made a small donation.

Even when better funded AIDS groups sponsor programs needed by women with HIV, they may set entrance criteria women can't meet. Even large groups like GMHC have restricted their client services to serve only those diagnosed with AIDS or AIDS-related conditions, as set by the male-oriented CDC definition; GMHC has long refused services to anyone still using drugs. Given the barriers women face getting diagnosed correctly, plus the high percentage who get AIDS from IV drug use, women are falling through the cracks even in community HIV service groups.

Some doctors are uneasy about women bringing new demands to the fray. They are critical of demands to include women's genital tract infections among AIDS-defining illnesses. "Some of these infections are very common," said Dr. Paula Shuman, infectious disease specialist at Wayne State University School of Medicine in Detroit. "It would terrify a lot of women into thinking it means they have HIV." No one wants to promote unnecessary anxiety, but viewing women as hysterics who would place extra demands on doctors is a common reason given to deny better research and medical care to women.

Women's organizations themselves are also guilty of ignoring the threat of HIV to women. Center for Women Policy Studies Executive Director Leslie Wolfe says her group will be pushing women's organizations to start giving AIDS priority, after years of groups insisting HIV is not a women's issue.

"If women don't fit some stereotype, HIV won't be considered," said Cohen of Chicago's Cook County Hospital. For women of color, the poor and IV drug users who are the majority of women with AIDS, HIV adds a grim dimension to the neglect they always have experienced; for middle-class European American women, HIV is often missed because AIDS is what happens to other people.

Older women also suffer from doctor biases. According to Dr. Mary A. Young, who sees scores of infected women at her office in the Georgetown University Medical Center in Washington, D.C., one 62-year-old was given cancer tests for a year before anyone thought to take her sexual history and recommend an HIV test. It was positive. "No one had considered this widow might be sexually active," Young said.

But women with HIV have been organizing among themselves to try to answer the questions that the AIDS establishment has ignored. Michelle Wilson, 39, a legal services aide from Washington, D.C., started a newsletter and an organization called "The Positive Woman" for women like herself who live with the virus. Sex is one of the toughest topics.

"Initially, it made me feel unclean," she said about trying to have sex after learning of her infection last year. "I felt like my husband couldn't touch me without infecting himself." For a while, he didn't wear a condom because he thought it would make her feel bad. "It was hard to relax and feel good. I couldn't keep feeling sexually aroused because I knew what that condom meant. But at some point, a coping mechanism kicks in and you feel, 'Now what a guy—our lovemaking remains unchanged because he really loves me'. And that keeps us a loving and sexual couple."

Wilson gets calls from around the country about the newsletter. Many women describe frustrations when they look for support from male-oriented service groups. "You're reluctant if you're in a room filled with men to raise your hand and say, 'I have lesions on my vagina,'" Wilson said.

Lesbians with HIV find their existence even more widely denied. Drug use, alternative methods of fertilization, blood transfusions, and sex with infected men are known routes of HIV into the lesbian population. As for lesbian sexual HIV transmission, several possible cases have been reported in letters to medical journals, but the risk remains unclear. CDC epidemiologist Susan Chu, the lead author of a recent report that looked for AIDS in lesbians, said she found no cases of female-to-female transmission.

But Chu states flatly her study did not rule out HIV risks in lesbian sex. Notably, the study used the CDC's narrow definition of AIDS, not a cross section of HIV-infected women. And the authors defined "lesbian" more strictly than would many lesbian women: they omitted any women mentioned in CDC AIDS reports through 1989 who had sex with men since 1977, leaving 79 lesbians, or 0.8 percent of all reported adult women with AIDS in the country. Almost all were intravenous drug users and 5 percent were described as infected through transfusions. This gives no help for lesbians who, for whatever reason,

are infected. The CDC has not found the question of lesbian risk significant enough to warrant safer sex guidelines.

As far as menstrual blood is concerned, Chu said she doesn't know if it is as HIV-laden as circulating blood in infected women. She could not say if sex during menses was riskier for one's sex partner, although the menstruating woman might be at more risk of infection herself, because her cervix is more open.

In trying to assess their own risk, women should probably consider the geographic prevalence of the virus where they or their sexual partners have had sex, shared hypodermic needles, had blood transfusions, maybe even had tattoos and electrolysis performed since the late 1970s. Perhaps most tangled is the daisy chain of sex tied to everyone's history that is both invisible and sometimes distorted by guilt.

The answer to uncertain risk—"just wear a condom"—ignores the fact that women don't wear condoms. Men do and most don't like it; some admit it gives them performance anxiety and others say it is "unnatural." For some, says Dooley Worth, Ph.D., an anthropologist and adviser to New York's Health and Hospitals Corporation, condoms are unwelcome symbols of extra-relationship activity. Worth also warns that no relationship is static and commitment to condom use can diminish over time. And condom campaigns ignore the real pressures in women's relationships that sometimes make unsafe sex seem the less risky alternative.

"Women may be getting battered, or fear the possibility of battery or of losing the relationship," said Sally Jue, the mental health program manager for AIDS Project Los Angeles. "For many Asian and Hispanic women, being assertive and getting their men to wear condoms is a ludicrous idea"

In one study of women in prostitution, only 4 percent of nearly 600 women reported they regularly had customers use condoms. In a more encouraging study, the Alan Guttmacher Institute recently reported that levels of condom use among Latino teenagers had tripled during the 1980s.

But if condoms are not known as perfect birth control, why are they so great when it comes to a question of life and death? After all, condom failure in pregnancy prevention ranges between 3 percent for older, white married women and 36 percent for younger, nonmarried women of color. With HIV protection, less is known. One study concluded that condom use reduces HIV infection risk for women by a factor of 10.

There are mixed recommendations about antiviral spermicides, containing nonoxynol 9, sodium oxychlorosene, or benzalkonium chloride. Although these are in the woman's control, they are less effective than condoms. Also, spermicides can irritate mucous membranes lining the vagina and anus, making them more vulnerable to infection.

As a long-term public health strategy, condoms are not the answer for women wanting control over their health. But federal officials were dumbfounded when Representative Constance Morella (R.-Md.) and other congresswomen asked what was being done to give women control of HIV protection "They have not been doing anything," said Morella, whose district includes the NIH's sprawling research campus.

The concept that women's health counts as much as men's is long overdue. Last summer, the Congressional Caucus for Women's Issues forced the formation of an Office of Research on Women's Health at NIH. The caucus also introduced the Women's Health Equity Act, which includes AIDS initiatives written by the Center for Women Policy Studies in Washington.

"The activists are right," said AmFAR's Krim. "But unless politicians also feel pressure from the mainstream, from groups like NOW and the League of Women Voters, they won't do it for women." Certainly, scientists and doctors, when asked to spend time and money on women's health, must stop reacting like men who have been asked to wear condoms.

Women cannot afford to let the Health Equity Act follow the path of the ERA. Unless true health equity is addressed, thousands and thousands of women, especially in the inner cities and gradually across the country, are sentenced to death as HIV in the U.S. begins to take on the global pattern of AIDS.

Ω

♀

Survey of States Reveals Lack of Policy on Women and HIV Disease
by the National Women's Health Network

The National Women's Health Network has released the first survey of state policies on women and AIDS. "Women, AIDS and Public Health Policies" reports the results of interviews conducted with AIDS officials in all fifty states, the District of Columbia, the U.S. territories, Indian Health Service and the military.

According to Executive Director Beverly F. Baker, the survey findings are cause for concern: "We were disheartened, although not surprised, to find so many areas without any written policy addressing women and AIDS. Without policy, there is no way to ensure that the needs of women affected by the HIV epidemic are being met."

Survey findings include:
- *Lack of women-specific policies*
  Nearly two thirds of the states had *no* policy specifically directed towards women;
- *Violations of women's rights*
  Two thirds of the areas surveyed have policies in place that violate women's rights. Many of the states do not protect the confidentiality of HIV antibody test results. Thirty-two states reported mandatory testing of at least one group of people; and
- *Treatment of women as "risk factors"*
  Typically, HIV prevention, education, and services are only offered to women who could potentially infect others. Only 11 areas provided any HIV-related services to women who were not pregnant or seeking birth control.

According to Baker, "It is past time for public health officials in our states, territories and jurisdictions to formulate women-specific HIV policies. 150,000 women are estimated to be infected with HIV, and tens of thousands more are caring for loved ones with HIV disease. Our state governments can't continue to ignore these women."

The report includes the following policy recommendations:
- Access to contraception, abortion, and childbearing services must be ensured and no coerced abortion or sterilization should be allowed;
- All women should have access to confidential or anonymous testing on a voluntary basis. State policy should ensure that testing is accompanied by effective pre- and post-test counseling;
- Areas should offer temporary foster care to children of HIV infected parents seeking needed medical or drug treatment. Children should not be permanently separated from families as a precondition for receiving care;
- Voluntary partner notification systems should be made available to everyone seeking testing for HIV antibodies;
- Clinical trials conducted in state-supported institutions should be required to include significant percentages of women; and
- A diagnosis of AIDS should not be required for eligibility for medical and other assistance. Services should be made available to everyone needing care who has tested positive for HIV antibodies.

With the publication of "Women, AIDS and Public Health Policies" the Network made an urgent call for the development of policy. Public health officials need to listen to the advice of the many community-based service organizations and national advocacy groups that are now developing recommendations for policy on women and HIV disease. The booklet is available for $3 from the NWHN, 514 10th St., N.W., Suite 400, Washington, DC 20004

From *The Network News*, (January/February 1991). Copyright © 1991 by National Women's Health Network. Reprinted by permission.

Ω

Spermicides, Virucides, and HIV

by Jane Juffer

Throughout the world women, are being infected with HIV, the virus that causes AIDS, at staggering rates—as a result of heterosexual sex with infected men. According to a recent report from the World Health Organization, by the year 2000 most of the newly infected will be women. Yet health professionals still promote the condom as women's main means of protection from HIV and other sexually transmitted diseases (STDs), even when virucides that kill STD-causing viruses might prove more effective.

Laboratory tests show that the condom may interrupt viruses like HIV in as many as 99 percent of sexual encounters. But what works in the lab doesn't seem to work in the bedroom. In research comparing the effectiveness of protection by condoms and by spermicides, Dr. Michael Rosenberg, president of a private research organization called Health Decisions, found that in real life condom effectiveness drops to 50 percent—a protection rate comparable to spermicides.

Rosenberg evaluated 5,681 visits by women to an urban STD clinic for chlamydia, trichomoniasis, and gonorrhea, the three most common STDs in women. The study, which was recently published in the *American Journal of Public Health,* found that, compared to women who used no contraceptives, women who used the sponge had a 71 percent reduction in gonorrhea, a 74 percent decrease in trichomoniasis, and a 13 percent drop in chlamydia; with a diaphragm, reductions were 65 percent for gonorrhea, 71 percent for trichomoniasis, and 72 percent for chlamydia. For women whose male partners used a condom, the decreases .were far lower: respectively, 34 percent, 30 percent, and 3 percent.

These figures suggest that condoms are less effective than diaphragms and sponges because they are used less, probably because of male resistance. This isn't a new finding for feminists. "AIDS prevention experts are singing a one-note song: condoms, condoms, condoms," says Vicki Legion, program coordinator for the Chicago Women's AIDS Project. "Rosenberg's study confirms that this doesn't play too well in the real lives of many women. Condoms put many of us in a cruel Catch-22: if you insist on condoms, you may get battered. If you don't, you might get infected with HIV."

While the diaphragm and sponge act as barriers that protect the cervix, thus inhibiting transmission of some STDs, researchers believe that the spermicides often used with them have the greatest potential in preventing HIV transmission. Barrier methods by themselves *may* inhibit HIV, says Rosenberg, but the bottom line is that much more research must be done on the mechanisms of heterosexual transmission—how and when women are infected via the reproductive tract—before barrier methods of contraception can be proven effective against HIV transmission. Does the virus attach itself to sperm to cause infection in the uterus? Does infection occur mainly on the vaginal surfaces or at the cervix?

An ideal means of protection for women would be a virucide (virus killer) against HIV that a woman could insert without her male partner's knowledge, and that would be effective whether inserted before or after intercourse, further increasing a woman's leverage. And it would not have to be discarded, but should dissolve.

Most of these criteria seem to be met in the form of a product now marketed as a contraceptive—the Vaginal Contraceptive Film, or VCF. The VCF is a small, thin square with a 28 percent concentration of nonoxynol-9. Inserted high into the vagina, close to the cervix, the film dissolves within minutes, remains active for about two hours, and washes away with body fluids.

Nonoxynol-9's effectiveness against HIV has been proven in laboratory tests on monkeys infected with simian immunodeficiency virus (SIV, a retrovirus closely related to HIV). In a recent study funded by the National Institute of Child Health and Human Development, only six out of 12 female monkeys treated with a contraceptive gel containing nonoxynol-9 became infected through vaginal transmission, compared to all six untreated control monkeys.

Many questions about nonoxynol-9 remain unanswered, however. It's not known, for example, how the different vehicles for spermicides—gels, creams, and foams—affect their ability to prevent HIV transmission. Also, what concentration of nonoxynol-9 is necessary to kill HIV in the vagina? Can nonoxynol-9 be used after intercourse and still be effective in killing viruses? Perhaps most critical is the fact that nonoxynol-9 can irritate the vaginal lining: results of recent studies conflict on whether and at what point irritation occurs—and the possible impact this may have on HIV transmission.

Clearly, nonoxynol-9 merits considerable research into its potential as a female-controlled virucide. "What struck me most in reading about the recent international AIDS conference in Amsterdam is that people are looking around for something new," says Rosenberg. "We're overlooking something that's been around since the turn of the century but needs more study. We may already have something to protect ourselves—nonoxynol-9."

From *Ms. Magazine,* Sept./Oct. 1992, pp. 74–75. Copyright © 1992 by Ms. Magazine. Reprinted by permission.

Jane Juffer, a free-lance writer, is currently attending the University of Illinois at Champaign/Urbana as a graduate student in English literature.

Funding, however, lags far behind the need; currently, for example, the Centers for Disease Control is not funding any efficacy studies on the female condom or on virucides. The National Institutes of Health is at least funding some studies of immediate relevance: in addition to a study on the effects of nonoxynol-9, NIH is spending $2.7 million over four years to investigate a spermicide-releasing diaphragm that is discarded after one use. NIH is also funding a project to test substances for spermicidal and virucidal potential; $285,000 has been spent in the last three years. Next year a $1.2 million study on spermicides and virucides will begin; let your congressional representatives know that this is not enough money to research such a potentially lifesaving substance.

The search for woman-controlled methods does not mean that women must take complete responsibility for prevention of STDs. Men must still be educated about their role in preventing HIV transmission, and women must still be empowered to negotiate condom use with their partners. But to recognize that condoms are an unlikely option for many women is to recognize that the need for women-controlled methods is—for an increasing number of women around the world—a matter of life and death.

Ω

♀

With or Without the Dam Thing: The Lesbian Safer Sex Debate

by Carol Camlin

I have a rare lesbian safer sex poster on my office wall that shows two young white women embracing, naked and wet, in a steamy public bath. One woman sits on a tiled ledge with her legs spread, hair tossed in her face, smiling blissfully. The other is on her knees, leaning into her lover's open thighs, her head arched back. The text, in lavender, reads: "Wet your appetite for safer sex."

As a lesbian HIV/AIDS educator at the AIDS Action Committee of Massachusetts, I pay keen attention to the few safer sex messages and images produced for lesbians by national and international HIV/AIDS service organizations. For one thing, this environment brimming with gay male erotic safer sex posters would make any healthy lesbian long for a few pictures of nude women. I also pay attention to keep abreast of the raging debate about lesbian sexual transmission of HIV—the so-called dam debate—among those who advocate either for or against the use of dental dams for oral sex (dental dams are small latex squares available at your local dental supply store: just masquerade as a dentist and ask for the 100-pak).

The lesbian safer-sex poster on my wall is different from gay male posters in one significant way. The scene evokes the eroticism of wetness, and seems to encourage comfort with bodily fluids. Wetness is sexy but, in the context of HIV, has come to seem dangerous. Although the poster would probably be a turn-on for most lesbians, I would imagine that The Terrence Higgins Trust (THT), the British AIDS service organization that produced the poster, has taken some flak for this one. The poster introduces the idea that there is such a thing as lesbian safer sex, without directly advocating the use of dental dams.

Carrying this message one step further, at the VIII International Conference on AIDS in July, THT unveiled a poster that directly advocates that lesbians *not* use dental dams. "Very low risk in oral sex," it advised, "so ditch those dental dams. Don't bother with gloves unless it turns you on."

The poster immediately unleased a storm of protest. Dozens of ACT UP members (most of them men) zapped the THT display booth, chanting "Shame!", spray painting it and modifying the poster with messages like "This poster is killing lesbians."

The intense controversy surrounding woman to woman sexual transmission of HIV is largely due to the fact that very little HIV-prevention education information is geared to lesbians, despite our involvement in all aspects of the epidemic.

How many lesbians either harbor exaggerated fears of HIV or assume they're at no risk of HIV infection (or any other sexually transmitted disease)? How many lesbians are tacitly restricting their sexual practices, and so their sexual pleasure, out of fear of the unknown? How many HIV-positive lesbians know what they can safely do with their HIV-negative girlfriends? How many HIV-negative lesbians worry about how to have sex with their HIV-positive girlfriends without putting them at risk of an immune- threatening infection? Why this dearth of information?

In her July 1992 *Herizons* article, "Dammed If You Do, Damned If You Don't," Lesli Gaynor of the AIDS Committee of Toronto argues: "The exclusion of lesbians and lesbian sexuality from AIDS education is not only a reflection of homophobia within mainstream education, but also a sign of the systematic sexism that exists within the gay community."

Lesbians need and deserve to get the facts about AIDS, but the rare attempts to define safer sex for lesbians have focused almost exclusively on the use of dental dams. As a result, many lesbians have a vague idea that they should be using these devices, yet as Nancy Solomon notes in her Spring 1992 *Out/Look* article, "Risky Business", very few women do—including lesbian safe sex educators who issue public pronouncements about dental dams.

Given the lack of availability of dental dams and their sexual unattractiveness, is it any surprise that we're not using them? I've heard the "damn dams" described as "about as sexy as a pair of rubber pants for the diaper wearing set" in Jenifer Firestone's "Memoirs of a Safe Sex Slut" (*Bad Attitude* no.__) and cunnilingus with a dam described as "chewing on a rubber tire."

Most lesbian health educators acknowledge that the three-inch-by- three-inch dental dams are small and difficult to use. How do you know when your spit ends and her fluids begin, unless you're really alert? Some educators advocate plastic wrap as an option for oral sex, because it's convenient, and it's larger. "Also," as one plastic-wrap aficionado puts it, "you can see through it, and that's nice."

Still others question barrier use in the first place. Louise Rice, a lesbian health educator and nurse at the AIDS Action Committee observes in her August 1992 *Sojourner* article, "Rethinking Dental Dams": "Barrier protection against HIV in vaginal fluids has no proven efficacy. Dental dams provide false security for an activity (going down) that already carries a relatively low risk."

Instead of broadening the topic of lesbian safer sex, the dam debate has sometimes obscured a deeper and more detailed discussion about the range of behaviors and activities which put lesbians at highest risk for infection with HIV and other STDs. After all, cunnilingus is not *all* we do. Do we focus on the use of dental dams because that's all we know how to talk about? Do we avoid discussion about the behaviors which put us at highest risk because of deep-seated taboos within the lesbian community?

Most HIV-positive lesbians became infected by sharing injection drug needles, or having sex with men without a condom. Several studies have shown that at least one-third of lesbians in the 20 to 35 year-old age group have slept with men, even after coming out. Simply having a lesbian identity does not make you "immune" to HIV: Our community must come to terms with the facts that lesbians sometimes use IV drugs and sometimes have sex with men.

Although these two risk factors are primarily responsible for the incidence of HIV among lesbians, it is possible for HIV to be transmitted sexually from woman to woman. Even those who aren't lesbian latex zealots agree that we are not "God's Chosen People." Lesbian sexual transmission of HIV is very rare—but just how rare, exactly how it happens, and how to prevent it are all points of debate.

The information available to lesbians about what constitutes safer sex for lesbians is ambiguous and diverse in opinion.

AIDS service organizations offer advice to lesbians ranging from "stock up on latex condoms or dams" to AIDS Committee of Toronto's provocative suggestion "a little more sex, a little more leather, a little more lace, a little LESS LATEX". Somewhere in the middle of this, a growing number of lesbian health educators argue that, well into the second decade of this epidemic, enough is known about HIV transmission to suggest that HIV prevention education for lesbians need not include the "dental dams at all times under all circumstances" message. What exactly are the HIV transmission risks with woman to woman sex?

Let's review the facts. For someone to get infected, HIV not only has to get OUT of one person, via an infected body fluid, it also has to get INTO another person's bloodstream, via the mucous membranes or a break in the skin.

How the virus leaves the body: The highest concentration of HIV can be found in blood, and the next highest in semen. In vaginal fluid and pre-seminal fluid (or pre-cum, the fluid that men emit before ejaculation), the concentration is much lower. In some fluids such as tears or saliva, the concentration of HIV is so low or non-existent that there's no risk of infection.

The chance of infection via oral contact with vaginal fluid is very low, and it depends on the presence of blood products. However, several factors can increase the likelihood of the presence of HIV: menstrual blood, vaginal infections (such as yeast) and sexually transmitted diseases (such as herpes and chlamydia) can elevate levels of HIV in vaginal fluid, because all would contain white blood cells which harbor HIV. In later stages of HIV disease all bodily fluids contain higher concentrations of HIV. Also, the pH, or level of acidity, of the vaginal fluid can influence whether HIV is present. The pH of vaginal fluid is normally low, or acidic, and "inhospitable" to HIV (the pH of semen, on the other hand, is higher, or alkaline—and therefore more "hospitable" to HIV). Vaginal fluid is more alkaline during menstruation and ovulation.

How the virus enters the body: You can become infected with HIV if someone else's infected body fluid enters your bloodstream via breaks in the skin or via mucous membranes. Mucous membranes line the rectum, vagina and mouth (and in men also the urethra and glans— the tip of the penis); they're also found in the inside of your nose and eyelids. Some mucous membranes are thick and strong, and others are thin, and easier for the virus to pass through. The rectum is the most vulnerable because the walls of the rectum are very thin and there are tiny blood vessels at its surface which are easily ruptured during anal intercourse. The walls of the vagina are tougher and thicker, therefore less vulnerable to fissures and tears (with well-lubricated penetration and trimmed fingernails). The mucous membranes in the mouth are thicker than either the rectum or the vagina. It's therefore difficult for HIV to enter the bloodstream through your mouth. Moreover, saliva has a neutralizing effect on HIV, making it harmless when present in a low concentration, such as in vaginal fluid.

Reducing Your Risks: "Lesbians do everything from nibbling on each other's ears to fisting—and in between there are a lot of things that are safe and some things that aren't," notes Amelie Zurn, Director of Lesbian Services at the Whitman-Walker Clinic in D.C. "The point is, risk is relative . . . for some people, any risk at all is unacceptable. For other people, more risk is okay."

The key to safer sex is communication: defining your limits and talking to your partner about what you want. To assess your risks and decide what to do, communicate with your partner.

Get to know your vagina: "Vaginal fluids have not been studied enough," Louise Rice acknowledges, "but women are capable of doing the studying. Getting to know your vagina, your discharges and smells, and those of a partner, can alert you to changes and potential infections. Unrecognized and untreated infections are a concern for all women, not just those with HIV. When HIV is present, an infection can quickly become disabling."

Get to know your mouth: Remember, even if you go down on a woman and she is menstruating or has a vaginal infection, the virus still has to find its way into your bloodstream. You may want to use a barrier under those circumstances—but if you don't there are ways to make oral sex even safer than it is, without having to use a barrier.

If you have a cold sore, or bleeding gums, or a cut on your tongue, "wait until you've healed so that you don't have to waste time or needless worry," Lesli Gaynor of Toronto advises. "If you have a contagious mouth condition like herpes, it's only courteous to consider the other person's health."

Gaynor offers an additional tip for safe licking: "Don't brush [or floss] your teeth before oral sex—use mouthwash to get that just-brushed fresh feeling." If your partner is HIV-positive, you may want to use mouthwash as a matter of course, to protect her from germs in your mouth.

You also may want to go down on your partner BEFORE you penetrate her with your hand or a sex toy. This will reduce the chance of there being blood present in the vaginal fluid.

Gaynor also suggests, "Take a closer look at what you're about to eat. If there are sores or areas of concern, don't panic but avoid contact. Kiss the surrounding areas lovingly."

Rimming: Oral contact with the anus isn't a risk for HIV transmission unless the rectum contains blood (such as following "rough" anal penetration, and even then bleeding may not necessarily occur). But, you could contract another kind of infection via rimming, such as hepatitis A or amoebas. It's a good idea to use a barrier for rimming.

Fingerfucking or using a dildo: HIV can be transmitted if menstrual or other blood of an HIV-positive woman gets into the vagina or anus of her partner. The safest option is to use your own toy. Wash thoroughly after each use

with soap and water. If you share toys, use a condom and put on a new condom (with plenty of water-based lubricant) before you share. Or, wash thoroughly before sharing.

Remember, **intact skin is a good barrier against HIV infection.** If you have open cuts on your fingers and she's menstruating or has a vaginal infection, use latex or vinyl gloves or finger cots when penetrating her. A message to all you "Lee-Press On" femmes: trim those finger nails if you're planning to fuck her! The lesbian fashion of trimmed, smooth fingernails is in place for good reason: you don't want to cut or tear the lining of the vagina.

If you or your partner is HIV-positive, latex or vinyl gloves serve the function of not exposing an HIV-positive woman to bacteria and other germs under the fingernails, and reducing the risk of a cut in your or her vagina which could allow the germs to pass through to the bloodstream.

Fisting: This can result in fissures or tears in the vaginal (or rectal) lining, which can result in both the presence of blood and access to the bloodstream. Fisting is an activity which can place both partners at risk, since tears may occur on the skin of the person doing the fisting. Use latex or vinyl gloves with plenty of water-based lubricant when fisting, and if you plan to go down on her, either do so before you penetrate her or use a barrier.

Piercing, cutting and other S/M activities: Let the above principles of HIV transmission, and common sense be your guide in assessing risks and taking precautions with S/M activities. Invest in your own favorite equipment: latex or rubber toys, leather goods or metal equipment. The surest and safest guide is to not share equipment at all. If, however, it's not possible for you to supply your own, every precaution should be taken by you and your partner to make sure that equipment is properly cleaned prior to any sexual scene: 1) wash your equipment thoroughly, 2) soak it for several hours in a solution of one-part bleach to ten-parts water, and 3) rinse it thoroughly several times to be sure that all the bleach has been removed. These guidelines are adapted from the brochure "AIDS-Safe S/M/," distributed by the AIDS Action Committee of Mass. For further information about S/M safety, see Pat Califia's *The Lesbian S/M Safety Manual: Basic Health and Safety for Woman-to-Woman S/M* Denver: Lace Publications, 1988.

Do I think cunnilingus is an effective way of spreading HIV? No . . . and the reason is that cunnilingus is not an effective way of spreading things which are much more infectious, like hepatitis B, which has **100,000 times more viral particles per cubic milliliter of blood than HIV.** There has never been a single reported case of woman-to-woman transmission of hepatitis B via oral sex. In addition, given the number of lesbians infected with HIV, we would be seeing many, many cases of women getting infected via oral sex with other women—and we aren't

When HIV/AIDS educators talk to gay men about oral sex, most say, "Oral sex is very low risk. You can make it safer by not taking his come into your mouth. To be absolutely safe, you can use a condom." Very few gay men use condoms for oral sex, yet studies have shown that only about two dozen gay men worldwide, of the millions infected with HIV, have become infected via oral sex—and in those cases, almost all the men had taken ejaculate in the mouth, there were usually severe dental or gum problems, and often a high number of sexual partners (in the hundreds).

Dental dam advocates argue that data on lesbian transmission is fragmentary, since the Centers for Disease Control (CDC) doesn't include woman-to-woman transmission among the risk factors they normally track. Any well-informed AIDS activist knows that the CDC AIDS surveillance system is faulty, because it is based on the identity rather than the behavior of the person with AIDS. The sexual orientation of a person with AIDS does not explain how they became infected. The category "male homosexual/bisexual" doesn't tell us, for example, whether a man had insertive or receptive anal sex. The "heterosexual" category doesn't differentiate between those who became infected via anal or vaginal intercourse.

Although the right questions are not asked, the surveillance data is based on a hierarchy of transmission grounded in medical research and the real experience of people who've become infected with HIV. Sharing injection drug needles will put you in the "IV Drug User" category whether you are a gay or straight woman. Having unprotected intercourse with a man will put you in the "Heterosexual" category even though you identify as a lesbian. Both of those behaviors are much more likely to have caused your infection with HIV than going down on your girlfriend, because HIV is transmitted very efficiently and easily via blood to blood or semen to blood contact. To know the scope of the epidemic in the lesbian community at large, we need among other things a national seroprevalence survey of self-identified lesbians.

Most lesbian health educators acknowledge that although lesbians with HIV haven't been studied well, several lesbian health studies do exist. In studies of hundreds of lesbians with AIDS, only four cases of woman-to-woman transmission of HIV via sex have been reported in the medical literature. In the first case, both partners reported oral, anal and vaginal contact with blood during sex (*Annals of Internal Medicine,* vol. 105, no. 6). The second case involved a woman whose female partner, an injection drug user, was in the late stages of HIV disease (*Annals of Internal Medicine,* vol. 111, no. 11). In the final two cases the HIV-positive lesbians' sexual partners were HIV-negative, and they reported no IV drug use or sex with men (*The Lancet,* 7/87 and *AIDS Research,* vol. 1, '84). The problem with these last three cases is that it is not reported exactly how the women became infected. There are several other anecdotal, word-of-mouth reports of sexual transmission of HIV between women. We may never know the full story with those cases, but we need only return to what we know about HIV transmission to be able to assess risks and make decisions about what we want to do sexually.

HIV prevention education for gay men is usually very sex-positive. Why do we reserve all of our sexual conservatism for lesbians, by passing out dams and gloves and issuing blanket statements to lesbians such as "oral sex on a woman is risky" and "putting your fingers inside her can be risky"? Most HIV/AIDS educators wouldn't dream of telling a heterosexual man to wear a glove when putting his fingers in his girlfriend's vagina.

Many lesbian educators and activists are feeling that lesbians already have so much stacked against our sexual pleasure and freedom: internalized homophobia, racism and sexual abuse drain our self-esteem and sexual power; sexism and the puritan tradition subtly pervade how we think about sexuality and our bodies; our parents inculcated sexual shame in most of us, and that shame and guilt is only multiplied when we realize that we are queer.

Coming out can be an explosion of that shame into delight and power—and yet well-publicized phenomena such as "Lesbian Bed Death" and the general perception that lesbians do it less than everybody else ("Bullshit!" some of us say; "Well, quantity and quality are two separate things," other of us say) are signs that these various forms of oppression have taken their toll on our community.

The implicit question asked by many lesbian educators is: Do we want to be a part of what's keeping lesbians from getting it on and enjoying themselves, by exacerbating fears and encouraging lesbians to restrict themselves sexually? Absolutely not. We do need to continue to get the information out about what's risky and what's not.

"Every day, women make decisions about the risk of different activities," Louise Rice noted, "Most of these activities (smoking or driving a car, for example) carry a far greater risk than cunnilingus. Thousands of lesbians' lives could be saved if we were to devote half the attention to mammograms and breast self-awareness that has been focused on dental dams."

Having put out all of this provocative information, I'd like to suggest that we turn our political focus outward and turn our activism towards improving the lives of ALL women with AIDS—not just lesbians with AIDS. In the United States, women with AIDS make up only 4 percent of all clinical trials, although women make up 13 percent of all people with AIDS (and that's an underestimate of about 28 percent). Fourteen million women still don't have access to health insurance. The CDC case definition of AIDS still doesn't include life-threatening gynecological manifestations of AIDS. The number-one HIV transmission risk for women is IV-drug use: We need to make clean needles available and drug treatment accessible. All of these issues are lesbian health issues. And we can achieve victories on many of these fronts if we ACT UP louder and in greater numbers. Meantime, let's talk about sex—and have as much as we want.

Ω

The Politics of Disease

1. One of the most rapidly growing groups of people infected with HIV is that of adolescents, many of whom become infected through heterosexual intercourse.

    a. If you were to design an educational program for high school students to help prevent transmission of HIV, what specific information would you want to include?

    b. What obstacles might there be to presenting this information in the public schools? Discuss how you might present an argument for inclusion of the prevention program.

    c. Discuss any ideas you might have for overcoming adolescents' belief in their own invulnerability ("It can't happen to me") when teaching about HIV/AIDS.

2. Fill in the chart below, showing what is available in terms of prevention, detection, and treatment for each of the three cancers listed.

Cancer	Prevention	Detection	Treatment
Breast			
Cervical			
Endometrial			

3. The separation of detection from treatment (biopsy from mastectomy or other surgery) with breast cancer has been considered a major victory of the women's health movement. Why was this change to a "two-step" procedure considered so important?

4. Why do you think it is dangerous for there to be confusion about prevention vs. treatment for cancers? How could health education and health policies emphasize *prevention?*

12

Violence Against Women

Many women define violence—both their actual experiences with violence and their fear of violence—as their number one health issue. It is certainly an issue which affects both our mental and physical health. Many women who have suffered severe physical pain from violence have said that the emotional and psychological scars from abuse take much longer to heal than the physical injuries.

This chapter looks at some of the many ways violence manifests itself in women's lives. Although each specific form of violence may be unique in its consequences and the knowledge needed to recognize it, respond to it, and prevent it, all forms of violence (against women) can be defined as issues of power and control where one person or a group takes advantage of their power and control over another individual or group. The power and control wheel (developed by battered women and formerly battered women to describe the violence in their lives) illustrates the many prongs of abuse including making someone feel emotionally, physically or financially dependent, using children, and isolating someone from other networks, with physical abuse being just one of the many forms of control. In contrast, the equality wheel (also developed by battered and formerly battered women) serves as an inspiring model of what we want to work for in creating healthy relationships, striving to equalize rather than use or abuse power. The continuum of family violence chart demonstrates the relationship of subtle forms of physical, verbal/emotional and sexual abuse, which society all too often tolerates and condones, to the forms more obviously recognized as serious and deadly. The more subtle forms can themselves have serious consequences and invariably lead to other means of control.

Women have not passively accepted violence as a part of our lives! Organizing against violence against women and developing an analysis of how violence is based on and perpetuated by patriarchal structures which work to maintain power and control over groups of women in much the same way as individual men abuse women in intimate relationships have been very visible parts of modern women's movements. For the last two decades, women have been putting much time, energy and resources into rape crisis centers, battered women's programs and incest survivor groups. Although social change work is always

slower than we imagine, in other ways it has been almost "revolutionary" in the impact that the violence against women movements have had on the legal system, the criminal justice system, and the general public's awareness that this is a serious issue.

The sexual harassment, acquaintance/date rape and sexual assault fact sheets, compiled by the Wisconsin Coalition Against Sexual Assault, are examples of the excellent information which is now produced and distributed by activist groups working to end violence in women's lives. The article, "A More Hidden Crime: Adolescent Battered Women" summarizes how much of the information gained by the battered women's movement must now be directed to the needs of younger battered women whose issues may actually be exaggerated while their resources and options are more limited.

Other articles in this chapter more specifically address the *new* issue of the health system's response to violence against women. Although women who were victims/survivors of violence have long identified violence as a major health issue and have been aware of how violence impacted on their mental and physical health, the health system has been notoriously poor at addressing violence issues and has actually played a dangerous role of revictimizing survivors of violence. As articles in this chapter demonstrate, the good news is that the health system has now "discovered" that violence against women is an issue the health system must respond to. Women's health activists and violence against women activists now face new challenges in helping the health system define appropriate vs. non-appropriate responses to victims/survivors of violence. We must be vigilant in making sure this is not one more aspect of women's lives which gets medicalized.

Evelyn Barbee's article, "Ethnicity and Woman Abuse in the United States" emphasizes that understanding the impact and intersection of sexism and racism is essential for health workers to appropriately serve the needs of abused women of color. Although her article is geared to nurses, many victims of abuse could be better served if all health workers were aware of Barbee's cautions about recognizing racism and classism: "The consequences of the nurse holding stereotypical beliefs while trying to assist an abused woman can be disastrous." and "If of the same ethnicity but different social class from the client, the nurse needs to be aware of when and whether the social class differences prejudice data collection."

In "Surviving the Incest Industry," Louise Armstrong, one of the first incest survivors to break the silence about incest (many years ago) examines the dangers of one more women's health issue being medicalized and she describes what has gone drastically wrong with the medical response to incest. In the "capitalism-compatible incest industry" Armstrong sees that this political issue has been personalized so that personal growth of the survivor not social change becomes the answer, and in a trend which sounds distinctly like the very popular co-dependency concept (see p. 136), the victim not the abuser is held responsible for violent behavior.

In their training of health workers to appropriately respond to sexual assault and domestic violence, both Ivy Schwartz (at the University of Arizona) and Nancy Worcester (at the University of WI-Madison and through-out Wisconsin) have worked to share the philosophy and understanding of violence of the sexual assault and battered women's movements with health care providers. This approach is summarized in their articles, "Sexual Violence Against Women: Prevalence, Consequences, Societal Factors and Prevention" and "The Unique Role Health Workers Can Play in Recognizing and Responding to Battered Women." Similarly, building on the analysis of the battered women's movement, Amanda Cosgrove and Kevin Fullin, M.D., of the Kenosha, Wisconsin Hospital Based Domestic Violence Project have changed the power and control and equality wheels into tools which health workers can use to determine whether their response to victims/survivors is abusing their power (medical power and control) or whether they are using their positions to advocate for women and help them end the violence in their lives.

Power and Control Wheel
by The Domestic Abuse Intervention Project, Duluth MN.

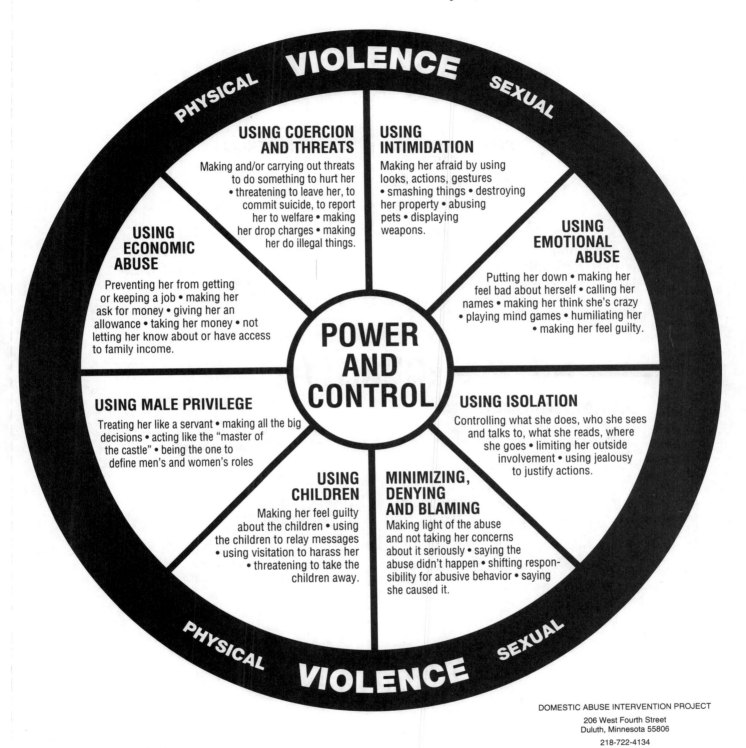

DOMESTIC ABUSE INTERVENTION PROJECT
206 West Fourth Street
Duluth, Minnesota 55806
218-722-4134

Equality Wheel
by the Domestic Abuse Intervention Project, Duluth, MN.

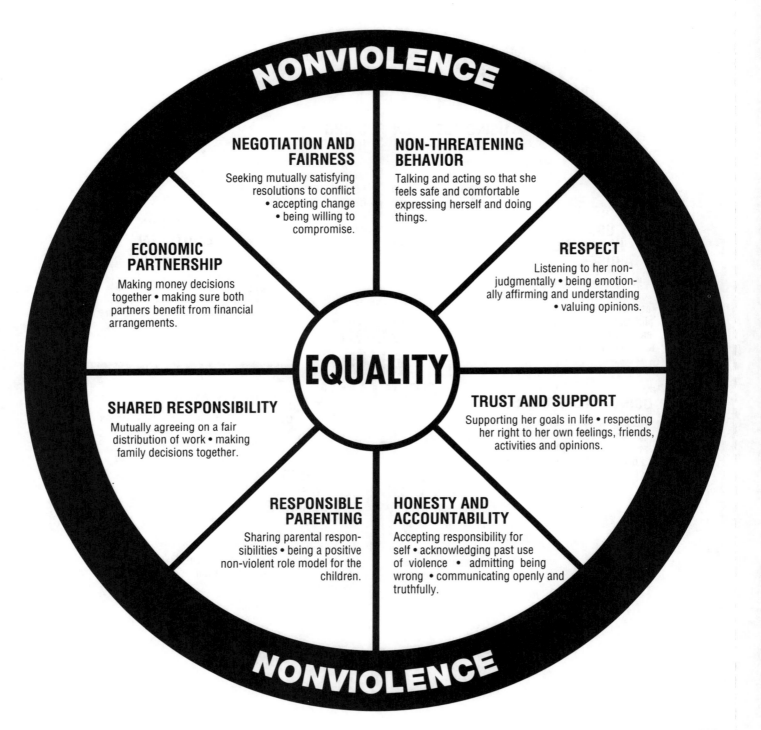

NONVIOLENCE

NEGOTIATION AND FAIRNESS
Seeking mutually satisfying resolutions to conflict • accepting change • being willing to compromise.

NON-THREATENING BEHAVIOR
Talking and acting so that she feels safe and comfortable expressing herself and doing things.

ECONOMIC PARTNERSHIP
Making money decisions together • making sure both partners benefit from financial arrangements.

RESPECT
Listening to her non-judgmentally • being emotionally affirming and understanding • valuing opinions.

EQUALITY

SHARED RESPONSIBILITY
Mutually agreeing on a fair distribution of work • making family decisions together.

TRUST AND SUPPORT
Supporting her goals in life • respecting her right to her own feelings, friends, activities and opinions.

RESPONSIBLE PARENTING
Sharing parental responsibilities • being a positive non-violent role model for the children.

HONESTY AND ACCOUNTABILITY
Accepting responsibility for self • acknowledging past use of violence • admitting being wrong • communicating openly and truthfully.

NONVIOLENCE

DOMESTIC ABUSE INTERVENTION PROJECT
206 West Fourth Street
Duluth, Minnesota 55806
218-722-4134

Continuum of Family Violence
from Alaska Dept. of Public Safety

PHYSICAL

pushing   punching   slapping   kicking   throwing objects   choking   using weapons   homicide/suicide → **DEATH**

VERBAL EMOTIONAL

name calling   criticizing   "you're no good"   ignoring   yelling   isolation   humiliation → **SUICIDE**

SEXUAL

unwanted touching   sexual name calling   unfaithfulness   false accusations   forced sex   hurtful sex → **RAPE**

Without some kind of help, the violence usually gets worse. The end result can be death.

Sexual Harassment Information Sheet

by Wisconsin Coalition Against Sexual Assault

What is Sexual Harassment?

The roots of sexual harassment lie in our misogynist culture which views women as sexual objects. It is part of the continuum of violence against women. Sexual harassment is the sexualization of an otherwise nonsexual relationship. It is an assertion by men of the primacy of a woman's sexuality over her role as a worker, colleague, student or human being. Additionally, sexual harassment includes harassment, not sexual in nature, that would not occur but for the sex of the person. It is not about sex, harassment is about power which serves to keep the victim "in her place." It is sexual victimization, an insidious form of sex discrimination, not a benign mating ritual.

How Often Does It Occur?

- All women have been sexually harassed at sometime or another, for sexual harassment can happen to us from the moment of birth until the moment of death and sometimes even after death (Wise and Stanley, 1987).
- Twenty million women in the U.S. labor force are victims of sexual harassment annually (Chapman and Chapman, 1984).
- 88% of the respondents to a 1976 survey reported having experienced one or more forms of unwanted sexual advances on the job (Redbook, 1976).
- Women are nine times more likely than men to quit jobs because of sexual harassment, five times more likely to transfer and three times more likely to lose jobs (Konrad and Gutek, 1986).
- 50% – 80% of American women will experience some form of sexual harassment during their academic or working life (Hughes and Sandler, 1986, 1987; U.S. Merit Protection Board 1987).
- Surveys on campus show that up to 30% of all female college students experience some form of sexual harassment (In Case of Sexual Harassment, 1986).
- 90% of sexual harassment victims are unwilling to come forward for two primary reasons: fear of retaliation and fear of loss of privacy (Klien, 1988).
- Sexual harassment costs a typical Fortune 500 company $6.7 million per year—a cost of $282.53 per employee; meaningful preventive steps can be taken for $200,000—a cost of $8.41 per employee. It is 34 times more expensive to ignore the problem (Klien, 1988).

Who Is Involved?

There are no 'typical' harassers. Harassers are found in all types of occupations, at all organizational levels, among college professors as well as in the business world, and among individuals who live otherwise exemplary lives. Most harassers are older than their victims (although some are younger), married (although some are single) and of the same race as their victims. Usually there is a pattern of harassment: one man harasses a number of women either sequentially or simultaneously, or both. In a typical sexual harassment case, the accuser becomes the accused, and the victim feels twice-victimized.

What Type of Activities Are Involved?

Sexual harassment may encompass a full range of coercive behaviors from subtle psychological force to physical abuse.

- Undressing a person with one's eyes
- Looking down a woman's shirt
- Caressing a person's hand
- Using sexually explicit language
- Picking lint or hair off of a person's clothing in a personal area
- "Accidently," brushing against someone
- Direct verbal abuse and propositions
- Hugging, grabbing, kissing or directly touching
- Coercion of sexual activity by threat of punishment
- Gross sexual imposition like touching, fondling, grabbing or assaulting
- Talking about sexually explicit movies or TV shows
- Asking sexual questions
- Inquiring and projecting about one's sexual interests
- Discussing the size of sexual organs
- Questioning a woman's judgement or decisions because "she's a woman"
- Devaluing a woman because "she has PMS"
- Creating a hostile work environment
- General sexist remarks and behavior
- Solicitation of sexual activity or other sex-linked behavior by promise of rewards
- Displaying pornography in the workplace

Ω

Acquaintance/Date Rape Information Sheet

by the Wisconsin Coalition Against Sexual Assault

Date/acquaintance rape is an extremely underreported crime, yet it is the most common type of sexual violence. The perpetrators may be: friends, relatives, employers, a date, or someone the victim/survivors recently met. What they have in common is a belief system which incorporates myths such as: women owe men sex if they spend money on her; some women play hard to get and say no when they mean yes; and women enjoy being pursued by an aggressive male. Additionally, perpetrators often do not identify as rapists. Frequently, perpetrators are not held responsible and victim/survivors are blamed for being raped.

Date/acquaintance rape is a coercive, manipulative form of sexual violence. It is NEVER the victim/survivors fault no matter what she wore, where she was, whether or not she fought back, or whether or not she was drinking. The perpetrators are 100% responsible for their actions. Rape is violence where sex is used as the weapon.

Individuals who have been assaulted by someone they know may feel guilty or responsible for the assault, feel betrayed, question their judgment and have difficulty trusting people. Recovery from an assault can be assisted by contacting an advocate who understands the needs of sexual assault victims. Many communities have rape crisis centers with 24-hour counseling and advocacy services.

Here Are the Facts:

- A woman has a 4 times greater chance of being raped by someone she knows than by a stranger (Warshaw, 1988).
- Only 17% of rapists are strangers; 83% of perpetrators are acquaintances (friends of the family, dates, boyfriends, relatives, authority figures). (Russell, 1986).
- Rape by acquaintances accounts for 60% of all rapes reported to rape crisis centers (Levy, 1991).
- 55% of rapes where the perpetrator is a stranger are reported to the police, while 19% of acquaintance rapes are reported. Of acquaintance rapes, only 2% of rapes were reported when the perpetrator was a friend of the family or a date (Russell, 1986).
- Women aged 16 to 24 are three times more likely to be raped than other women (US Dept. of Justice, 1991).
- Approximately 50% of all sexual assault offenders are under 25 years old (FBI, 1989).
- 5% to 16% of adolescent males sexually assault each year (Ageton, 1983).
- 27% of girls aged 15 to 19 have been victims of rape or attempted rape. 84% of these victims knew their attacker. (Warshaw, 1988).
- 75% of men and 55% of women involved in acquaintance rapes reported using alcohol or other drugs prior to the incident (Warshaw, 1988).
- Studies indicate that dating violence affects at least 1 in 10 teen couples. It is one of the major sources of violence in teen life (Levy, 1991).
- Young women between the ages of 14 and 17 represent an estimated 38% of those victimized by date rape (Warshaw, 1988).
- Over 50% of high school boys and 42% of high school girls believe that there are times when it is "acceptable for a male to hold a female down and physically force her to engage in intercourse." (Warshaw, 1988).
- 1 in 4 women report being the victims of rape or attempted rape during their years in college (Warshaw, 1988).
- 75% of these women did not identify their experience as sexual assault (Warshaw, 1988).
- 47% of college-age women report having been sexually assaulted by first or casual dates or by acquaintances at some time in their life (Warshaw, 1988).
- 1 in 12 college-age men admit having fulfilled the prevailing definition of rape or attempted rape, yet virtually none of these men identify themselves as rapists (Warshaw, 1988).
- 60% of male college students "indicated some likelihood of raping or using force in certain circumstances." (Briere and Malamuth, 1983).
- Only 19.7% of reported campus sexual assaults in 1989–1990 resulted in criminal penalties; 38.8% resulted in campus penalties (Towson State University, Campus Violence Prevention Center, 1988 National Campus Violence Survey).
- There have been more than 75 *documented* cases of gang rape on college campuses in recent years. The number is most likely much higher (Ehrhart & Sandler, 1985).

Ω

By the Wisconsin Coalition Against Sexual Assualt (WCASA), 1400 East Washington Ave., Suite 148, Madison, WI 53703, (608) 257–1516. Copyright © 1992 by the Wisconsin Coalition Against Sexual Assault. Reprinted by permission.

♀

Sexual Assault Information Sheet

by Wisconsin Coalition Against Sexual Assault

Sexual assault is an act (verbal and/or physical) which breaks a person's trust and/or safety and is sexual in nature. The term "sexual assault" includes: rape, incest, sexual harassment, child sexual assault, marital rape, exposure, and voyeurism.

Sexual assaults are acts of violence where sex is used as the weapon. Assaults are motivated primarily out of anger and/or a need to feel powerful by controlling, dominating, or humiliating the victim. Victims/survivors of sexual assaults are forced, coerced, and/or manipulated to participate in unwanted sexual activity. Victims/survivors do not cause their assaults and are not to blame. Offenders are responsible for the assaults.

Here Are the Facts:

In the United States

- People from 2 months to 97 years have been raped (Benedict, 1984).
- 1 in 3 women will be raped in her lifetime (Los Angeles Commission on Assaults Against Women, 1985).
- 1 in 4 girls will be sexually assaulted before the age of 18 (Russell, 1983).
- 1 in 7 boys will be sexually assaulted before the age of 18 (Russell, 1983).
- In 1989, 94,504 rapes were reported in the U.S. Based on reports to the police, 16 rapes are attempted and 10 women are raped every hour in the U.S. (FBI Uniform Crime Report, 1989).
- In 1990, rape rose faster than any other reported violent crime in the U.S. The number of rapes reported to the police exceeded 100,000 for the first time. It is estimated that the actual number of rapes was between 1.3 and 2 million which makes the U.S. rape rate the world's highest (Senate Judiciary Committee Study on Violence Against Women, March 1991).
- Rape is the most underreported violent crime, with only 5% to 20% reporting (Helen Benedict, Recovery; How to Survive Sexual Assault, 1985).
- 83% of raped adolescents, 71.4% of raped young adults, and 68.4% of raped adults did not report their assault to the police (Kilpatrick, 1990).
- Victimization rates are highest among women aged 16–34 (U.S. DOJ, 1988).
- A woman's risk of being raped by someone she knows is 4 times greater than being raped by a stranger (Warshaw, 1988).
- An estimated 60–80% of all rape is date or acquaintance rape (Koss, 1988; Russell, 1990).
- 1 in 7 women reported that they had been raped by their husbands (Russell, 1985).
- For years following a rape, 60% of rape victims experience post traumatic stress disorder and 16% still suffer with emotional problems 15 years following the rape (HRS Rape Awareness Program, Tallahassee, FL, 1987).
- White victims were raped by white perpetrators 81.5% of the time. Black victims are raped by black perpetrators 85.3% of the time (U.S. DOJ, 1988).

In Wisconsin

- 6,366 sexual assaults were reported to law enforcement agencies in 1990.
- 93% of victims are female.
- 98% of offenders are male.
- The majority of rapes were perpetrated by someone known to the victim; 58% of offenders were friends or acquaintances of the victim; 16% were family members.
- Average age of the victim is 18.
- Average age of the offender is 25.

Ω

A More Hidden Crime:
Adolescent Battered Women

by Nancy Worcester

Domestic violence has often been referred to as our nation's most hidden crime. However, after 15 years of activism and the establishment of more than 1000 battered women's shelter programs around the country, the battered women's movement has made many people and community services aware of the fact that huge numbers of women are entrapped in relationships of ongoing abuse of power, control, and physical coercion. The FBI estimates that a woman is battered every 15–18 seconds in this county and that approximately one of every three women experiences some physical violence in her long-term relationship(s). The pervasiveness of the violence may be best represented by the statement that one of every five women probably experiences five or more serious battering incidents each year.

Just as there is finally a public consciousness of the magnitude of the problem of women being battered, we are discovering an even more hidden, perhaps even more prevalent crime—violence against adolescent women. It turns out that most of the understanding of the dynamics of power and control in intimate relationships gained from the battered women's movement applies as much to adolescent women in dating relationships as it does to adult women. Tragically, the ramifications of violence for younger women are often exaggerated by a number of factors, but there are far fewer resources and options available to adolescent than adult women who are trying to end the violence in their lives.

Working to prevent violence in young people's lives must be a highest priority for any of us committed to creating a better world for the next generation and to helping young women maximize on their full potential. The isolation and lowered self-esteem which are so often a *consequence* of violence will have exaggerated ramifications for a young woman if they cause her to limit or eliminate skill-building, career opportunities or educational opportunities which could affect the rest of her life. (It is important to emphasize that the isolation, lowered self-esteem, and unhealthy coping mechanisms which are often observed in abused women are predictable *consequences* of violence and are not the *cause* of the violence. Confusing a consequence of violence with a cause can lead to dangerous, victim-blaming misunderstandings of the violence.)

If a woman is experiencing violence in her dating relationship(s), it will almost certainly be related to many other issues in her life. Anyone working with adolescents will benefit from seeing the connections between violence and the issues they already address. Why she is not always able to show up for study group, why she "had to go" to a concert instead of studying the night before an important exam, why she is no longer best friends with "the nice girl who seemed to have such a positive influence on her" or why she "suddenly" started dressing in a way which always *or* never shows off her figure may be explained by knowing that a young woman is in a relationship where someone else is taking control over almost all aspects of her life. Health educators need to recognize that many women are beaten up if they try to insist that male partners wear a condom or abstain from sexual activity. Because battering so often starts or accelerates during pregnancy and because sexual assault and other forms of violence are so intimately connected, anyone who works with adolescent pregnancy or sexual assault issues needs to be aware of the connections.

Ironically, many women learn about motherhood and battering at exactly the same time. Retrospective studies show that 25% of battered women experienced their first physical abuse during a pregnancy and that 40–60% of battered women were abused during a pregnancy or during pregnancies. The consequences are a much higher rate of miscarriage, stillbirth, premature delivery, and low birth weight infants in battered than non-battered women. The problem may be even more exaggerated in pregnant teens. A study looking specifically at physical abuse during teen pregnancy found that 26% of pregnant teens reported they were involved with a man who physically hurt them and 40–60% said that the battering had begun or escalated since their boyfriends knew they were pregnant. This study also provides an urgent reminder that services are not addressing the issue of violence for adolescent women: 65% of pregnant teens had not talked to *anyone* about the abuse.[1]

Looking at the continuum of violence issues (The Power and Control and Equity Wheels by the Duluth Domestic Abuse Intervention Project (see pp 347 & 348) and the Continuum of Family Violence Chart from Village to Village (see p 349), by the Alaska Dept. of Public Safety are particularly useful), it becomes apparent how a range of forms of violence—physical, verbal, emotional, and sexual—are used by abusers to dominate their partners. The more subtle forms of sexual violence (unwanted touching, sexual name calling, unfaithfulness or threat of unfaithfulness, saying "no one else will ever love you", false accusations) are clearly emotionally as well as sexually controlling. These need to be identified as "violence issues" which are related to, and can escalate into, unwanted sex, unprotected sex, hurtful sex and other forms of sexual assault. Sexual violence is often the expression of violence which is the most painful for a woman to discuss. Emotional abuse is almost always present if there are other forms of abuse in a relationship but a clever abuser may achieve sufficient control by emotional abuse without ever resorting to other forms. Women consistently say that emotional abuse is the hardest form to identify (Is this really happening? Is this abuse? Am I making too much of this?) but recognize it as the form of abuse which has the most impact on their lives and their view of themselves. Many women who have been in life-threatening situations say, "The physical battering was nothing compared to the daily emotional abuse." Helping young women see the interconnectedness of verbal, emotional, physical and sexual power and control issues may be the most useful information in empowering them to end *all* forms of violence in their lives.

By the time adolescents start experimenting with their own dating relationships, they have been bombarded with messages that violence against women is tolerated and even encouraged and that dominance, aggression, and abuse of power and control are appropriate masculine behaviors which are rewarded by society. Today's young people have been exposed to a tolerance and perpetuation of male violence which is unique to this generation. They grew up in the era when the average child was watching 24 hours of television a week with children's programming averaging 15.5 violent acts per hour. By the time they reach 18, the average US adolescent has witnessed approximately 26,000 murders, in their own homes, via the tv screen.[2]

The role of television in sex-role socialization and the perpetuation of male violence has been grossly exaggerated for today's young people because changes in federal regulations, in the early 1980s, allowed the sale of toys directly connected to tv shows, removed regulations limiting the amount of advertising allowed on children's programming, and ruled that product-based shows were legal. The result was a totally new integration of the tv and toy industries. By 1986 all of the ten best selling toys had shows connected with them and by 1988, 80% of children's tv programming was produced by toy companies. Parallel marketing promoted definitions of masculinity and femininity as clearly defined as the distinct lines of boys' toys vs. girls' toys. Because of the new integration of tv and toys, today's young people did not learn to explore their own creativity or imagination in healthy ways but instead learned to "act out their scripts" as dominant and competitive *or* caring, helpless, and concentrating on appearance, either as GI Joe or Ghostbusters vs. Barbie or My Little Pony.[3]

With electronic video games, an even newer and unstudied phenomena, young people get to act out and be rewarded for playing their violent roles. The direct participation in "performing" the violence of video games is predicted to magnify whatever effect more passive tv viewing has on one's acceptance or perpetuation of violence. In a violence promoting and accepting culture, it is not surprising to find that *most* video games are very violent (a sampling of 120 machines in three arcades in Madison, Wisconsin, found that more than 70 involved either hand-to-hand combat or shooting to kill enemies) and that the most popular games in an arcade are the most violent.[4]

Consequently, *unlearning* the tolerance of violence and *learning* how to achieve violence-free, equal relationships are skills which are now as crucial to *teach* young people as reading, writing, math and the use of computers. The way people learn, in their earliest experimentation, to be in intimate relationships can set the pattern for what they expect in future relationships. It is a time when the highest standards should be set! Adolescents need to see models of healthy, equal, violence-free relationships, in order to aim for that in their own lives and *to be able to model that for their peers.*

At this stage, many teens do not have the knowledge or skills to prevent or react against violence in their own lives or in their friends' lives. In fact, exactly the opposite is much more likely. Many young women have said that even when they have told friends they were being hurt by their boyfriends, the response was that they were lucky to have boyfriends. There is enormous peer pressure not to break up. Many teens regard violence as a normal part of dating and have no idea they deserve better. Extreme possessiveness, jealousy, dominance, and not being "allowed" to break up get wrongly identified as desirable, positive signs of caring, love and commitment, rather than strong warning signs that they are in an unhealthy, potentially dangerous relationship.

Figuring out what to expect in relationships may be particularly confusing for anyone who grew up in a home where there was violence. Many young men only see abusing males (in reality *and* in the media) as role models. Many young women who told their mother about being hurt by their boyfriend, have heard, "you have to learn to take the bad and the good in a relationship to make it work."

Many teens who have grown-up in violent homes face the difficulty of trying to figure out how they want to be in their own young adult relationships while they are still learning (or not learning) to cope with being affected by the violence with which they grew up. The battered women's movement has very effectively identified that when a woman is battered, the children are almost always affected by the violence. Seventy-five percent of women who are battered in this country have children living at home. Children in homes where domestic violence occurs are physically abused or seriously neglected at a rate 1500% higher than the national average in the general population.[5] Even witnessing domestic violence can have a tremendous impact on young people and may result in symptoms very similar to those seen in people who have been abused.[6] Helping these young people learn healthy relationship skills can be particularly challenging as many teens do not recognize the impact the violence in their homes has had on them and many teens do not want to talk about witnessing or experiencing abuse.[7]

Particularly crucial to how we help young people learn relationship skills *and* acknowledge that violence in their lives may have already influenced their attitudes and behaviors is how we address the impact of the "intergenerational transmission of violence." There is a confusing body of work which examines how the cycle of violence can be passed on through the generations. We now know the old "dad beats mom, mom beats the children, and the children beat the pets" picture was much too simplistic and inaccurate. Increasingly, it is being shown that the person beating mom may also be the one beating the children[8] and protecting the mother is often the best way to protect the children.[9] Although research is inconsistent in documenting the rates of intergenerational transmission of violence, there is a consistent trend which shows that boys who witness domestic violence as children are more likely to batter their female partners as adults than are men from non-violent homes.

How we use this information can be a key factor in determining whether we help break the intergenerational transmission of violence or actually contribute to its perpetuation. Too much of the literature deals with this data as if were inevitable. Central to breaking the pattern is addressing and researching a different set of questions. *If* 30% of boys who witness violence become abusers, the question must be asked, "What can we learn from the 70% who witness violence but do not become abusers?" What factors help young people who have witnessed violence learn to resist violent behavior? Young people from violent homes who have experienced the ugliness of violence and have learned to value non-violent relationships can be exactly the people most committed to breaking the cycle of violence and can be incredibly effective peer leaders.

Most important, young people must *never* learn that violence is inevitable. Many dating violence resources (including some of the materials I highly recommend on other aspects) include information on the intergenerational transmission of violence without making it clear that the cycle can be broken. Information on warning signs of potential abusers almost always include "boys who grew up in violent homes". What does it feel like to see that information if you are a young man who witnessed violence at home? We must make certain that none of our materials or our messages ever contribute towards a young man feeling that he is destined to be violent.

Studies on dating violence consistently show that many teens in violent relationships have not talked to *any* adults about the violence in their lives. We need to start identifying the barriers which have made us so ineffective on this issue and acknowledge that we are only starting to have the language and tools for opening a dialogue on dating violence.

The good news is that a wide range of excellent resources, curricula, and videos have been produced on dating violence issues and violence-free relationships in recent years. It's a very exciting stage to be working on this issue because no one needs to "start from scratch". However, work needs to be done to make the excellent resources and services available to, and appropriate for, many more teens. Few of the resources address the issue in a way that has any meaning for lesbian, gay or bisexual teens or for young people of color. Many of the materials seem to have the underlying assumption that children grow up in homes where there is one male and one female adult. Special issues for teens with disabilities need to be addressed because of both the high rate of sexual assault of people with disabilities and the complexities of dating which arise from the myth that people with disabilities are "asexual". The obsession with body image and a very narrow definition of attractiveness can also be particularly cruel and abusive in adolescence.

"You deserve to be treated with respect."

"You are not alone if someone is hurting you. There are excellent resources to help you end the violence in your life."

These messages which we have been giving adult battered women for the last 15 years are now the same messages we have to give to much younger women.

References

1. "Violence During Teen Pregnancy: Health Consequences for Mother and Child" by Judith McFarlane, in *Dating Violence*, edited by Barrie Levy, Seal Press, 1991, pp. 136–141.
2. *Boys Will Be Boys (Breaking the Link Between Masculinity and Violence)* by Myriam Miedzian, Doubleday, New York, 1991.
3. *Who's Calling the Shots? How to Respond Effectively to Children's Fascination with War Play and War Toys* by Nancy Carlsson-Paige and Diane E. Levin, New Society Publishers, Santa Cruz, CA, 1990.
4. "Decapitate Your Enemy for 50 Cents", "Most Violent Games Draw Most Attention", and "Researcher Says TV Programs Undoubtedly Affect Children" by Nathan Seppa, in *Wisconsin State Journal* January 3, 1993, pp 1A & 7A.
5. National Women's Abuse Prevention Project, Washington, D.C.
6. A video of Susan Schechter speaking on "Battered Women and Abused Children: Interests in Common or Interest in Conflict?" is available from the WI. Domestic Violence Training Project.
7. Ann Brickson, Briarpatch, Madison. WI.
8. "Exploring the Complexities of Working on Children's Issues" by Nancy Worcester, in *Wisconsin Coalition Against Domestic Violence Newsletter*, December 1988.
9. *Health Care Services for Battered Women and Their Abused Children* (manual about the AWAKE—Advocacy for Women and Their Kids in Emergencies Program), Boston's Children's Hospital, 300 Longwood Avenue, Boston, MA 02115 ($22), 1992.

A list of resources is available from the Wisconsin Domestic Violence Training Project, 623 Lowell Hall, 610 Langdon St., Madison WI 53703. Barrie Levy's books *In Love and In Danger* (A Teen's Guide to Breaking Free of Abusive Relationships), *Dating Violence—Young Women in Danger* and her curriculum, *Skills for Violence-Free Relationships* are particularly recommended.

Power and Control and Equality wall charts are available ($6@) from the Minnesota Program Development, Inc. 206 W. 4th St., Duluth, MN 55806 and the "Continuum of Family Violence" is available in *Domestic Violence—A Guide for Health Care Professionals* ($10) from the New Jersey Department of Community Affairs, Domestic Violence Prevention Program (CN–0801), 101 S. Broad St., Trenton, NJ 08625–0801.

Ω

♀

Ethnicity and Woman Abuse in the United States

by Evelyn L. Barbee

Introduction

"You Black bitch, I'll beat the shit out of you!" Those were the words that began my nightmarish experience with a violent encounter on the streets of New York City. Usually a chapter like this begins with an overview of the problem and definition of terms. However, as I thought about my task it occurred to me that a more appropriate way to introduce the subject of ethnicity and woman abuse was to share an experience, that I, as an African-American woman, had with abuse. I chose to share this experience for two reasons. First, I believe that the experience demonstrates the type of abuse to which African-American and other women of color are subjected. Second, the experience is also illustrative of Euro-American attitudes about violence that are directed toward women of color.

When I was a master's student in nursing education at Teachers College, Columbia University, I had an apartment in Greenwich Village. It was a beautiful spring day and a friend called and suggested that I take a break from writing my master's project to meet her for lunch. We decided to meet at the Chock Full O'Nuts restaurant because it was next door to her supermarket job and around the corner from my house. At the appointed time I grabbed my sunglasses, keys, and change purse and ran downstairs to meet her. On the way to the restaurant, I noticed two young White males soliciting food for Biafra outside the supermarket. My friend was late; it was a sunny day, so I decided to wait for her outside. Sixth Avenue is a very busy Greenwich Village street, so I stepped into a doorway in order to change from regular glasses to sunglasses.

While I was changing glasses, a Black male came by and demanded that I give him some money. His clothing

was filthy, and he smelled. His eyes were glazed and bloodshot. Perhaps I was irritated because my friend was late. I know that I was tired of strangers asking my for money. So I said, "Do I look like a bank to you?" That is when he snarled, "You black bitch, I'll beat the shit out of you!" and moved towards me. My first thought was: "He's serious! I've got to get out of this doorway. He can kill me in here." As I moved out of the doorway, I had several thoughts. The first one was of Kitty Genovese, a 28-year-old Euro-American woman who was stabbed to death in a middle-class neighborhood in Queens, New York, in 1964. None of the 38 witnesses to her stabbing called the police until after she was dead (Rosenthal, 1964). And now, here I was a Black woman being assaulted by a Black man on a busy street full of White pedestrians. I knew that I was on my own.

Lest one think that I was exaggerating, let me share another experience. This took place the previous summer on the same street. On this occasion I witnessed an argument between a Black woman and her Black male partner. Across the street, laughing and talking, stood four White New York City police officers. When the couple's argument deteriorated from verbal disagreements to threats of bodily harm, I crossed the street and approached the police officers. I asked if they believed that the police had a role in the prevention of crime. They replied, "Yes." Then I asked why they were ignoring the increasing volatile situation with the couple across the street. I wrote down their badge numbers and said that if the man harmed the woman then at least I had the badge numbers of the police officers who witnessed the crime. Two of them proceeded to go across the street. Given that the police would only intervene in an altercation between an African-American couple when threatened, I felt that I had good reason to believe that the citizenry would offer little or no help to me.

My second thought was that I had to keep this man from hitting me. I recalled the boxing lessons my brothers had given me when I first started working on psychiatric units.

From VIOLENCE AGAINST WOMEN: NURSING RESEARCH, EDUCATION, AND PRACTICE ISSUES. Copyright © 1992 by Taylor & Francis, Inc. Reprinted by permission.

The author acknowledges Audre Lorde who encouraged her to put her experience in print.

So there we were in the middle of Sixth Avenue, people walking by, this stranger throwing hard punches at me, and me circling and blocking them. His inability to hit me had two results. He became more angry and my arms felt like they were going to fall off. Realizing that I could not block any more of his punches, I ran into Chock Full O'Nuts. He tried to come in after me but was unable because I held the door. While I was holding the door, five or six White men came up to enter the restaurant. They became irritated with me and moved away when they saw what was happening.

I looked for a weapon. A quick glance ascertained what I thought before I ran inside: I could not defend myself with sugar packets. So, I let go of the door and he flew backwards. More enraged, he charged toward me. I remember thinking, "What ignominy. I'm going to die in Chock Full O'Nuts!" Fortunately, I was saved by an elderly White woman with a cane. She approached him and said: "If you think you're a man because you can hit a woman, then hit me." The White men who were waiting outside the door suddenly mobilized, and my assaulter ran across the street. She turned to me and said: "You don't know him, do you dear." I said, "No." She then said, "I didn't think so." I thanked her profusely and walked next door to the supermarket. The two young White men soliciting food for Biafra outside of the supermarket asked me to "Remember the people of Biafra and buy an extra can to donate." I asked them how could they have the nerve to ask me to donate anything to them when they stood there and watched while this man tried to kill me. Their response, "We thought you knew him." I said: "Why? Because we're both Black?"

I recount this story for several reasons. First, it is a concrete example of the factors that affect the risk of violence to ethnic women of color in this country. These factors, racism and sexism, are important aspects that need to be dealt with whenever the subject is violence and African-American women in the United States. Second, my situation is an example of how deeply ingrained racist and sexist attitudes are in this society. Although I was rescued from bodily harm, it is ironic that both action and nonaction were based upon individual perceptions of whether I "knew" my assailant. Quite obviously, for the bulk of people who chose not to respond to my dilemma, I must have known this man because we were both Black and he was attacking me.

In a sense their perceptions more accurately reflect the nature of violence against women because it is usually committed by someone the woman knows. At the same time, there is tacit approval of the violence because she "knows" him. Fortunately for me, a physically vulnerable person, an elderly White woman who walked with a cane, came to my defense because she decided that I did not know my attacker. Later I wondered what would have happened if I had known him and what gave anyone the right to assume it is all right for a woman to be attacked by a man that she knows. Obviously, it was not all right for him to attack my rescuer. Simply put, in this White patriarchal, racist society, it was all right for him (a Black man)

to hit me (a Black woman) but wrong for him to strike her (an older White woman). As hate crimes of violence escalate against people because of their race, ethnicity, sexual orientation, gender, or religion, the history of and structural conditions that contribute to violence against "the other" in this society receive less attention. Yet the fact remains that violence against people of color, particularly women, is a historical reality.

Ethnicity, Culture, and Violence

Although there are numerous definitions of ethnicity, this chapter uses a social science definition of ethic group. This definition of ethnicity refers to a cultural orientation or participation that is shared by a large group of people. Included in this cultural orientation are common customs and traditions. The above definition allows us to recognize African-Americans as an ethnic and cultural rather than a racial group. The definition further enables us to recognize the common cultural orientation of Latinas in a way that the term Hispanic does not.

Culture and Violence

A common theory that has been used to explain violence cross-culturally is the "culture of violence." The culture of violence theory is based upon cultural patterning theory (Levinson, 1989). Cultural patterning theory, in turn, incorporates aspects of social learning theory to explain how people learn certain cultural values. The cultural patterning theory suggests that through socialization, either as a member of a violent family or as a member of a violent society, people learn that the use of violence is an appropriate means of achieving goals. In terms of families, socialization into violence underlies research that suggests that victims of child abuse are more likely to become child abusers than nonvictims of child abuse. As applied to families, the culture of violence theory has been challenged by Cazenave and Straus (1979), and Hampton (1987a) who points out that structural/social (poverty, unemployment) and situational (chemical dependency) conditions, rather than cultural values, may influence family violence. Furthermore, recent research on Latinos in California suggests that despite their poverty and deprivation, they do not demonstrate the traits usually found in the violent underclass (Winkler, 1990).

At the societal level, the cultural pattern model underlies those studies that use the cultural spillover hypothesis (Levinson, 1989). The cultural spillover hypothesis points to a positive correlation between a society's endorsement of the use of physical force to meet certain social ends (e.g., crime control, political hegemony) and generalization of force to other areas of social life (e.g., rape, family violence) (Baron & Straus, 1983, cited in Levinson, 1989). Unfortunately discussions of cultural patterning tend to neglect the influence of social structural conditions on violence. Social structure refers to the relationships between individuals and groups within a society. Social structure is maintained because it is governed by laws, rules, norms, and practices. Two structural conditions that are seldom acknowledged in regard to ethnicity and violence in this country are the patriarchy and racism. As a major structural component of this society, the patriarchy has been used to condone violence against women of color.

Although the traditions and customs of ethnic groups of color sometimes come into conflict with those of Euro-American values, for ethnic women of color the importance of the patriarchy is usually revealed in situations of violence. Across the country there are examples of men using culture, custom, and tradition as excuses for perpetrating violence against women. For example, Findlen (1990) reported two cases of violence against Asian women. In the first case, an Asian man in New York City was sentenced to five years probation for bludgeoning his wife to death. In the second a Hmong man was acquitted of kidnapping, sexual assault, and menacing after abducting a 16-year-old girl. The use of an anthropologist in one case and a cultural defense in both cases simply serves to maintain the status quo of the patriarchy because in both cases the men were viewed as following patriarchal customs.

Racism and Image

Violence toward women of color in this country cannot be fully understood without some understanding of the impact of racism and sexism on attitudes toward women of color and violence. The racist and sexist attitudes toward women of color are best found in the images that are developed by White men. The following discussion of racism and image specifically refers to African-American women; however, the process of devaluation is applicable to Latinas, Native American, and Asian women.

Although, woman abuse cuts across racial, ethnic, social, and economic boundaries, the situation of African-American women in this patriarchal society is particularly unique. As Christensen (1988, p. 191) pointed out "No other woman has suffered physical and mental abuse, degradation, and exploitation on North American shores comparable to that experienced by the Black female." The devaluation of African-American women began with the sexual exploitation of these women during slavery and continues today. Many of the historical incidents of sexual abuse of African-American women during and after slavery are discussed in Lerner (1973, Ch. 1, 3). Today as in the past, the treatment of African-American women is based on a racist and sexist ideology.

In pointing out that race, class, and gender oppression depend on powerful ideological justification for their existence, Collins (1990) identifies four externally defined, controlling images that are applied to African-American women. These images are mammy, the faithful, obedient domestic servant; matriarch, the overly aggressive, emasculating, strong, independent, unfeminine woman; the welfare mother, a breeder who produces children for the state to support; and the Jezebel, a sexually aggressive woman. Although each of these images contributes to society's and consequently nursing's view of abused

African-American women, this chapter will only deal with the latter three.

The promiscuous stereotype of African-American women serves several functions. Historically and currently, the sexually promiscuous stereotype is used to contrast African-American women with the "virtuous" White women. Furthermore, the sexually promiscuous stereotype was used by White men as a reason for sexually abusing African-American women (Hooks, 1981). The view of African-American women as sexually promiscuous is also promoted by the scientific literature. Wyatt, Peters, and Guthrie (1988, p. 290) commented that dated research on African-American women's sexuality is used to "place some of the more controversial aspects of the sexual behavior of white women in perspective." The use of research findings in this way underscores Collins' (1990) point that one purpose of defining African-American women as outsiders is that these women can serve as the point from which other groups define their normality.

Further "evidence" of African-American women's "promiscuous" behavior is found in the research on age of coitus. Wyatt et al. (1988) note most sexuality research concludes that African-American women begin coitus at a younger age than Euro-American women. However, using a multiethnic sample of 248 women between 18 and 36 years of age, Wyatt (1989) found that ethnicity was not significantly associated with the strongest predictors of first intercourse. For both groups, the predictors for an older age at first coitus were stronger parental than peer influence during adolescence, and being in love and ready for sex (Wyatt, 1989).

In addition to being portrayed as sexually promiscuous, another predominant image of African-American women is that of matriarch. As Collins (1990) points out, viewing African-American women as matriarchal allows the dominant group in this society to blame these women for the success or failure of their children. Another effect of this image is that it allows "helping" professionals to not recognize when African-American women need assistance. (Whenever I have pointed out to Euro-American nurses that their unquestioned acceptance of African-American women as strong and independent, allows them to ignore that African-American women have feelings, the response has been silence.)

The problem that arises when the White patriarchal image of African-American women as matriarch is accepted without question is well documented by publications like Shahrazad Ali's *Blackman's Guide to Understanding the Blackwoman*. This undocumented polemic blamed the problems of African-Americans on the ethnic group's women. Moreover, it recommended the beating of African-American women (Ali, 1990, p.169). Unfortunately, the book received the type of publicity usually reserved for a major work. Although negatively reviewed, the publication of such reviews in *Newsweek* (Wilson, 1990) and several other major magazines and newspapers imparted a credibility the book did not deserve.

Equally damaging is the welfare mother image. This is essentially an updated version of the slavery created breeder image (Collins, 1990). As Collins notes, the breeder image allowed slave owners and others to depict African-American women as being more suitable for bearing children than White women. As a result slave owners felt they were justified in interfering with the reproductive rights of enslaved women. Today, welfare mothers are viewed as being too lazy to work and content to sit around and collect their checks. This current objectification of African-American women as welfare mothers serves to label as unnecessary and dangerous to the values of the country the fertility of women who are not Euro-American and middle class (Collins, 1990). The net result of these externally produced, controlling images is that African-American women's bodies are viewed as expendable (Hooks, 1990).

The Abuse of African-American Women

Homicide

Of all forms of interpersonal violence, homicide has some of the most devastating effects. Homicide is the leading cause of death in African-American women between 15–34 years of age. African-American women have a 1 in 104 chance of being a homicide victim. African-American women are more likely to be killed by their husband/partner during the course of a verbal argument (Bell, 1990). Using 1976– 1979 data from the Federal Bureau of Investigation—Uniform Crime Reporting Program (FBI–UCR), Jason, Strauss, and Tyler (1983) found that African-Americans were more involved in acquaintance homicide incidents than stranger incidents.

Wife Abuse

Unlike the homicide statistics of African-American women, the statistics on wife abuse are contradictory. For example, Straus, Gelles, and Steinmetz (1980) in their study of family violence in 2,143 African-American, White, Jewish, and other both spouse present families, found that a greater percentage of African-American wives were abused than any other group. Wife abuse was nearly 400% more common in African-American than White families. On the other hand, Coley and Beckett (1988), in a review of battered women research that included African-American women, suggest that likelihood of greater spousal wife abuse of African-American women and other minority women is a myth. In terms of social class, Cazenave and Straus (1979) indicated that wife abuse was less common among middle income African-Americans than middle income Euro- Americans. They also reported two cultural findings that lessened African-American wife abuse: embeddedness in a network of family and friends and the presence of nonnuclear family members in the home.

Sexual Abuse and Assault

In commenting upon the link between the rape of African-American women and the White patriarchy, Carby (1987) noted:

Rape has always involved patriarchal notions of women being, at best, not entirely unwilling accomplices, if not outwardly inviting a sexual attack. The links between Black women and illicit sexuality consolidated during the antebellum years had powerful ideological consequences for the next 150 years. (p.39)

An estimated 1 out of 10 sexual assaults is reported to the police. A low report rate combined with the poor police, public, and media response to sexual crimes against women of color make it very difficult to assess the incidence of sexual assault in African-American communities. The recent differential media circuses that surrounded the Tawana Brawley and the "Central Park Jogger" may only serve to decrease African-American women's sexual assault reports.

In November 1987, Tawana Brawley, a 15-year-old African-American girl, reported that she had been kidnapped, held captive for 4 days, and assaulted by six white men. She was found dazed, semi-conscious, and smeared with feces and semen in a trash bag. The words "KKK" and "nigger" were written on her body (Gillespie, 1988). After a series of investigations, a New York grand jury concluded that she had fabricated her report of kidnap and sexual abuse ("Evidence points," 1988). Her name and photograph were printed by newspapers and seen on television.

On April 19, 1989, a 28-year-old Euro-American female investment banker was beaten, sodomized, and raped while jogging in New York City's Central Park ("Youth rape," 1989). Eventually six African-American and Latino boys were indicted and sentenced for this heinous crime. Both the savagery of the attack and the social class of the victim made the crime national news, yet the jogger's name was not revealed by the New York Times (Mosedale, 1989; Harrison, 1989).

These two victims were treated very differently by the media. One, the "Central Park jogger," was treated with respect and dignity. The other, a minor, was treated like a criminal.

Child Abuse

Statistics from 1984 demonstrate that of 100,000 substantiated cases of child sexual abuse, 78% involved a girl (Wyatt & Powell, 1988). Frequently reported long-term effects of child sexual abuse "are self-destructive behavior, anxiety, feelings of isolation and stigma, poor self-esteem, difficulty in trusting others, a tendency toward revictimization, substance abuse, sexual maladjustment and psychological problems" (Wyatt & Powell, 1988, pp. 13–14).

Ethnic differences have been found among African-American, Latinos, and White abused children in regard to age of victim, family income, type and severity of abuse, and perpetrator (Hampton, 1987b). In terms of physical abuse, African-American victims who suffered more serious injuries were in the 6–12 age group, resided in urban areas, and had mothers who had not completed high school. Girls had higher rates of physical, sexual, and emotional abuse than boys (Hampton, 1987b). Russell, Schurman, and Trocki (1988) in a comparison study of African-American and White incest victims found that African-American women victims were more likely to report being extremely upset by the abuse and suffered from greater long-term effects. The African-American women also reported that their abuse was at the very severe level (i.e., involving oral, anal, or vaginal intercourse; that the abuse was more likely to be accompanied by force; that their perpetrators were more likely to be middle-aged; and that they were more likely to be abused by their uncles [Russell et al., 1988]).

The Nursing Process with Abused African-American Women

Assessment

The assessment data that are gathered by the nurse in the area of abused African-American women is largely dependent upon where the nurse encounters the women. It has been found that African-American women are more likely to use medical facilities than they are shelters, law enforcement, or human service personnel (Minnesota Department of Corrections, 1982).

Regardless of where the woman is encountered, there are certain general principles that all nurses need to heed. First, the nurse needs to have a strong awareness of how much she/he believes in the myths, beliefs, and stereotypes that surround African-American women. Although most nurses deny holding deleterious beliefs, as members of this society most nurses are prone to the myths and behaviors that contribute to the oppression of African-American women (Christensen, 1988). The consequences of a nurse holding stereotypical beliefs while trying to assist an abused woman of color can be disastrous. For example, in the case of African-American women, if the nurse believes that they are strong matriarchal figures, there may be less sensitivity to the human fragility of the client. On the other hand, the same belief may lead to the inference that the woman did something to "deserve" the abuse. If of the same ethnicity but different social class from the client, the nurse needs to be aware of when and whether these social class differences prejudice data collection.

Most of nursing literature does not deal with woman abuse and ethnicity, therefore, the nurse needs to become familiar with literature that does deal with these subjects. White (1989) contains several chapters that explore African-American women's experiences with and responses to abuse. Two publications that specifically discuss woman abuse among the two largest ethnic groups of color in this country are White (1985) and Zambrano (1985). *Chain, Chain, Change* (White, 1985) is specifically written for abused African-American women. *Mejor Sola Que Mal Accompanada: For the Latina in an Abusive Relationship* (Zambrano, 1985) is a guide for Latinas who are in abusive relationships. Both books use culturally relevant language and situations. Although written for laypersons, these books are valuable references for professionals.

Euro-American nurses also need to become knowledgeable about the different approaches that are being advocated for those who work with African-American clients. One approach that is gaining increased acceptance among African-American professionals is the Afrocentric perspective. *Afrocentrism* is a sociocultural perspective approach advocated by African-American researchers, scholars, and professionals who are concerned with positively influencing the lives of African-American people. Consequently, these researchers argue that the appropriate theoretical approach used with African-American people is one that is based upon their background and experiences. Essentially, those who are concerned with the problems of African-American violence argue that taking on the Euro-American value system with its emphasis on individual autonomy, materialism, and segmentation of all aspects of reality has been detrimental for a people whose cultural roots place importance on the interrelatedness and interdependence of all things (Bell, 1986; Myers, 1987, 1988, 1990).

Ashbury, (1987) uses the Afrocentric perspective to examine specific factors that influence battered African-American women seeking help. The special factors that influence this are:

1. the number of domestic shelters available in African-American communities

2. the amount and nature of the friend and family support system

3. the level of social isolation African-American women may feel in a shelter that is dominated by Euro-Americans

4. reluctance to expose an African-American man as a batterer because of his more vulnerable position in the larger society

5. reluctance to seek help is she has internalized common media stereotypes of African-American women

6. given the lack of African-American men available, she has concern about endangering her relationship.

Since there is a strong association between violence and other forms of abuse, if possible, data on previous abuse should be gathered. Given the importance of family and friends, the strengths of these networks should be assessed. Nurses should understand that African-American women are socialized to *not* share their concerns and problems outside of the family/friend network. The African-American phrase for telling strangers your problems is "Putting your business in the streets." Often this reluctance to discuss family and personal problems is misinterpreted as strength. For example, professional counselors, Bingham and Guinyard (1982) reported most of the African-American women, including the battered ones, that they saw in their practices "seemed to be strong and able to handle their problems" (Bingham & Guinyard, 1982, cited in Coley &

Beckett 1988, p. 268). It would appear that Bingham and Guinyard endorse the matriarchal image of African-American women.

Intervention

Often nurses assume because they are not working with abused women that the problem of woman abuse is not their concern. At other times nurses are unsure how to handle a problem that touches so many women. The type of assistance the nurse can offer is dependent upon where the victim of woman abuse is encountered, the type of abuse, and the level at which the nurse chooses to intervene. In terms of African-American woman abuse, there are four levels of intervention: structural, organizational, institutional, and individual.

Interventions at the structural level require that the nurse begin to understand the consequences of the Euro-American patriarchy upon which this society is based. An ongoing assessment of personal attitudes, beliefs, and stereotypes about African-American women will assist the nurse in understanding the role that racism plays in supporting the abuse. Other structural level interventions include becoming familiar with and supporting local, state, and national legislation that deals with woman abuse. Organizational level interventions include supporting women's organizations that focus on the problem of woman abuse and assessing the position of district, state, and national nurses organizations toward it. At the educational level, nursing curricula content in terms of amount and types of material on abuse and African-American women should be monitored.

At the individual level, the appropriate basic intervention strategies that are used for victims of violence should be engaged. Also, some intervention strategies may be more culturally appropriate for African-American women. Culturally appropriate interventions at the individual level should be based upon the recognition that African-American women have been socialized not to talk about their problems; do not usually seek mental health services for their problems; are aware of the poor treatment given to African-American women by law enforcement, media, and health professionals; may be reluctant to prosecute the involved man; and typically value the importance of family and friend networks.

African-American women do not usually seek mental health services; therefore, establishing rapport is especially critical if the nurse decides that mental health referral is necessary. If the nurse has abused African-American women as mental health clients a major role may be to assist the women in making the private public. Regardless of setting, the nurse should assist the women in overcoming their distrust of law enforcement officers and encourage the women to press charges against the male perpetrator. Given the importance of family and friend networks to African-American women, the nurse should endeavor to include concerned family/friends in interventions (e.g., shelter). If the woman is in a shelter, it may be because of weak or nonexistent family/friend networks. In this case, the intervention would be to assist the women in strengthening or developing networks.

Since most African-American women are more likely to be killed by their husband/partner during the course of a verbal argument, the potential for violence in the home needs to be reduced. Homicide prevention strategies should emphasize exploring alternative means of dispute resolution. In these instances, the nurse needs to work with the woman and her husband/partner or refer them to the appropriate agency.

Summary

This paper explored some of the social and cultural factors that affect the risk of violence for women of color in general and African-American women in particular. Unfortunately, most of the nursing literature does not deal with African-American women in any capacity. Although they may deny it, as members of this society, nurses are just as influenced by the White male stereotypes and negative images of African-American women as any other group. Four levels of intervention strategies and examples of intervention are discussed.

In addition, an approach advocated by African-American professionals, the Afrocentric approach, was explored. Until there are enough African-American nurses to use the Afrocentric approach, Euro-American nurses need to engage in ongoing assessment of how their own attitudes, beliefs, and stereotypes influence their treatment of abused African-American women. However, unless the White patriarchy's externally generated images of these women and the wholesale acceptance of these images by Euro-Americans and some African-Americans changes, violence against African-American women will continue to be supported.

References

Ali, S. (1990). *Blackman's guide to understanding the black-woman.* Philadelphia: Civilized Publications.

Ashbury, J. (1987). African American women in violent relationships: An exploration of cultural differences. In R.L. Hapton (Ed.). *Violence in the Black family* (pp. 89–105). Lexington, MA: D.C. Heath.

Baron, L., & Straus, M.A. (1983). *Legitimate violence and rape: A test of the cultural spillover theory.* Unpublished paper, Family Research Laboratory, University of New Hampshire.

Bell, C. (1986). Impaired Black health professionals: Vulnerabilities and treatment approaches. *Journal of the National Medical Association, 78,* 1139–1141.

Bell, C. (1990). Black on Black homicide: The implications for Black community mental health. In D.S. Ruiz, (Ed.), *Handbook of mental health and mental disorder among Black Americans* (pp. 191–207). New York: Greenwood Press.

Bingham, R.P. & Guinyard, J. (1982, March). *Counseling Black women: Recognizing social scripts.* Paper presented at the annual meeting of the Southeastern Psychological Association, Atlanta, GA.

Carby, H. (1987). *Reconstructing womanhood: The emergence of the Afro-American woman novelist.* New York: Oxford University Press.

Cazenave, N.A., & Straus, M.A. (1979). Race, class network embeddedness and family violence: A search for potent support systems. *Journal of Comparative Family Studies, 10,* 281–300.

Christensen, C.P. (1988). Issues in sex therapy with ethnic and racial minority women. *Woman & Therapy, 7,* 187–205.

Coley, S.M. & Beckett, J.O. (1988). Black battered women: A review of the empirical literature. *Journal of Counseling and Development, 66,* 266–70.

Collins, P.H. (1990). *Black feminist thought: Knowledge, consciousness and the politics of empowerment.* Boston: Unwin Hyman.

Evidence points to deceit by Brawley. (1988, September 27). *New York Times,* pp. A1, B4–5.

Findlen, B. (1990, September/October). Culture: A refuge for murder. *Ms: The World of Women,* p. 46.

Gillespie, M. (1988, April). A crime of race *and* sex. *Ms. Magazine,* vol. 16, p.18.

Hampton, R. (1987a). (Ed.). Family violence and homicides in the Black community: Are they linked? *Violence in the Black family* (pp. 135–156). Lexington, MA: D.C. Heath.

Hampton, R. (1987b). (Ed.). Violence against Black children: Current knowledge and future research needs. *Violence in the Black family* (pp. 3–20). Lexington, MA: D.C. Heath.

Harrison, B.G. (1989). The jogger: Running for her life. *Madamoiselle,* Vol. 95, August, p. 122.

Hooks, B. (1981). *Ain't I a woman: Black women and feminism.* Boston: South End Press.

Hooks, B. (1990, April). *Representing Blackness: The culture marketplace (fashion, film, and television).* Paper presented at the University of Wisconsin-Madison.

Jason, J., Strauss, L.T., & Tyler, C.W. (1983). A comparison of primary and secondary homicides in the United States. *American Journal of Epidemiology, 117,* 309–319.

Lerner, G. (1973). (Ed.). *Black women in White America: A documentary history.* New York: Vintage Books.

Levinson, D. (1989). *Family violence in a cross-cultural perspective.* Newbury Park, CA: Sage Publications.

Minnesota Department of Corrections Program for Battered Women. (1982). *Data Summary Report.* St. Paul, MN.

Mosedale, L. (1989). The Central Park rape: Has it made us angry? Scared? or Smart? Glamour, vol. 87, pp. 212–213, 274–275.

Myers, L.J. (1987). The deep structure of culture: Relevance of traditional culture in contemporary life. *Journal of Black Studies, 18,* 72–75.

Myers, L.J. (1988). *Understanding an Afrocentric world view: Introduction to an optimal psychology.* Dubuque, IA: Kendall/Hunt.

Myers, L.J. (1990). Understanding family violence: An Afrocentric analysis based upon optimal theory. In D.S. Ruiz (Ed.), *Handbook of mental health and mental disorder among Black Americans* (pp. 183–189). New York: Greenwood Press.

Rosenthal, A.M. (1964). *Thirty-eight witnesses.* New York: McGraw-Hill.

Russell, D.E.H., Schurman, R.A., & Trocki, K. (1988). The long-term effects of incestuous abuse: A comparison of Afro- American and White victims. In E. Wyatt & G.J. Powell (Eds.), *Lasting effects of child sexual abuse* (pp. 119–134). Newbury Park, CA: Sage Publications.

Straus, M.A., Gelles, R.J., & Steinmetz, S.K. (1980). *Behind closed doors: Violence in American families.* New York: Doubleday.

White, E. (1985). *Chain, chain, change: For Black women dealing with physical and emotional abuse.* Seattle: The Seal Press.

White, E. (1989). (Ed.), *The Black women's health book: Speaking for ourselves.* Seattle: The Seal Press.

Wilson, L. (1990, September 3). This is understanding? *Newsweek,* p. 77.

Winkler, K.J. (1990). Researcher's examination of California's poor Latino population prompts debate over the traditional definitions of underclass. *Chronicle of Higher Education, 6,* A5, A8.

Wolff, Craig. (1989, April 21). Youths rape and beat Central Park jogger. *New York Times,* p. B1.

Wyatt, G.E., & Powell, G.J. (1988). (Eds.), Identifying the lasting effects of child sexual abuse. *Lasting effects of child sexual abuse* (pp. 11–17). Newbury Park, CA: Sage Publications.

Wyatt, G.E., Peters, S.D., & Guthrie, D. (1988). Kinsey revisited, Part II: Comparisons of the sexual socialization and sexual behavior of Black women over 33 years. *Archives of Sexual Behavior, 17,* 289–332.

Wyatt, G.E. (1989). Reexamining factors predicting Afro-American and White women's age at first coitus. *Archives of Sexual Behavior, 18,* 271–298.

Zambrano, M.M. (1985). *Mejor sola que mal acompanada: For the Latina in an abusive relationship.* Seattle: The Seal Press.

Ω

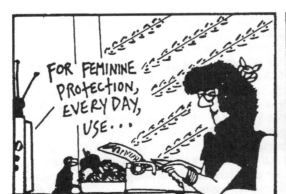
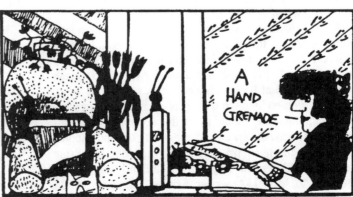

Reprinted from MA, CAN I BE A FEMINIST AND STILL LIKE MEN by Nicole Hollander, by arrangement with St. Martin's Press, Inc. Copyright © 1980 by Nicole Hollander.

Surviving the Incest Industry

by Louise Armstrong

Survivors of child sexual abuse spoke out about their experiences in order to expose this hidden aspect of male violence and destroy it. Louise Armstrong argues that their accounts have been reduced to fodder for a burgeoning 'incest industry' which individualises and medicalises survivors and marginalises feminist politics.

It is a dozen years since feminists first spoke out on the issue of incest, of repeated sexual violation of children by males—fathers, step-fathers, grandfathers, uncles. A dozen years later—survivors continue to speak out. Their writings, which I will call "I-story" books, have become a small sub-genre of the burgeoning incest literature (framed by books on healing yourself and, for professionals, books on healing others). When taken note of by the feminist press, "I-story" books tend to be dealt with gingerly, with delicacy, concerned to maintain a proper comportment in the face of anguish.

I will now proceed to be somewhat indelicate, to speak out—as it were—on speaking out.

Without in any way intending to diminish the genuine feeling which imbues these works or, in some cases, their literary qualities, I think the institutionalisation of speaking out on incest needs re-examination. I think we have been bamboozled.

Since I was among the first to break the silence, and since speaking out was one of the fundamentals of feminism, this may smack of the politically—not only incorrect, but outrageous. Since a central purpose of those speaking out is to help others know they are not alone, and since those who speak do so with great pain, this may smack of the callous. I do not think all that smacking applies. Bear with me.

What I want to show is that the context of speaking out has been altered so radically in these past dozen years that it changes the meaning of what is being said.

When we first exploded the news that this crime against children was routine and widespread, we did so within a feminist framework of the exposure of multiple, licensed violences against women and children: battering, rape, marital rape . . . Our analysis, our understanding, placed child sexual abuse squarely within this framework, identifying it as a historical permission, a male right: as normal, not deviant. The goal was to raise society's consciousness: to try for a consensus which—it seemed in that climate of feminist optimism—might now say, hey, let's revoke the license!

Oh, we did not expect the world to simply cry: 'good, glad you told us, we'll just cut that out'. But what we had learned, from talking, from listening, was so clearcut, so eminently *reasonable*—that men did not do this despite the fact they knew it was wrong, but because they believed it was their right— that it seemed possible the public would react at least to the embarrassing absurdity of so many fathers suddenly spotlighted playing doctor (and much worse) with their three-year-olds. Just because they wanted to. Just because they could. Ours was an exuberance that anticipated a healthy fight for which we felt properly armed.

There was no fight. If we expected to be told to shut up, we were wrong. If we expected to be told we were wrong that abuse was so common, we were wrong. If we expected to be told we were wrong about the sexual politics—we were wrong as well.

On this last point, we were simply ignored.

The Message-Suppressors

It was not the forces of repression that were sent in to meet us. It was battalions of newly minted mental health professionals. And they were so sure we were *not* wrong about the incidence, and so sure we were *not* wrong about the entrenched license, that they were willing to stake their careers on it: to enter a new specialty, "incest expert". We had agitated the public. They believed that they had the balm to peddle which would calm them. Being professionals, they banked on the fact that their calm-balm would prevail over our call for social change. They were right.

Almost from the start, the media carried our stories— and their analysis. Minutes after first opening our mouths, our message was first muffled, then obliterated.

We spoke of male violence and deliberate socially accepted violation. They spoke of family dysfunction. We spoke of rage. They named rage a stage. We spoke of social change. They spoke of personal healing. We spoke of political battle. They spoke of our need to hug the child within.

If our speaking out was an effort to litter the landscape with our cry for reform, they were message-suppressors, sent in by the powers that be, the sanitation engineers. Overt argument would have lent vigour to the fight. Converting the issue to a non-issue, they spoke in pieties of the horrors of incest—all the while often crying for the human advance which would be represented by de-criminalising

From TROUBLE AND STRIFE (Britain), No. 21, Summer 1991, pp. 29–32. Copyright © 1991 Louise Armstrong.

Louise Armstrong is the author of numerous books including *Kiss Daddy Goodnight,* and the forthcoming (Fall, 1994, Addison-Wesley) *Rocking the Cradle of Sexual Politics: What Happened When Women Said Incest.*

it. What they were after was medicalisation, making child-rape an individual emotional problem (the child's). This not only de-issued the issue, it gave birth to a lucrative incest industry—counselling programmes, prevention programmes (including a Spiderman comic so kiddies could know Spiderman had been "touched inappropriately" too)—all of which was terrifically capitalism-compatible.

We'd been dialing the cops. Who answered was a social worker. These new social police not only tidied up after us, they all but wiped out any trace that we had ever been there. The odd leaflet, the odd flyer, the odd piece in an increasingly limited feminist press were all that remained.

Now, having long since been quashed as a political issue, even incest-the-novelty-social-disease shows signs of going limp. (And this is one brilliance of the strategy of converting the personal-is-political into the political-as-personal: it palls so nicely.)

War on Women and Children

For a while there was some renewed vibrance as woman after woman, doing as she was told, believed her child's saying daddy'd raped her (or him), and sought protection—only to find herself vilified as vindictive and deprived of custody, often even of visitation. In the USA it is mothers who are regularly labelled as 'the real abusers'. Case after case described its arc across the horizon so predictably that it didn't seem even the shallowest of wit could fail to catch on to what was passing:

See Susie (or Johnny) tell. Now see mommy shocked. See mommy act: Pick up the phone, report the abuse, call her attorney, seek to protect the child, to end time spent with the alleged perpetrator.

Now see the court (the very court which would have convicted her of neglect had someone other than herself reported the abuse) react with disbelief. See daddy get access. See mommy take psychological tests. See daddy take them. See mommy's test label her hysterical. See daddy's anoint him as stable. See her anger called pathological. See his called righteous. See mommy lose custody. See mommy fight. See the court order her to be silent. See her argue. See mommy lose access. (And then, in America, see mommy take Susie and run. Run, mommy, run. Now see the FBI run after her . . .)

It did not seem possible that even the most stupid of the species could miss the fact that courts which would summarily remove a child from a mother for neglect based on *possible harm* were now consistently ruling for fathers in consideration of *possible error*. It did not seem possible to miss the idea that, while speaking out about abuse in the past did nothing to disturb the status quo, speaking out about abuse in the *present* was tantamount to a declaration of war. And the other guys had the army.

But the mainstream media continued insistently to term these cases "custody disputes". And the public, befuddled, looked on dimly. Interest waned.

Incest as Illness

The combination of medicalisation of the issues for survivors, alongside the open declaration of war on women and children in the present, is what I mean when I say the context of speaking out, of telling personal stories, has changed. This is what throws into question the idea a great many survivors embrace, that theirs is an "illness" from which they must "heal"; and that their speaking out about their "journeys" to "empowerment" in itself constitutes a political act. Each individual who has suffered socially sanctioned oppression feels individual pain from that oppression—may suffer "symptoms", emotional as well as practical. Whose purpose is served when the onus is on the oppressed to become well-adjusted (even as the oppression continues)? What goals are served by allowing the focus to be shifted to that pain, those symptoms which result? Absent emphasis on the root cause? All this does is to ensure business-as-usual—all the while converting a potentially uppity portion of the community into a new consumer group.

Medicalisation, personalisation of the *issue* of incest, has otherwise served to provide diversion. For a while multiple personalities (dubbed "multiples") kicked in, and suddenly—like would-be Miss Teenage Americas competing for Most Personality, survivors competed for The Most Personalities. That now appears to have topped out at ninety-two (with the book *When Rabbit Howls*). Multiples, I am told by counsellors, are out of fashion. So what will be next?

Retreats for survivors, often run by private for-profit psychiatric institutions charging exorbitant prices, have become a fad. Retreats? What we need are *attacks*.

"Gender neutrality" has triumphed. Equal emphasis on female offenders (who are statistically negligible in every study) obviates the fact that female sexual violence is *not* equally routine and equally normative within the culture. Worse than that. It means that to speak of sexual politics, of *male* violence, seems not only retrograde, but actually gauche and insulting and bigoted—so firmly is the subject now rooted in terms of the individual-psychological-emotional. And so we are now silenced by ourselves.

"Incested"—the conversion of a noun to a verb ("I was incested when I was five"). This struck me when I first heard it as truly horrific, deserving of ongoing remark. (Doesn't it sound like a rite of passage? I was baptized? I was confirmed?) But—it occasioned no remark.

Survivors, the "incested", continue to speak out.

Many of the "I-story" books now carry an introduction or endorsement by mental health professionals attesting that this is one brave woman's story of her journey through the stages of healing. Thus, the survivor is made into a case history, fodder for the professionals: pre-fabricated notions. Incest-as-illness has so successfully suffused the culture that the personal— illustrative of pathology— emerges truncated, stunted: personal. In effect, the stories illuminate not the need for social change, but only the need for personal growth. Childhood rape is presented as an opportunity: a challenge to your courage—to heal.

Detoxifying Feminism

In fact, the arc described by the issue of incest should provide, for feminists, a textbook case of the social system's newly refined techniques for detoxifying feminist protest. Unquestionably, the motives of survivors remain genuine—to help others. But placed side by side with the ongoing blatant threat that "abused children become abusers", the promise of 'healing' bears an uncanny resemblance to that of salvation from hellfire and damnation.

Witness this: speak out today, and here are some of the twelve steps that may be provided for your recovery:

- Admit you are powerless over your early experience and that your life has become unmanageable.
- Come to believe that a power greater than yourself can restore you to sanity.
- Make a decision to turn your will and your life over to the care of God as you understand Her/Him.
- Admit to God, yourself and another human being the exact nature of your wrongs (yes, yours).
- Be entirely ready to have God remove these defects of character (yes, *yours*).
- Humbly ask Her/Him to remove your shortcomings.
- Make a list of all persons you have harmed and become willing to make amends to them all . . .

I ask you. If this were a 12-step designed by rapists, could they have improved on this programme of sin and redemption? (Sin, yours. Redemption task, yours.)

Why (one does not know whether to bang the table with one's fists or one's forehead)—*why* have so many survivors so readily bought into this "model" in which their childhood rape becomes the fuel driving an ongoing industry? Why have they been so ready to embrace the recommended teddy bear, rather than embracing their rage?

Many, many survivors came to consciousness after that brief light shone on the politics of incest. However all of their experience since then has taken place within the context of incest-as-illness. They have been courted by a cadre of helpers; given codewords and buzz phrases; had an emotional universe custom-designed, their feelings predicted and pre-articulated, their path delineated. In embracing their identity as "survivors" they are granted belonging in a community which celebrates the primacy of Feelings.

To be fair: they have been horribly threatened. Abused children become abusers. On your head be it. Take the cure, or else.

And—to be fair: the most perceptive of them must ask why, if feminists were so right, we made so little headway. And who better placed to know that when you challenge such a power-invested centre; attempting to storm, as it were, the very room where the king is diddling his daughter, the guards will do something nasty indeed to you should you get in. Those victimised as children by fathers must know more surely than any the threatened price of defiance.

Incest and Identity

But perhaps most importantly incest-as-illness offered survivors support—an item noticeably in short supply in the feminist movement in recent years. By the time incest arose as an issue, the women's movement had already become a loose collection of the single-issue identified: the battered women's contingent, the anti-pornography contingent, reproductive rights . . . It had already begun to splinter into a zillion often-antagonistic identity groups: Black, Jewish, Hispanic, lesbian, Marxist, socialist, communalist, spiritualist, vegetarian . . . Individuals were deriving their identities from these identifications. "Survivor" became a ticket, a passport, a membership card.

It was hardly survivors' faults that, in placing their primary identities in incest, they colluded with the medicalisers in their own clientisation.

And, of course, this ghettoising of the issue served to corroborate the more general feminist population's sense that the issue was off bounds for any but card-carrying victims.

Is the issue re-claimable as a feminist one? Can the greatest number of survivors yet be brought within a political base, and can their energies be converted to activism? I am told not by counsellors: that they are too weakened, and too emotionally fragile. I do not know this. I do not know anymore how much of the fragility is intrinsic and how much is fed by the prevailing wisdom.

I do suspect that nothing can change without concerted energy on the part of feminists as a whole, nor unless we can offer a satisfactory belonging and sense of community and purpose. What survivors are buying into presently is, after all, profoundly respectable. In a world in which people are volunteering wholesale to identify themselves as addicted to anything-you-name-it, to confess to an illness and subject themselves to a cure, those embracing incest as their illness seem positively wholesome (in the social sense).

The goals served by the illness model are deeply opposed to feminist goals. To fight on behalf of feminist goals is to focus attention on child-rape as a crime and on men and male power as the problem. The goal of most therapies is *forgiveness* of offenders. As with religious goals of enemy forgiveness. This is a beautiful way of containing the anger of an oppressed population by fostering an unholy delusion: that the oppressor gives a damn one way or the other; that your power to forgive is any kind of power at all.

Perhaps, ironically, a first step now is to speak out about all this. Perhaps now is the time to break the *real* silence.

Ω

Sexual Violence Against Women:
Prevalence, Consequences, Societal Factors, and Prevention

by Ivy L. Schwartz, MD

Sexual assault of women in the United States may have a prevalence rate of 25% or more. Moreover, the majority of survivors of sexual assault know their assailants. Consequences of assault may be severe and long-term, including fear and anxiety, depression, suicide attempts, difficulties with daily functioning and interpersonal relationships, sexual dysfunction, and a whole range of somatic complaints. Recent evidence implicates societal factors, such as acceptance of rape myths, rigid sex role stereotyping beliefs, and acceptance of violence as a legitimate means for obtaining compliance in interpersonal relationships, in the etiology of sexual violence against women.

I present a model for primary, secondary, and tertiary prevention of rape. Primary prevention represents a program of anticipatory guidance in a developmental framework. Secondary prevention entails identification of and early intervention in dysfunctional families. Tertiary prevention consists of the appropriate treatment of the survivor of sexual assault to prevent or minimize subsequent physical and psychological problems. This preventive framework may be incorporated in the practice of clinical preventive medicine and primary care. [Am J Prev Med 1991;7:363–73]

Sexual violence is a widespread and serious problem in American society. Recent data suggest that sexual violence against women is considerably more common than previously thought. Moreover, in the majority of sexual assaults, the attack is evidently perpetrated by a man known to the woman.

Research suggests that the "acceptability" of rape relates to cognitive factors, such as sex role stereotyping beliefs, acceptance of rape myths, and acceptance of interpersonal violence as a means for obtaining compliance in personal relationships. These same factors appear to predict self-reported likelihood of committing rape, as well as the occurrence of sexually coercive behavior.

Several governmental agencies address the problem of sexual violence, including the Center for the Study of Antisocial and Violent Behavior (of the National Institute of Mental Health) and the Violence Epidemiology Branch of the Centers for Disease Control's Center for Health Promotion and Education. However, only minimal attention has been directed toward the means by which sexual assault and its consequences may be effectively treated by health care providers,[1–3] much less toward how sexual violence might be prevented.

This article summarizes the prevalence of rape, its medical and psychological consequences, societal factors identified by recent research, and the implications these hold for prevention. I present a model for primary, secondary, and tertiary prevention of rape, which may be incorporated into the practice of clinical preventive medicine and primary care.

Definition of the Problem

To determine the extent of sexual violence against women in the United States, one must define terminology clearly. The legal term "forcible rape" embodies three aspects: (1) lack of consent (including the inability to give consent through impaired mental functioning as a result of alcohol or drug use, sleep, or unconsciousness), (2) use of force through physical violence or the threat of bodily harm, and (3) oral, vaginal, or anal penetration.[3] There is variability in definition among legal and law enforcement jurisdictions. For example, FBI Uniform Crime Reports exclude oral and anal intercourse, statutory and marital rape, and inability to give consent through altered mental functioning. Twenty-one states continue to hold statutes containing spousal exclusion clauses; thus, a woman cannot be raped by her husband under the law.[4]

In recent years many state statutes have adopted more inclusive terminologies (e.g., sexual assault, sexual battery, criminal sexual conduct). These statutes have broadened the range of forcible and coercive acts, recognized that coercion and intimidation may be as powerful as physical force in obtaining submission, and emphasized the assaultive (rather than sexual) nature of the offense.[4]

When working with patients and their families, the clinician should note that sexual coercion may take many forms (Appendix 1).[5] In addition, sexual coercion may be manifested along a continuum of sexual activity, from kissing and fondling to intercourse. Similarly, a continuum of intimacy of relationship exists between victim and assailant. Recent studies suggest that the majority of rapes are perpetrated by nonstrangers.[6] Nonstranger assailants include acquaintances, dates or romantic acquaintances, husbands/long-term partners, and family members (typically, fathers, stepfathers, uncles or brothers). The nature

Schwartz, "Sexual Violence Against Women: Prevalence, Consequences, Societal Factors, and Prevention", *American Journal of Preventive Medicine* 7(6) : 363–373 (1991).

Portions of this paper were presented at PREVENTION 88, Atlanta, Georgia, April 14–17, 1988, and at the annual meeting of the American Public Health Association, Boston, Massachusetts, November 13–17, 1988.
I thank Dr. Mary P. Koss for references and for critical review of this manuscript and Dr. Cheryl Ritenbaugh for her helpful comments.

of the relationship, as well as degree of force and type of sexual activity, holds implications for the consequences of the assault on the survivor.

Extent of Sexual Assault

Historically, estimates of rape have been derived from law enforcement sources. These methods have greatly underestimated incidence and prevalence through severe underrrporting and the use of restrictive definitions of rape. In addition, the use of the word "rape" in these surveys represents a serious problem, as nearly three-quarters of women may not use the word "rape" to describe a sexual assault experience that legally qualifies as such.[7] (This situation has implications beyond giving the mistaken impression that rape is an infrequent event. "Unacknowledged" rape victims are less likely to report their experiences to police, a rape crisis center, a hospital emergency room, friends or family. They suffer equally severe social and psychological consequences of the rape and may in fact have greater difficulty in their efforts toward healing as a result of their isolation.)[8]

Table 1 summarizes the prevalence of sexual violence reported by women, as cited in the literature to date.[5,9–14] Of these studies, those using a more behaviorally specific approach to questioning have yielded the highest prevalence rates.[15]

Similarly, several investigators have documented sexual aggression acknowledged by men.[16–18] The most extensive study was a national sample of 2,972 male college students.[5] Men were asked to report the most severe form of sexual aggression perpetrated. Of these students, 25.1% admitted sexually aggressive acts: 7.7% of men admitted to rape or attempted rape (Ohio legal definition; see Table 1), 7.2% reported sexual intercourse following the use of menacing verbal pressure or misuse of authority, and 10.2% acknowledged fondling or kissing following the use of menacing verbal pressure, misuse of authority, threats of harm, or actual physical force. Although each study has methodological limitations,[15] it is apparent that coercive sexual behavior is very common in the United States.

Consequences of Rape

The acute and long-term consequences of sexual violence are variable. The following discussion summarizes recent research evaluating the medical and social consequences for women who have experienced forcible rape, as previously defined (with the exception of Burnam et al.,[19] as noted).

Pepitone-Rockwell states, "Rape is a violent act which for most women is a major and unforgettable crisis."[1] Its impact is based upon the personal experience of each woman, including the nature of her relationship with the assailant. Rape by an acquaintance (including a romantic intimate), which may represent three-quarters or more of all rapes,[20] tends to cloud the issue of consent for many women and for society in general.[21] Rape in marriage is particularly devastating, resulting in substantial disillusionment and feelings of betrayal and may occur in up to 10%–14% of all marriages.[22–24]

Table 1. Studies of sexual violence in the United States

Author/year reported	Source of data	Definition	Prevalence rate per 100 women
Geroge and Winfield-Laird, 1986[9]	ECA[a] study interview, 1,779 rural and urban women, North Carolina	"sexual assault" with no definition	4.6 lifetime
Kilpatrick et al., 1985[10]	Telephone survey, 2,004 women, Charleston County, SC	"forcible rape"[b]	5.0 lifetime
Kilpatrick et al., 1987[11]	Interview, 391 women, Charleston County, SC	"forcible rape"[b]	23.3 lifetime
Koss, et al., 1987[5]	In-person survey, national sample, 3,187 female college students	Ohio legal[c]	27.5 since age 14
Koss et al., 1991[12]	Mailed survey, 2,291 female patients of health maintenance organization	Ohio legal[c]	21.3 since age 14
Russell, 1982[13]	Interview, 930 women, San Francisco, CA	1978 California legal[c]	24.0 lifetime
Sorenson et al., 1987[14]	ECA[a] study interview, 1,660 women Los angeles, CA	"pressured or forced to have sexual contact" (includes attempts)	16.7 lifetime

[a]Epidemiologic Catchment Area.
[b]Nonconsenting anal, oral, or vaginal penetration, through the use of force or threat of bodily harm.
[c] Same as forcible rape (above), except includes inability to give consent through mental impairment, intoxication, sleep, unconsciousness.

Burgess and Holmstrom[25] first described a constellation of physical and psychological symptoms that they called the Rape Trauma Syndrome. Symptoms include fear, helplessness, shock and disbelief, guilt, humiliation and embarrassment, anger and self-blame. Flashbacks of the rape, difficulty concentrating, "seeing the assailant everywhere," and nightmares retraumatize the rape survivor, maintaining a high level of anxiety. Over the long term, the survivor of rape may suffer from depression, insomnia, sexual dysfunction, difficulties with relationships, fear and phobias, and a return of nightmares.

More recently, the Los Angeles Epidemiologic Catchment Area study[19] found that women who had experienced sexual assault (defined as forced or pressured sexual contact) had a two- to fourfold increased risk of subsequent depressive, anxiety, or substance abuse disorders. In addition, Kilpatrick et al.[11] found that 57% of women who had been raped suffered from posttraumatic stress disorder after the rape.

One prospective study of 93 women followed for 12 months after rape indicated that their greatest difficulties were impairment of functioning at work and problems with family relationships.[26] In another study,[27] nearly half of the women lost their jobs or were forced to quit in the year following the rape.

Social isolation, depression, and suicidal ideation are common after rape,[27,28] and nearly one in five women attempts suicide.[10] Frequently, family members refuse to discuss the rape.[27] Up to 50% of women may tell no one of their rape experience.[8,27]

Sexual dysfunction is a common problem after rape and may continue for years.[28,29] Disruption of pre-existing heterosexual relationships is often severe, with termination common.[27,30] Husbands or boyfriends may initially react with anger, then avoidance and anxiety, and later depression associated with guilt and sexual difficulty.[31]

The experience of rape holds implications beyond the discipline of mental health. In a cross-sectional study of primary care patients of a health maintenance organization,[12] women who had been raped rated themselves as significantly less healthy, visited a physician nearly twice as often, and incurred medical costs over twice as high as women who had not experienced any criminal victimization. Severity of criminal victimization was a significant predictor of perception of health, number of physician visits, and medical costs, after the effects of demographic variables (age, marital status, ethnicity, family income, education) and other stressful life events were statistically controlled. In fact, the level of violence the woman had experienced was a more powerful predictor of medical services use than demographic variables, other life stressors, self-perceived physical health, or injurious health habits. An analysis over five years (two years before the crime, the year of the crime, and two years after the crime) revealed that the number of outpatient visits of women experiencing rape doubled in the two years after the rape; their visits per year before the rape were not significantly different than those of the nonvictimized women, whose health services use did not change over the five-year period.[12] A prospective study is needed to further delineate the relationships among the experience of violence, perception of health, and medical services use and costs.

Length of recovery from rape is variable. In one study, 37% of women reported that recovery took several years, and 26% felt they had not yet recovered four–six years after being raped.[29] The authors noted that spontaneous comments showing self-esteem, conscious use of defense mechanisms and coping strategies, high levels of activity in daily life, and partnership stability were associated with faster recovery, whereas alcohol and drug use and suicide attempts were maladaptive. Self-blame is also related to poor outcome.[32]

Clearly, stressful life events can promote growth. Nadelson et al.[28] noted positive adaptational outcomes in 44% of women interviewed nearly two years after rape. These women reported being stronger and more serious, careful, and self-reliant.

More recently, Burt and Katz[33] have presented a framework for defining how women grow and change in constructive ways through their efforts to recover from rape. They hypothesize an "integrative" phase of recovery, which follows the more acute, symptom-reduction phase and may be delayed for many years. The landscape of integration encompasses a redefinition of self and one's life and involves a self-ascribed change in attitudes and behavior: understanding of one's needs and how to meet them, assertiveness, independence, competence, self-worth, and awareness of the sociopolitical context of rape in society.

In summary, there is a wide spectrum of medical and social consequences of sexual violence. Although severity and time to recovery are variable, the impact is substantial for nearly all women. For this reason, tertiary preventive efforts are particularly important. Health care providers, counselors, friends, and family members can play a key role in facilitating the recovery process and in encouraging the personal growth of the survivor of rape.

Societal Factors Related to Rape

Preventive efforts require the elucidation of variables that increase the risk for women of experiencing rape and for men of perpetrating rape. This section will discuss (1) the misconception of blaming the woman for her rape, (2) factors that may increase the risk of experiencing rape for a particular woman, and (3) attitudinal and behavioral variables that appear to increase the risk for men of perpetrating sexual violence.

Rape has traditionally been defined by experts and the lay public as a sexual crime, and the behavior, appearance, or character of the victim often has been blamed for its occurrence.[34] Victim-blaming is a key feature of such rape myths as "she asked for it" and "nice girls don't get raped." This has been referred to as "secondary victimization" and may result in a lack of support and even condemnation of the rape survivor.[35]

Unfortunately, many Americans blame women for rape. In a random sample of 598 Minnesota adults, more than 50% agreed with such statements as "a woman who goes to the home ... of a man on the first date implies she is willing to have sex" and "in the majority of rapes, the victim was promiscuous or had a bad reputation."[36] Professionals who assist rape victims may blame the woman as well. For example, Feild[37] found that police and convicted rapists share many beliefs about rape. Even female student nurses viewed a woman as responsible for her rape when she was perceived as careless in her actions.[38] McGuire and Stern[39] surveyed more than 500 physicians about their experience with and attitudes toward rape victims. Nearly one half felt that 40% or more of rape victims "increased their likelihood of being attacked by behavior such as wearing revealing clothes or behaving in a suggestive manner." However, only a subsample of physicians answered this question, making interpretation difficult. Finally, Popiel and Susskind[40] found that rape survivors regarded physicians as less helpful than friends, their boyfriend/partner, other family members, police, or nurses. As the care the rape survivor receives is likely related, in part, to that provider's attitudes toward rape, all health providers should examine their attitudes toward rape, in order to better serve their patients.

Evidence is inconclusive that certain women are uniquely vulnerable to sexual assault. Koss[8] found no evidence of attitudinal or personality differences between victims and nonvictims of rape. Recently, white college women with higher than average levels of sexual activity and alcohol use, "liberal" sexual attitudes, and a history of childhood sexual abuse were found to be at higher risk of rape.[41] Others have documented the association of rape as an adult with childhood sexual abuse. In a probability sample of 930 adult women, Russell[42] found rape/attempted rape prevalence rates of 33%–68% among child sexual abuse survivors compared to a prevalence of 17% among women who had not been abused as children. The highest prevalence rates were among those women who experienced the most severe childhood sexual abuse (e.g., incestuous rape/attempted rape). Her data yield an odds ratio for rape or attempted rape among childhood incestuous sexual abuse survivors of 3.4.[43] Finkelhor and Browne[44] theorize that childhood sexual abuse results in traumatic sexualization, betrayal, powerlessness, and stigmatization. These factors may result in a preoccupation with sex, leading to behavior perceived as seductive by older children and adults; an aversion to sex in intimate relationships; an impaired ability to correctly judge others' trustworthiness; socialization into the role of victim; and feelings of guilt, shame, a sense of being different from others; and impaired self-esteem. All of these effects may render one vulnerable to future sexual exploitation. In addition, the knowledge by potential abusers of prior childhood sexual abuse may disinhibit their abusive tendencies, increasing the risk of revictimization.[43] Further study of this association is crucial. Since the vast majority of women who had been raped could not be distinguished from those who had not, Koss and Dinero[41] suggested that future research should address the possibility that the primary difference between women who had been raped and those who had not may be that the raped women had encountered a sexually aggressive man.

In the past decade, there has been a substantial accumulation of data implicating sociocultural factors, such as acceptance of interpersonal violence, adversarial perception of heterosexual relations, acceptance of myths about rape, and sex role stereotyping beliefs, in the etiology of sexual violence against women. A summary of these research findings will be useful because they hold clear implications for prevention.

Goodchilds et al.[45] interviewed 432 male and female adolescents, ages 14 through 18, recruited through a youth employment program in Los Angeles. Their sample was one-third white, one-third black, and one-third Hispanic representing a broad range of socioeconomic groups. Most participants were still in school, and 66% expected to attend college. The majority (61%) were sexually active and 49% came from father-absent homes. Respondents were asked, "Under what circumstances it is okay for a guy to hold a girl down and force her to have sexual intercourse?" Although 72% initially responded that force was never justified, when presented with nine specific scenarios, the percentage responding that force was definitely not acceptable in any circumstances fell to 44% of girls and 24% of boys. Force was seen as most acceptable "when a girl gets a guy sexually excited," "when she says she's going to have sex then changes her mind," and "when she's led him on." Although not representing a random sample of adolescents, these results are consistent with the findings of other investigators, as discussed below.

Fischer[46] surveyed 823 undergraduate students and found that students' acceptance of date rape was positively correlated with traditional attitudes toward women. In a sample consisting of both college students and nonstudent employed men and women, belief in myths about rape was associated with stereotypical sex role beliefs.[47] These findings were replicated in England, West Germany, and Israel.[48] Similarly, in a random sample of 598 adults, 46.6% of the variability in rape myth acceptance was statistically predicted by acceptance of interpersonal violence, sex role stereotyping beliefs, and an adversarial view of heterosexual relations.[36]

A number of researchers[49–51] have investigated males' self-reported likelihood of raping, using a five-point scale ranging from (1) "not at all likely" to (5) "very likely." Subjects, mostly college students living in California and Canada, were asked if they personally would rape "if assured they would not be caught and punished." This question was asked in a variety of settings (e.g., after reading a fictionalized account of a rape, viewing a videotaped interview with an actual rape victim, or without any prior "exposure treatment"). These studies consistently found that one-third of men indicated some likelihood of raping (at least a two on the scale), and 20% indicated a higher likelihood of raping (three or greater on the scale).

In a similar study, of 301 college males classified as sexually nonaggressive by self-reports, 21% indicated some likelihood of forcing a woman into sexual acts, and another 14% reported some likelihood of raping.[52] Those reporting a higher likelihood of raping believed rape myths, held a more sympathetic view of the rapist, blamed the victim, felt that other men would be likely to rape, held adversarial sexual beliefs, and accepted violence as legitimate.[49,52] They also scored lower in self-reported femininity than other men, supporting the association of attitudes toward rape and sex role stereotyping beliefs.[49] Although not representing random samples of males, the consistency of these findings obtained in a variety of settings argues against selection bias as an important explanation for these results.

A number of studies have investigated sexual arousal to depictions of rape in the laboratory. Results have indicated that arousal to forced sex is statistically correlated with self-reported likelihood of raping, an ideology of male dominance, sex role stereotyping beliefs, and acceptance of sexual and nonsexual violence.[50,51,53] In addition, sexual arousal was found to be disinhibited by anger, alcohol, and the perception that the rape was enjoyed by the woman.[51,54]

Recently, several studies have explored the relationship between attitudes and actual aggressive behavior. Malamuth[55] found that rape myth acceptance, acceptance of interpersonal violence, and sexual arousal to accounts of rape in the laboratory predicted laboratory aggression against a female confederate, accounting for 43% of the variance in aggressive behavior. College men who admitted to sexual violence viewed women as adversaries and thought that aggression is legitimate behavior.[52] Additionally, in a national sample of male college students, severity of self- reported sexual aggression could be statistically predicted based upon the following variables: early childhood sexual experiences (forced and voluntary), hostility toward women, acceptance of aggression as legitimate behavior, frequent use of alcohol, use of violent pornography, and membership in a peer group that sexually objectifies women.[56]

Finally, a growing body of research is defining the detrimental impact of exposure to mass media that portray violent sexuality on attitudes toward sexual and nonsexual violence, sexual arousal to rape, self-reported likelihood of raping, and aggressive behavior. Although it is beyond the scope of this article to address this issue in detail, I will summarize the salient aspects. (For detailed reviews, see Malamuth and Briere, Russell, Bowen, and Mulvey and Haugaard.[57–60])

In this discussion, pornography is defined as sexually explicit material that represents or describes degrading or abusive sexual behavior, for the purpose of the sexual arousal of the consumer (Russell[58]). Through this definition, pornography may be violent or nonviolent. Erotica, on the other hand, represents sexually explicit material premised on equality and mutual respect between partners.

A number of studies have evaluated the effects on attitudes of exposure to violent pornography in both laboratory and naturalistic settings. Compared to control groups, male subjects exposed to media depictions of sexual violence (1) perceived less victim trauma on viewing subsequent rape portrayals,[61] (2) reported greater acceptance of interpersonal violence against women,[62] (3) viewed rape as less debasing and degrading and viewed the victim as more worthless,[63] and (4) viewed rape victims less sympathetically, felt less empathy, and rated the women's injury as less severe during a subsequent videotaped reenactment of a rape trial.[64] The portrayal of the woman as initially resisting, but secretly desiring and eventually enjoying the assault, which is common in pornographic depictions of rape,[57] appears to have a particularly powerful effect on attitudes.[61,62] In addition, subjects appeared to become desensitized to this material, perceiving the films as less violent and less degrading to women and reporting a decrease to baseline levels of anxiety and depression (which initially rose after the first film), by the end of the viewing period.[64]

Check and Guloien[65] found that after viewing a video of either nonviolent or violent pornography, male subjects reported significantly greater likelihood of raping than those who had not viewed either video. In addition, self-reported likelihood of raping was associated with the belief that the women previously seen in the pornographic material, as well as women in general, derived pleasure from rape.[51, 61]

Others have investigated sexual arousal to rape depictions in the laboratory. When presented with material in which the woman is portrayed as "enjoying" rape, male subjects (1) reported greater arousal than when the rape is portrayed as not pleasurable to the woman,[66] (2) reported greater arousal to a subsequent realistic rape depiction (with subjects' arousal increasing as their perception of the victim's pain increased), compared with those who had read an erotic story,[51] and (3) reported greater use of violent sexual fantasies, compared to those who had previously seen a depiction of consenting sex, when subsequently asked to achieve as high a level of arousal as possible using only fantasy.[67] In addition, among subjects who previously reported a low likelihood of raping, depictions of rape in which the woman "enjoyed" the rape were equally arousing as depictions of consenting sex; among subjects who previously reported a higher likelihood of raping, depictions in which the woman "enjoyed" the rape were more arousing than consenting sex depictions.[68]

There are fewer data on the relationship between exposure to violent sexual material and actual aggressive behavior. Male subjects shown a film depicting violent sexuality (1) were subsequently more aggressive to a female (but not male) confederate of the experimenter than those who viewed a film with sex only or a neutral film,[69,70] (2) displayed more aggression against a female confederate whether the woman in the film was portrayed as "enjoying" the rape or not, when they had been made angry before viewing the sexually violent material,[70] and

(3) displayed increased aggression against the female confederate after viewing a film which portrayed the woman as "enjoying" the rape, whether the subjects were angered before viewing the film or not.[70]

The Report of the Surgeon General's Workshop on Pornography and Public Health[60] concludes that (1) material "that portrays sexual aggression as pleasurable to the victim increases the acceptance of the use of coercion in sexual relations," (2) "the acceptance of coercive sexuality appears related to sexual aggression," and (3) "in laboratory evidence measuring short-term effects, exposure to violent pornography increases punitive behavior toward women." These effects are found as long as violence is presented in a sexual context; sexually explicit depictions do not appear to be required.[60]

Because these data reveal significant trends, those providing primary or preventive care to young people might prudently caution them (and their parents) about the probable harmful effects of materials that depict violent or abusive sexuality. As the findings in these studies show, the sheer prevalence of rape; the large numbers of Americans who see rape as "acceptable"; the likelihood that many men would rape (by their own self-report) if assured they would not be punished; the interwoven relationships among acceptance of rape myths, sex role stereotyping beliefs, adversarial perceptions of heterosexual relationships, acceptance of violence as legitimate behavior, sexual arousal to depictions of rape, and actual aggressive behavior; and the mirroring of these values and attitudes in the mass media, taken together, refute the notion that sexual violence is an uncommon event perpetrated by a small psychopathic minority of men. Rather, the evidence suggests that sexual coercion, for many Americans, constitutes a standard of behavior, or norm, for heterosexual relations.[2,33,71]

Clinical Prevention of Rape

Health care providers have a unique opportunity and responsibility to incorporate the increasing recognition of the prevalence of sexual aggression and its related sociocultural factors into the practice of clinical prevention. The following discussion presents a model for the clinical prevention of rape, based upon the previously described research findings. This discussion is organized within the three traditional levels of prevention: primary prevention of rape represents a program of anticipatory guidance in a developmental framework, secondary prevention focuses on dysfunctional behavior and relationships to prevent future sexual violence, and tertiary prevention outlines appropriate attention to the needs of the woman with a history of sexual assault.

Primary prevention. The goal of primary prevention is to prevent rape. Although this may seem an impossible task, Sanday[72] has shown in her cross-cultural analysis of sexual violence that there are (and have been) nearly rape-free societies. However, attaining this goal will require commitment and a good deal of education. The following educational approach is designed to address several basic themes relevant to the perpetration of sexual violence against women, as previously discussed: (1) rigid sex role stereotyping beliefs, (2) acceptance of violence as a legitimate method for resolution of conflict, and (3) pairing of violence and sexuality in sexual relations. Although these strategies are meant to address sexual violence against teenaged and adult women, other forms of interpersonal violence (e.g., wife battering and child abuse) may be preventable by employing similar strategies. The long-range goal of the health care provider is to help promote healthy interpersonal relationships and noncoercive sexuality.

This educational approach may be conceptualized developmentally, targeting parents and parents-to-be, children, and adolescents and young adults. Optimally, strategies and programs would be incorporated into the provision of preventive and primary heath care at the appropriate times in a longitudinal fashion, thereby reinforcing prior educational efforts.[73]

Prenatal care. A beneficial time to begin the educational process in the health care setting is before having a child. Prenatal care provides an opportunity to talk with the pregnant woman, and her partner if possible, about what will promote the healthy growth and development of the child. Routine discussions of parenting skills, strategies to avoid burn-out, and partners' help in parenting are valuable. Within these discussions, sex role stereotyping beliefs may become apparent and can then be discussed. Appendix 2 is an example of an exercise that clinicians can encourage parents (and parents-to-be) to do at home to stimulate discussion about sex role expectations. These issues may be further explored during a subsequent prenatal visit.

Issues concerning decision making, stress, and conflict may be explored. The Conflict Tactics Scale[74] may be used to assess conflict resolution methods. (Providers should recognize that both partners may minimize the extent of violence in the relationship.[75]) The Family APGAR may be used to explore relationship satisfaction.[76] These screening tools will be unfamiliar to most parents. Consequently, the provider can emphasize that pregnancy and the arrival of a new child is stressful to all family members and that thinking about these issues before the birth of the child may be helpful. The importance of resolving conflict in the home in a creative and nonviolent manner[75] may be discussed, as needed. Parents can be made aware of resources available in the community, including parent support groups, parenting skills classes, and conflict resolution programs. Optimally, a foundation is laid for considering these issues again after the birth of the child.

Well-child care. The provision of well-child care allows the opportunity to reinforce previous discussions concerning parenting, sex roles, and conflict resolution skills in a structured fashion. Health providers can display nonsexist books and toys in the office or clinic to provide examples to parents of flexible sex role socialization. To discuss child sexual abuse with parents is important, including prevention strategies and effective and age-appropriate parent-child communication on this issue.[77]

A number of researchers have investigated the relationship between watching violence on television and aggressive behavior in children. Viewing violence in the laboratory increases aggression among experimental subjects.[78] Field studies have demonstrated a positive correlation, but the direction of causality is unclear.[79] (One reason is that aggressive individuals are likely to watch more violent television than nonaggressive individuals.) Most of the evidence from longitudinal studies supports a causal relationship.[80] Although the preponderance of data suggests causality,[81] psychological variables, parental aggressiveness, and other factors likely moderate the effects of viewing violence on later aggression in children and as adults.[80]

Strategies that parents can employ to mitigate any harmful effects include controlling children's viewing habits, providing negative evaluation to children of aggressive acts viewed together on television, promoting games to increase children's creativity and imagination, discussing the unacceptability of aggressive behavior with children (including behaving like an aggressive television character), refuting the realism of television portrayals, increasing the viewing of programs with prosocial content, developing games to model prosocial behaviors, and helping children develop critical viewing skills.[82]

Childhood health promotion. Health promotion strategies during childhood encourage the physical and emotional well-being of youngsters. Primary providers who care for children can model flexible sex role behaviors and attitudes, including encouraging boys to honor and express feelings, and encouraging girls to be physically strong, active, and assertive. Interestingly, women who successfully resisted rape were more likely to have played sports as a child and to engage regularly in sports as adults.[83] This association provides further support (in addition to the more established reasons of prevention of obesity, cardiovascular disease, etc.) for the promotion of physical exercise in childhood.

Children are empowered when a provider routinely asks permission to examine their bodies, even to look in their ears. Children should learn that their bodies are their own, and no one has the right to touch them in a way that they do not want or that makes them feel uncomfortable. Wherever possible, parents can teach their children to distinguish good touch, bad touch, and confusing touch.[77] Talking about these experiences and feelings gives children permission to feel good, bad, or confused about being touched. This is the basis for prevention of sexual assault of children. Building on this understanding holds promise for the prevention of sexual coercion in adolescents and young adults. An environment that encourages talking about experiences of sexual aggression becomes part of prevention by removing the need to hide the experience.[84]

Adolescence and young adulthood. Koss's study[8] of the hidden rape victim emphasizes the importance of early educational efforts. One way to begin to explore such issues is a "What If" exercise, which my be used in a clinical setting with adolescents or their parents. Two examples are "You are at a party with a guy you think is nice but you don't know him very well. He tries to kiss you but you don't want to be kissed. What do you do?" and "Another guy is boasting that he had sex with his girlfriend even though she didn't want to. What do you say or do?" These exercises provide an opportunity for teens to think ahead of time about confusing or compromising situations and to explore their values and feelings about sexuality and power.

Discussions of rape myths are particularly worthwhile beginning in early adolescence, as issues concerning dating arise. Some myths that are important to refute include "She asked for it," "She seduced him," "Nice girls don't get raped," "Women secretly want to be raped," and "Women mean 'yes' when they say 'no.'" In addition, research suggests that adolescent girls interpret the way people dress and act in a less sexualized way, while boys' interpretation is more sexualized.[45] Consequently, it is important to discuss these differences with adolescents and their parents and emphasize the need for clear verbalization of impressions and intentions regarding sexual activity to avoid misinterpretation among adolescents.

To initiate such discussions with teenaged children may be difficult for parents. Fortunately, available resources help parents to define the issues and suggest approaches that will facilitate honest and supportive communication (e.g., Adams et al.[85]).

Health promotion for young people should incorporate education about the typical setting of acquaintance or date rape, warning signs in dating relationships, and limit-setting for sexual activity. Strategies for resisting peer pressure may be explored. For young women, important components of this education include assertiveness training, self-defense, and leadership skills building. For young men, an important component is encouraging sensitivity to one's feelings and willingness to express them verbally. The healthy expression of anger and frustration[75] is particularly vital. Young women can be taught methods to avoid rape successfully, including discrimination of cues of impending coercion, early and active resistance,[86,87] and use of multiple assertive strategies of resistance (e.g., yelling, kicking, fleeing, fighting back).[83]

Young people must understand the dangers of the fusion of sex and violence. Anticipatory guidance regarding media depictions of sexual violence must begin early, since the mean age of boys' first exposure to magazines such as *Playboy* is 11 years, and the mean age of their first exposure to sexually oriented R-rated films is 12.5 years (Bryant, 1985, cited in Russell[58]). Health providers can take this opportunity to discuss male and female sexual responses and emphasize that sexual arousal to violence is neither normal nor healthy. The impact of media violence and sex role rigidity on teens' attitudes concerning what is appropriate behavior may be explored as well. Parents can be encouraged to discuss sex as a mutually pleasurable activity between equal partners, not a power game or competition between adversaries. Finally, concrete methods may be taught by health providers and parents for the nonviolent resolution of conflict and anger control.[75] Young people can employ these in the family setting,[88] at school,[89] and in interpersonal romantic relationships. This knowledge is vital to breaking the link between acceptance of violence and sexual coercion.

Secondary prevention. Secondary prevention classically refers to the screening of individuals for the presence of early disease or dysfunction, with the goal of reversal or retardation of its progression. In the secondary prevention of sexual violence, individuals and families are routinely screened for dysfunctional patterns which increase the risk of future sexual coercion (e.g., alcohol or other drug abuse, sexual abuse of children, extreme jealousy or dependence, and abusive methods of conflict resolution, both psychological and physical). For example, a woman in a dysfunctional relationship (particularly a battering relationship) may be at risk for sexual violence at the hands of her spouse/partner.[24] In these homes, children learn unhealthy messages about power, control, sexuality, and appropriate means for resolution of conflict, which influence future attitudes and behavior. In addition, childhood sexual abuse puts boys at increased risk of perpetrating and girls at increased risk of experiencing sexual aggression as adults.

The following findings, albeit of limited specificity, may be clues that a relationship or family system is not functioning in a healthy manner. A child's problems with peers, parents, or other adults may represent past or current abuse, alcohol or drug dependence in a family member, or other difficulties. Symptoms may take the form of social incompetence, fearfulness or aggression with peers, dependence, lack of curiosity, self-reproach, disruptive or provoking behavior, depression, anxiety, alcohol or drug use, or frank psychiatric disturbance.[90] Similarly, one or both adult partners may present to the health care setting with a host of emotional or physical complaints, reflecting an underlying family or relationship problem. The key issues may be uncovered through gentle and persistent questioning.

The framework for intervention depends upon the particular problem areas identified and their severity. Clinicians may explore with parents ways to promote flexible sex role socialization in the family. Health care providers can support the efforts of teachers and counselors working with children having difficulties in school. They may also serve as mediators in family disputes[91] or refer families to community mediation programs. Evaluation of one parent-child mediation program found an improvement in relationships, with less fighting and arguing, better understanding of others' point of view, and more positive ways of handling conflict after participation in the mediation process.[88] Parents may benefit from help in defining

appropriate nonabusive disciplinary strategies, including how to guide adolescent decision-making and growing autonomy. In families suffering from tension and conflict, clinicians can train both parents and children in anger control techniques and effective communication skills.[75] In growing numbers of schools across the United States, peer mediation programs are being established. McCormick[89] reported a 47% decrease in officially reported aggressive conflicts, a 51% decrease in students' self-reported aggressive conflicts, less severe conflictive situations (e.g., twice the rate of "talking it out"), and half as many conflicts remaining unresolved three months after the training of 25 students as peer mediators in one junior high school. These results are consistent with those of other school peer mediation programs.[92] In addition, student mediators have been noted to exhibit greater personal responsibility and self-esteem, and so-called "troublemakers" have expressed a desire to be trained as mediators.[89]

Clinicians can provide information and encourage involvement with other community resources, including parenting groups, alcohol and drug abstinence support groups, and support groups for battered women. Families with drug, alcohol, or violent behavior problems, including child abuse, should be referred to treatment programs, and battered women referred to shelters. In a growing number of communities, therapeutic groups are available for abusive men as well. Children with ongoing behavioral or emotional problems should be referred with the parent(s) for counseling. However, the primary care provider should maintain close contact with these families to provide continuity of care and support and to periodically reassess the situation and recommend changes in the treatment plan as needed.

Tertiary prevention. Tertiary prevention focuses on the woman who has had the experience of sexual assault at some time in her life. It is not the function of health care providers to determine whether a woman has been raped, as legally defined.[93] Rather, the importance lies in the perception of that individual that she has been violated. Consequently, assessing the meaning of rape for that individual woman is necessary.

The assumption underlying tertiary preventive efforts is that early detection of a history of sexual violence will lead to improved clinical outcomes. As previously discussed, women may experience medical, psychological, social, and sexual difficulties for many years after rape. In one randomly assigned controlled study of therapeutic methods with rape survivors, women in the treatment groups reported significantly less depression, anxiety, and general distress than the women in the no treatment (i.e., control) group.[94] Apparently, spontaneous recovery from rape may, for many women, be minimal. Offering support and providing counseling to women having difficulties are likely to be therapeutic.

Most women will not volunteer the information that they have been assaulted, especially if the assault occurred long before. Thus, the provider must always think of assault as a possibility. Problems that may be related to a history of assault include depression, sexual dysfunction, fear or suspiciousness of others, anxiety, difficulties at work, difficulties with relationships, drug or alcohol dependence, self-derogating behavior, and a host of chronic or nonspecific physical complaints. These encompass a large number and variety of concerns that people bring to the health care setting. As these symptoms or difficulties are not specific to the experience of rape, successful identification of the woman with a history of rape requires a high index of suspicion.

Health care providers can begin to break the silence surrounding sexual aggression in the health care setting by asking about past experiences of sexual violence or coercion. This questioning may be done when there is no suspicious presenting complaint as well. Including open-ended questions as part of a battery of lifestyle questions in health promotion is is another way to break the silence. The development of a health history questionnaire that includes screening questions concerning childhood experiences of abuse, family or relationship conflict, and physical or sexual abuse as an adult will facilitate these efforts.

Some clinicians may think that patients may find these questions inappropriate or may be resistant to discussing these issues, particularly in the absence of symptoms. There are only limited data addressing this concern. In an analysis of 316 (mostly female) family practice patients' attitudes toward a wide variety of psychosocial issues, the vast majority endorsed at least some family physician involvement in such areas as spouse abuse, rape, alcoholism, and child abuse.[95] Similarly, among injured women presenting to an emergency room, those who had not been abused "did not appear to mind being asked if someone had hurt them," and those who had been abused "appeared relieved that someone had directly asked them how they had been hurt."[96] Future work should specifically examine physician and patient attitudes regarding the discussion of sexual violence in the clinical setting.

DiVasto[97] has developed an instrument for measuring common symptoms after sexual assault that may be employed with a woman presenting with acute or ongoing sexual abuse. In addition, assessing the safety of a woman (and her children) who is in an ongoing abusive relationship is imperative.[98,99] Referral to a rape crisis center, battered women's shelter, or experienced counselor for psychological counseling is important. The counselor can also provide information on the legal aspects of the woman's situation and refer her to an attorney or to law enforcement personnel, as desired by the woman.

Health care providers can play an important role in providing support and promoting healing. Clinical research provides insights into what goals to work toward with the survivor of sexual assault:[33] (1) provide accurate information about sexual assault, focusing on societal rather than self-blame, (2) promote healthy relationships and social support systems, (3) encourage positive actions that the woman can take on her own behalf, (4) help the woman set goals for herself and follow through on those goals, and (5) emphasize that you understand the challenges posed by the rape experience and that recovery from rape yields personal growth, increased strength, and self-reliance for the majority of women.

Providing a safe place to talk about feelings and to work through some of these issues may be all that is needed. Information on community resources, including support groups and counselors, can be provided. Collaboration between professional and volunteer helpers is very important; it is empowering for the survivor of rape to identify with a peer who has shared her experiences and is strong and self-reliant. Stress reduction techniques have been helpful for many women. To maintain frequent contact is important, assuring the woman that support and information are always available. Finally, consider intervention with the family or partner as needed, so that their sense of victimization will not interfere with the recovery of the woman.[100]

In conclusion, the extent of sexual violence against women is astounding. Much research remains to be done to (1) further delineate risk factors for sexual violence, (2) develop instruments for sensitive and specific identification of those at risk for experiencing or perpetrating sexual violence, (3) develop a valid and reliable instrument to identify individuals with a history of violence, (4) further define and evaluate preventive and therapeutic intervention modalities, (5) explore practitioner and patient attitudes toward the implementation of preventive strategies in the clinical setting, and (6) assess medical school and postgraduate curricular content regarding interpersonal violence. In addition, barriers to the incorporation of health promotion into primary care medicine (e.g., the structure of the medical care encounter, reimbursement for preventive services, the disease-oriented model of medical care, and others) must be resolved.[73]

However, research in the past 10 years has succeeded in providing a much greater understanding of the causes and consequences of sexual violence than was previously possible. This understanding has clear implications in the area of prevention. Preventive medicine and primary care specialists have the opportunity to employ preventive strategies to reduce the risk of sexual violence against women in American society.

Appendix 1

Coerced Sexual Activity

Menacing verbal pressure	Misuse of authority	Induce mental impairment	Threat or use of physical force
threats	teachers	alcohol	
promises	employers	drugs	
lies	family	sleep	

Appendix 2

Sex Role Expectations Exercise

The most important thing in life for a woman is _____
The most important thing in life for a man is _____
The "human" in me wants to _____

	I am required to_____	I am allowed to_____	I am forbidden to_____
Since I am a woman (man) _____			
If I were a woman (man) _____			

References

1. Pepitone-Rockwell F. Patterns of rape and approaches to care. *J. Fam Pract* 1978;6:521–9.
2. Burgess A., Hartman C. Rape and sexual assault. *Background paper prepared for the Surgeon General's Workshop on Violence and Public Health*. Leesburg, Virginia: Centers for Disease Control, U.S. Public Health Service, 1985.
3. Kobernick M, Seifert S, Saunders A. *Emergency department management of sexual assault victims*. J Emerg Med 1985; 2:205–14.
4. Largen M. Rape-law Reform: an analysis. In: Burgess A, ed. *Rape and sexual assault II*. New York: Garland, 1988;271–92.
5. Koss M., Gidycz C, Wisniewski N. The scope of rape: incidence and prevalence of sexual aggression and victimization in a national sample of higher education students. *J. Consult Clin Psychol* 19875; 5:162–70.
6. Koss M. The scope of rape: implications for the clinical treatment of victims. *Clin Psychol* 1983;36:88–91.
7. Koss M. Hidden rape: sexual aggression and victimization in a national sample of students in higher education. In: Burgess A. ed. *Rape and sexual assault II*. New York: Garland, 1988;3–25.
8. Koss M. The hidden rape victim: personality, attitudinal, and situational characteristics. *Pschol Women Q* 1985;9:193–212.
9. George L. Winfield-Laird I, *Sexual assault: prevalence and mental health consequences. Final report*. Rockville, Maryland: National Institute of Mental Health, 1986.
10. Kilpatrick D, Best C, Veronen L, Amick A, Villeponteaux L, Ruff G. Mental health correlates of criminal victimization: a random community survey. *J. Consult Clin Psychol* 1985;53:866–73.
11. Kilpatrick D, Saunders B, Veronen L, Best C, Von J. Criminal victimization: lifetime prevalence, reporting to police, and psychological impact. *Crime Delinquency* 1987;33:479–89.
12. Koss M, Koss P, Woodruff WJ. Deleterious effects of criminal victimization on women's health and medical utilization. *Arch Intern Med* 1991;151:342–7.
13. Russell D. The prevalence and incidence of forcible rape and attempted rape of females. *Victimol* 1982;7:81–93.
14. Sorenson S, Stein J, Siegel J, Golding J, Burnam M. Prevalence of adult sexual assault: the Los Angeles Catchment Area Study. *Am J Epidemiol* 1987;126:1154–64.
15. Koss M. Is there a rape epidemic? Paper presented at the American Association for the Advancement of Science annual meeting, San Francisco, California, January 16, 1989.
16. Kirkpatrick C, Kanin E. Male sexual aggression on a university campus. *Am Social Rev* 1957;22:52–8.
17. Rapaport K, Burkhart B. Personality and attitudinal characteristics of sexually coercive college males. *J Abnorm Psychol* 1984;93:216–21.
18. Koss M, Oros C. Sexual experiences survey: a research instrument investigating sexual aggression and victimization. *J Consult Clin Psychol* 1982;50:455–7.
19. Burnam M, Stein J, Golding J, Siegel J, Sorenson S, Forsythe A, Telles C. Sexual assault and mental disorders in a community population. *J Consult Clin Psychol* 1988;56:843–50.
20. Koss M, Dinero T, Siebel C, Cox S. Stranger and acquaintance rape: are there differences in the victim's experience? *Psychol Women Q* 1988;12:1–24.
21. Hall E, Gloyer G. How adolescents perceive sexual assault services. *Health Soc Work* 1985;10:120–8.
22. Weingourt R. Wife rape; barriers to identification and treatment. *Am J Psychother* 1985;39:187–92.
23. Russell D. *Rape in marriage*. New York: Macmillan, 1982.
24. Hanneke C, Shields J, McCall G. Assessing the prevalence of marital rape. *J Interpersonal Violence* 1986;1:350–62.
25. Burgess A, Holmstrom L. Rape trauma syndrome. *Am J Psychiatry* 1974;131:981–6.
26. Resick P, Atkeson B, Ellis E. Social adjustment in victims of sexual assault. *J Consult Clin Psychol* 1981;49:705–12.
27. Ellis E, Atkeson B, Calhoun K. An assessment of long term reactions to rape. *J Abnorm Psychol* 1981;90:263–6.
28. Nadelson C, Notman M, Zackson H, Gornick J. A follow-up study of rape victims. *Am J Psychiatry* 1982;139:1266–70.
29. Burgess A, Holmstrom L. Adaptive strategies and recovery from rape. *Am J Psychiatry* 1979;136:1278–82.
30. Holmstrom L, Burgess B. Rape: the husband's and boyfriend's initial reactions. *Family Coordinator* 1979;28:321–30.
31. Bateman A. Rape: the forgotten victim. *Br Med J* 1986;292:1306.
32. Meyer C, Taylor S. Adjustment to rape. *J Pers Soc Psychol* 1986;50:1226–34.
33. Burt M, Katz B. Dimensions of recovery from rape. *J Interpersonal Violence* 1987;2:57–81.
34. Brownmiller S. *Against our will: men, women, and rape*. New York: Simon and Schuster, 1975.
35. Williams J. Secondary victimization: confronting public attitudes about rape. *Victimol* 1984;9:66–81.
36. Burt M. Cultural myths and supports for rape. *J Pers Soc Psychol* 1980; 38:217–30.
37. Feild H. Attitudes toward rape: a comparative analysis of police, rapists, crisis counselors, and citizens. *J Pers Soc Psych* 1978;36:156–79.
38. Damrosch S. How perceived carelessness and time of attack affect nursing students' attributions about rape victims. *Psychol Rep* 1985;56:531–6.
39. McGuire L, Stern M. Survey of incidence of and physicians' attitudes toward sexual assault. *Public Health Rep* 1976;91:103–9.
40. Popiel D, Susskind E. The impact of rape: social support as a moderator of stress. *Am J Community Psychol* 1985;13:645–76.
41. Koss M, Dinero T. Discriminant analysis of risk factors for sexual victimization among a national sample of college women. *J Consult Clin Psychol* 1989;57:242–50.
42. Russell D. *Sexual exploitation: rape, child sexual abuse, and workplace harassment*. Newbury Park, California: Sage, 1984.
43. Russell D. *The secret trauma: incest in the lives of girls and women*. New York: Basic Books, 1986.
44. Finkelhor D, Browne A. The traumatic impact of child sexual abuse: a conceptualization. *Am J Orthopsychiatry* 1985;55:530–41.

45. Goodchilds J, Zellman G, Johnson P, Giarrusso R. Adolescents and their perceptions of sexual interactions. In: Burgess A, ed. *Rape and sexual assault II*. New York: Garland, 1988:245–70.

46. Fischer G. College student attitudes toward forcible date rape: cognitive predictors. *Arch Sex Behav* 1986;15:457–66.

47. Costin F. Beliefs about rape and women's social roles. *Arch Sex Behav* 1985;14:319–25.

48. Costin F, Schwarz N. Beliefs about rape and women's social roles. A four nation study. *J Interpersonal Violence* 1987;2:46–55.

49. Tieger, T. Self-rated likelihood of raping and the social perception of rape. *J Res Pers* 1981;15:147–58.

50. Check J, Malamuth N. Sex role stereotyping and reactions to depictions of stranger versus acquaintance rape. *J Pers Soc Psychol* 1983;45:344–56.

51. Malamuth N, Haber S, Feshbach S. Testing hypotheses regarding rape: exposure to sexual violence, sex differences, and the "normality" of rapists. *J Res Pers* 1980;14:121–37.

52. Malamuth N. A multidimensional approach to sexual aggression combining measures of past behavior and present likelihood. *Ann New York Aca Sci* 1988;528:1233–32.

53. Malamuth N, Check J, Briere J. Sexual arousal in response to aggression: ideological, aggressive, and sexual correlates. *J Pers Soc Psychol* 1986;50:330–40.

54. Barbaree H, Marshall W, Yates E. Alcohol intoxication and deviant sexual arousal in male social drinkers. *Behav Res Ther* 1983;21:365–73.

55. Malamuth N. Factors associated with rape as predictors of laboratory aggression against women. *J Pers Soc Psychol* 1983;45:432–42.

56. Koss M, Dinero T. Predictors of sexual aggression among a national sample of male college students. *Ann New York Aca Sci* 1988;528:133–47.

57. Malamuth N. Briere J. Sexual violence in the media: indirect effects on aggression against women. *J Soc Issues* 1986;42:75–92.

58. Russell D. Pornography and rape: a causal model. *Political Psychol* 1988;9:41–73.

59. Bowen N. Pornography: research review and implications for counseling. *J Counseling Dev* 1987;65:345–50.

60. Mulvey E, Haugaard J. *Report of the Surgeon General's Workshop on Pornography and Public Health*. Washington, DC: U.S. Department of Health and Human Services, Office of the Surgeon General, 1986.

61. Malamuth N, Check J. Penile tumescence and perceptual responses to rape as a function of the victim's perceived reactions. *J Appl Soc Psychol* 1980;10:528–47.

62. Malamuth N, Check J. The effects of mass media exposure on acceptance of violence against women: a field experiment. *J Res Pers* 1981;15:436–46.

63. Donnerstein E. Pornography: its effects on violence against women. In: Malamuth N, Donnerstein E, eds. *Pornography and sexual aggression*. Orlando, Florida: Academic, 1984;53–79.

64. Linz D, Donnerstein E. Penrod S. Effects of long-term exposure to violent and sexually degrading depictions of women. *J Pers Soc Psychol* 1988;55:758–68.

65. Check J, Guloien T. The effects of repeated exposure to sexually violent pornography, nonviolent dehumanizing pornography, and erotica. In: Zillman D, Bryant J, eds. *Pornography: recent research, interpretations, and policy considerations*. Hillside, NJ: Erlbaum, 1988.

66. Malamuth N, Heim M, Feshbach S. Sexual responsiveness of college students to rape depictions: inhibitory and disinhibitory effects. *J Pers Soc Psychol* 1980;38:399–408.

67. Malamuth N. Rape fantasies as a function of exposure to violent sexual stimuli. *Arch Sex Behav* 1981;10:33–47.

68. Malamuth N, Check J. Sexual arousal to rape depictions: individual differences. *J Abnorm Psychol* 1983;92:55–67.

69. Donnerstein E. Aggressive erotica and violence against women. *J Pers Soc Psychol* 1980;39:269–77.

70. Donnerstein E, Berkowitz L. Victim reactions in aggressive erotic films as a factor in violence against women. *J Pers Soc Psychol* 1981;41:710–24.

71. Johnson A. On the prevalence of rape in the U.S. *Signs: J of Women in Culture and Society* 1980;6:136–46.

72. Sanday P. The socio-cultural context of rape: a cross-cultural study. *J Soc Issues* 1981;37:5–27.

73. Nutting P. Health promotion in primary medical care: problems and potential. *Prev Med* 1986;15:537–48.

74. Straus M. Measuring intrafamily conflict and violence: the Conflict Tactics Scale. *J Marriage Fam* 1979;41:75–88.

75. Stordeur R, Stille R. *Ending men's violence against their partners*. Newbury Park, California: Sage, 1989.

76. Smilkstein G. The family APGAR: a proposal for a family function test and its use by physicians. *J Fam Pract* 1978;6:1231–9.

77. Wurtele S. School-based sexual abuse prevention programs: a review. *Child Abuse Negl* 1987;11:483–95.

78. Friedrich-Cofer L. Huston A. Television violence and aggression: the debate continues. *Psychol Bull* 1986;100:364–71.

79. Freedman J. Effect of television violence on aggressiveness. *Psychol Bull* 1984;96:227–46.

80. Turner C, Hesse B, Peter-Lewis S. Naturalistic studies of the long-term effects of television violence. *J Soc Issues* 1986;42:51–73.

81. Pearl D, Bouthilet L, Lazar J, eds. *Television and behavior: ten years of scientific progress and implications for the eighties*. Department of Health and Human Services, National Institute of Mental Health. Washington, DC: U.S. Government Printing Office, 1982.

82. Eron L. Interventions to mitigate the psychological effects of media violence on aggressive behavior. *J Soc Issues* 1986;42:155–69.

83. Bart P. A study of women who both were raped and avoided rape. *J Soc Issues* 1981;37:123–37.

84. Roark M. Preventing violence on college campuses. *J Counsel Dev* 1987;65:367–71.

85. Adams C, Fay J, Loreen-Martin J. *No is not enough: helping teenagers avoid sexual assault*. San Luis Obispo, California: Impact, 1984.

86. Amick E, Calhoun K. Resistance to sexual aggression: personality, attitudinal, and situational factors. *Arch Sex Behav* 1987;16:153–63.

87. Bateman P. Let's get out from between the rock and the hard place. *J Interpersonal Violence* 1986;1:105–11.

88. Merry S, Rocheleau A. *Mediation in families: a study of the Children's Hearing Project*. Cambridge, Massachusetts: Children's Hearing Project, 1985.

89. McCormick M. *Mediation in the schools: an evaluation of the Wakefield pilot peer-mediation program in Tucson, Arizona*. Washington, DC: American Bar Association, Standing Committee on Dispute Resolution, Fund for Justice and Education; Government Affairs Group, Public Services Division; 1988; Dispute Resolution paper series; 5.

90. Kaplan A. How normal is normal development? Some connections between adult development and the roots of abuse and victimization. In: Straus M, ed. *Abuse and victimization across the life span*. Baltimore: Johns Hopkins University Press, 1988:127–39.

91. Veltkamp L, Miller T. Family mediation: clinical strategies in mediating child custody. *Fam Med* 1986;18:301–5.

92. Davis A. Dispute resolution at an early age. *Negotiation J* 1986;2:287–97.

93. Mezey G. Rape—victiminological and psychiatric aspects. *Br J Hosp Med* 1985;33:152–8.

94. Ledray L. *The impact of rape and the relative efficacy of guide to goals and supportive counseling as treatment models for rape victims.* Unpublished doctoral dissertation, University of Minnesota, 1984.

95. Schwenk T, Clark C, Jones G, Simmons R, Coleman M. Defining a behavioral science curriculum for family physicians: what do patients think? *J Fam Pract* 1982;15:339–45.

96. McLeer S, Anwar R. A study of battered women presenting in an emergency department. *Am J Public Health* 1989;79:65–6.

97. DiVasto P. Measuring the aftermath of rape. *J Psychosocial Nurs* 1985;23:33–5.

98. McLeer S, Anwar R. The role of the emergency physician in the prevention of domestic violence. *Ann Emerg Med* 1987;16:1155–61.

99. Campbell J. Nursing assessment for risk of homicide with battered women. *Adv Nurs Sci* 1986;8:36–51.

100. Castleman M. *Sexual solutions: an informative guide.* New York: Simon and Schuster, 1980.

Ω

♀

The Unique Role Health Workers Can Play in Recognizing and Responding to Battered Women

by Nancy Worcester

"Battering appears to be the single most common cause of injury to women—more common than automobile accidents, muggings and rapes combined.[1]"

Many women identify violence in their lives, and their fear of violence, as the number one health issue they face. For health workers responding to battering, it is important to remember that battering is *much* more than the physical injuries. Violence serves as an excellent reminder that mental and physical health issues cannot be separated. For a woman being abused, physical violence is but one of the tools that her abuser uses to have power and control over many, or all, aspects of her life. Many formerly battered women who have even suffered life-threatening injuries say that the physical violence was nothing compared to the psychological and emotional abuse they endured.

Now that many states have mandatory arrest laws, battered women have been quick to remind us that stopping abuse in a home is much more complex than simply stopping the hitting. Women have noted that a result of abuser counselling can be that abusers learn they can no longer get away with hitting their partners. However, unless larger issues of power and control are also addressed, the abuser may learn to shift to psychological/emotional forms of abuse and the woman continues to be battered even if she is no longer physically injured.

A wide range of chronic health issues including headaches, backaches, sleep disorders, anxiety, abdominal complaints, eating disorders, depression and chronic pain are particularly common in battered women and are clearly related to the stress of living in a violent relationship.

You See Battered Women Everyday

The FBI estimates that a woman is beaten every 15–18 seconds in this country. Violence affects women of all social groups, ages, races, rural and urban environments, and affects both rich and poor and both heterosexual and lesbian women. Many health workers and health workers' partners live with violence as a part of their lives.

Battered women regularly call upon the health system even though health workers have a poor record of identifying them. Studies have shown that abused women have more health problems than non- abused women[2], so those who trust the health system and have insurance probably seek health care at disproportionately high rates. Studies have shown that 22–35 percent of all women who use emergency room services are battered women and because the same women may need to return time and time again, almost half of all injuries presented by women in emergency rooms may be a result of abuse.

Although health workers do not regularly ask about battering during pregnancy, it is more common then and has as serious consequences (increased rates of miscarriage, stillbirth, low birth weight babies, and risk of homicide) as the conditions routinely tested for in prenatal care. Retrospective studies of battered women have found that 40–60 percent were abused during pregnancy; 25 percent of battered women say they were beaten for the first time during a pregnancy. The problems may be even more exaggerated in pregnant teenagers. One study[3] found that 26 percent of pregnant teens were currently in a relationship with a man who was abusive; many stated that the abuse had started when they discovered they were pregnant. Most alarming, 65 percent of the battered teens had not talked to *anyone* about the violence in their lives.

Health Workers Can Play a Key Role

Many battered women would like to tell someone about the violence in their lives and would greatly benefit from knowing that their situation is not unusual and that there are a range of excellent resources available to them. Understanding common patterns of domestic violence makes it obvious that health workers who do recognize battered women and empower them to explore their options can play a key role in helping women end the violence in their lives.

Isolation

Isolation is a primary weapon that one person can use to gain control over another person's life. Battered women describe how abusers gradually isolate them from their other social/emotional support networks so that eventually the abuser is the main person in the abused woman's life giving her information about her own value. Messages like "No one else will ever love you" and "You deserve to be beaten" become very powerful when a woman is not hearing any other messages. Understanding that isolation is a *consequence (not* a cause) of battering can help health workers recognize that what they say to battered women can be extremely important. Health workers aware of power imbalances in health worker-patient relationships can see why this can be exaggerated when the patient is an abused woman. A health worker who implies that the woman is "the problem" will reinforce the messages she gets at home; the health worker who says "You don't deserve to be hit" will be giving a crucial, different message.

The Cycle of Violence

The cycle of violence is a pattern that most battered women start to recognize in their lives. The battering incident seldom comes from "nowhere," but is the expected "explosion" from a period of increasing tension. Women describe the stress of living in the tension-building stage, the waiting for the straw that will finally provoke the battering, as so awful that some women remember when even a severe battering was almost a welcome "release" from the unbearable tension.

Particularly in the early years of abusive relationships, the battering incident is almost always immediately followed by a good stage which some women call the "honeymoon stage." The honeymoon stage is the wonderful stage we *all* want in relationships. Understanding the importance of the honeymoon stage in battering relationships can help us understand the complexities of these (and all!) relationships. This is the stage at which abusers say (and think they mean) that they are very sorry and it will

never happen again. This is the stage when loving sex, extravagant presents, and a renewing of dreams and life long plans/goals can be very enticing.

If the battering is severe enough to cause injuries, the health worker, particularly emergency service providers, may see the woman immediately after the battering and before the "honeymoon stage." This is a key time to make sure the woman knows her options and resources, because she may be the most open to exploring alternatives to staying in a violent relationship. Once the "honeymoon stage" begins, the woman may be "hooked" into another cycle, convinced that if only she tries harder the violence will end.

Escalation

Unless there is intervention (and a sincere commitment from the abuser to learn totally new ways of communicating in the relationship), battering relationships tend to escalate over a period of time. The battering incidents become more frequent and often increase in severity. (Battered women describe the "honeymoon stage" as being less of a "hook" in long-term battering relationships than are the enormous social and economic pressures which keep them in relationships they know are unhealthy.) Because battered women may be seeing health workers long before they turn to other services, good medical records with clear notes, and even photographs, of injuries and chronic health problems that may be related to domestic violence are essential. These can help health workers who will see the records in the future, and the battered woman herself, to see the emerging pattern.

Revictimizing the Battered Woman

Even though health workers are not good at identifying battered women, studies have found that health workers do treat battered women differently than non-battered women and that the treatment actually contributes to the consequences of battering.

Unless there is an understanding of battering, a woman who calls upon the health system regularly, with a range of symptoms and injuries, may be seen as a frustrating patient by health workers who pride themselves on being able to diagnose and treat specific conditions. Only 5–10 percent of battered women in emergency services are identified as such by physicians on their records. Instead, the ground-breaking work on this by Stark, Flitcraft and Frazier,[4] found that medical records included the labels "neurotic," "hysteric," "hypochondriac" or "a well-known patient with multiple vague complaints" for one in four battered women compared to one in 50 non-battered women. One in four battered women were given pain medications and/or minor tranquilizers compared to one in ten non-battered women. This "treatment" has the same effect as paying fire fighters to *push* people back into burning homes! Medication and victimizing labels reinforce the woman's feeling that she is the problem and may contribute to depression, drug and alcohol abuse, and the high rate of suicide attempts seen as a consequence of battering.

Empowering Battered Women

Excellent resources are now available for health workers spelling out specific ways to identify and respond to battered women and to help them end the violence in their lives. Responding more appropriately to battered women does not necessarily mean more work for the health care provider. It means *starting* to ask about violence ("Since so many women are hurt by their partners, we ask every patient with injuries like yours whether they've ever been hit/kicked/hurt by their partner.") and documenting it, making sure safety issues are addressed for a woman before she returns to the situation that caused the mental or physical injuries, giving women information about community resources, and *stopping* treating abused women by providing only labels and tranquilizers.

Battered women must be empowered to make their *own* decisions at their *own* pace. Outside intervention, certain behaviors, or trying to leave at the "wrong" time can escalate the violence. Thirty percent of women murdered in this country are killed by the men they had loved. Most of these murders occur when women are trying to get out of a relationship. Understanding the complexities of *leaving* battering relationships is central to serving battered women's needs.

Health workers will seldom know the impact of their responses to battered women. Saying "You don't deserve to be treated like this" or "Here is a list of community resources" may be the medical advice that saves more lives and does more for the mental health of patients than do other more "medical" skills.

Hospital Protocols Now Required

Effective January 1, 1992, all accredited hospitals are required to have protocols in place describing how they respond to battered women and how health professionals are trained on this issue. This is the ideal time for health workers and battered women's advocates to work together to make sure that protocols serve to empower battered women. There are over 1,000 programs in the U.S. specifically serving battered women. These "experts" can help a woman with the legal, safety, housing and support services she needs.

References

1. "Domestic Violence Intervention Calls for More Than Treating Injuries" by Teri Randall, *Journal of the American Medical Association*, volume 264, no. 8, August 22–29, 1990, pp. 939–940.
2. "Abused Women and Chronic Pain" by Joel D. Harber, *American Journal of Nursing*, volume 85, September, 1985, pp. 1010–1012.
3. "Violence During Teen Pregnancy: Health Consequences for Mother and Child" by Judith McFarlane, pp. 136–141, in *Dating Violence* edited by Barrie Levy, Seal Press, 1991.
4. "Medicine and Patriarchal Violence: The Social Construction of a 'Private' Event" by Evan Stark, Anne Flitcraft & William Frazier, *International Journal of Health Services*, volume 9, no.3, 1979, pp. 461–493.

Ω

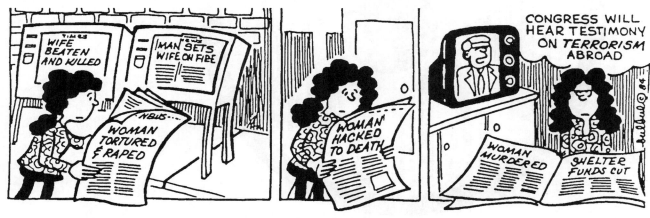

Reprinted with permission from bulbul, *Feminist Connection*, Madison, WI. December, 1984.

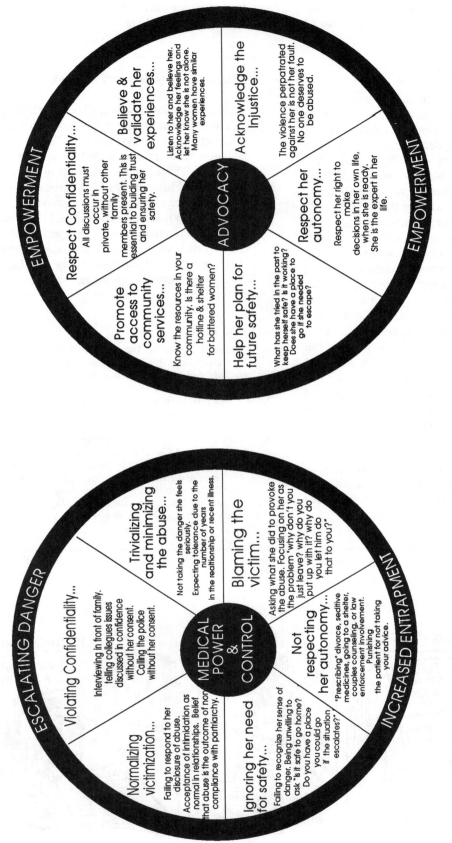

The Empowerment Wheel

EMPOWERMENT

ADVOCACY

Believe & validate her experiences...
Listen to her and believe her. Acknowledge her feelings and let her know she is not alone. Many women have similar experiences.

Respect Confidentiality...
All discussions must occur in private, without other family members present. This is essential to building trust and ensuring her safety.

Acknowledge the Injustice...
The violence perpetrated against her is not her fault. No one deserves to be abused.

Promote access to community services...
Know the resources in your community. Is there a hotline & shelter for battered women?

Respect her autonomy...
Respect her right to make decisions in her own life, when she is ready. She is the expert in her life.

Help her plan for future safety...
What has she tried in the past to keep herself safe? Is it working? Does she have a place to go if she needed to escape?

EMPOWERMENT

"The Empowerment Wheel"

The Medical Power and Control Wheel

ESCALATING DANGER

MEDICAL POWER & CONTROL

Trivializing and minimizing the abuse...
Not taking the danger she feels seriously. Expecting tolerance due to the number of years in the relationship or recent illness.

Violating Confidentiality...
Interviewing in front of family, telling colleagues issues discussed in confidence without her consent. Calling the police without her consent.

Blaming the victim...
Asking what she did to provoke the abuse. Focusing on her as "the problem "why don't you just leave? why do you put up with it? why do you let him do that to you?"

Normalizing victimization...
Failing to respond to her disclosure of abuse. Acceptance of intimidation as normal in relationships. Belief that abuse is the outcome of non compliance with patriarchy.

Not respecting her autonomy...
"Prescribing' divorce, seditive medicines, going to a shelter, couples counseling, or law enforcement involvement. Punishing the patient for not taking your advice.

Ignoring her need for safety...
Failing to recognize her sense of danger. Being unwilling to ask "is it safe to go home? Do you have a place you could go if the situation escalates?"

INCREASED ENTRAPMENT

"The Medical Power and Control Wheel"

Based on the "Power and Control Wheel" and the "Equality Wheel" by the Domestic Abuse Intervention Project. Developed by the Domestic Violence Project, Inc., 6308 8th Ave., Kenosha, WI. 53143, (414) 656–8502. Reprinted by permission.

Worksheet - Chapter 12

Violence Against Women

I. Societal Responsibility for Violence Against Women

How do men get the message that "it's ok", "it's socially acceptable" for men to be violent towards women? Give examples of ways in which men are given this message. (Use examples from advertising, t.v., literature, movies, etc.)

II. Violence Against Women is NOT Funny

But, violence against women is a common theme of stand-up comedians, cartoons, lectures, jokes. Collect examples of violence-as-fun material.

Think of positive ways one can work against violence being considered as suitable material for laughs.

III. Continuum of Violence

Sexual harassment at school or work, pornography, child sexual abuse, date rape, sexual assault, wife battering, and elder abuse are all part of a continuum of ways in which violence against women gets expressed.

Choose any two of the above mentioned forms of violence. Show ways in which these two forms of violence are similar, what they reflect about attitudes towards women, how they limit women's role in society, and why they are mental and physical health issues.

IV. Myths about Violence

Myths prevent us from really understanding violence against women and serve to perpetuate it.
Using the chart below, identify some of the myths which support violence against women.
Think about the answers and see if you can fill in the chart without help. If you get stuck, refer to the chart on page 134 of THE NEW OUR BODIES, OURSELVES. If you use the book, fill in the chart using your own words.

Myths which help perpetuate violence against women

| Type of Myth | How the myth gets applied to each specific form of violence | | | |
	Rape	Battering	Sexual Harassment	Child Sexual Assault
Victim-blaming				
Not a common problem or not a real issue				
Male perpretrator isn't responsible for his actions				
Racist assumptions				

V. Health workers recognize and respond to violence
Several articles in this chapter address the importance of health workers' response to violence.

a. Have you ever had a health worker ask you about violence issues? If you can remember the approach used (exact words, attitude, etc.), describe the situation and whether it felt appropriate to you.

b. If you were involved in training health workers to recognize and respond to violence, what specific recommendations would you give them?

Chapter

13

Food and Body Image

We are what we eat. This last section explores how social, cultural, and economic factors impact upon the basic physiological process of feeding our bodies. The relationship of women to food is as complex as any other phenomenon examined in this collection of articles.

"Nourishing Ourselves" pulls together many of the multi-layered interrelationships between women's roles as the world's food producers, how women's inferior status and internalized sexism may affect women's access to the very food they have produced, and the tragic short and long term individual and societal costs of females being undernourished. Placed within a global context, the similarities are drawn between malnutrition in poor countries/poor communities and in richer communities where societal pressure to be thin similarly deprives girls and women of the quality of diet they need for maximum mental and physical health. This leads to the ultimate question of whether the relationship to food is so different between women and men that it actually becomes a factor in determining gender differences.

Although women are held responsible for providing healthy diets for their families, "The Obesity of the Food Industry" shows it is actually the food industry which chooses the "choices" available and how this results in a trend towards a less healthy and more fattening pattern of eating.

The next articles concentrate on the ramifications, particularly for women, of learning to hate fatness in others and especially in ourselves. "Fatphobia" looks at one of the most prevalent, yet uncriticized, forms of prejudice in our society. "Dieting is Dangerous to Your Health" and "Mental Health Issues Related to Dieting" discuss mental health consequences of this cultural obsession with trying to be thin. "We'll Always Be Fat But Fat Can Be Fit" expresses a much healthier attitude towards one's nonskinny body.

The worksheet, "The Continuum of Women and Food Relationships" is a study guide to thinking through how the so-called "eating disorders" are exaggerated manifestations of the ambivalent relationship most women have to their bodies and their food.

To end on a lighter note, "A Feminist Perspective on the Latke-Hamentash Debate" uses food to bring together most of the issues tasted in this reader.

Nourishing Ourselves

by Nancy Worcester

What could be more ironic? Nourishing others is a fundamental part of women's lives but that very role itself limits the ability of women to take care of their own nutritional needs.

Women are the world's food producers and throughout the world, within a wide range of family units, women have responsibility for purchasing and/or preparing the daily food. Yet, both globally and within families, women are much more likely than men to be malnourished. Nearly universally, wherever there is a shortage of food or a limited supply of quality food, women's diets are inferior to men's quantitatively and qualitatively. Even when food supply is adequate or abundant, women's diets may be nutritionally inferior to men's.

It matters! At some level we all have a feel for how important a good diet is: "We are what we eat." If we feed our bodies the basic nutrients, the healthy body is amazingly clever at being able to take care of itself. An adequate diet is obviously important for *every* man, woman and child. However, both societally and individually, a terrible mistake is being made when women's diets are inferior to men's.

A woman's diet must be more "nutrient-concentrated" than a man's in order to be nutritionally adequate. Most women require considerably less energy than most men. For example, the US Food and Nutrition Board recommends an intake of 1600–2400 Calories per day for women age 23–50, compared to 2300–2700 Calories per day for the same age men. A US Food Consumption Survey showed that the average 23 year old woman consumes only two-thirds as many Calories as the average 23 year old man, 1600 compared to 2400.[1] However, women's requirements for many specific nutrients are identical or greater than men's. The ramifications for this are most serious for calcium and iron. US Food and Nutrition Board Recommended Daily Allowance (RDA)[2] for calcium is the same for men and women. The RDA of 15 mg. of iron per day for reproductive aged women is 50% higher than the 10 mg. RDA for men.

Picture a woman and a man sitting down to consume their daily nutritional needs. The man's pile of food will be 50% bigger than the woman's but in the woman's smaller pile she will need to have the same amount of calcium and 50% more iron. Each bite the woman takes must contain 50% more calcium and twice as much iron! Put another way, even if a man does not have a particularly nutrient-rich diet, he will probably be able to meet his body's needs and he will even get away with consuming quite a few empty-calorie or low-quality foods whereas a woman's diet must be of a relatively higher quality. A man's diet can be nutritionally inferior to a woman's and still be adequate for his needs. The world and millions of individuals are paying a high price for the fact that women's diets are often inferior to men's.

Sex Differential in Food Distribution and Consumption

The trend to feed boys better than girls gets established early in life. In Kashmir, girls are breastfed for only 8–10 months but boys are allowed to suckle for three years or longer.[3] In Arabic Islam, girls are breastfed for only 1—1-1/2 years while it is common for a boy to be nursed until the age of 2—2-1/2.[4]

A recent Italian study also showed differences in the patterns of feeding baby boys and girls—girls are breastfed less often and for shorter periods; girls are weaned an average of three months earlier than boys. Additionally, it was observed that boys were more irritable and upset before feeding but went to sleep immediately after feeding. In contrast, the girls were less aggressive in asking for food but settled down less easily after feeding.[5]

Throughout the world, men and boys get feeding priority. In many cases, men literally eat first and women and children get what food is left-over, such as in Bangladesh where the tradition of sequential feeding means adult men are served first, followed by male children, then adult women and female children. Ethiopian women and girls of all classes must prepare two meals, one for the males and a second, often containing no meat or other substantial protein, for the females.[6] Boys' better access to food based on a gender defined division of labour can get started early in life. For example, in Alor, Indonesia, very young boys are encouraged to do "masculine" work and food serves as an important incentive and reward for that work. Boys receive "masculine" meals as guests of adult men for whom they have performed some service. In contrast, young girls do less valued work like weeding and get a lower quality vegetable lunch.[7]

In whatever way a particular society works it out, there is a nearly universal pattern of men getting fed more and better. Most women recognize this pattern and can identify ways in which they feed their children and their partners better than themselves. Although this may mean nothing more serious than taking the burnt slice of toast or the least attractive piece of dessert for oneself, in times of shortage this pattern means that women are the most likely to be malnourished.

Family members may not even be aware of the sacrifices the woman is making. A British woman who fed her husband and her children even when she could not feed herself during the 1930s remembered, "Many a time I have had bread dripping [animal fat on bread] for my dinner before my husband came home and I said I had my dinner as I would not wait."[8] That pattern is becoming prevalent again as many families do not have enough food. How many women say they are on a diet when in fact they would love some of what they are serving up to their family?

Hilary Land's study of large families in Britain concluded, "It was very evident that the mother was the most likely to go without food for she was the most dependent on meals provided at home. . . It was clear that the father's needs were put first, then the children's and finally the mother's." Over half of the women had no cooked meal in the middle of the day. A quarter had no breakfast and nothing more than a sandwich for lunch. One in twelve women *never* had a cooked meal.[9]

Studies in both Britain and the US have shown that poor parents go without food in order to leave enough food for their children. A British survey found that children were generally better and more regularly fed than their parents. "Only" 15% of the children had fewer than three meals during the previous twenty- four hours in contrast to 75% of the parents having had fewer than three meals, 50% having had two meals and 25% having had only one meal in the twenty-four hour period.[10] A 1983 New York study interviewed people at various sites including emergency feeding centers, food stamp offices, health centers and community centers. When asked, "Do your children eat and sometimes you're unable to?", over one-third of all respondents answered yes and 70% of the parents interviewed at the emergency feeding sites said yes.[11] (These studies did not look for different impacts on mothers and fathers.)

The feminization of poverty means that women in singleheaded households are often the worst affected. A Northern Ireland survey of 700 lone parents found that food was the item on which economies were most likely to be made and inevitably the savings were made by the mother herself going without food.[12] An English woman living on Supplementary Benefits describes the stark "choice" between her needs and the children's:

It has to be me cutting down on what I eat. It's the only way to find the extra money you need. The rest of it, they take it before you can get your hands on it really. So it's the food. It's the only thing I can cut because I use as little heating as I can and I don't smoke.[13]

Providing food for the children is such a worry for women who are the only parent that they may actually deprive themselves more than is necessary. Marsden's study of 116 lone mothers found that they hoarded food to be able to feed the children. He observed a stress reaction to living on low income in which the caregivers economized on their own food more than the size of their income required.[14]

Efforts specifically designed to improve women's diets are not successful if programmes are not planned around the recognition that women feed their families before they feed themselves and that men tend to get the high status foods. For example, a very ambitious 86 million dollar (US dollars) World Food Programme (WFP) project set up to improve the nutrition of pregnant and nursing mothers and their young children in Pakistan has had practically no nutritional impact. The major problem with the programme was that food was rationed so that each woman would receive an individual dietary supplement of 850 Calories per day, but, of course, the women shared the extra food with their families. The average family had six people so one-sixth of the supplement, less than 150 Calories a day, did not make a significant improvement in women's diets.

The acknowledgement that women do not give themselves priority in food allocation posed new problems for evaluators of the Pakistan WFP project:

Another possibility that has been mentioned is to simply accept the realities of family structure and food habits in Pakistan and expand the rations given to the women so that they are enough to provide supplements to the entire family. Obviously, a major drawback to this approach is that the same amount of food would then supply fewer women because of the increased ration size and not nearly as many women would be drawn to the centers.[15]

Judit Katona-Apte, consultant to the World Food Programme (but apparently not terribly influential!), suggests that one way to make certain that women benefit from food aid is to provide foods which are nutritionally-rich but less desirable than traditional foods. In such situations, the high status traditional foods will be given to the men and the newer, less desirable but nutritional foods will be relegated to the members of low status in the household—the women and children![16]

The differential access to food is often exaggerated by food taboos, which have more impact on women that men. Food habits, including rituals and taboos are an integral part of defining cultures ("we" versus "others"). Food taboos serve the function of reinforcing social status differences between individuals and social groups and symbolize the place one has in society. Taboos characteristically involve the prohibition of the highest quality protein foods. Jelliffe and Jelliffe suggest that, "The reservation of the best foods for the males reflects the ancient situation where it was imperative that hunters be well fed." However, Trant's explanation seems more to the point, "Widespread prohibitions applied to women against the eating of flesh foods may have partly derived from the male wish to keep the foods for themselves."[17] Those Italian baby boys aggressively demanding their food are just perpetuating a very ancient pattern!

Overall, it seems that most permanent taboos and avoidances have little effect on the nutrition of individuals practicing them because the group's diet will have evolved so that other foods supply the nutrients found in prohibited foods. However, temporary avoidance, particularly at crucial periods of the life cycle can have grave consequences.

Such limited duration taboos particularly affect women because they occur at the most nutritionally sensitive periods. For example, hot and cold or yin and yang classifications of food are common throughout the world and are especially important in Latin America and parts of Asia. Although hot and cold and yin and yang are defined differently in diverse cultures, in all cultures practicing these classifications, the balancing concept is closely tied to women's reproductive cycles. So, however menstruation, pregnancy and lactation get defined, it will be particularly important that women avoid certain "unbalancing" foods during those times. The foods which must be avoided are often foods of high nutritional value. Some Puerto Rican women consider pregnancy to be a hot state so avoid hot foods and medications, including vitamin and iron supplements, to prevent babies from being born with a rash or red skin. Bangladeshi women must not eat meat, eggs, fish or hot curries for several days after childbirth because those foods are believed to cause indigestion. Women are expected to eat only rice, bread, tea and cumin seed for those nutritionally-demanding post-partum days.[18]

There are two more points to consider in looking at the impact of food taboos and avoidance on women's nutrition. First, food taboos, as a cultural construct, are a part of the values of the society which are taught to people as they grow up. People learn those taboos as patterns of behavior which are right, normal, best. Other ways of doing things are viewed as wrong, misguided, or irrational. Understanding and appreciating another culture will require getting to know the food habits and vice versa. Second, sound nutritional practices can, with thought and planning, be developed and reinforced within the context of most existing food patterns.

This relates to an important theme I am introducing here which I will then weave throughout this chapter. I am suggesting that our society's fear of fat and obsession with dieting play a role in limiting women's access to optimum nutrition similarly to the way food taboos can affect women's nutrient intake in more traditional cultures. Dieting certainly has more impact on women than men, reinforces social status differences, and leaves more food for others. As a cultural phenomenon, there can be no denying that women from many parts of the world would find the notion of purposefully restricting food intake to lose weight to be "wrong" or "misguided". Imagine trying to explain the pattern of American college women who intentionally skip meals to save calories for snacking and beer drinking at parties to Western Samoan women who exaggerate the amount they eat on diet surveys because, "The more they could say they had eaten... the more powerful that meant the village was in being able to amass lots of food."[20,21] When we hear that many nine year old girls are already on slimming diets, we must recognize dieting to be a part of the values which our society now teaches to young women. Because much dieting is erratic behavior, "a temporary drastic measure just to take off a few pounds" (repeatedly performed!), it is more similar to temporary taboos with the potential for grave consequences than to permanent taboos for which people have learned to compensate. Just as one can eat a nutritionally adequate or even nutritionally superior vegetarian or vegan diet if one knows animal products are going to be consciously avoided or unavailable, it is certainly possible to consume nutrient-rich low calorie or weight-maintenance diets. But, that is not how the dieting taboo is usually practiced in this society.

Nutritional Consequences of Sex Differentiation

Clearly there is no way to summarize the effects of sex differentiated nutrition. Nutritional vulnerabilities vary enormously from one part of the world to another, from one region to another, and between classes in the same small community. Malnutrition, of course, is not inevitable and is totally preventable. There is enough food and land available to feed the world's population if our governments considered that to be an important priority.[22] Factors such as cultural food preferences, storage and transport facilities, the soil the food is grown in and the value placed on equal food distribution within a community will have more influence on one's chances of being malnourished than whether one is a woman or a man. But, a pattern emerges which shows that universally malnutrition is far too common and that it affects girls and women more than boys and men.

Hunger affects whole regions and classes of people and sweeps men as well as women into its nets. It seldom happens that the male members of a family are well-fed or overfed while the females starve. The differentials are narrow, and the question is that of which sex first crosses the line between health and sickness. In general, those who skate closest to the margin of deprivation are the most powerless—the very young, the old, and, everywhere, the women.[23]

Nutritional studies do not always look for or find sex differences in nutritional deficiencies. However, when nutritional sex differences are found it is almost always in the direction of the higher occurrence being in females. *Women and Nutrition in Third World Countries*[24] summarizes hundreds of nutritional studies in poor countries and concludes:

Calorie intake is often low among women, although a few populations show adequate intake (Mexico, Tarahumaras, Korea) or excessive (Micronesia) ones. Deficiencies in caloric intake are common, regardless of physiological status...where intakes are reported by income, low-income women appear to consume less than their middle and high income counterparts. Not only do women consistently eat less than men, in a number of studies, they consume, on average a smaller percentage of their recommended daily intake...Women often consume lower quality, vegetable protein while men receive the larger share of whatever animal protein is available...On the basis of quantity alone, women often consumed a smaller percentage of their protein requirements than did men.

The adequacy of vitamin intake varies greatly by culture. Riboflavin intakes are adequate in almost every country reviewed. The adequacy of vitamin A varies considerably, while most women (except those in Singapore, Iran, and the Tarahumara Indians) are deficient in their vitamin C intakes.

Calcium and iron are the two minerals most commonly studied and in a majority of the countries reviewed, women are seriously deficient in their intakes of both.

The particular ramifications of women's iron and calcium deficiencies will be recurring themes in this book.

Iron is vital to the oxygen-carrying capacity of the blood and muscles but iron deficiency anaemia is the most common nutrition problem in rich and poor countries and in rich and poor people. Iron is available in many foods including meats, eggs, vegetables (especially greens), cocoa powder, apricots, breads and cereals, but in light of the prevalence of iron deficiency, the United Nations Committee on Nutrition recommends that more priority be given to iron fortification and supplementation.[25]

Reproductive age women are particularly vulnerable to iron deficiency because iron lost through menstruation must be replaced and highly increased circulatory requirements of pregnancy must be supplied in addition to the body's other needs for iron. Iron deficiency anaemia's incapacitating physiological and psychological effects influence the lives of women three or four times as much as men in many parts of the world. In low income countries, about half of non-pregnant women and nearly two-thirds of pregnant women show signs of iron deficiency anaemia.[27] Bangladesh is the most extreme example where a national survey discovered abnormally low iron (measured as blood haemoglobin) levels in 95% of rural women.[28]

Serious anaemia increases the risks of difficulty and death in childbirth of these women. While the consequences of iron deficiency anaemia are usually less severe in richer countries, the debilitating condition is far too common. Anaemia was identified in 40% of pregnant women in New Mexico's Women, Infant, and Children (WIC) Program and in 33% of poor pregnant women in Minneapolis, Minnesota. Black children show consistently higher rates (often more that twice as high) of anaemia than white children, so the effects of anaemia are probably even more exaggerated for Black than white US women.[29]

The consequences of sex differentiated nutrition become most obvious at the vulnerable times just after weaning and during the childbearing years. These are the two stages of life at which the female to male sex ratios take a dive.[30]

Biologically, it seems females are stronger than males. In general, life expectancy in females is greater than that in males. More males than females are conceived (120–150 males: 100 females), seemingly to "prepare" for the male biological vulnerability. More male fetuses are spontaneously aborted or stillborn, so the male to female ratio is down to 103–105:100 at birth.[31] Fifty-four percent more males die of birth injuries, 18% more males die of congenital malformations, and males account for 54% of all infant deaths in the first year of life.

Given the apparent biological advantage of females, a fascinating exercise is to try to identify the biological versus social and political causes of sex differences in death rates. Obviously, the fact that 68% of the US deaths at age 21 are male is more related to societal messages about who should play with guns and drive fast cars than a biological difference. Whether the supposedly higher rate of coronary heart disease in middle aged men than in women is more related to different roles in society, women's higher oestrogen levels, or a difference of who gets diagnosed, is a much more complex debate. Wherever there is a higher death rate for males, there may be a combination of biological and social factors working. Higher death rates for females clearly indicate that there are social, political or economic conditions overriding the female biological advantage.

The most marked sex discrimination in nutrition occurs after disasters in which there is a food shortage. Although physiological differences between males and females suggest that figures would show an excess mortality among males, statistics which exist consistently show that it is females and especially girl children who are at highest risk.[32] In the economic disasters after flooding in West Bengal, girls under five had a 60 percent higher incidence of third-degree malnutrition than the same age boys.[33]

A number of studies in South Asia have shown dramatic differences in the food and health care available to girls and boys. Preferential treatment of boys begins at birth when the birth of a boy is almost always viewed as a splendid occasion. Attitudes to the birth of a baby girl are at best ambivalent. While explicit female infanticide is no longer commonly practiced, the withholding of food and health care resources from girls can be viewed as a modern day version of female infanticide. The end result is the same: female mortality exceeds male mortality by as much as 50 percent in the 1–4 year age groups in rural Bangladesh.

A detailed study of six rural Bangladeshi villages pinpoints how this happens.[34] Intrafamily food distribution surveys carried out by 130 families showed that energy and protein intakes were consistently higher for males than females in all age groups.

Protein consumption in males compared to females was 14% higher in 0–4 year olds, 22% higher in 5–14 year olds, 25% higher in 15–44 year olds, and 53% higher in males over 45. Malnutrition rates reflected the intrafamily distribution pattern. Of 882 children surveyed, 14.4 percent of girls were classified as severely malnourished compared to 5.1 percent of boys.

There is usually a distinct, almost synergistic relationship between malnutrition and infection. Malnutrition severely compromises the body's ability to resist infection, and resisting or succumbing to infection increases the body's nutritional needs, thus enhancing the degree of malnutrition. The effects of malnutrition will usually be exaggerated by this malnutrition—infection—increased malnutrition cycle and malnourished children can die from normally non-lethal diseases like measles.

Surprisingly, the six village rural Bangladesh study found rates of infection among female children were consistently lower than among males, although the differences were small and statistically insignificant. (More proof of the biological strength of little girls!) The tragedy was that girls were valued so much less than boys that health resources were made available to ill boys but not to ill girls *even when transport and health care was provided for free.* Despite nearly comparable incidence levels of diarrhea, boys exceeded girls at the treatment center by 66 percent: diarrhea treatment rates averaged 135.6 per 1000 for male children in comparison to 81.9 for female children.

Studies from India show even more starkly the consistent and systematic discrimination against females in the allocation of food and health care resources. Kwashiorkor (protein-calorie malnutrition) is four to five times more common among girls than boys. Though girls were more likely to be suffering from this life-threatening form of malnutrition, boys outnumbered girls at the hospital for treatment by a ratio of 50:1. When treated, children of both sexes responded equally well, but the mortality rate was considerably higher in girls due to both a lack of food and a lack of health care.[35,36]

Male-preferential distribution of food and other resources is certainly not a phenomenon only in poor households. Excess female to male mortality in 1–4 year olds is observed even among wealthy landowning families in Bangladesh, demonstrating that competition for scarce, insufficient resources does not explain all the disparity. It is not known whether this pattern is more marked in poor families when there is simply not enough for everyone so less valued members must be "sacrificed" for the sake of others or whether it is exaggerated in wealthier families where the social role of rich women is even more inferior in comparison to the status of rich men. In Bangladesh, excess female mortality is higher in rich households some years but other years excess mortality is higher in poor families.[37]

Intergenerational Consequences of Female Malnutrition

Malnutrition in girls and women can have long term and intergenerational repercussions, because of women's reproductive role. Any nutritional deficiency, such as rickets, which interferes with the physical development of little girls can cause problems, including maternal and infant death, decades later in pregnancy and childbirth.

The most profound and long term effect of women's malnutrition is demonstrated by the link between poor maternal height and weight and low birth weight babies. Low birth weight babies, defined as weighing less than 2500 grams (five and one-half pounds) at full gestation, have a much higher mortality rate and are more susceptible to illness throughout childhood than normal weight babies. A Sri Lankan study found an average maternal height of 150 cm (4'9") for low birth weight babies and a modal maternal height of 155 cm (5'1") for well-grown babies.[38]

Poor maternal height and weight can be a reflection of the mother's own intrauterine growth retardation and inadequate childhood nutrition. Healthy diets for *all* potential mothers from pre-conception through pregnancy can be seen as a high societal priority when one realizes that *it takes at least two generations to eliminate the effect of stunted maternal growth on future generations of women and men.*

Reversing the effect of malnutrition brings new challenges. When a basic nutritionally-adequate diet for everyone becomes a national priority, young women with a family history of malnutrition will have access to a healthy diet after their own development has been stunted. In revolutionary China, as a consequence of major improvements in food production and distribution, birth weights rose dramatically within one generation. In order to maximize on its nutritional achievements, China's health services had to be able to cope with an increased rate of complicated deliveries as there was a generation of small mothers producing relatively large babies.[39]

While the relationship of women's malnutrition to generations of limited development may be most exaggerated in the poorest countries, it is certainly also an issue for wealthier countries. Some figures will help us follow through the impact of restricted nutrition on poor women in Britain and the U.S. but one has to be critical of categories of analysis. Not by accident, measures of social class such as wealth, income, education and job classification are seldom recorded on US records such as death certificates.[40] Britain is much better at recognizing/not hiding the importance of social class information but the information is more appropriate to men than to women. Women's social class is based on husband's occupation. Even when categorization is based on the woman's own job, as with unmarried heterosexual or lesbian women, women's jobs certainly do not sum up women's lives.[41]

In Britain, 41 percent of wives of professional men have a height of at least 165 cm (5'5") compared to only 26 percent of wives of manual workers. Similarly, in the US, women in low income families have an average height of 160.4 cm (5'3") compared to 163.4 cm (5'4") for women in higher income families.[42] Heights for US children have, on average, been increasing throughout the last century, but the average height for poor children lags behind that for nonpoor children by more than a generation. The average height of ten year olds from families above poverty level is now significantly higher than the average height of ten year olds living below poverty. (This is not a race difference, for the average height of Black children is slightly higher than that of white children of the same income.) Sweden has recently managed to eliminate growth differences between social classes and is probably the only country with this achievement.[43]

In Britain, low birth weight babies and stillbirths are nearly twice as common in poor families (social classes IV and V) as in wealthier families (classes I and II). In the US, infant mortality rate is thirty times higher in low birth weight babies than normal weight babies.[44] Infant mortality rate (IMR = the number of babies per thousand live births who die in the first year of life) is an invaluable tool for comparing the health status of groups because it is a figure which is calculated similarly all over the world and is an excellent reflection of maternal and infant nutrition, as well as general standard of living and access to preventative and curative health care. IMR is 50 percent higher for US whites living in poverty areas than for US whites living in nonpoverty areas and IMR is at least 2.5 times higher in poor than in wealthy families in the UK. The intersection of poverty and racism is obvious from national (US) figures showing IMR more than twice as high for Black babies as white babies. Blacks in poor areas have a far higher IMR than Blacks in nonpoor areas although Black IMR is higher than white IMR in both income areas.[45,46]

The potential for change with an improved standard of living, including an emphasis on nutrition and access to health care, is most striking when IMRs are compared for small geographical areas. The Physician Task Force on Hunger in America contrasts the New York City IMRs of 5.8 in the Sunset Park section of Brooklyn with the 25.6 rate for Central Harlem and the Houston, Texas IMRs of 10.0 in the Sunnyside areas versus 23.5 in the Riverside Health Center community.[47] When we see that two or four times as many babies are dying in one part of town than in another, little guessing is needed to figure out where the poor, malnourished people live in New York City or Houston.

Malnutrition: Cause and Effect on Women's Role in Society

It is women not men who are unequally distributing food within the family, giving men and boys more than their share of what is available for the household. Women depriving themselves and their daughters of life-sustaining nourishment is the ultimate example of internalized sexism. Men do not need to discriminate against women or carry out nasty plans to "keep women in their place" if women are sufficiently well socialized to their inferior role that they themselves perpetuate keeping women in inferior roles.

A profoundly intermeshing relationship exits between women's status in society and the responsibility for food production and distribution. Women's responsibility for domestic work, especially food production, is so undervalued that women internalize that low value and starve themselves literally or figuratively. Although millions of women and girls die each year as a result of malnutrition, that number is a mere fraction of the number of women and girls who cannot maximize on their full potential because of undernutrition and because their responsibilities for feeding others do not leave them food, time or energy to nourish and nurture themselves.

Women's role as food producer can actually restrict a woman's ability to feed herself and others. How often have

we observed a woman who eats practically nothing herself after spending hours preparing a meal for others? How often have we seen a woman so busy serving others that she barely sits down herself? A woman's standards for feeding herself may be totally different than those she holds to for her family. For example, a (London) *Daily Mirror* survey showed that even though mothers of school-age children make sure their children have breakfast, a fifth of mothers do not take time to eat breakfast themselves.[48]

Charmian Kenner's interviews with English women who have survived times of economic hardship show how the family's dependence on mum's food can make mum so ill that she cannot feed them:

There was a vicious circle in which sickness bred further sickness. Lacking food, women had less resistance to infections. And when a woman fell ill and especially needed better food nobody else could take over and stretch the budget. Some women did not even feel able to set aside valuable time to teach their children to help them.[49]

It is exactly the women who face the most demanding food preparation tasks who have the least time and energy for this work. The woman who can afford the latest food processor and microwave may also be able to afford to buy easy-to-cook or partially prepared nutritious foods when she is too busy to cook. The woman who has to work overtime to have money to buy beans may not be able to buy a pressure cooker to reduce cooking time. Before or after a long day, she may have to decide between spending several hours on food preparation and eating less nutritional foods.

In many agricultural communities, it is *because* women have put all their time and energy into growing and harvesting the food that they may not be able to take the final steps, often extremely time and energy consuming, of turning the raw products into an edible form so that they can feed themselves and others.

One report speaks of African women "sitting about hungry with millet in their granaries and relish in the bush" because they were too exhausted to tackle the heavy, three-hour work of preparing the food for eating.[50]

The seasonal nature of agriculture exacerbates this. Peak periods for women's work in the fields are normally at planting, harvesting and post-harvesting processing times when the working day can average fifteen hours. This coincides with the food supply being scarcest, most expensive, least varied and least well prepared. As a consequence, it has been noted that in Gambia, pregnant women actually lose weight during the peak agricultural time and, in Thailand, there is a marked increase in miscarriages and an early termination of breastfeeding during the rice planting and harvesting seasons.[51,52]

The relationship between productivity and nutrition works in several ways. Not only does extreme work keep women from feeding themselves, but also undernutrition is clearly a factor limiting women's productivity. Intensity of work, the productive value of work activities selected, and labour time are all dimensions of productivity which have been shown to be affected by nutrition. If women are not able to maximize on their productivity, food production is limited; several studies have identified women's labour input as the critical constraint on crop production. Although the value of women's productivity is universally and consistently *not* recognized, any signs of poor performance are definitely used to prolong women's low status.

The case of Sri Lankan women tea workers illustrates the cycle whereby low status affects diet, then malnutrition perpetuates low status. Tea workers' poor social and economic position is reflected by high morbidity and maternal mortality rates. Due to poor diets and hook worm manifestation, the women also have high rates of iron deficiency anaemia (measured as low haemoglobin levels). Studies found that this iron deficiency restricted work performance; a significant relationship was found between haemoglobin levels and various treadmill tests of physiological capacity. (Iron deficiency anaemia affects work intensity by decreasing the blood's oxygen transporting capacity.) After the women were given iron supplements for one month, significantly more tea got picked! These studies were of particular interest to the Sri Lankan government because tea has been the main asset for foreign exchange and the poor nutritional status of the female labour force was seen as having far reaching socio-economic consequence. Assuming women's increasing productivity was appropriately financially rewarded, one can see where something as seemingly simple as iron supplements can be an important step to improved economic status for some women.[53,54]

This specific example suggests an even bigger question: How much does the image and reality of the malnourished woman as weak, lethargic and not maximizing on her potential become the generalized description for "women" which then justifies and perpetuates women's inferior status?

Worldwide the high incidence of iron deficiency anemia has to be seen as a major, often unrecognized, component of women's low status. We know that this one nutrition issue affects as many as 95 percent of women in some communities and has profound physiological and psychological repercussions, including impaired work capacity, lassitude, lowered resistance to infection, and increased complications of pregnancy and childbirth. The Sri Lankan tea workers' example is worth remembering as a positive example of both how easily some consequences of iron deficiency can be reversed and the need to make sure our governments become better educated about what they have to gain from a well nourished female labour force.

A wide range of other nutrition problems also have an impact on women's status. As an illustration which has nearly universal ramifications, low Calorie diets serve as an important example of undernutrition which, for very different reasons, can interfere with women maximizing on their potential and limiting their role in society in both rich and poor countries and for both rich and poor women. It is well known that low energy intakes restrict work potential and conversely that Calorie supplementation significantly increases work intensity and capacity.[55] The body, of course, has to work equally hard at coping with the limitations of a low Calorie diet whether that restriction is imposed because of a natural disaster food shortage or the fact that someone "chooses" to diet down to a smaller size. Research from poor countries indicates that the body does have adaptation mechanisms for adjusting to *permanently* restricted food intake but the body has a particularly chaotic job adjusting to great dietary fluctuations such as erratic food supply or yo-yo dieting.

What price do individuals and society pay for women's undernutrition caused by lifelong dieting? Hilde Bruch, psychiatrist respected for her groundbreaking work on eating disorders, describes "thin fat people" as people (usually women) who routinely eat less than their bodies require in order to stay at a weight which is artificially low for themselves. Very often these women are tense, irritable and unable to pursue educational and professional goals as a direct result of their chronic undernutrition. But, if they never allowed themselves to eat properly they do not recognize the signs that these limitations are due to undereating rather than personal weaknesses. Characteristic signs of malnutrition—fatigue, listlessness, irritability, difficulties in concentration and chronic depression— often escape correct professional diagnosis because the starved appearance (and especially average weight appearance in someone meant to be heavy) is a matter for praise rather than concern by our fatphobic society. "It has become customary to prescribe tranquilizers for such people; three square meals a day would be more logical treatment, but one that is equally unacceptable to physicians and patients because they share the conviction that being slim is good and healthy in itself."[56]

Is it possible that the relationship to food is sufficiently different between women and men that it helps determine gender differences in how women and men operate in the world? What if our scientific studies which "prove" that men are superior at performing certain tasks are actually measuring men's superior ability to fulfill their nutritional requirements rather than measuring task performing abilities? How would we even begin to start to think about or "measure" such things?

Claire Etaugh and Patricia Hill have started on some fascinating research to test their theory that gender differences in eating restraint (dieting) influence previously reported gender differences in cognitive restructuring tasks. Their initial study found that gender differences were in fact eliminated on one of two tasks when men and women were matched for eating restraint. On the other task, eating-restricted females performed the task more poorly than unrestricted females, thus exaggerating the male-female difference.[57] This work certainly confirms the need for eating restraint to be a factor which must be controlled in any study which attempts to measure gender differences. This research builds on previous work which showed that many differences found between fat and thin people are actually differences between restrained eaters (dieters) and non-restrained eaters (non-dieters). Even without further research, we know that some cognitive restructuring task gender differences disappear when dieting is controlled for and we know that dieting can result in poorer performance on a range of tests. What more proof do we need that dieting can prevent women from maximizing on their potential?

Although we have started to explore how the nearly universal pattern of men and boys getting fed more and better than women and girls can play a part in perpetuating women's inferior social and economic roles, it is hard to imagine all the many subtle and unnoticed ways in which this may manifest itself.

Hamilton, Popkin and Spicer suggest that nutritional status affects one's selection of work activities. Only well-nourished workers would be expected to qualify for the higher paying jobs if they are more physically or mentally demanding. Conversely, they suggest, individuals adapt to low energy intakes by being involved in less demanding occupations.[58]

Not surprisingly, most studies concentrate on nutrition-productivity relationships in men. Much less is known about the interaction of nutrition and productivity in women and, of course, even less is known about how nutrition affects women's roles outside the paid labour force. One study reported that supplementation of women's diets improves the mother-child interactions and enhances child development by providing women with greater energy and increasing their potential capacity for physical effort and active time for interaction with the children.[59] A study of Guatemalan peasants found that women who receive dietary supplements spent more leisure and market time in physically active tasks than women who did not receive supplements. Sixty-seven percent of the supplemented group were considered "fully active" compared to only five percent of the unsupplemented group.[60]

The long term and intergenerational costs of the malnutrition-low status relationship in girls is just starting to be recognized. It is now known that cognitive development is dependent on both adequate nutrition and intellectual stimulation. Ten year follow-up studies of children who were treated for severe protein-calorie malnutrition showed no significant difference in mental performance when compared to their siblings or controls. But, there was a strong correlation between their intellectual achievement and years of schooling. It was noted that malnourished children sometimes took a few years to recover from any mental consequences of early childhood malnutrition and that the normal curriculum might not be appropriate during that time. This finding has particular significance for girls since in many communities girls will have already been withdrawn from school before the recovery time and thus girls will be deprived of the educational opportunity even if they were lucky enough to be treated for malnutrition.[61]

Several studies have now demonstrated the crucial importance of female education as a factor contributing to lower child mortality even when family income is controlled.[62] These studies do not try to explain the complex mechanisms through which improved female education operates to reduce child mortality, but they help emphasize that women, their children, and society are deprived when women do not get to explore their educational potential.

The relationship of girls' undernutrition and girls' not being able to maximize on their mental development and educational capabilities obviously has enormous ramifications for what women can contribute to society, what women are expected or encouraged to do, and the recognition they are given for their achievements. We saw how a child's birth weight, and thus "good start in life", was influenced by the mother's height and weight which was affected by the grandmother's nutrition (p. 389). We now see the vital link among childhood nutrition, female educational opportunities and child mortality. Although this may be two different ways of looking at similar information, it is also a reminder of how these social and economic factors work together and exaggerate each other.

Consequently, the low value of females can cause the mothers to feed boys better than girls so that boys are less apt to be malnourished and more likely to be capable of benefitting from, and having access to, educational opportunities. Boys will then be far more likely to be the "well-nourished workers to qualify for the higher paying, higher status, physically or mentally demanding jobs" than their undernourished sisters. In one generation, in one community, the pattern could be clear cut—the boys worked to their potential more than the girls and the boys have more status than their sisters. When the sisters have their own children, how equally will they distribute the food and will they be aware of the unequal distribution if they give more to their sons than their daughters? In the extreme Bangladesh example (p. 388), women tended to deny unequal distribution except when male child preference was expressed in relation to marked food shortages or in reference to sex differentials with regard to food quality.[63]

Does this extreme but not exaggerated example give us clues to how this process may operate more subtly? Having seen that cognitive development is dependent on both adequate nutrition and intellectual stimulation and having seen gender differences disappear (in one test) when men and women were matched for eating restraint, what significance is there in the fact that many nine year old girls are now dieting? We know the physical abilities of girls and boys are pretty evenly matched until age 10–12 when social pressure discourages young women from developing their physical potential. We know that many girls excel in maths at an early age but then internalize the "girls aren't good at maths" idea by adolescence. In what ways do these messages which limit young women from maximizing on their potential now get exaggerated by the pressure on them (and their mothers) not to let themselves get fat?

A young woman's nutritional needs are among the highest of her life when she is 11–14 years: an average 100 pound girl uses up 2400 Calories a day and needs a very vitamin and mineral concentrated diet. This is also one of life's most crucial times for making educational decisions which will influence future choices. If individuals or society wish to improve the role of women in society, this is the worst possible stage for young women to start practicing their lives as "thin fat people"!

References

1. Judith Willis, "The Gender Gap at the Dinner Table", *FDA Consumer,* June, 1984, pp. 13–17.
2. 1989 RDA
3. Mary Roodkowsky, "Underdevelopment Means Double Jeopardy for Women", *Food Monitor,* September/October 1979, pp. 8–10.
4. Lisa Leghorn and Mary Roodkowsky, *Who Really Starve? Women and World Hunger,* New York: Friendship Press 1977, p. 20.
5. Colin Spencer, "Sex, Lies and Fed by Men", *Guardian,* November 4–5, 1989, p. 11.
6. Leghorn and Roodkowsky, *op. cit.*
7. E.M.Roenberg, "Demographic Effects of Sex Differential Nutrition" in N.W.Jerome, R.F.Kandel and G.H. Pelto (ed.) *Nutritional Anthropology—Contemporary Approaches to Diet and Culture,* Redgrave Publishing co. 1980, pp. 181–203.
8. Charmian Kenner, *No Time for Women—Exploring Women's Health in the 1930s and Today,* London:Pandora 1985, p. 8.
9. Hilary Land, "Inequalities in Large Families: More of the Same or Different?" in Robert Chester and John Peel (ed.) *Equalities and Inequalities in Family Life,* New York: Academic Press 1977, pp. 163–175.
10. Hilary Graham, *Women, Health and the Family,* Brighton, Sussex: Wheatsheaf Books 1984, pp. 120–135.
11. Ruth Sidel, *Women and Children Last—The Plight of Poor Women in Affluent America,* New York: Viking 1986, p. 149.
12. E.Evason, *Just Me and the Kids: A Study of Single Parent Families in Northern Ireland,* Belfast: EOC 1980, p. 25, quoted in Graham, *op. cit.*
13. "Food for All?" *London Food News,* no.4-Autumn 1986, p.l.
14. D.Marsden, *Mothers Alone: Poverty and the Fatherless Family,* Harmondsworth, Middlesex: Penguin 1973, p. 43, quoted in Graham, *op.cit.*
15. Neil Gallagher, "Obstacles Curb Efforts to Improve Nutrition", *World Food Programme Journal,* no.3, July- September, 1987, pp. 19–22.
16. Judit Katona-Apte, "Women and Food Aid—A Developmental Perspective", *Food Policy,* August, 1986, pp. 216–222.
17. Paul Fieldhouse, *Food and Nutrition: Customs and Culture,* London: Croom Helm 1986, pp. 168–169.
18. *Ibid.,* pp. 41–54.
19. *Ibid.*
20. Betsy A. Lehman, "Fighting the Battle of Freshman Fat", *The Boston Globe,* September 25, 1989, pp. 23,25.
21. Joan Price, "Food Fixations and Body Biases—An Anthropologist Analyzes American Attitudes", *Radiance,* Summer 1989, pp. 46–47.
22. See for example the excellent resources of the Institute for Food and Development Policy, 1885 Mission Street, San Francisco, CA. 94103 (USA) or Oxfam, 274 Banbury Rd., Oxford OX2–7DZ (England).
23. Kathleen Newland, *The Sisterhood of Man,* London: W.W.Norton 1979, pp. 47–52.
24. Sahni Hamilton, Barry Popkin and Deborah Spicer, *Women and Nutrition in Third World Countries,* South Hadley, Massachusetts: Bergin and Garvey Publishers 1984, pp. 22–26.
25. United Nations Administrative Committee on Coordination—Subcommittee on Nutrition, *First Report on the World Nutrition Situation,* Rome, Italy: FAO Food Policy and Nutrition Division 1987, pp. 36–39.
26. UNICEF News Fact Sheet printed in Leghorn and Roodkowsky, *op. cit.*
27. Hamilton, Popkin and Spicer, *op. cit.* p. 55.
28. Shushum Bhatia, "Status and Survival", *World Health,* April, 1985, pp. 12–14.
29. Physician Task Force on Hunger in America, *Hunger in America—The Growing Epidemic,* Middletown, Connecticut: Wesleyan University Press 1985, pp. 119–120.
30. Newland, *op.cit.*
31. Ethel Sloane, *Biology of Women,* 2nd Edition, New York: John Wiley 1985, pp. 122–123.
32. J.P.W.Rivers, "Women and Children Last: An Essay on Sex Discrimination in Disasters", *Disasters,* 6(4), 1982, pp. 256–267.
33. Amartya Sen, "The Battle to Get Food", *New Society,* 13 October, 1983, pp. 54–57.
34. Lincoln C. Chen, Emdadul Huq and Stan D'Souza, "Sex Bias in the Family Allocation of Food and Health Care in Rural Bangladesh", *Population and Development Review,* vol. 7, no.1, March, 1981, pp. 55–70.
35. Newland, *op. cit.*
36. Bhatia, *op. cit.*
37. Chen, Huq and D'Souza, *op. cit.*
38. Priyani Soysa, "Women and Nutrition", *World Review of Nutrition and Dietetics,* vol.52, 1987, pp. 11–12.
39. Discussions with Chinese health workers and the All China Women's Federation, March 1978 and March 1983.
40. Victor W. Sidel and Ruth Sidel, *A Healthy State—An International Perspective on the Crisis in United States Medical Care,* New York:Pantheon 1977, p. 15.
41. Jeannette Mitchell, *What Is To Be Done About Illness and Health?* Harmondsworth, Middlesex:Penguin 1984, p. 22.
42. Soysa, *op. cit.*
43. Sidel and Sidel, *op. cit.,* p. 26,
44. Physician Task Force on Hunger in America, *op. cit.,* p. 99.
45. Melanie Tervalon, "Black Women's Reproductive Rights" in Nancy Worcester and Mariamne H. Whatley (ed.) *Women's Health: Readings on Social, Economic and Political Issues,* Dubuque, Iowa: Kendall/Hunt 1988, pp. 136–137.
46. Sidel and Sidel, *op. cit.,* p.17.
47. Physician Task Force on Hunger in America, *op. cit.,* p. 109.
48. Kenner, *op. cit.,* p. 10.
49. *Ibid.,* p. 8.
50. Ester, Boserup, *Women's Role in Economic Development,* London: George Allen and Unwin 1970, p. 165 quoted in Barbara Rogers, *The Domestication of Women—Discrimination in Developing Societies,* London:Tavistock 1981, p. 155.
51. Hamilton, Popkin and Spicer, *op. cit.* p.45.
52. Ellen McLean, "World Agricultural Policy and Its Effect on Women's Health", *Health Care for Women International,* vol.8, 1987, pp. 231–237.
53. Hamilton, Popkin and Spicer, *op. cit.,* pp. 20– 21.

54. Soysa, *op. cit.*, pp. 35–37.
55. Hamilton, Popkin and Spicer, *op. cit.*
56. Hilde Bruch, "Thin Fat People" in Jane Rachel Kaplan (ed.) *A Woman's Conflict—The Special Relationship Between Women and Food,* Englewood Cliffs, New Jersey:Prentice-Hall 1980, pp. 17–28.
57. Claire Etaugh and Patricia Hall, "Restrained Eating: Mediator of Gender Differences on Cognitive Restructuring Tasks?", *Sex Roles,* vol.20, nos.7/8, 1989, pp. 465–471.

58. Hamilton, Popkin and Spicer, *op. cit.*
59. *Ibid.*
60. *Ibid.*
61. Soysa, *op. cit.*, pp. 13–14.
62. Chen, Huq and D'Souza, *op. cit.*
63. *Ibid.*

The Obesity of the Food Industry

by Nancy Worcester

It is ironical that while women in Europe and North America are intentionally starving themselves in order to lose weight and better fit the prized slim image, in other parts of the world (e.g., parts of Africa) the daughters of rich families are sent to special fattening houses, fed rich foods and allowed no exercise. The fatter a girl grows, the more beautiful she is considered.[1] Wherever there is a limited food supply or an unequal distribution of resources, fatness and obesity become status symbols because only the wealthy or powerful have access to ample food supplies.

The food industry makes certain that we have access to an abundance of food, but in the process of making itself a fat profit, the food industry also ends up making us fat.

In our affluent society, we are assured a steady, plentiful food supply. We have more nutritional information than ever before and have a clearer understanding of the relationship of food to health. We should be eating the healthiest diet* of all time. Instead we are now eating too much of the wrong foods and our pattern of food consumption is a major cause of ill health and death. Incongruously, the change in the balance of nutrients which is recommended to us today to promote health and prevent illness is very similar to the pattern which was consumed at the turn of the century (see Table 1) before the food industry became so influential in determining food habits.

Table 1. Nutrition Recommendations vs. Reality. **(Percent of Diet from Different Nutrients)**

	1909–1913	Current	Dietary Goals*
Protein	12%	12%	12%
Fat	32%	42%	30%
Carbohydrate	56%	46%	58%

*Dietary Goals for the US, 1977. Senate Select Committee on Nutrition and Human Needs

With an increased awareness of what is good for us, there is a tendency to blame the individual, or more specifically the woman of the family, for not choosing the healthiest foods. Such 'victim blaming' ignores the tremendous pressure on everyone to eat in certain ways and overlooks the fact that consumers have little voice in choosing the choices available to them.

The food industry simply sets out to make a profit, but the food industry has a peculiar problem.[2] Unlike other consumer industries, the food industry cannot count on us buying more of their products as our incomes rise. Even if we are encouraged to overeat and are wasteful of food, there is a limit to the amount of food we can consume. In order to maximize their profits, the food companies must gain a greater share of the market and entice us to buy the foods with the highest profit margin.[3]

To gain the greatest share of the market, the food industry is now dominated by monopolies. For example,

---

"The Obesity of the Food Industry" is an excerpt from WOMEN AND FOOD, by Nancy Worcester, being written for Pluto Press, London, England. Copyright © Nancy Worcester.

*Note: Diet is used as a term to denote one's usual pattern of eating and does not refer to a slimming diet unless specifically stated. Consistent with common usage of the word, dieting will be used to indicate the process of being on a reducing diet.

three corporations, Kelloggs, Weetabix and the National Biscuit Company control nearly 90% of the breakfast cereal market in the UK.[4] Similarly, Kelloggs, General Mills, and General Foods dominate over 90% of the breakfast cereal market in the USA.[5] Food companies are now a part of giant multinationals so ITT executives are making decisions about Hostess CupCakes, Wonder Bread and Morton Frozen Foods, and Beatrice Foods owns Dannon yogurt, LaChoy oriental foods and Samsonite luggage.[6] The health implications are obvious: the food industry gets further removed from consumers and is less and less responsive to the quality or quantity of foods which consumers want or need. Monopoly power results in extra profits for the food industry at our expense. Frances Moore Lappé, in *Diet for a Small Planet*, estimates that every single North American overpays $90 per year for food compared to what prices should be in a more competitive food economy.[7]

In order to increase sales, a food company offers a number of variations of the same products, and they benefit whether we choose product A or B. In the 1950's, UK consumers had 1500 lines of processed foods from which to choose.[8] Today there are more like 12,000 lines of processed foods. Whether being able to choose between bar-b-qued, sour cream, and au gratin flavored potato chips improves the quality of one's life may be a matter of debate: it certainly does not improve our access to healthy foods.

In an article on 'Women and Food' (Women may have freed themselves from the kitchen, but at what cost?) Joan Dye Gussow comments, 'The average supermarket has more than 12,000 items, the purpose of many of which would be unclear if it were not explained by advertising.'[9] Through advertising, the food industry manages to exert a tremendous influence on food habits, aggressively promoting those foods which are most profitable. It is no coincidence that Quaker Oats was the first reputable industry to appoint a fulltime advertising manager. In the late 1800's, Quaker introduced the use of trademarks to establish brand loyalty. This denoted a radical change in the marketing of foods. 'Food was no longer something people simply needed; for the first time it was defined as something people needed to be persuaded to buy.'[10] More is spent on advertising food products than any other product category. In the UK, 42 percent of the total advertising expenditure is spent advertising food, drink, and tobacco; nearly one-quarter of all advertising is especially for food products.[11] In the USA, the food industry spends three percent of the cost of the food directly on advertising and promotion, another 13 percent of the food cost goes for packaging which can be viewed as another form of advertising.[12] If we ate foods in proportion to the amount spent on advertising them, our diet would be made up of sweet foods, breakfast cereals, margarine, and potato chips.[13] A USA study found that ads for presweetened breakfast cereals outnumbered ads for meat, vegetables, milk, or cheese by a ratio of 1,800 to 1 on daytime television.[14] This puts tremendous pressure on women to buy unhealthy foods for their children.

Advertising turns out to be a major source of nutrition information for many people. This is a shame because advertising at its best is a poor source of nutrition information. At its worst, it deliberately confuses the consumer, exaggerates small differences between products without addressing real nutritional issues, and employs clever techniques to stay within the guidelines established to prevent false advertising. For example, enormous quantities are spent confusing the consumer about the benefits of polyunsaturated fatty acids compared to saturated fatty acids, trying to get the consumer to switch between butter and margarine or different types of margarine (usually all made by the same company). The urgent message which intentionally gets lost is that we need to cut down on *both* butter and margarine in order to reduce total fat consumption.

The consumer is deliberately encouraged to believe that there is little agreement about what constitutes a good diet and that so-called experts totally disagree with one another. Consumers are left feeling that they need not bother trying to modify their food habits because nutritional theories may change tomorrow. While there remain a number of nutritional questions which are being researched and debated, there is in fact overwhelming agreement between nutritionists, scientific, health, and governmental agencies about major constituents of a healthy diet. There is general agreement that for a healthier diet, we must [15]

- eat a variety of foods
- increase consumption of complex carbohydrates (starch and fiber)
- restrict sugar intake
- restrict fat intake (especially saturated fat)
- restrict cholesterol intake
- restrict salt
- use alcohol in moderation
- maintain a good body weight.

Those most influenced by food advertising are exactly the same people who could most benefit from getting the maximum nutritional value from their money. Tests gauging nutrition knowledge have found the worst scores among those with the lowest income and in the highest age groups. (Though overall nutrition knowledge is disappointingly low in *most* groups.) The effects of poverty and lack of education tend to exaggerate each other, so it is not surprising to find the US Senate Select Committee on Nutrition and Human Needs stating, 'It is likely that those most influenced by food advertising are low-income and elderly consumers.'[16]

We know there are class differences in health patterns and access to health care. Poor people have less chance of being healthy than middle class or wealthy people. There are good reasons to believe that class differences in health patterns are related to diet. Poor people consume a less healthy diet than middle class people. The 1980 Household

Food Survey (UK), compared poor and middle class families. Individuals in the poorer families were found to consume only 75 percent as many fresh vegetables, only 56 percent as much fresh fruit, but 150 percent more sugars as individuals in the better off families.[17] One can guess how much the influence of food advertising contributes to this situation.

The high profit foods are those with inexpensive ingredients and a long shelf life. Sugar and wheat are promoted by the food industry because they are cheap and easy to handle. White flour is more profitable than brown because the bran (fiber) and germ which have been removed can be sold separately and white flour products are less satisfying to the appetite, so people consume more of them.[18] Processing of food inevitably increases the profit margin even though nutrients are inevitably lost in the process. Salt adds to the taste and coloring adds to the appearance without adding much cost to the industry. People have learned to like the flavors carried by fats and the texture of fats, so it is particularly profitable to process foods in a way which increases the fat content. (Adding animal fats inevitably means also adding cholesterol.) Food additives are an inexpensive way of prolonging shelf life. So, we end up with a diet low in fiber, high in sugar, salt, fat, cholesterol and food additives even though we know that a healthy diet is high in fiber, and low in sugar, salt, fat, cholesterol, and food additives. A diet low in fiber and high in fat will lack bulk and will be very concentrated—literally will not take up much space. This is exactly the kind of diet which encourages one to eat more than one's body needs.

The fat story is a good one to use as an illustration of how we end up eating a diet which may make us unhealthy and fat while the food industry simply works at making its profit. Table 2 compares the price we pay for potatoes marketed in different ways and the caloric value of each style of potato. In each case, the added fat is responsible for the added Calories. Calories are a unit of measure for the energy content of food. Fats are the most concentrated form of energy. Every ounce of pure fat we eat gives us a whopping 250 Calories compared to the 112 Calories per ounce in any carbohydrate or protein. This is why every *good* slimming diet works by directly or indirectly cutting down on the amount of fat consumed. People gain weight when the energy (Calorie) intake is greater than the energy being used by the body. It is easy to see how simply increasing the fat content of the diet (without increasing our energy output) has been the equivalent of sending us all to special fattening houses. Unfortunately, our high fat diet also seems to be a cause of heart disease, breast and colon cancer.

The food industry certainly does not set out to deliberately sell us unhealthy foods. In truth, no one would be happier than the food industry if they could manage to get us to pay $3.18 per pound for baking potatoes without their increased costs of adding fat, processing, and packaging. They are as willing to make money from healthy foods as from any other product line.

Table 2. Paying a Lot for Fat!

Product	Price/pound	Calories/ounce
Baking Potatoes	20¢	23
French Fried Potatoes	99¢	68
Sour Cream Potato Chips	$2.85	90
Stacking Potato Chips	$3.18	117

The response of the food industry to the interest in healthier foods has been a good way to see how food companies actually work. They spend large sums on research trying to predict health trends which can be exploited as new markets. Nearly twenty years ago, doing product development for a food company, I was working to create 'nutritious instant breakfast products children can fix for themselves.' Market research had indicated that an increase in the number of mothers working outside the home combined with increased nutrition awareness could create a demand for such products.

Indeed the so-called health food market has turned out to be a big money-maker for the food industry though there is usually a gigantic gap between what the industry labels as health foods and what a nutritionist would identify as healthy eating. Much of what is passed off as health foods are merely variations of regular processed foods with a new packaging image emphasizing naturalness, purity, and old fashioned goodness, and a new price tag. The choice of which vitamins and minerals are added to products are more often based on what 'sounds good' (e.g., for which the consumer will pay a disproportionally higher price) rather than which nutrients are low in the diet or have been removed in processing that particular foodstuff.

The food industry was especially quick in offering a huge range of products to fit in with information showing the advantages of a high fiber diet. Why not? They already had the fiber which *they* had removed in processing. Instead of looking for another buyer, the manufacturer simply had to add it back, label the product 'high in fiber' or 'added fiber' and charge the consumer. Consumers have been willing to pay extraordinary amounts for high fiber foods because they finally hit upon a way to improve their diet without having to make any basic changes in their eating patterns. As an added attraction, on a high fiber diet the body gives immediate feedback that the changes in the diet are having the desired effect. (Bowel movements become larger, softer, and are easily eliminated indicating the absorbed water has facilitated the waste products to smoothly pass through the digestive tract. In the long term, this process probably helps prevent diverticulosis, colon cancer and other diseases.) In contrast, one has to be satisfied with only *knowing,* not seeing, the beneficial effects of reducing saturated fats, reducing cholesterol, or giving up cigarettes. The fact that it is difficult to find high fiber foods without sugar is a reminder that the consumer is being offered this new range of supposed health foods because it sells well rather than for health reasons.

This all leads up to a look at how the food industry benefits as much as anyone from the obsession for slimming. In fact we will have to question the role that the food industry has in specifically creating the obsession for slimming. In a pattern which should now sound familiar, the food industry makes huge profits on special slimming products. The same companies which have encouraged us to buy fattening foods now offer us virtually the same products, with a slightly reduced fat content and calorie information, at a higher slimming product, lite-version, price.

References

1. Hilde Bruch, *Eating Disorders—Obesity, Anorexia Nervosa. and the Person Within,* New York: Basic Books 1973 pp. 14–15.
2. The Politics of Health Group, *Food and Profit—It Makes You Sick,* London: POHG, 1980, p. 7.
3. Chris Wardle, *Changing Food Inhabits in the U.K.,* London: Earth Resources, 1977, p. 29.
4. Wardle, *op. cit.* p. 25.
5. Frances Moore Lappé, *Diet for a Small Planet,* New York: Ballantine Books 1982, p. 43.
6. Brett Silverstein, *Fed up! The Food Forces That Make You Fat, Sick, and Poor,* Boston, MA: South End Press 1984, pp. 4–5.
7. Lappé, *op. cit.*
8. Wardle, *op. cit.* p. 26.
9. Joan Dye Gussow, 'Women and Food', *Country Journal,* February, 1985, pp. 52–57.
10. Naomi Aronson, 'Working Up an Appetite' in Jane Rachel Kaplan (ed.) *A Woman's Conflict—The Special Relationship Between Women and Food,* Englewood Cliffs, NJ.: Prentice Hall 1980, pp. 215–216.
11. Wardle, *op. cit.* p. 31–33.
12. Letitia Brewster and Michael F. Jacobson, *The Changing American Diet,* Washington, D.C.: Center for Science in the Public Interest, 1978, p. 2.
13. POHG, *op. cit.* p. 11.
14. Aronson, *op. cit.* p. 216.
15. Marion Nestle, *Nutrition in Clinical Practice,* Greenbrae, CA.: Jones Medical Publications, 1985 pp. 42– 44.
16. U.S. Senate Select Committee on Nutrition and Human Needs, *Eating in America—Dietary Goals for the United States,* London: MIT Press 1979, p. 63.
17. Ministry of Agriculture, Fisheries and Food, *Household Food Consumption and Expenditure,* 1980, Table 20, pp. 104–106, quoted in Hilary Graham, *Women Health and the Family,* Brighton, Sussex: Wheatsheaf Books 1984, p. 124.
18. POHG, *op. cit.* pp. 6–7.

Ω

Fatphobia
by Nancy Worcester

We learn not to like fat people, then we internalize that as anxiety of gaining weight ourselves or self-hatred if we are already overweight. Both English and American studies consistently show that excess body fat is the most stigmatized physical feature except skin color.[1,2] Fatphobia differs from racism in that being overweight is thought to be under voluntary control. Anti-fat attitudes are well established before a child reaches kindergarten. 'Even at that young age, children attribute negative characteristics to the heavy physique, do not want to be like that themselves, and choose a greater "personal space distance" between themselves and a heavy child than from other children.'[3]

The animosity towards fat people is such a fundamental part of our society, that people who have consciously worked on their other prejudices have not questioned their attitudes towards body weight. People who would not think of laughing at a sexist or racist joke, ridicule and make comments about fat people without recognizing that they are simply perpetuating another set of attitudes which negatively affect a whole group of people.

The pressure to look like the 'ideal' is so strong that we do not question the implications behind teaching that routinely instructs young women on how to make their bodies look 'as perfect as possible'. Home economics classes teach young women that horizontal stripes make one look wider, vertical stripes make one look thinner. I was so well socialized by such instruction that I still find it hard to be comfortable in horizontal stripes, unless, of course, they are strategically placed so as to make the chest look larger! Even after years of criticizing the pressure on women to look thin, instead of admiring a large woman who has the courage to wear the "wrong" stripes, I still find myself wondering, 'But, doesn't she know . . . ?'

Although the prejudice against fat people affects both men and women, its impact is most exaggerated on women and their lives. Women put on body fat more easily than men for a number of social and physiological reasons. Of course, every topic in this book is a part of the explanation. The physical abilities of females and males are identical until puberty, but by that time socialization in most western cultures discourages physical fitness in young women thus encouraging weight to be put on as fat rather than as muscle. (At the age of 25, body fat content averages 14% for men and 23% for women.[4]) Although both females and males have a mixture of the sex hormones estrogens and androgens, the average female tends to have higher levels of estrogens than androgens and this influences the deposition of fat. Times of hormonal changes, adolescence, going on oral contraceptive pills, pregnancy, and menopause, are all times when some women notice that they put on fat easily.

Women are judged by appearance far more than men and a much wider range of sizes and shapes is considered attractive in men. For example, a 1982 study of the most popular North American television programs, found that of male characters, less than one-fifth were slim and more than one-quarter were plump, whereas of the female characters, over two-thirds were slim and only one-tenth were plump.[5] Women, not men, are bombarded with information that the size and shape of their bodies is central to who they are and if it is less than perfect they should be working to try to change it. Comparing the most popular of men's and women's magazines, we see that articles and advertising relating to body weight and dieting appear 17 times more often in women's magazines.[6]

At any moment in history, the ideal female figure is quite precisely defined. Studies have shown that both men and women judge women's bodies by how closely they measure up to that supposed ideal. The more a woman deviates from that 'norm', the more her appearance will adversely affect her social life, her acceptance at college, her employment, and her status.

In both England and North America, obesity is more common in working class women than in women of higher socio-economic groups. With men, the relationship of class and body weight is not so well defined.[7,8]

It seems relevant to suggest that the relationship between social class and obesity is not as simple as just the fact that poor people have less access to healthy, non-fattening foods. It is both poor women and men who have less access to these foods so we would expect that the relationship of class to obesity to be more consistent for both women and men. I am not convinced that differences in manual labor provide an explanation. (It has been suggested that working class men offset a tendency to obesity by doing more physical labor than middle class men. This explanation does not take into account that middle class men have more access to leisure exercise opportunities and facilities than do working class men and that working class women are also more likely to be involved in physically active jobs than middle class women.)

Is it possible that in our society a woman's body build is a factor in *determining* her socio-economic status? Nearly twenty years ago, a paper on the stigma of obesity concluded that, 'Obesity, especially as far as girls is concerned, is not so much a mark of low social economic status as a condemnation to it.'[9] A study of 1660 adults in Manhattan observed that overweight women compared to non-obese women are far less likely to achieve a higher socio-economic status and are much more likely to have a lower socio-economic status than their parents.[10] This relationship was not found in men. A now classical study of the late 1960's found that non-obese women were more likely to be accepted for college than obese women even though the obese and non-obese women did not differ on intellectual ability or percentage who applied for college admission.

If obese adolescents have difficulty in attending college, a substantial proportion may experience a drop in social class, or fail to advance beyond present levels. Education, occupation, and income are social-class variables that are strongly interrelated. A vicious circle, therefore, may begin as a result of college admission discrimination, preventing the obese from rising in the social-class system.[11]

As long as women are valued and rewarded for their roles as sex objects, and the non-skinny woman is not seen as fitting this image, it is easy to see how the stigma of excess weight limits a woman's status through job discrimination, apparently less marriage to high-status men (sic!) and fewer social and economic opportunities. The discrimination against fat women should serve as a reminder to all of us that we need to change the basis upon which the worth of all women is determined by society. Tragically, instead of viewing fatphobia as *society's* problem, many women internalize the fear and intolerance of fat as their *individual* problem. Instead of trying to change the world, women end up trying to change themselves.

In this era, when inflation has assumed alarming proportions and the threat of nuclear war has become a serious danger, when violent crime is on the increase and unemployment a persistent social fact, 500 people are asked by pollsters what they fear the most in the world and 190 of them answer that their greatest fear is 'getting fat'.[12]

References

1. S.J. Chetwynd, R.A. Stewart, and G.E. Powell, "Social Attitudes Towards the Obese Physique" in Alan Howard (ed.) *Recent Advances in Obesity Research: 1,* London: Newman Publishing 1975, pp. 223–225.
2. Susan C. Wooley and Orland W. Wooley, "Obesity and Women—I. A Closer Look at the Facts", *Women's Studies International Quarterly,* vol. 2, 1979a, pp. 69–79.
3. Orland W. Wooley, Susan C. Wooley, and Sue R. Dyrenforth, "Obesity and Women—II. A Neglected Feminist Topic", *Women's Studies International Quarterly,* vol. 2, 1979b, pp. 81–92.

4. Marion Nestle, *Nutrition in Clinical Practice,* Greenbrae, California: Jones Medical Publications 1985, p. 222.
5. Brett Silverstein, *Fed Up—The Food Forces That Make You Fat, Sick and Poor,* Boston: South End Press 1984, p. 107.
6. Silverstein, *op. cit.*
7. Wooley, 1979b, *op. cit.*
8. J. Yudkin, "Obesity and Society", *Biblthca Nutri Dieta,* vol. 26, 1978, p. 146.
9. W.J. Cahnman, "The Stigma of Obesity", *Sociological Quarterly,* vol. 9, 1968, pp. 283–299, quoted in Wooley, 1979b, *op. cit.*
10. P.B. Goldblatt, M.E. Moore, and A.J. Stunkard, "Social Factors in Obesity", *Journal of the American Medical Association,* vol. 192, 1965, pp. 1039–1044.
11. H. Canning and J. Mayer, "Obesity—Its Possible Effect on College Acceptance", *New England Journal of Medicine,* vol. 275, 1966, pp. 1172–1174.
12. *San Francisco Chronicle,* January 17, 1981, quoted in Kim Chernin, *Womansize—The Tyranny of Slenderness,* London: The Women's Press 1983, p. 23.

Ω

Dieting Is Dangerous to Your Health

by Judy Norsigian

Chronic dieting wreaks havoc with women's health. A ten-billion dollar diet industry, largely aimed at women, plays on our cultural obsession with thinness to ensure continued allegiance to its myriad programs and products. Let's take a look at women's magazines for one measure of this increasing obsession with thinness. From 1959–78 the number of articles on dieting and losing weight in six popular women's magazines increased from 17.1 per year in the first decade to 29.6 per year in the second. At the same time, eating problems, such as anorexia nervosa and bulimia, are on the rise, among women of all ages, racial groups and socio-economic classes, making for a tyranny of thinness.

This tyranny is couched in erroneous myths. For example, there is a common belief that fat people eat more than thin people. False. Many studies have shown that fat people do not on the average eat more than thin people. Many researchers now believe there is a "setpoint" for body fat, that is, a level of fatness that the body strives to maintain, which may be determined by heredity. To go far above or below this point requires extraordinary measures. A study recently reported in the New England Journal of Medicine revealed that adopted persons closely resembled their birth parents in weight, regardless of their eating habits, and the strongest link was found between mothers and their biological daughters. This does not mean that there is nothing individuals can do, but low calorie, starvation diets will not improve our health or fitness.

Another myth is that dieting is a good way to lose weight. In fact, it doesn't work for 99 percent of those who try. Most people regain lost weight within five years, 95 percent of them ending up heavier than before they dieted.

Even slow-loss diets don't work permanently. Your body interprets not satisfying hunger over a period of several days as starvation, responding by conserving energy and using calories more sparingly. To satisfy its energy and protein needs, your body also burns up muscle, including heart muscle. Fat is burned only as a second resort because muscle provides fuel that the body prefers. Because fat requires fewer calories to maintain than muscle, when you go off your diet, you'll acquire more fat and are likely to gain additional pounds.

Going on and off diets repeatedly stresses the heart and other organs. Some dieters have even died of heart failure. In addition, even with vitamin and mineral supplements, it is probably impossible to take in adequate nutrients on less than 1500 or 1600 calories a day. The amount of time, money and energy women spend trying out one diet after another might well win a presidential election. There is a huge distinction, however, between going on a reducing diet and changing one's diet to eat more nutritiously. Paying attention to our diets by eating more whole grains and vegetables, more iron and calcium-rich foods, and less sugar and salt-laden, high fat, highly processed foods could produce innumerable health benefits.

There are certainly health risks associated with excessive fatness, including an increased risk of uterine cancer, high blood pressure, and diabetes. But an improved diet, not a reducing diet, along with exercise frequently helps those conditions. Many problems may be unfairly blamed on fatness, since so many studies have included only those fat people who have been on constant diets. It is not clear in those instances whether we are measuring the risks of being fat as opposed to the risks of chronic dieting. Many fat people who do not diet, but who do exercise regularly, are extremely healthy people.

There are also risks associated with thinness. The major reason why unusually thin people tend to die young is

Reprinted with permission from *The Network News,* National Women's Health Network, Washington, D.C., May/June, 1986.

because of increased cancer risk. Thinner people are also more susceptible to lung diseases such as emphysema, fatal infections such as tuberculosis, and other problems such as ulcers, anemia, and osteoporosis. Also, thin women are much more likely to give birth to premature or underdeveloped babies.

Little research has been done on the connection between underweight and illness, but one researcher (P. Ernsberger) believes that poor health is not caused by natural thinness, as in a person with thin parents and grandparents. Instead, he suggests that the thin people who are unhealthy are probably starving themselves to stay that way. (This hypothesis remains to be tested.)

What about the benefits of extra body fat? First, we survive trauma better because of more body reserves. Second, menopause may be a gentler transition because of the estrogen production which takes place in fat tissue. Third, carrying around some extra weight can help to prevent osteoporosis because of the bone strengthening caused by the extra body mass. In one famous study (Framingham heart study), the women with the lowest mortality rates were 10–30 percent over the ideal weights on the insurance tables. So being thin may not be so healthy after all!

All this is easy to say, but unless the prevailing media messages and cultural attitudes change, women will still be under enormous pressure to be thin. We will be discriminated against on the job and ridiculed on the streets and in our homes. Ironically, the psychological stress associated with being fat in a "fat phobic" society and the stress from constant yo-yo dieting may well be far more damaging to our health than simply being fat. Furthermore, fear of ridicule keeps many fat women from exercising in front of others and regular exercise may be the major key to looking and feeling better for most of us.

Even if we don't lose weight, through regular exercise we may become smaller because we increase the proportion of lean body weight and reduce the proportion of fat. Very simply, fat tissue, pound for pound, takes up more space than muscle or lean tissue, so through exercise alone we may look thinner while not actually losing weight. And if we do lose weight, as some women do, it will not come from starving our bodies or resorting to risky procedures like stomach stapling, surgical fat removal, or even taking diet pills.

Clearly when we look at what desperate actions women are willing to resort to in order to avoid the stigma of being fat, we know we are a long way from changing attitudes about fatness. The Madison Avenue ideal is still deeply imbedded in the minds of all of us. But we can begin with small gestures and hope for a cumulative effect. Instead of dieting, we might put our energy into finding enjoyable ways to exercise, perhaps with a friend. When we hear comments that equate thinness with good health or raves about a newly publicized diet, we might take the opportunity to do a little health education of our own. We can write to women's magazines which carry frequent articles on dieting and ask that they provide more responsible reporting. And we can protest when we see others discriminated against simply on the basis of how fat they are.

If women didn't go on low-calorie starvation diets, and instead took a brisk half-hour walk every day or two, we might well prevent illness and promote health on an impressive scale. It would be terrific if more of us could adopt the attitude expressed in the title of an article in *MS. Magazine*: "I may always be fat, but fat can be fit."

Ω

Mental Health Issues Related to Dieting

by Nancy Worcester

The assumption is that if anyone is overweight they must be trying to lose weight and if they are not trying to lose weight, they certainly should be. The slimming industry has sold us this assumption and it is time that we stop swallowing it. The dieting experience is pretty disastrous for many women. We need to be more aware of the mental hazards of slimming and figure out ways to be more supportive of women who choose not to lose weight.[1] The more that women discover that they can live in large bodies without having to torture themselves with endless slimming diets, the less pressure there will be on all women to carve themselves down to smaller sizes.

1. Women Feel Guilty if They Are Not Slimming

The most liberating gift many women can give themselves is the decision that they are not going to try to lose weight. Until that decision is made, it is tempting to put off everything else and meanwhile dislike oneself both

"Mental Health Issues Related to Dieting" is an excerpt from WOMEN AND FOOD, by Nancy Worcester, being written for Pluto Press, London, England. Copyright © Nancy Worcester.

because of the fat itself and because the fat becomes symbolic of an unfulfilled goal.

As long as someone is thinking about changing her body, she is not going to be putting energy into learning to like her body the way it is.

As long as someone is postponing accepting and liking her body, there is a tendency not to work at making that body healthy and fit. This is a part of a self-perpetuating cycle. The more 'out-of-shape' one is, the more dissatisfying (and hard!) it is to undertake even ordinary exercise, the less exercise the body has the worse it feels and fewer calories will be burned up. This, of course, contributes to the tendency to gain weight and feelings of sluggishness.

See 'We'll Always Be Fat But Fat Can Be Fit'[2] which takes a positive approach to accepting one's body weight and improving both mental and physical health.

2. Dieting Makes a Person More Aware of Food

We have all heard of someone who works through lunchtime without realizing they have not eaten or the person who loses weight because they are too busy to eat regularly.

One of the primary purposes of food advertising is simply to keep food on the mind so that the consumer is aware of her appetite. Secondly, of course, advertising aims to influence which particular product is on the mind.

In much the same way, the very act of dieting works to keep food on the mind. The constant preoccupation with not overeating (or more often, not eating normally) makes food take on a new significance. Thus, paradoxically, the most unmanageable time to restrict food consumption is when one is consciously attempting to limit food intake. Can you imagine committed dieters working through a lunchtime without realizing it or being so busy that they did not eat regularly?

Old studies claimed that a difference between fat people and thin people was that fat people ate according to external cues—set meal times, attractive foods, social situation—whereas thin people ate in response to internal cues such as hunger signals. Thus, this explanation implied, thin people were less likely to eat more than their bodies needed. This work is now being reinterpreted.[3] It seems that dieting is a major factor in determining whether one responds to external or internal signals. A dieter cannot respond to internal cues saying she is hungry because dieting creates a state of almost constant hunger. The old studies simply overlooked the fact that fat people are far more likely to be dieting than thin people. Instead of looking at the differences between fat and thin people, researchers were looking at the differences between dieters (restrained eaters) and non-dieters (non-restrained eaters). Dieting makes people unable to listen to their own body signals.

Dieting may be responsible for setting up a vicious cycle which increases the need for further dieting. Once a dieter's restraint is broken, the dieter can easily move in the opposite direction and 'overeat'. Depression and anxi-

ety are emotions likely to break a dieter's restraint. Yet, dieting itself can cause anxiety, depression, and apathy.[4]

In attempting to change food habits, we are embarking upon changing one of our most conservative behaviors, something often intricately related to our inner sense of security. Food habits are the last patterns to change even when a person is living in a new environment and living a new lifestyle, e.g., immigrant food habits often more nearly resemble the diet of the homeland than of the new country even years after settling.

Additionally, changing one's pattern of food consumption presents a uniquely arduous challenge in that one has to deal with it daily, at regular intervals throughout the day. Difficult though it is, someone who is concerned about their smoking or drinking habits may choose to give up cigarettes or alcohol. Someone concerned about their eating habits does not have the option of giving up food.

These problems are all distinctly exaggerated for a woman responsible for others. She does not have the luxury of escaping from thoughts of food. While trying to ignore her own preoccupations with food/hunger, she will need to be making grocery lists, shopping in environments filled with visions and aromas of food, preparing food, serving food to others, and then cleaning up after the meals.

Such a seemingly unappetizing task as clearing up after a meal can be an immense challenge for the dieter. Keeping food intake records for nutrition classes, my students with young children have often discovered that a high percentage of their calorie intake comes from cleaning up the children's plates. They find themselves constantly torn between their lines not to waste food and their waistlines.

A major reason why women are somewhat less successful at losing weight than men is because their domestic responsibilities are so directly contradictory to the optimum conditions for dieting. Responsibility for food preparation is the worst imaginable antidote for the diet-induced obsession with food.

3. Dieting Often Fails

Few people would encourage a loved one, a friend, or a professional client to embark upon an activity which they knew was destined for failure. Yet, knowing that most dieting fails (probably 90%–98% in the long term), people in all types of capacities are constantly advising and cajoling each other to 'try to lose some weight', to check out the newest slimming gimmick, or to try the most recent bestselling diet.

While it may be an overstatement to say that it is sadistic to encourage someone else to diet, it is time to acknowledge that it is often irresponsible to influence someone else to diet. The act of encouraging dieting needs to carry with it the obligation to support the dieter practically and emotionally through the challenges of the dieting process and to nurture the dieter if the attempt to lose weight is not successful. How many people would be willing to commit themselves to something so risky and potentially demanding? There would be far less pressure on people to diet if such pressure had to be accompanied by appropriate supportive commitments.

No one likes failure in any aspect of their life. Too often failure at dieting can take on a significance unexpected and unrecognized by the dieter and her friends. Media bombardment of fictitious slimming success stories completely nullifies the fact that only one to ten percent of dieting is 'successful'. Therefore dieting gets experienced as 'something anyone should be able to do' and is not seen as a particularly ambitious goal. Failing at such a seemingly simplistic task can be especially disheartening.

Because of all the factors which influence body weight and the unpredictable ease with which one can or cannot lose weight, body weight is one of the most difficult areas of one's life to control. But, because body image is so central to a woman's self-image and confidence and is so related to her actual experiences in the world, a woman's inability to lose weight too often becomes symbolic for her of her failure to be in control of her own life.

4. Dieting May Be 'Successful'

If a woman is successful at losing weight, she will lose the advantages of being fat.

Advantages of being fat are imperceptible to most dieters. Yet having managed to lose weight, many women are shocked to discover that the expectations of a slim woman are different than those of a fat woman in this society. I have stopped being surprised by how regularly I meet women who have purposefully gained back weight because they found that 'sexual attractiveness' and not being taken seriously as thin women were so problematic. *Fat Is a Feminist Issue* has been immensely popular because it explores the meaning of being fat or thin in our society and enables women to discover why they may be subconsciously choosing to stay fat.

My fat says 'screw you' to all who want me to be the perfect mom, sweetheart, maid, and whore. Take me for who *I* am, not for who I'm supposed to be. If you are really interested in *me,* you can wade through the layers and find out who *I* am.[5]

Food can be an invaluable tool for relieving tension, coping with stress, or rewarding oneself. Successful dieting inevitably means changing those food habits that one has developed over a number of years. Additionally, the stress of dieting itself may undermine even the most well established coping mechanisms. Ingenuity is necessary in providing oneself with healthy alternatives to the role that food has played in keeping life in balance.

Education against child abuse is increasingly suggesting that adults hit a pillow or eat something to relieve tension involved in some adult-child interactions. This is a questionable and simplistic approach to decreasing child abuse, but it is a reminder of the role that food can play in defusing tension which could lead to physical violence or verbal confrontation with a child or an adult. Eating, even if that means overeating, will often be the healthiest way of dealing with immediate distress. We need to be alert to the dangers of dieting blocking that outlet.

There is also an obvious problem with the inverse relationship between cigarette smoking and weight. Women have been encouraged to use cigarettes as a means of weight control since the American Tobacco Company introduced the slogan "Reach for a Lucky instead of a sweet" in 1928.[6] Probably because of the way the cigarette smoking affects metabolic rate, most people gain some weight when they stop smoking. Fear of weight gain is a major reason why women are less successful than men at quitting smoking.[7] Thus, lung cancer has now surpassed breast cancer as the leading cause of death in middle-aged women (in the USA).[8] Women are paying with their lives for their success in keeping off a few pounds.

5. Suicide is Less Common in Obese

A most intriguing figure never gets explained. Hidden near the bottom of all the charts showing the differences in mortality for obese and non-obese are the figures for suicide. Suicide rates are noticeably lower in both obese men and women. If obese and non-obese committed suicide at the same rate, suicide rates for obese would be recorded as 100% of actual expected deaths. Instead, the figure is only 73% for obese women and 78% for obese men.[9]

There seems to be at least one mental health advantage of obesity that is overlooked and not understood.

References

1. Many of the ideas in this section have grown out of discussions of *Fat Is a Feminist Issue* with students and women's groups. (Susie Orbach, *Fat Is a Feminist Issue,* London: Paddington Press, 1978.)
2. Carol Sternhell, "We'll Always Be Fat But Fat Can Be Fit", *Ms,* May, 1985, pp. 66–68 and 142–154.
3. William Bennett and Joel Gurin, *The Dieter's Dilemma,* New York: Basic Books, 1982, pp. 34–45.
4. Valerie S. Smead, "Anorexia Nervosa, Buliminarexia, and Bulimia: Labeled Pathology and the Western Female", *Women and Therapy,* vol. 2, no. 1, 1983, pp. 19–35.
5. Susie Orbach, *Fat Is a Feminist Issue,* London: Paddington Books, 1978, p. 21.
6. Bennett and Gurin, *op. cit.,* pp. 92–93.
7. Bobbie Jacobson, *The Ladykillers—Why Smoking Is a Feminist Issue,* London: Pluto Press, 1981, pp. 14–15.
8. *1986 Cancer Facts and Figures,* American Cancer Society, 90 Park Avenue, New York, N.Y. 10016.
9. Jean Mayer, "Obesity" in Robert S. Goodhart and Maurice E. Shils (ed.) Febiger Press, 1980, pp. 721–740.

Ω

We'll Always Be Fat But Fat Can Be Fit

by Carol Sternhell

Sometimes I think we've all gone crazy. Sometimes I feel like a feminist at a Right-to-Life conference, an atheist in Puritan New England, a socialist in the Reagan White House. Sometimes I fear that fat women have become our culture's last undefeated heretics, our greatest collective nightmare made all too-solid flesh. I worry—despite our new ethos of sexual freedom—that female bodies are as terrifying and repulsive as ever, as greatly in need of purification and mortification. Certainly these days, when I hear people talking about temptation and sin, guilt and shame, I know they're referring to food rather than sex. When my friend Janet calls me up and confesses "I was bad today," I don't wonder whether she committed adultery (how archaic that sounds!); I know she merely means she ate dessert. When posters quoting Mae West appeared recently on Manhattan buses ("When choosing between two evils, I always like to take the one I've never tried before"), I wasn't surprised to find her remark illustrated with a picture of two different ice cream sundaes. (As I recall, however, when Mae West talked about evil, she generally wasn't thinking of hot fudge.) Kim Chernin, in *The Obsession: Reflections on the Tyranny of Slenderness* (Harper & Row), compares the language of diet books to "The old fire-and-brimstone sermons, intended to frighten men and women away from the delights and pleasures of sexual experience of their bodies." The sins of the flesh have been redefined, but the message is the same; a tremendous fear that women's natural appetites, uncontrolled, will bring about destruction.

Everything in this world, for women, boils down to body size.

We all know the story—the ugly duckling transformed into swan after years of liquid protein, the virtuous but oppressed stepdaughter whose fairy godmother appears with a pumpkin and a lifetime membership in Weight Watchers. Our fantasies of transformation are desperate, thrilling; when women imagine changing our lives, we frequently begin with our weight. "I always feel as if real life will begin tomorrow, next week, sometime after the next diet," said one friend, a talented writer who has been cheerfully married for 12 years and a mother for five. "I know it's crazy, but I won't be happy until I lose these fifteen pounds." So far her efforts—like 98 percent of all diets—have been unsuccessful. A few years ago, when public opinion pollsters asked respondents to name their greatest fear, 38 percent said "getting fat." Even very slender women believe that their lives would be better if only they could take off five pounds, or three, or two. In a

Reprinted with permission from *Ms.* Magazine, May, 1985, pp. 66–68; 141–154.

recent survey conducted for *Glamour* by Susan Wooley, an associate professor in the psychiatry department of the University of Cincinnati College of Medicine, 75 percent of the 33,000 women who replied said that they were "too fat," including, according to Wooley, "45 percent who in fact were underweight," by the conservative 1959 Metropolitan Life Insurance Company Height and Weight Table. (By the revised 1983 table, which set generally higher levels of up to 13 pounds for desirable weights, these women would be even more underweight.) Wooley, who is also codirector of the university's Eating Disorders Clinic, sees our contemporary obsession with weight in part as a perversion of feminism. "This striving for thinness is striving to have a more masculine-type body," she points out. "As we join men's worlds, we shouldn't be cashing in women's bodies. We have to reclaim the right to have female bodies and still be respected. Thinness has become the cultural symbol of competency—if we buy that symbol and foster it ourselves, that's a very self-mutilating stand to take."

Everything in this world, for women, boils down to body size.

Cinderella's unfortunate stepsisters cut off chunks of their feet in order to fit into the prince's slipper. He knew they were impostors when he saw their blood oozing insistently over the delicate glass. These days women merely wire their jaws, staple their stomachs, and cut off chunks of their intestines in their effort to win the prince. "Stomach stapling" operations—50,000 are reportedly performed each year, 80 to 95 percent of them on women—can have side effects, such as abdominal pain, severe malnutrition, nausea and vomiting, osteoporosis, brain damage, and possibly even cancer. "Weight-loss surgery, including intestinal bypass operations, has probably already killed well over a hundred times as many people as the toxic shock syndrome, and has caused more than ten times as many deaths as AIDS," notes Paul Ernsberger, a postdoctoral research fellow at Cornell University Medical College. "More Americans have died in the surgeons' War on Fat than died in the Vietnam War." Yet desperate fat women—veterans of Stillman and Atkins, Scarsdale and Beverly Hills, diet camps and amphetamines—gratefully welcome the surgeon's knife, perhaps dreaming of old fairy tales. "I sometimes wish I had cancer," said a large, pretty woman in her early twenties at a diet workshop I once attended in San Francisco. "I sometimes think I wouldn't mind dying, if only I could die thin."

Everything in this world, for women, boils down to body size.

I still remember those little girls drinking diet soda and waiting for the miracle. I was 14 years old and 145 pounds that summer, at Camp Stanley for overweight girls, but many of the campers were younger, chubby little kids who already knew their bodies were their shame. When some of us failed to lose weight even on the camp's low-calorie regime, we were put on a special plan: three scoops of cottage cheese a day and all the diet soda we could drink. I remember the hunger (I would roll my pillow up under my stomach at night, trying to fill the hollow so I could sleep), the dizziness, but also the exhilaration; I felt like a secular saint, virtuous, disembodied, utterly pure. We sat around, starving, and talked about food, food we recalled from our profligate pasts. We talked about the new lives we would inhabit in the fall, transmuted all into magical swans.

I lost 15 pounds that summer and felt quite swanlike for a while, particularly among my relatives, who often seemed to admire weight loss the way other families might esteem an Olympic medal. By Christmas, however, when a group of campers gathered for a mini-reunion, every one of us had recouped our loses, and then some. We talked about the new lives we would inhabit in the spring, after the next diet had made us swans.

After the next diet, of course, most of us were fatter than before. Not only do almost all diets fail; according to Kim Chernin, "ninety percent of those who have dieted 'successfully' gain back more than they ever lost." This is not because "overweight" people are weak-willed compulsives, unable to pull our faces out of the Haagen-Dazs. (The medical profession may still disagree, but the medical profession, remember, once advised women that our reproductive organs would shrivel if we made the mistake of obtaining a higher education.) In fact, observes Wooley, "On the whole fat people eat no more than thin people—often women who believe they're compulsive eaters are trying to deny the need to eat at all." The one thing fat women do more than other people is *diet*—and continual dieting, we now know, actually causes weight gain. "Repeated starvation can encourage fatness at the same time it destroys somebody's health," explains Ernsberger. "Cutting calories turns out to be the great fattener. The body—threatened with famine—overcompensates and creates new fat cells when normal eating is resumed. The cells may even double in number, and these new fat cells are forever. The body can now store more fat—the next diet will be harder."

A decade or so after my summer at Camp Stanley, I failed at a much more ambitious diet. This time I felt like a swan humiliatingly transformed into an ugly duckling. Even worse, I felt like a criminal; I was wearing my scarlet letter for all to see. My shame was intense—but as Wooley has remarked, "If shame could cure obesity, there wouldn't be a fat woman in the world."

During this period while attending graduate school in California, I sampled a variety of weight-loss groups. Two in particular were so disturbing that they made me question for the first time my own obsession with slimness. At the first, an Overeaters Anonymous meeting in Palo Alto, a depressed group of middle-aged people—mostly large and mostly women—sat on uncomfortable chairs in a chilly church basement and acknowledged that they were helplessly controlled by food. Only the aid of their "Higher Power" could save them, they agreed. At the height of the meeting one sad, gray-haired women got up to tell us that she "really was shit." She didn't understand why, now that she'd lost weight, her husband had left her, but she said she was sure it must be for the best because everything—of course—was part of her Higher Power's plan. She said again and again that without the guidance of her HP she was "a piece of shit," and many group members murmured that they were too.

Then, in a San Francisco workshop ironically titled "Fat Liberation"—a supposedly progressive approach to weight loss in which participants "got in touch" with their feelings about fat and food—a group of women, almost all slender (but feeling fat), sat in a circle and imagined meeting a fat person in the street. "You were huge, gigantic, obese," one women wrote, "a man or a woman, androgynous in fat. I feel uncomfortable around you, and guilty. I avoid looking at your body, I feel sorry for you, threatened—you don't have to look like that. Under the surface you have nothing. I follow you to a dark room; you go in alone and sit. I leave you sitting there in the dark. When I leave, I am happy, whistling." We then sat on the floor and told a pile of food that it couldn't scare us any more.

After this workshop I bought a new political button: "How Dare You Presume I'd Rather Be Thin?" I've never had the nerve to wear it.

Fat women are continually told to lose weight in order to improve our health—but, in fact, we are likely to damage our health while trying to lose weight. Women don't drink liquid protein, pour saccharin in our coffee, and staple our stomachs in order to be healthy; instead, women risk death in order to be thin. According to Dr. Faith Fitzgerald of the University of California at Davis, "Obesity, as we commonly use the term, may be more of an aesthetic and moral problem than one of physical health." Certainly our horrified revulsion at the sight of a fat body springs from deeper sources than a disinterested concern for that body's well-being. If it did, the billions of dollars poured into the diet industry each year would be transferred to an anti-smoking campaign.

"In general, the healthiest eaters we see are fat women," adds Susan Wooley. "Most would have to be on a starvation diet their whole lives to get them down to a weight the culture considers normal, and the physical and emotional effects of starvation are much worse than the effects of overweight."

Nevertheless, most Americans—including most medical professionals—believe that fatness and good health are antithetical. A panel convened by the National Institutes of Health recently proclaimed obesity a "killer" disease. The 14-member panel set the danger point at a level of 20 percent or more above "desirable" body weight, but said that even five to 10 pounds above recommended weights could pose increased health risks to those people

404

susceptible to or suffering from diseases like high blood pressure, adult onset of diabetes, and some cancers. A woman of my height, five feet four, would be 20 percent overweight at about 160, 40 pounds less than I weigh. The health charge is disturbing. No one—however terrific, energetic, and attractive she may feel—wants to walk around with a "killer" disease.

According to Ernsberger, the NIH report is simply wrong. "Fatness is *not* associated with a higher death rate," he says. "In fact, in every given population examined, the thinnest people have the highest death rate." The new NIH panel "flatly contradicts" previous reports of the same data, the well-known Framingham Heart Study, he adds. "The fact is the very fattest women in Framingham had a lower death rate than women who were at their 'correct' insurance table weights." The heaviest Framingham women, ranging from 40 percent to 172 percent over the 1959 tables, had lower mortality than both underweight women and women within a few pounds of their "desirable" weight. The *lowest* death rates, Ernsberger points out, occurred in women who were between 10 percent and 30 percent over the insurance tables. About 30 controlled studies correlating mortality and weight have reported similar findings. Dr. Ancel Keys of the University of Minnesota, a cardiovascular researcher, coordinated such studies in 16 different geographical areas with an emphasis on risk factors leading to heart attacks. He concluded that "in none of the areas of this study was overweight or obesity a major risk factor for death or the incidence of coronary heart disease."

"Cancer deaths actually decrease with increasing fatness," says Ernsberger. "Only one study, the study cited in the NIH report, showed an increase in cancer rates," he adds, "while five or six that I know of show a decrease with increasing fatness." The NIH panel chose to ignore the decreased overall cancer rate in obesity, mentioning only that a single type of cancer, uterine cancer, is more common in obese women.

Wooley concurs. "A person can definitely be fat and healthy," she says. "My reading of the literature tells me that for women there's a very sizable weight range in which extra weight does *not* constitute a risk in mortality." Wooley notes that some studies have shown that women can weigh up to 200 pounds, without increased mortality risks, and even after that point, she says, being overweight may be healthier than dieting.

Many of the health problems commonly associated with fatness are probably caused by fat people's incessant pursuit of thinness, Ernsberger points out. Thus the "yo-yo syndrome"—that deadly cycle of weight loss and weight regain—may cause hypertension; diet pills can also cause high blood pressure and amphetamine psychosis; low carbohydrate diets can raise cholesterol; and liquid protein diets have led to heart disease and sudden death. "We don't know how unhealthy overweight is in and of itself because most overweight people have been doing these things," Ernsberger comments.

Furthermore, fat people receive terrible health care, partly because doctors see them as "bad patients" and partly because the overweight person herself tends to give up in despair. "We've had it drummed into our heads that the *only* route to fitness is through weight loss," explains Nancy Summer, member of the board of directors of the National Association To Aid Fat Americans (NAAFA), a nationwide fat rights organization based in New York. Summer, a dynamic blond who weighs more than 300 pounds, swims twice a week on Long Island with a group of large women. "Many of us have developed an all-or-nothing attitude. If we can't be thin, we may as well not worry about nutrition or exercise—we are going to die young anyway. I think it's time we reject that concept."

The medical evidence may be contradictory—obesity "experts" may disagree—but the message to me as a self-accepting fat woman is fairly simple. People come in lots of different sizes, and our frantic struggle to squeeze—all of us—into the thinnest 10 percent of a once-normal bell-shaped curve is driving us all crazy (and at the same time making us fatter). Self-hatred and cultural stigmatization doesn't do anyone any good; indeed, many of the diseases frequently associated with overweight are stress-related illnesses. Even, if all the other things being equal, it is "healthier" to be thin, weight-reduction programs fail 98 percent of the time, according to Chernin. Therefore I have two choices: I can be fat and unhealthy or I can be fat and healthy. I can find a new miracle diet, or I can eat sensible food (fruit and veggies, fiber, not too much fat, sugar, or salt), avoid cigarettes, and get plenty of exercise.

I'll still be fat, but fat can be fit.

The six women flash brightly colored tights and leotards, shake to a driving rock beat, smile at their reflections in shiny mirrors, bend and stretch, tap some feet. It's just another Manhattan exercise class, but here all the women look like Rubens' models, ranging in size from perhaps 150 pounds to well over 200. At the Greater Woman, "New York's first exercise studio for the large woman," clients are expected to be at least 30 pounds over their "ideal" weight—some weigh nearly 300 pounds—but the program emphasizes fitness and self-esteem rather than weight loss.

"There's a great difference between fitness and skinniness," says Mary Sams, a family psychotherapist who heads the studio. "Women are told that fat is immoral, that everyone who is overweight is out of control, consuming massive amounts of food. That's garbage."

According to Sams, the purpose of Greater Woman "is not to get people to lose weight, but to help people become fit and healthy and change their feelings about themselves. A lot of women come here wanting to get thinner," she adds, "but three weeks into the program they're thinking entirely differently." Clients are likely to lose inches rather than pounds. "Over several months, their dress sizes may go down," says Greater Woman's nutritionist, Jeannette Harris, "but they don't see a decrease on the scale." "Fitness isn't a scale measurement," agrees Sams. "Our goal is to increase lean body mass and raise the metabolic rate."

In order to accomplish this, the studio has developed exercise classes specifically tailored to the needs of larger women. "The only exercise that really increases metabolic rate is aerobics," explains Sams. "We have learned to choreograph aerobic dances that are very lively but don't involve pounding exercises, which put too much stress on the knees and back."

The class members I speak with seem genuinely enthusiastic, and sometimes amazed to find themselves moving about so vigorously. One, a psychiatric social worker who has lost 30 pounds in the last year, explains earnestly, "People don't come here to lose weight, just to feel human about their bodies."

Remember the old fairy tales, the ugly ducklings and crippled stepsisters and hungry little girls all waiting for their miracle? Well, it's not exactly the story I'd imagined, but my transformation finally took place. My chronicle has a happy ending, but it's an ending with a twist, for as Susan Wooley once remarked, "When it comes to weight, people can't accept a happy ending that leaves us different shapes and sizes. To me, a happy ending is when someone can accept her body as it is."

My fairy godmother showed up after all, but she didn't change my body: she changed my mind.

Resources

Shadow on a Tightrope: Writings by Women on Fat Oppression, edited by Lisa Schoenfielder and Barb Wieser, foreword by Vivian Mayer (*Aunt Lute Book Company. Iowa City*). The best feminist collection I know of on the subject of fat. Includes much material from the original Fat Underground, a feminist fat liberation group that formed in Los Angeles in 1973.

The Obsession: Reflections on the Tyranny of Slenderness, by Kim Chernin (*Harper Colophon Book*). A subtle, well-written, and sometimes brilliant dissection of our cultures' frenzied pursuit of thinness, and its terror of female flesh.

The Dieter's Dilemma, by William Bennett, M.D., and Joel Gurin (*Basic Books*). A thoughtfully presented and scientific case against dieting as a means of weight control.

Such a Pretty Face: Being Fat in America, by Marcia Millman, with photographs by Naomi Bushman (*Norton*). A sociologist's investigation of what it is like "to live as a fat person in our society." Much of the material is drawn from interviews with fat people and from observations of organizations like NAAFA and Overeaters Anonymous.

Fat Is a Feminist Issue: a Self-Help Guide for Compulsive Eaters, by Susie Orbach (*Berkley*). Some feminists have found Orbach's discussion helpful, but it disturbs me because its emphasis is still on achieving thinness. Here fatness is seen not as a sin, but as a means of adapting to a sexist society. When women learn better ways of coping with sexism, Orbach believes, they will become slim. She also makes the mistake of confusing fatness with compulsive eating. They are two distinctly different conditions.

Big & Beautiful: How To Be Gorgeous on Your Own Grand Scale, by Ruthanne Olds (*Acropolis Books*). A fashion guide for women size 14 and up.

BBW: The World's First Fashion Magazine for the Large-Size Woman. Six-issue subscription is $13 from BBW (*Suite 214. 5535 Balboa Blvd. Encino. Calif. 91316*). A fashion magazine published six times a year. BBW stands for Big Beautiful Woman.

NAAFA—The National Association To Aid Fat Americans (*P.O. Box 43. Bellerose. N.Y. 11426*). The country's premier fat rights organization, active since 1969. Call 516-352–3120 or write for information. Sponsors both political action and social events.

The Greater Woman (*111 East 65 St., N.Y., N.Y. 10128; telephone: 212–737–4889*). Exercise classes for the larger woman.

Ω

A Feminist Perspective on the Latke-Hamentash Debate
by Mariamne H. Whatley

Presented February 27, 1983

The Latke-Hamentash Debate is an annual event in which experts from different academic disciplines debate the merits of two traditional Jewish foods. The latke is a potato pancake, usually associated with Chanukah, and the hamentash is a three-cornered filled pastry, associated with Purim. In the debate in Madison, Wisconsin, in 1983, two men, a former mayor and the chair of a university department, debated the issue, each supporting the case of one of these foods. After they debated, a Women's Studies faculty member presented a third view—a feminist perspective on the debate.

My invitation to speak in this debate came at an opportune moment. I am currently working on an introduction

to a book, *Our Kitchens, Ourselves,* by the Midwest Women's Cooking Collective, to be published by Vashti Feminist Press. Part of my talk today will be from that introduction. First, though I am not a separatist, I was rather surprised to find men participating in this debate. In fact, historically it has been mostly men who have debated this issue, though usually as consumers and not as producers. When I was discussing the issue with a member of our collective, Dr. Earth Moonstar Saradaughter, she told me her theory:

Men who prefer hamentashen are trying to possess what they clearly lack—I don't need to elaborate since you have all seen the Queen Esther setting of Judy Brooklyn's "The Noshing Party."

Those men who are on the latke side, on the other hand, suffer menstruation envy. Since latke production often involves knuckle grating, eating latkes is an attempt to participate in women's ability both to bleed and create.

Enough of Dr. Saradaughter's theories. You can read more in her book, *Braided Loaves: Women, Creativity, and the Challah.*

As we all know from Women's Studies 101, those in power define and the powerless are defined. As women we are defined by men as the makers of knishes, blintzes, latkes, and hamentashen. As can be seen from a history of these debates, male experts have produced the knowledge about women's work. Women are the objects of this knowledge, not the knowers. Just as there have been male medical experts defining the childbirth experience for women, there are male gastronomic experts defining women's experience in the kitchen. For years we have accepted the patriarchal definitions and our own voices and experiences have been silenced.

This point is illustrated by the brilliant feminist short story, "I'm Not Hungry; I Had a Bite to Eat in the Kitchen," the only writing produced by an anonymous maker of latkes. In this story, the unnamed narrator subtly undermines the knowledge men believe they have about women's lives and kitchens. In the movie made from the story, the sound track is dominated by sounds of grating and the narrative punctuated by close-ups of onion-induced tears. These scenes are interspersed with flash forwards to the narrator's husband, father and sons commenting on the flavor and texture of the large pile of latkes in front of them. I suggest you see this film when it shows at the Majestic next month in a benefit for our collective.

Where does a politically correct feminist stand in the latke-hamentash debate? Clearly, feminism is an argument for choice, for the rights of women to make our own decisions and control our lives. Men have always defined the traditions and we have carried them out. We are defined in terms of men's pleasure—in bed or at the table. (For a more complete discussion, read the feminist classic, *Stovetop Politics* by Kate Kasha and the weak rebuttal, *Prisoner of Food* by Norman Mensch.) We must now be actively involved in the decision-making processes that affect our lives directly. This is truly an issue of informed consent. Women must have all the information about the risks, side-effects, contraindications, and benefits of making latkes and hamentashen, so that we can make decisions based on that knowledge—and that knowledge must come from the makers, not the eaters. That is why we have written *Our Kitchens, Ourselves.* We gathered information on all the major cooking procedures and illustrated them with clear line drawings and photographs. In each section, there are personal accounts representing the diversity of women's cooking experience, in terms of race, class, ethnicity and sexual preference. In addition, the Berkeley Women's Cooking Collective has just published *A New View of a Woman's Kitchen,* including a brilliant redefinition of the stove in a feminist context.

It is time we turn to our sisters for support in making decisions about what to produce in our kitchens and not rely on male expertise—from friends, relatives, Chef Tell, or the distinguished male debaters. We must create our own definitions and make our own choices. We cannot relinquish our decision-making power on issues as important as what we cook or bake.

Clearly, then, the rest of this debate was irrelevant.

Ω

Food and Body Image
The Continuum of Women and Food Relationships

by Nancy Worcester

This study guide is designed to help us see the similarities among a wide range of behaviors which get labeled as "eating disorders".

The so-called "eating disorders" feel less threatening to us if we can view them as extreme cases which have nothing to do with us. However, even if we look at how common the extremes are, we must already face the fact that eating disorders are very much a part of our lives.

It may be more helpful to understanding the ambivalent relationship almost all women (in most western countries) have to their bodies and their food if we look at a wide range of eating patterns as a part of a continuum. If anorexia, bulimia, and compulsive eating are seen as only exaggerated manifestations of dieting, we may be better able to both understand how our society encourages "eating disorders" and the unnaturalness and unhealthiness of most dieting.

1. Make a list (collect examples from magazines, television, conversations, jokes) of messages women get about what they should look like. Make a list (collect examples from magazines, television, conversations, on-street advertising) of messages women get about delicious food available to them to eat or prepare.

    What is contradictory about these messages? How do women internalize these confused messages?

2. Read the definitions for all the eating disorders (pp. 412–413). Look for similarities between the different patterns.

    Being creative (!), think of a way to show the similarities between different patterns by connecting them with overlapping circles or lines. You may want to photocopy the page and do a "cut and paste" job. You may want to use several different colors to identify themes which keep occurring.

3. Reread definition #9 for "unnatural relationship to food and eating". Do you think this description of women for a body image study reflects *all* women or is peculiar only to women concerned with body image? Can you name ten women you know who are not concerned about body image? Can you think of ten women you know who are not very conscious of food/weight/exercise issues? Do you think body image issues are the same or different for white women and women of color?

4. If extremes get labeled as eating disorders, what is considered "ordered eating"? What would you identify as a normal, healthy eating pattern? What changes could help encourage normal, healthy eating patterns?

The Continuum of Women and Food Relationships

Starving[16]   Large for years[15]

Anorexia[1]   Subgroup of   Weight   Up and down dieters[14]
                     weight preoccupied[2] preoccupied[3]

          Anorexia-like symptoms[4]   Compulsive eater[13]

          Chronic anorexia[5]   Dieter
                                                                 ex-"normal eater"[12]

          Recovered anorexic[6]   Bulimorexic[8]

                                                                 Thin fat people[11]

     Ex-anorexic difficulties resolved[7]   Used to living on
                                                        semi-starvation diet[10]

                         Unnatural
                         relationship
                         to food and eating[9]

1. Anorexic—Try to avoid eating as far as possible. Often have a distorted view of their bodies seeing themselves as grotesque and enormous instead of thin. Tend to be extremely close mouthed about their eating but observe others closely. (Orbach, 1984, p.30)

2. Sub-group of weight pre-occupied women. This group scored high or higher than the anorexia nervosa group on all Eating Disorder Inventory (EDI) subscales. (The EDI is designed to assess the cognitive and behavioral dimensions characteristic of anorexia and to differentiate between patients with anorexia and those without the disorder.) "It is likely that at the very least, they suffer from a subclinical variant of the disorder." (Garner, 1984, pp. 255–266.)

3. Weight preoccupied women. This group was compared to women with anorexia by the EDI (see 2). Weight preoccupied women and anorexic women were comparable on body dissatisfaction, bulimia, perfectionism, and maturity fears subscales. The EDI subscales which best differentiated weight preoccupied women from anorexics were ineffectiveness and interreceptive awareness. (Garner, 1984, pp. 255–266)

4. Women with anorexia-like symptoms. College women who scored high on Garner and Garfinkel's Eating Attitudes Test. This group was similar to the anorexia group in the proportion of subjects reporting binge eating and self-induced vomiting. This group did not show distress on a psychiatric symptom checklist. "These findings indicate that food and weight preoccupations common in anorexia nervosa do occur on a continuum, but the milder expression was not associated with psychosocial impairment." (Thompson and Schwartz, 1982, quoted in Garner, 1984)

5. Chronic anorexic—anorexic makes a partial recovery, gains enough weight to keep her alive but maintains it at an artificially low level, sometimes for years. Her life continues to be utterly dominated by the desire to avoid food. (Lawrence, 1984, p. 108)

6. Recovered anorexic—a sizeable proportion of ex-anorexics are able to live creative and independent lives but still retain some elements of their preoccupation with food and weight. (Lawrence, 1984, p. 108)

7. Ex-anorexic—difficulties resolved. "The woman is no longer vulnerable to further anorexic episodes and *is no more neurotic about food than anyone else.*" (Lawrence, 1984, p.109)

8. Bulimorexic—women often of average size, but weekly, daily, sometimes hourly, they binge on substantial amounts of food which they bring up. Very few feel comfortable talking about their way of coping. Feel purging after gorging is the only way to stay slim. (Orbach, 1984, p.30) Estimated 15–20% of USA college women have bulimia. Only 44% sought professional help. (Potts, 1984, p. 32–35)

9. Unnatural relationship to food and eating. For body image study, "I sought subjects with no history of psychiatric illness or eating disorder. It immediately became clear that it is a rare woman in this culture who is not eating disordered or who does not experience herself as struggling with food and weight issues. Of 114 women screened for this study 109 reported an unnatural relationship to food and eating. Of those selected as subjects—whose weights all fell within the normal range—only 1 woman was not actively waging a war against fat. This astonishing statistic suggests that weight and eating issues are inseparable from body image struggles in today's woman. "Although describing themselves as eating disordered . . . most women reported eating patterns typical of the culture as a whole, patterns that in men would never be labeled as pathological. These women are for the most part suffering not from eating disorders but from labeling disorders" (Hutchinson, 1982, p. 61)

10. Used to living on semi-starvation diet. Having grown up with the concept that thinness is identical with beauty and attractiveness . . . these women have grown used to living on a semi-starvation diet, never eating more than their bony figures show. Never having permitted themselves to eat adequately, they are unaware of how much their tension, bad disposition, irritability, even inability to pursue educational and professional goals is the direct result of chronic undernutrition. (Bruch, 1980, p. 19)

11. Thin fat people—people who stay reduced but who cannot relax. They seem as preoccupied with weight and dieting after they have become slim as before. (Bruch, 1980, p. 18)

12. "Diets turn 'normal eaters' into people who are afraid of food." (Orbach, 1984, p. 29)

13. Compulsive eating means eating without regard to physical cues signalling hunger or satisfaction. Feels out of control about what she eats. (Orbach, 1984, p. 29)

14. Women who go up and down the scale (maximum of 60 lbs), diet from time to time and binge irregularly. Open about talking about food problems. Feel that things would be better for them if they were thin. "The largest group of women." (Orbach, 1984, p. 30)

15. Women who have been large for years, who feel themselves to be fat, but are despairing about ever being able to lose weight. Experience their eating as chaotic. Discuss the topic openly. Feel things would be a lot better if they were slim. (Orbach)

16. Both starvation and dieting may produce many of the behaviors associated with anorexia. Both obese humans and starving organisms demonstrate thrifty metabolism, heightened preference for sweets and inhibition of satiety mechanisms. (Smead, 1983)

References

Bruch, H., "Thin Fat People" in Kaplan, J.R. (ed) *A Woman's Conflict: The Special Relationship Between Women and Food,* Prentice Hall, New York, 1980.

Garner, D.M., Olmstead, M.P., Polivy, J., and Garfinkel, P.E., "Comparison Between Weight-Preoccupied Women and Anorexia Nervosa", *Psychosomatic Medicine,* Vol. 46, No. 3, 1984, pp. 255–266.

Hutchinson, M.G., "Transforming Body Image: Your Body, Friend or Foe?", *Women and Therapy,* Vol. 1, No. 3, 1982, pp. 59–67

Lawrence, M., *The Anorexic Experience,* Women's Press, London, 1984.

Orbach, S., *Fat Is a Feminist Issue 2,* Hamlyn Paperback, London, 1984.

Potts, N.L., "Eating Disorders—The Secret Pattern of Binge/Purge", *American Journal of Nursing,* Vol. 84, No. 1, 1984, pp. 32–35.

Smead, V.S., "Anorexia Nervosa, Bulimarexia, and Bulimia: Labeled Pathology and the Western Female", *Women and Therapy,* Vol. 2, No. 1, 1983, pp. 19–35.

Resource Information

The following resources have been used in drawing together this collection of readings and are examples of the wide range of publications which now cover women's health issues

(NOTE: *Feminist Connection, Healthsharing—A Canadian Women's Health Quarterly, Science for the People, and Spare Rib* are no longer being published and some of the groups (Bread and Roses, The Coalition for the Medical Rights of Women and the New Mexico Affiliate of the National Women's Health Network) which produced articles reprinted here are no longer actively meeting.)

American Journal of Preventive Medicine
Oxford University Press
Journals
200 Madison Ave
New York, NY 10016

Changing Men
Feminist Men's Publications
306 N Brooks St
Madison, WI 53715

Common Ground - Different Planes (The Women of Color Partnership Program Newsletter)
100 Maryland Avenue, NE
Washington, DC 20002

COPE
Pulse Publications Inc
Box 1700
Franklin, TN 37065

Council on Interracial Books for Children
1841 Broadway, Room 500
New York, NY 10023

Domestic Abuse Intervention Project
206 West Fourth Street
Duluth, MN 55806

Domestic Violence Hospital-Based Project
6308 8th Avenue
Kenosha, WI 53143

FDA Consumer
Dept HHS, FDA
5600 Fishers Lane
Rockville, MD 20857

Feminist Review
11 Carleton Gardens, Brecknock Road
London N19 5AQ, England

Frontiers: A Journal of Women's Studies
Mesa Vista Hall #2142
University of New Mexico
Albuquerque, NM 87131

Glamour Magazine
Conde Nast Publications
350 Madison Ave
New York, NY 10017

Health Letter (Public Citizen Health Research Group)
2000 P Street N.W.
Washington, DC 20036

Health/PAC Bulletin
47 West 14th Street
3rd Floor
New York, NY 10011

Health Values
PNG Publications
Box 4593
Star City, WV 26504-4593

In Health (currently published as *Health*)
275 Madison Ave Suite 1314
New York, NY 10016

JAMA: Journal of the American Medical Association
515 N State St
Chicago, IL 60610

Journal of Sex Education and Therapy
Guilford Publications Inc
72 Spring St 4th Floor
New York, NY 10012

Journal of Women's Health
1651 Third Avenue
New York, N.Y. 10128

Lilith
250 West 57th Street
Suite 2432
New York, NY 10107

MS Magazine
Lang Communications
230 Park Ave
New York, NY 10169

The Nation
72 Fifth Avenue
New York, NY 10011

National Latina Health Organization Newsletter
c/o National Latina Health Organization
PO Box 7567
Oakland, CA 94601

Network News (Newsletter of the National Women's Health Network)
514 10th Street, N.W.
Suite 400
Washington, D.C. 20004

New Internationalist
PO Box 1143
Lewiston, NY 14092

New York Times
229 West 43rd Street
New York, NY 10036

The Progressive
409 East Main Street
Madison, WI 53703

SIGNS
University of Chicago Press
Journals Division
5720 S Woodlawn Ave
Chicago, IL 60637

Social Policy
Union Institute
25 W 43rd St
New York, NY 10036

Sojourner (The Women's Forum)
42 Seaverns Avenue
Jamaica Plain, MA 02130

Teaching Forum
c/o The Undergraduate Teaching Improvement Council
University of Wisconsin System
1642 Van Hise Hall
1220 Linden Drive
Madison, WI 53706

Trouble and Strife
PO Box 8
Diss
Norfolk IP22 3XG
England

Wisconsin Coalition Against Sexual Assault (WCASA)
1400 E. Washington (Suite 148)
Madison, WI 53703

Women & Health
The Haworth Press, Inc
10 Alice St
Binghamton, NY 13904

Women and Therapy
Haworth Press, Inc
10 Alice Street
Binghamton, NY 13904

Women's Institute for Childbearing Policy
c/o Jane Pincus, Box 72
Roxbury, VT 05669

The Women's Health Data Book
Jacobs Institute of Women's Health
409 12th Street SW
Washington, DC 20024

Women's Studies International Forum
Pergamon Press Inc
Journals Division
660 White Plains Rd
Tarrytown, NY 10591-5153

WomenWise
c/o Concord Feminist Health Centers
38 So. Main Street
Concord, NH 03301

World Health Forum
World Health Organization
1211 Geneva 27
Switzerland

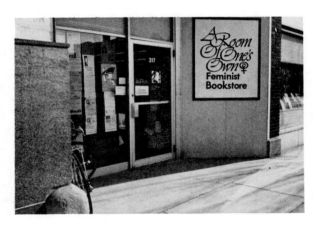

Feminist Bookstore, Madison, WI.